Jörg M. Steiner (ed.)

Small Animal Gastroenterology

Jörg M. Steiner (ed.)

Small Animal Gastroenterology

with

Karin Allenspach · Roger M. Batt · Thomas Bilzer · Andrea Boari · John V. DeBiasio · Olivier Dossin · Frédéric P. Gaschen · Lorrie Gaschen · Alexander J. German · Edward J. Hall · Carolyn J. Henry · Johannes Hirschberger · Ann E. Hohenhaus · Albert E. Jergens · Michael S. Leib · Terry L. Medinger · Lisa E. Moore · Reto Neiger · Keith P. Richter · Jan Rothuizen · Craig G. Ruaux · H. Carolien Rutgers · Jan S. Suchodolski · David C. Twedt · Shelly L. Vaden · Robert J. Washabau · Elias Westermarck · Michael D. Willard · David A. Williams

schlütersche

© 2008, Schlütersche Verlagsgesellschaft mbH & Co.KG, Hans-Böckler-Allee 7, 30173 Hannover
E-mail: info@schluetersche.de

Printed in Germany

ISBN 978-3-89993-027-6
10 05476200

Bibliographic information published by Die Deutsche Bibliothek

Die Deutsche Bibliothek lists this publication in the Deutsche Nationalbibliografie; detailed bibliographic data are available in the Internet at http://dnb.ddb.de.

Contents

Part I Diagnosis of Gastrointestinal Disorders

1 Diagnostic Tools

Authors

Karin Allenspach Dr. med. vet., FVH, PhD, DECVIM-CA
    (Internal Medicine)
Lecturer in Small Animal Internal Medicine
Veterinary Clinical Sciences
Royal Veterinary College
University of London
Hawkshead Lane
North Mymms
Herts., AL97TA
UK

Roger M Batt BVSc, MSc, PhD, FRCVS, DECVIM-CA
Professor
Batt Laboratories Ltd.
University of Warwick Science Park
The Venture Centre
Sir William Lyons Road
Coventry CV4 7EZ
UK

Thomas Bilzer Dr. med. vet., Dr. habil.
Professor
Institut für Neuropathologie
Heinrich-Heine-Universität Düsseldorf
Moorenstr. 5
40225 Düsseldorf
Germany

Andrea Boari DVM
Professor and Head of Department
Department of Veterinary Clinical Sciences
University of Teramo
Viale f. Crispi 212
64100 Teramo
Italy

John V. DeBiasio DVM
Resident in Small Animal Internal Medicine
Department of Veterinary Small Animal Clinical Sciences
College of Veterinary Medicine
Texas A&M University
College Station, TX
USA

Olivier Dossin DVM, PhD, DECVIM-CA
    (Internal Medicine)
Assistant Professor of Small Animal Internal Medicine
University of Illinois at Urbana-Champaign
Department of Veterinary Clinical Medicine
College of Veterinary Medicine
1008 Hazelwood Drive
Urbana, IL 61802
USA

Frédéric P. Gaschen Dr. med. vet., Dr. habil., DACVIM
    DECVIM-CA
Associate Professor and Section Chief,
    Companion Animal Medicine
Veterinary Clinical Sciences
School of Veterinary Medicine
Louisiana State University
Baton Rouge, LA 70803
USA

Lorrie Gaschen DVM, Dr. med. vet., PhD, Dr. habil.,
    DECVDI
Associate Professor
Veterinary Clinical Sciences
School of Veterinary Medicine
Louisiana State University
Baton Rouge, LA 70803
USA

Alexander J. German BVSC (Hons), PhD, certsam,
    DECVIM-CA, MRCVS
Royal Canin Associate Professor in Small Animal Medicine
Department of Veterinary Clinical Sciences
University of Liverpool
Small Animal Teaching Hospital
Chester High Road, Neston, Wirral, CH64 7TE
UK

Edward J Hall MA, VetMB, PhD, DECVIM-CA
Professor of Small Animal Internal Medicine
University of Bristol
Department of Clinical Veterinary Science
Langford House
Langford
Bristol BS40 5DU
UK

Carolyn J. Henry DVM, MS, DACVIM (Oncology)
Associate Professor of Oncology
900 E. Campus Drive
Department of Veterinary Medicine and Surgery
University of Missouri
Columbia, MO 65211
USA

Johannes Hirschberger, Dr. med. vet., Dr. habil.,
    DECVIM-CA (Internal Medicine), DECVIM-CA
    (Oncology), Hon. DECVCP
Professor
Medizinische Kleintierklinik
Clinic of Small Animal Medicine
Universität München
Veterinärstr. 13
80539 München
Germany

Ann E. Hohenhaus DVM, DACVIM
    (Oncology and Internal Medicine)
    Chairman, Department of Medicine
    The Animal Medical Center
510 East 62nd Street, NY, NY 10065
USA

Albert E. Jergens DVM, PhD, DACVIM
Professor and Staff Internist
Department of Veterinary Clinical Sciences
CVM, Iowa State University
Ames, IA, 50010
USA

Michael S. Leib DVM, MS, DACVIM
C.R. Roberts Professor
Virginia Maryland Regional College of Veterinary
    Medicine
Virginia Tech
Blacksburg, VA 24061
USA

Terry L. Medinger DVM, MS, DACVIM (SA)
Department Head Internal Medicine
VCA Aurora Animal Hospital
2600 W. Galena Blvd.
Aurora, IL 60506
USA

Lisa E. Moore DVM, DACVIM
    (Small Animal Internal Medicine)
Staff Internist
Affiliated Veterinary Specialists
9905 South US Highway 17-92
Maitland, FL 32751
USA

Reto Neiger Dr. med. vet., PhD, DACVIM, DECVIM-CA
Professor of Small Animal Internal Medicine
Small animal clinic
Justus-Liebig-University
Frankfurter Straße 126
35392 Gießen
Germany

Keith P. Richter DVM, DACVIM
Hospital Director and Staff Internist
Veterinary Specialty Hospital of San Diego
10435 Sorrento Valley Road
San Diego, CA 92121
USA

Jan Rothuizen DVM, PhD
Professor of Internal Medicine
Chair, Department of Clinical Sciences of
    Companion Animals
Faculty of Veterinary Medicine
University Utrecht
P.O. Box 80.154, 3508 TD Utrecht
The Netherlands

Craig G. Ruaux BVSc, PhD, MACVSC
Research Associate
Dept of Clinical Sciences
Magruder Hall, College of Veterinary Medicine
Oregon State University
Corvallis, Oregon 97331
USA

H. Carolien Rutgers DVM, MS, MRCVS, DACVIM,
    DECVIM-CA, DSAM
Consultant for Scientific Writing
4 Prestwood Gate
Sandridge Road
St Albans
Hertfordshire AL1 4AE
UK

Jörg M. Steiner Dr. med. vet., PhD, DACVIM,
    DECVIM-CA
Associate Professor of Small Animal Internal Medicine
    and Director of the GI Lab
Gastrointestinal Laboratory
Department of Small Animal Clinical Sciences
College of Veterinary Medicine and Biomedical Sciences
Texas A&M University
4474 TAMU
College Station, TX 77843-4474
USA

Jan S. Suchodolski Dr. med. vet., PhD
Research Assistant Professor & Associate Director
Gastrointestinal Laboratory
Department of Small Animal Clinical Sciences
College of Veterinary Medicine and Biomedical Sciences
Texas A&M University
4474 TAMU
College Station, TX 77843-4474
USA

David C. Twedt DVM, DACVIM
Professor
Department of Clinical Sciences
College of Veterinary Medicine and Biomedical Sciences
Colorado State University
Fort Collins, CO 80523
USA

Shelly L. Vaden DVM, PhD, DACVIM
Professor, Internal Medicine
North Carolina State University
College of Veterinary Medicine
4700 Hillsborough St., Raleigh, NC 27606
USA

Robert J. Washabau VMD, PhD, DACVIM
Professor of Medicine and Department Chair
Department of Veterinary Clinical Sciences
College of Veterinary Medicine
1352 Boyd Avenue
University of Minnesota
St. Paul, Minnesota 55108
USA

Elias Westermarck DVM, PhD, DECVIM-CA
Professor of Small Animal Internal Medicine
Tammitie 1
02270 Espoo
Finland

Michael D. Willard DVM, MS, DACVIM
Professor of Small Animal Internal Medicine
Department of Small Animal Clinical Sciences
College of Veterinary Medicine and Biomedical Sciences
Texas A&M University
4474 TAMU
College Station, TX 77843-4474
USA
2806 Rayado Court North
College Station
TX 77845
USA

David A. Williams MA, vetmb, PhD, DACVIM,
    DECVIM-CA
Professor and Department Head
Veterinary Clinical Medicine
1008 West Hazelwood Drive
Urbana IL 61802
USA

Abbreviations

^{13}C-OBT	^{13}C–octanoic acid breath test	cTLI	canine trypsin-like immunoreactivity
5-ASA	5-aminosalicylic acid	CVP	cyclophosphamide, vincristine, and prednisone
5-HT$_3$	5-hydroxytryptamine		
6MP	6-mercaptopurine		
		Da	Dalton
α_1-PI	alpha$_1$-proteinase inhibitor	DDAVP	desmopressin acetate
		DIC	disseminated intravascular coagulation
AC	adenocarcinoma	DOB	dose over baseline
ACh	acetylcholine	DSH	domestic shorthair cat
ACTH	adrenocorticotropic hormone		
AgNOR	argyrophilic nucleolar organizer region	EBDO	extrahepatic bile duct obstruction
ALP	alkaline phosphatase	ECG	electrocardiogram
ALT	alanine aminotransferase	ECL	enterochromaffin-like
APUDoma	tumors of cells of the amine precursor uptake and decarboxylation system	ED	equilibrium dialysis
		EE	eosinophilic enteritis
ARD	antibiotic-responsive diarrhea	EEG	electroencephalogram
AST	aspartate aminotransferase	EGE	eosinophilic gastroenteritis
AT-III	antithrombin-III	EGEC	eosinophilic gastroenterocolitis
		EGF	epidermal growth factor
BIPS	barium-impregnated polyethylene spheres	ELISA	enzyme-linked immunosorbent assay
		EPEC	enteropathogenic *E. coli*
BUN	blood urea nitrogen	EPI	exocrine pancreatic insufficiency
BW	body weight	ERCP	endoscopic retrograde cholangio-pancreatography
BZ	benzodiazepine		
		ETEC	enterotoxigenic *E. coli*
CAV1	canine adenovirus-1		
CBC	complete blood count	FeCoV	feline coronavirus
CCK	cholecystokinin	FeLV	feline leukemia virus
CCNU	lomustine	FIP	feline infectious peritonitis
CD	Crohn's disease	FIV	feline immunodeficiency virus
cDNA	complementary DNA	FNA	fine needle aspiration
CDV	canine distemper virus	FO	foreign object
CFU	colony-forming units	FOS	fructo-oligosaccharides
CIBDAI	canine inflammatory bowel disease activity index	FPA	fecal proteolytic activity
		fPLI	feline pancreatic lipase immunoreactivity
CK	creatinine kinase	FPV	feline parvovirus
CLO	*Campylobacter-like organism*	FRLBD	fiber-responsive large bowel diarrhea
CNS	central nervous system	fTLI	feline trypsin-like immunoreactivity
COX	cyclooxygenase		
CPE	*Clostridium perfringens enterotoxin*	GABA	gamma-aminobutyric acid
cPL	canine pancreatic lipase	GALT	gut-associated lymphoid tissue
cPLI	canine pancreatic lipase immunoreactivity	G-CSF	granulocyte colony stimulating factor
CPSS	congenital portosystemic shunt	GDV	gastric dilatation-volvulus
CPV	canine parvovirus	GER	gastroesophageal reflux
CRI	constant rate infusion	GERD	gastroesophageal reflux disease
CRT	capillary refill time	GES	gastroesophageal sphincter
CRTZ	chemoreceptor trigger zone	GGT	γ-glutamyl transferase
CSF	cerebrospinal fluid	GHLO	gastric *Helicobacter*-like organisms
CT	computed tomography	GhRH	growth hormone releasing hormone

GI	gastrointestinal	PAA	pancreatic acinar atrophy
GIT	gastrointestinal tract	PABA	para-aminobenzoic acid
GN	glomerulonephritis	PAFANT	platelet activating factor antagonist
GSE	gluten-sensitive enteropathy	pANCA	perinuclear antineutrophilic antibodies
		PAS	periodic acid Schiff
H&E	hematoxylin and eosin	PCR	polymerase chain reaction
H_2-RA	histamin$_2$-receptor antagonists	PCV	packed cell volume
HAS	hemangiosarcoma	PEG	percutaneous endoscopic gastrostomy
HE	hepatic encephalopathy	PGE_1	prostaglandin E_1
HGE	hemorrhagic gastroenteritis	P-gp	P-glycoprotein
HGF	hepatocyte growth factor	PI	pulsatility index
HLA	human leukocyte antigen	PIVKA	proteins induced by vitamin K antagonism
Htc	hematocrit		
HUC	histiocytic ulcerative colitis	PLE	protein-losing enteropathy
		PLI	pancreatic lipase immunoreactivity
IBD	inflammatory bowel disease	PLN	protein-losing nephropathy
IBS	irritable bowel syndrome	PO	per os
IEL	intraepithelial lymphocyte	PPI	proton pump inhibitor
IF	intrinsic factor	PP	Peyer's patch
IFA	immunofluorescence assay	PSS	portosystemic shunt
IFCR	intrinsic factor-cobalamin receptor	PSTI	pancreatic secretory trypsin inhibitor
IFN-γ	interferon γ	PT	prothrombin time (i.e., one-stage prothrombin time)
IGF	insulin-like growth factor		
IHC	immunohistochemistry	PTT	partial thromboplastin time (i.e., activated partial thromboplastin time)
IL	interleukin		
KCS	keratoconjunctivitis sicca	PU/PD	polydipsia
KIT	CD117		
		q	(*quodque*) every
L/R ratio	lactulose/rhamnose ratio	Q-PCR	quantitative polymerase chain reaction
LES	lower esophageal sphincter		
LI	large intestinal	RAST	radio-allergosorbent test
LP	lamina propria	RBC	red blood cell
LPC	lymphocytic-plasmacytic colitis	RI	resistive indice
LPE	lymphocytic-plasmacytic enteritis	RIA	radioimmunoassay
LSA	lymphosarcoma	ROS	reactive oxygen species
		RT-PCR	reverse transcriptase polymerase chain reaction
MAb	monoclonal antibody		
MALT	mucosal associated lymphoid tissue		
MCT	mast cell tumors	SAF	sodium acetate/acetic acid/formaldehyde
MCT	medium-chain triglyceride		
MEN	multiple endocrine neoplasia	SAME	S-adenosyl methionine
MER	maintenance energy requirement	SBA	serum bile acids
MHC	major histocompatibility complex	SI	small intestinal
MRI	magnetic resonance imaging	SIBO	small intestinal bacterial overgrowth
MST	median survival time	sIgA	secretory IgA
MVD	microvascular dysplasia	SLE	systemic lupus erythematosus
		SND	superficial necrolytic dermatitis
NET	neuroendocrine tumor	SNP	single nucleotide polymorphisms
NK_1	neurokinin$_1$	SPF	specific pathogen free
NME	necrolytic migratory erythema	spp.	species
NO	nitric oxide	SRS	somatostatin receptor scintigraphy
NPO	nothing per os	sst2	somatostatin receptor subtype 2
NSAID	non-steroidal anti-inflammatory drug	STEC	Shiga-toxin-producing *E. coli*
NTZ	nitazoxanide	SUCA	serum unconjugated cholic acid

T4	thyroxine	UA	urinalysis
TAP	trypsinogen activation peptide	UC	ulcerative colitis
TFF	trefoil factor		
TGF	transforming growth factor	VIPoma	vasoactive intestinal polypeptidoma
Th1	T-helper cell, type 1	VLDL	very low density lipoproteins
Th2	T-helper cell, type 2	vWF	von Willebrand's factor
THV	terminal hepatic veins		
TLI	trypsin-like immunoreactivity	WSAVA	World Small Animal Veterinary Association
TNF	tumor necrosis factor		
TPMT	thiopurine methyltransferase	X / M ratio	xylose / 3-O-methylglucose ratio
TRD	tylosin-responsive diarrhea		
TS	total solids	ZSC	zinc sulfate concentration centrifugation
		ZSFC	zinc sulfate fecal centrifugation

Dedication
This book is dedicated to Edward Anthony Kane.

Preface

While much still remains to be discovered, our understanding of gastrointestinal diseases in dogs and cats is steadily progressing. This book aims to highlight and consolidate recent advances.

It has taken several years to complete this project and I feel very fortunate to have worked with such a fantastic group of authors from around the globe. Our goal was a textbook that is both scientific and practical. To that end, in addition to discussing gastrointestinal diseases, diagnostic modalities and common clinical problems are discussed separately. We have tried to keep the material brief, but have provided pertinent references for readers wishing to evaluate the scientific evidence behind our observations.

We hope that this book helps you care for your patients, as ultimately, it was written for their benefit.

College Station, January 2008   *Jörg M. Steiner*

Part I

Diagnosis of Gastrointestinal Disorders

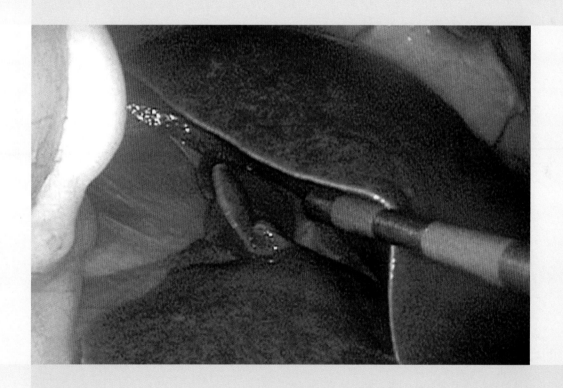

1 Diagnostic Tools

1.1 Clinical History

Olivier Dossin

1.1.1 Introduction

For most clinical problems, acquiring an accurate history can be as important as the clinical findings on physical examination. This is especially true for gastrointestinal disorders since they are usually expressed by clinical signs that cannot be observed during the clinical examination but are only reported by the owner. Therefore, the clinician must be skilled in obtaining the most accurate information by questioning the owner, which needs to be adapted to each case.

The steps and general guidelines for a good history are shown in the Tables 1.1 and 1.2. The observations of the owner, which are valuable, must be differentiated from his or her conclusion or interpretation, which may be misleading. For example, the terms vomiting and regurgitation may be used synonymously by the owner. In order to avoid confusion, it is essential to ask the owner to describe the patient's symptoms with his or her own words.

The signalment can be helpful as some age or breed predispositions (Tables 1.3 and 1.4) have been proposed for various gastrointestinal disorders. Also, a complete vaccination and drug history is important. Many drugs can induce gastrointestinal disturbances (e.g., NSAIDs can cause gastric ulcers and some antibiotic agents can be associated with diarrhea). Intolerance of anesthetic agents has been reported in patients with hepatic disorders, especially in those with portosystemic vascular anomalies.[1]

Written records of the history are essential for the follow-up. As a general rule, everything that can be quantified during history taking should be, as this could be beneficial for the assessment of the severity of the problem or for the follow-up.

1.1.2 History of specific gastrointestinal signs

This section focuses on the main specific gastrointestinal signs, but other, less specific signs, such as anorexia, weight loss, or polyuria/polydipsia should also not be overlooked.

Table 1.1: Steps for taking a history in patients with gastrointestinal signs[2,7,8]

Parameters addressed

- Signalment
- Chief complaint
- Present medical history (including chronology and treatments)
- Past medical history
- Systems review
- Current health status (including environment and dietary history)

Table 1.2: Guidelines for history acquisition in patients with gastrointestinal signs[10,11]

Guidelines for history acquisition

- always begin with the chief complaint
- start by asking broad questions
- ask narrow questions (questions that can be answered with few words such as "yes", "no", or "I do not know") to confirm previous answers
- try to use the owner's words to avoid confusion about what the owner means
- do not bombard the owner with questions
- avoid combining questions
- try to be reassuring when necessary
- try to focus owner on the main points of the history
- avoid categorical answers or judgments at the time of history collection
- avoid external interruptions

1.1.2.1 Dysphagia and regurgitation

Dysphagia, which is defined as difficult or painful swallowing, can be classified as oral, pharyngeal, or esophageal. A good history can help the clinician to characterize the type of dysphagia. An owner questionnaire has been evaluated for characterization of dysphagia and was shown to be useful for exclusion of oral dysphagia and for the detection of pharyngeal dysphagia; however, it was less sensitive and specific for the assessment of esophageal dysphagia.[2]

Oral dysphagia is characterized by the dropping of food, leaking of water, or abnormally interrupted chewing followed by rejection of food during the meal. Oral dysphagia is associated with disorders of the oral cavity, or with neuromuscular or osteo-articular disorders that impair normal chewing.

Abnormal, repeated swallowing efforts followed by periprandial regurgitation of an alimentary bolus mixed with saliva are

1

Table 1.3: Suspected or confirmed breed predispositions for gastrointestinal diseases in dogs[3,6,12]

Breed	Disease predisposition
Australian Cattle Dog	Portosystemic vascular anomalies
Basenji	Immunoproliferative lymphoplasmacytic enteritis
Bedlington Terrier	Copper-associated chronic hepatitis
Belgian Shepherd	Gastric carcinoma
Brachycephalic breeds	Hiatal hernia, pyloric stenosis
Border Collie	Selective cobalamin malabsorption
Boston Terrier	Pyloric muscular stenosis, vascular ring anomalies
Bouvier des Flandres	Muscular dystrophy associated dysphagia
Boxer	Histiocytic ulcerative colitis, eosinophilic enteritis, lymphoplasmacytic colitis, pyloric muscular stenosis
Cairn Terrier	Portosystemic vascular anomalies
Cocker Spaniel	Chronic hepatitis and cirrhosis
Dalmatian	Copper-associated chronic hepatitis
Doberman Pinscher	Parvoviral enteritis, eosinophilic enteritis, chronic hepatitis
English Bulldog	Vascular ring anomaly, constipation, fecal incontinence
German Shepherd	Exocrine pancreatic insufficiency, megaesophagus, parvoviral enteritis, lymphoplasmacytic enteritis, eosinophilic enteritis, idiopathic hepatic fibrosis, vascular ring anomaly, perianal fistula, small intestinal bacterial overgrowth
Giant Schnauzer	Selective cobalamin malabsorption
Great Dane	Gastric dilation volvulus
Irish Setter	Megaesophagus, gastric dilation volvulus, gluten-sensitive enteropathy, vascular ring anomaly
Irish Wolfhound	Portosystemic vascular anomalies (intrahepatic shunt)
Labrador Retriever	Megaesophagus, portosystemic vascular anomalies, chronic hepatitis
Lhasa Apso	Hypertrophic pyloric gastropathy
Maltese	Hypertrophic pyloric gastropathy, portosystemic vascular anomalies
Miniature Schnauzer	Pancreatitis, portosystemic vascular anomalies
Norwegian Lundehund	Protein-losing enteropathy, lymphangiectasia
Pekingese	Hypertrophic pyloric gastropathy
Rottweiler	Parvoviral enteritis, eosinophilic enteritis
Rough Collie	Exocrine pancreatic insufficiency, gastric carcinoma
Shar Pei	Hepatic amyloidosis, hiatal hernia, protein-losing enteropathy, lymphoplasmacytic enteritis, eosinophilic enteritis, cobalamin deficiency
Shi Tzu	Hypertrophic pyloric gastropathy
Skye Terrier	Copper-associated chronic hepatitis
Soft-coated Wheaten Terrier	Protein-losing enteropathy and/or nephropathy
Standard Poodle	Lobular dissecting hepatitis
West Highland White Terrier	Copper-associated chronic hepatitis
Yorkshire Terrier	Acute pancreatitis, portosystemic vascular anomalies, intestinal lymphangiectasia, hypertrophic pyloric gastropathy

the hallmarks of pharyngeal dysphagia. The swallowing efforts are frequently associated with coughing or choking, and also with gagging at rest.

Esophageal dysphagia is associated with regurgitation, which is a passive process during which an undigested food bolus is thrown up. Sometimes, the food bolus has a cylindrical sausage shape and is covered with mucus (Figure 1.1). The time elapsed between the swallowing of the food and regurgitation of the bolus is variable but can be quite long, especially when severe esophageal dilation is present. The time period is usually shorter in patients with esophagitis, esophageal stenosis, or esophageal obstruction. In contrast to pharyngeal dysphagia, esophageal dysphagia is usually not associated with swallowing attempts.[3] The history may also reveal respiratory signs such as coughing or nasal discharge, even as the primary complaint. A main task of history taking is to differentiate regurgitation from vomiting (Table 1.5).

Table 1.4: Suspected or confirmed breed predispositions for gastrointestinal diseases in cats[3,6,13]

Breed	Disease predisposition
Abyssinian	Hepatic amyloidosis
Manx	Fecal incontinence, constipation
Oriental Shorthair	Hepatic amyloidosis
Persian	Portosystemic vascular anomalies
Siamese	Megaesophagus, hepatic amyloidosis, pyloric stenosis, intestinal tumors

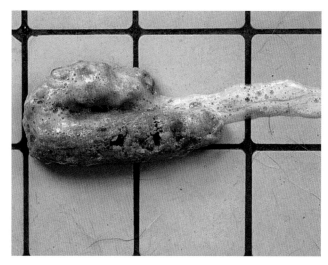

Figure 1.1:
Regurgitated food. This figure shows regurgitated food from a dog with esophageal stenosis following general anesthesia for spaying. Note the mucus surrounding a sausage-like bolus of food.

1.1.2.2 Gagging

Gagging is defined as swallowing attempts without the presence of an alimentary bolus. Gagging can be a clinical manifestation of dysphagia in patients with pharyngeal disease, but it can also be associated with certain respiratory disorders of the nasal passages, larynx, trachea, or bronchi. Gagging can be associated with ptyalism or retching due to activation of the pharyngeal vomiting receptors.

1.1.2.3 Vomiting

Vomiting is not always linked to a primary gastrointestinal tract disorder. It must be differentiated from regurgitation and coughing as discussed before (Table 1.5). Vomiting is an active process with prodromal clinical signs and has three phases. The first phase, nausea, is frequently associated with hypersalivation, agitation or depression, yawning, lip licking, or repeated swallowing attempts. The second phase, retching, appears as a vomiting effort with abdominal wall contractions but without ejection of vomitus and can be associated with belching. The last phase, vomiting, is the forceful ejection of gastric contents, which is associated with very repetitive strong abdominal wall contractions.

Vomiting can be classified as acute or chronic, with chronic being defined as lasting for more than 3 weeks. Also, the content of the vomitus should be described, especially concerning the presence of food, parasites, or foreign bodies. Hematemesis is blood-tinged vomitus containing either fresh blood or digested blood, resembling coffee grounds. Hematemesis is associated with gastric or duodenal erosions and should always be considered as a sign of severe disease. However, small amounts of fresh blood are sometimes related to capillary rupture linked to the rise in venous pressure during vomition.[4]

Gastritis may be associated with the vomiting of bile on an empty stomach or vomiting of food usually shortly (30 minutes to a few hours) after a meal.[4,5] Vomitus consisting of large volumes of fluid can be associated with ileus, small intestinal obstruction, or hypersecretory states such as gastrinoma.[4]

Table 1.5: Differentiation of regurgitation and vomiting[3,5,6]

Clinical sign	Regurgitation	Vomiting
Abdominal effort	Absent	Present
Bolus in the neck	Possible	Absent
Prodromal signs (nausea, retching)	Absent (except rare salivation)	Present
Character of ejected material	Undigested	Can be partially digested (depending on time between ingestion and vomiting)
	Bile absent	Bile can be present
	pH variable	pH <5
	Can be tubular shape	Variable shape
Time of ejection	Not reliable	Not reliable
Pain on swallowing	Can be present	Absent

Vomitus that smells like fecal material can sometimes be observed in patients with intestinal obstruction or chronic small intestinal bacterial overgrowth. Vomiting associated with bile that occurs in the morning can be due to duodenal reflux gastritis in small breeds. Vomitus containing food that is produced more than 8 to 12 hours after a meal is highly suggestive of a gastric emptying disorder.[3,5] Projectile vomiting can be observed in patients with a gastric outlet obstruction, but may also simply reflect violent vomiting due to any cause.[6]

1

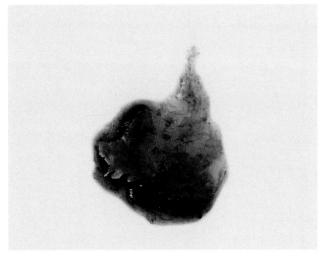

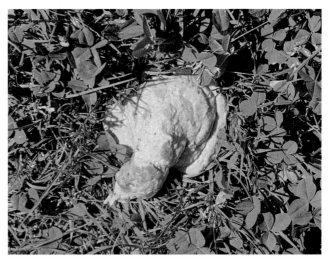

Figure 1.2:
Mucoid stool. This figure shows mucoid stools from a dog with severe colitis due to whipworm infestation. Note that the stool is almost exclusively composed of mucus and blood.

Figure 1.3:
Exocrine pancreatic insufficiency (EPI). Cow-patty yellowish stools from a dog with EPI.

Whenever possible, the number of vomiting episodes should be quantified. This is helpful to plan fluid therapy in patients with acute vomiting and also for the assessment of disease severity (canine IBD activity index; CIBDAI) in patients with chronic vomiting due to inflammatory bowel disease.[7]

1.1.2.4 Retching

Retching is defined by repetitive efforts to vomit without any expulsion of vomitus. Diagnostically, retching should be approached like vomiting. However, in some instances, even a good history can not differentiate retching or the regurgitation of saliva or mucus from coughing and/or expectorations. In patients that present with acute retching and abdominal distension, gastric dilation/volvulus (GDV) should be ruled out immediately.[4]

1.1.2.5 Diarrhea

Diarrhea is defined as the passage of feces that contain more water than normal, which increases daily fecal weight. As for vomiting, the first step is to classify whether the diarrhea is acute or chronic. The next step is to describe the fecal character by asking questions about any blood, foreign material, undigested food particles, or mucus in the feces (Figure 1.2). The color, volume, odor, and consistency of the feces might also be helpful, narrowing the list of differential diagnoses. For example, rancid smelling, large volume, grayish brown, and cow-

patty stools may suggest exocrine pancreatic insufficiency or another condition associated with maldigestion (Figure 1.3). The number of bowel movements per day should also be quantified. The main concern is to localize the origin of the diarrhea either to the small or to the large intestine. The characteristics that may be helpful for localization of the cause of diarrheal disease are shown in Table 1.6. However, these characteristics are not absolute by any means and patients with clinical signs of large bowel disease may have more significant small bowel disease. The use of photographic fecal scoring charts may be helpful for the characterization of the diarrhea (Figure 2.4).

1.1.2.6 Other stool abnormalities

Melena is characterized by black and tarry stools (Figure 1.4) and is sometimes associated with diarrhea. Melena is a sign of the presence of blood in the GI tract. The blood usually comes from the GI tract itself, but it can be swallowed in patients that are bleeding into the respiratory tract. Melena is mostly associated with bleeding of the upper gastrointestinal tract, but the black color and tarry consistency are due to the transit of the blood through the intestinal tract.[3] Therefore, blood from the upper parts of the large intestine can also be black and tarry, and blood coming from the small intestine can be fresh if the transit time does not allow for the digestion of the blood.[3] Some medications, such as metronidazole, ferrous sulfate, or bismuth or some food ingredients (liver, spinach) can also produce dark stools that can sometimes be confused with melena. Asking about ulcerogenic medications, especially NSAIDs,

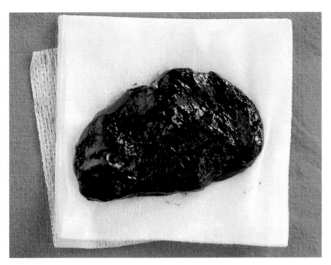

Figure 1.4:
Melena. This figure shows melena in a dog with severe gastric bleeding.

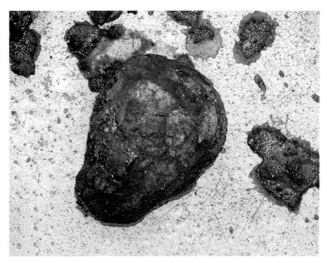

Figure 1.5:
Perineal herniation. Round stools that look like "horse manure" from a dog with perineal herniation.

anticoagulant exposure (e.g., rodenticide), or recent trauma is also important.

Fresh blood that is adherent to the feces is called hematochezia and is consistent with large bowel or recto-anal bleeding. Hematochezia can be associated with local disorders (colitis, proctitis, foreign body, or neoplasia) or coagulopathy. It is not always associated with dyschezia or straining to defecate and is therefore sometimes not observed by the owner.

Ribbon-like stools are observed in conditions associated with a narrowing of the colonic, rectal, or anal passage and frequently lead to dyschezia or constipation. Sometimes, round or ball-like feces looking like horse manure (Figure 1.5) are observed with perineal herniation or anal diverticula.

Acholic feces are clay-like feces that can be observed in patients with extra-hepatic bile duct obstruction or destructive choloangiolitis.[1]

1.1.2.7   Flatulence and borborygmus

Flatulence and borborygmus (rumbling of the gastrointestinal tract) are ultimately due to the presence of large amounts of intestinal gas that can occur in association with many digestive disorders. Excessive gas can also be associated with abdominal discomfort. A dietary history is important in these patients since certain types of foods commonly lead to the formation of excessive gas in the intestinal lumen (e.g., legumes, soybeans, or excess fat).

Table 1.6: Characterization of small and large bowel diarrhea[3,5,6,11]
Please note that none of these parameters is absolute.

Parameter	Small intestine	Large intestine
Feces		
Volume per defecation	Increased	Decreased or normal
Mucus	Absent (except in ileitis)	Frequently present
Melena	May be present	Rarely present
Hematochezia	Absent except in acute hemorrhagic diarrhea	Frequently present
Steatorrhea	Present in patients with maldigestion or malabsorption	Absent
Defecation		
Frequency	Usually slightly increased up to 4 times per day but can be severely increased in severe acute enteritis	Increased (many defecations with small volume)
Dyschezia	Absent	Present
Tenesmus	Absent	Frequently present
Urgency	Absent; except in severe cases	Usually present; sometimes with indoor soiling
Other signs		
Flatulence / borborygmus	May be present	May be present
Weight loss	May be present	Rare
Anal pruritus	Absent	May be present
Vomiting	May be present	May be present in acute colitis

1

1.1.2.8 Dyschezia

Dyschezia is defined as difficult or painful defecation characterized by straining to defecate with or without defecation. Dyschezia can be observed in association with large bowel diarrhea but also with some other conditions such as constipation, rectal disease, anal disorders such as anal furunculosis or anal gland sacculitis, or prostatomegaly in male dogs.

Tenesmus is straining to defecate and is a clinical manifestation of either dyschezia or colonic and recto-anal discomfort.

1.1.2.9 Constipation

Constipation is defined by the passage of dry, hard feces and is associated with a decreased number of bowel movements and straining to defecate. In cases of suspected constipation, it is important to ask about urination behavior as urinary straining can be confused with straining to defecate in some patients, especially in cats with lower urinary tract obstruction. Straining before defecation is usually associated with obstructive or functional disorders inducing constipation. In contrast, straining throughout defecation or persisting after defection has been completed is frequently associated with diarrhea of inflammatory disorders of the colon and/or rectum.[3]

Sometimes, the constipated patient is presented for diarrhea. The diarrhea perceived by the owner is due to a small quantity of liquid fecal material passing around the fecal bolus lodged in the colon and/or rectum.

1.1.2.10 Fecal incontinence

Fecal incontinence is characterized by uncontrolled loss of feces without crouching to defecate. It must be differentiated from urgency to defecate by carefully questioning the owner as these two causes of fecal soiling are frequently confused. In patients with true fecal incontinence, the stools are usually normal and loss of feces frequently occurs during excitation or coughing. The owner should be questioned about the presence of controlled and normal defecation to assess whether the neuro-muscular control of defecation is functional. A history of trauma (especially tail trauma in cats) as well as medical or surgical conditions of the perianal area are frequently associated with fecal incontinence.

1.1.2.11 Anal pruritus

Anal pruritus is manifested by perineal licking or biting, anal scratching, or scooting. It is usually associated with recto-anal diseases such as anal furunculosis, anal gland disorders, or *Dipylidium* infestation, but can also be a manifestation of food allergy, constipation, or inflammatory bowel disease.

1.1.2.12 Abdominal pain

The owner may report certain behaviors such as a saw horse stance or prayer position (stretching out the forelimbs with the sternum in contact with the floor and standing on the hindlimbs), which are strongly suggestive of cranial abdominal pain.[4] Bruxism (teeth grinding) or restlessness can also sometimes be associated with severe abdominal pain in dogs and cats. Restlessness can sometimes be observed during the first stages of gastric dilation/volvulus.[8] In cases of extreme abdominal pain, the pet may be severely depressed or even aggressive.

1.1.3 Dietary history

A complete dietary history can be very important in the diagnosis of gastrointestinal disease and should include specific commercial foods that are being fed, commercial snacks or treats, supplements and chewable medications, chewable toys, human foods (especially leftover foods from human meals), access to other sources of food (ask about other pets in the household or about people who may give extra food to the pet).[9] Many medical supplements or certain drugs contain proteins or additives that may elicit allergic or other adverse reactions (especially vitamins, fatty acids, or dermatological supplements). It is also important to try to identify any possible correlation between clinical signs and certain types of food, supplements, or medications.

Abnormal feeding patterns should be documented. Coprophagia can be observed in any disorders causing polyphagia such as exocrine pancreatic insufficiency or high-dose corticosteroid treatment. Also, coprophagia or pica can be observed in patients with nutritional deficiencies or those with behavioral problems. Eating grass is frequently reported in dogs and cats, and is of concern when it is followed by nausea or vomiting.[5] Eating grass could either be the cause or more commonly a consequence of a gastrointestinal problem.

🔑 Key Facts

■ Acquiring an accurate history is essential to further characterize the clinical signs related to digestive diseases.
■ Differentiation between regurgitation and vomiting is necessary to determine an optimal workup for each patient.
■ In cats constipation must not be mistaken for urinary straining.
■ Dietary history is a cornerstone in the diagnosis and management of digestive diseases.

References

1. Rothuizen J, Meyer HP. History, physical examination and signs of liver disease. In: Ettinger SJ, Feldman EC (eds.), *Textbook of veterinary internal medicine, 5th ed.* Philadelphia, WB Saunders, USA, 2000; 1272–1277.
2. Peeters ME, Venker van Haagen AJ, Wolvekamp WThC. Evaluation of a standardised questionnaire for the detection of dysphagia in 69 dogs. *Vet Rec* 1993; 132: 211–213.
3. Guilford WG. Approach to clinical problems in gastroenterology. In: Guilford WG et al (eds.), *Strombeck's small animal gastroenterology, 3rd ed.* Philadelphia, WB Saunders, USA, 1996; 50–76.
4. Elwood C. Investigations and differential diagnosis of vomiting in the dog. *In Practice,* 2003; 25: 374–386.
5. Tams TR. Gastrointestinal symptoms. In: Tams TR (ed.), *Handbook of small animal gastroenterology, 2nd ed.* Philadelphia, WB Saunders, 2003; 1–50.
6. Hall E. Introduction to investigating gastrointestinal diseases. In: Thomas D et al (eds.), *BSAVA Manual of Canine and Feline Gastroenterology, 1st ed.* Shurdington, UK, BSAVA, 1996; 9–19.
7. Jergens AE et al. A scoring index for disease activity in canine inflammatory bowel disease. *J Vet Intern Med,* 2003; 17: 291–297.
8. Houston DM. Clinical examination of the alimentary system – dogs and cats. In: Radositits OM, Mayhew IGJ, Houston DM (eds.), *Veterinary Clinical Examination and Diagnosis.* Philadelphia, WB Saunders, 2000; 349–369.
9. Roudebush P, Guilford WG, Shanley KJ. Adverse reactions to food. In: Hand MS et al. (eds.), *Small Animal Clinical Nutrition, 4th ed.* Topeka, USA, Mark Morris Institute, 2000; 431–453.
10. Drosman DA, Chang L. Psychosocial factors in the care of patients with gastrointestinal disorders. In: Yamada T (ed.), *Textbook of Gastroenterology, 4th ed.* Philadelphia, Lippincott Williams and Wilkins, 2003; 636–654.
11. Rijnberk A. The History. In: Rijnbberk A, de Vries HW (eds.), *Medical History and Physical Examination in Companion Animals.* Dordrecht, Netherlands, Kluwer Academic Publishers, 1995; 49–56.
12. Hoskins JD. Congenital defects of the dog. In: Ettinger SJ, Feldman EC (eds.), *Textbook of Veterinary Internal Medicine, 5th ed.* Philadelphia, WB Saunders, 2000; 1983–1996.
13. Hoskins JD. Congenital defects of the cat. In: Ettinger SJ, Feldman EC (eds.), *Textbook of Veterinary Internal Medicine, 5th ed.* Philadelphia, WB Saunders, 2000; 1975–1982.

1.2   Physical Examination

ANDREA BOARI

1.2.1   Introduction

By far the most important diagnostic tool that veterinarians can utilize is their ability to obtain a complete history and conduct a thorough physical examination. The objective of the physical examination is to recognize and describe gross deviations of the patient's physical appearance and behavior from those recognized as normal for the animal's species, breed, age, sex, and sexual status.

The trend toward an increased use of laboratory tests and instrumentation has added diagnostic capabilities, but such techniques are useful adjuncts for diagnosis only when a careful physical examination has been carried out. Thus, information gathered from laboratory and diagnostic imaging procedures must be considered a supplement to, but not a substitute for, hands-on examination. Inspection of the patient, palpation, percussion, and auscultation, all have a place in every examination. Only acute life-threatening situations require a shorter initial examination, until the animal's condition can be stabilized. In fact, if the patient is in shock or hemorrhaging, or has gastric dilation/volvulus, it is essential to initiate supportive care immediately and obtain a complete history with careful examination afterwards.

The physical examination of the gastrointestinal tract, as described in this chapter, is part of the methodical and standardized physical examination first developed at the School of Veterinary Medicine of Bologna University.[1]

In this chapter, the discussion is mainly limited to parameters of the physical examination that are specific and directly related to the gastrointestinal system, but it is important to note that the clinician should examine all body systems when presented with an patient that manifests signs of gastrointestinal disease. Ophthalmic and neurological examination, not included in this chapter, should not be forgotten because they can sometimes provide invaluable clues to the cause of a gastrointestinal dysfunction.

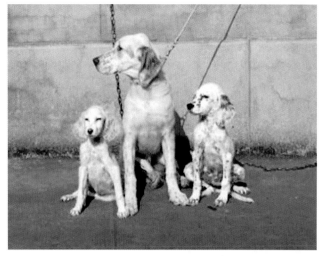

Figure 1.6:
Exocrine pancreatic insufficiency. This picture shows the failure to grow in two puppies with exocrine pancreatic insufficiency compared with a healthy littermate shown in the middle (these dogs are described in detail in: Boari A. et al. Observations on exocrine pancreatic insufficiency in a family of English setter dogs. *J Small Animal Practice* 1994, 35: 247–250).

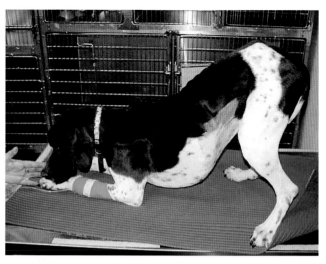

Figure 1.7:
"Prayer" position. This picture shows a dog with acute abdominal pain due to acute pancreatitis. This dog has assumed the "prayer" position with his front legs and sternum on the floor and his hind legs standing.

1.2.2 General physical examination

1.2.2.1 Skeletal growth and development

A failure to grow in dogs and cats, often seen with endocrinopathies such as hyposomatotropism and hypothyroidism, can also result from vascular ring or other esophageal anomalies, malabsorption, or portosystemic shunts (Figure 1.6).

1.2.2.2 Body condition

Measurement of body weight is inexpensive, easy, and very useful. Weight loss can be caused by inadequate nutrient assimilation (anorexia, regurgitation, vomiting, maldigestion, or malabsorption), increased loss of nutrients (protein-losing nephropathy [PLN] and/or protein-losing enteropathy [PLE]), and/or increased energy demand, as it occurs in hyperthyroid cats or febrile patients. Cachexia associated with fever can be due to infectious (e.g., FIP, FeLV), inflammatory (e.g., pancreatitis and others), or neoplastic (e.g., gastrointestinal neoplasia, lymphoma) causes.

Weight loss is unusual in patients with diarrhea due to large bowel disease, but it can be seen in patients with severe, longstanding colitis such as histiocytic ulcerative colitis (HUC), cecocolic intussusception, or diffuse colorectal neoplasia.[2]

However, it could also be caused by the tendency of owners to fast a pet with diarrhea.

It is very important to remember that an acute decrease in body weight can be due to water loss (i.e., vomiting and/or diarrhea) and that measurement of body weight will allow an accurate assessment of the level of dehydration.

1.2.2.3 Mental status

Depression or stupor can be related to abnormal brain function caused by metabolic (e.g., hepatic encephalopathy or acid-base and osmolality imbalances), inflammatory (e.g., canine distemper, FIP, sepsis), and vascular (e.g., coagulopathies, hypertension) disorders.

1.2.2.4 Abnormalities in posture and locomotion

In the cat, neck ventroflexion can be a sign of hypokalemia that can be caused by gastrointestinal loss of potassium due to vomiting, diarrhea, or anorexia. Abnormal posture, such as arching of the back or adoption of the "prayer" position (Figure 1.7), is a characteristic sign of abdominal pain, which needs to be differentiated from back pain.[3]

1.2.2.5 Mucous membranes

Mucous membrane color and capillary refill time (CRT) are used to estimate peripheral perfusion. A slower CRT suggests either dehydration or high peripheral sympathetic tone and vasoconstriction. Both are associated with low cardiac output. In a patient presented for vomiting, diarrhea, and/or anorexia, it is very important to address the patient's overall hydration status. To that end, the clinician should assess body weight, skin turgor or pliability, moistness and color of the mucous membranes, CRT, position of the eyes in their orbits, and the pulse and respiratory rates and their characteristics.

Pale mucous membranes are a manifestation of either decreased red blood cell mass or decreased peripheral perfusion. In the latter case, shock (i.e., hypovolemic, cardiogenic, or vasomotor shock) can cause hypovolemia, cardiac insufficiency, and vasoconstriction. As a result pallor is a hallmark of shock. In patients with endotoxemic shock, the mucous membranes may become cool to the touch.

Pale mucous membranes can also be associated with hepatobiliary disease due to increased consumption and/or as an effect of non-regenerative anemia due to chronic disease. Peptic and neoplastic gastric ulceration may also lead to anemia. Acute blood loss into the abdomen due to visceral hemangiosarcoma (HSA), which occurs much more frequently in dogs than cats, can also cause pale mucous membranes, weakness, abdominal distension, and increased pulse and respiration rates. The CRT is normal for anemic patients unless hypoperfusion is also present.

Also, the oral and ocular mucous membranes are often the first sites where jaundice can be seen. Yellow oral mucus membranes are almost always observed in cases of severe icterus and can be caused by immune-mediated hemolytic anemia or hepatobiliary disease.

A septic patient often has injected, highly vascular mucous membranes (brick-red) as can also occur in polycythemic patients, or those with acute hepatic and pancreatic disease, or severe azotemia. Congestion of mucous membranes may occur in patients with gastrointestinal disease, usually as a manifestation of dehydration. Mucous membranes should also be checked for signs of hemorrhage. Superficial bleeding into the skin or mucous membranes, and scleral and vitreal hemorrhage are often common manifestations of abnormalities of primary hemostasis. In addition to petechiae or ecchymoses, the animal may also present with hematemesis and melena as well as hematuria. Although infrequent, patients with severe hepatic disease can show bleeding diathesis due to coagulation factor deficiency, disseminated intravascular coagulation (DIC), or portal hypertension. Because of the multiple hemostatic defects present in patients with DIC, they may experience hemorrhage of any type and in any location (cavitary or superficial).

1.2.2.6 Peripheral lymph nodes

Mandibular, prescapular, and popliteal lymph nodes are usually palpable and they should be evaluated for size, shape, and consistency. The axillary and superficial inguinal lymph nodes are not always discernible. Given the close proximity of the mandibular lymph nodes and submaxillary salivary glands, it is essential that the clinician be able to distinguish between the two. Especially in cats, the surrounding subcutaneous fat may make the popliteal lymph nodes seem larger than their actual size. On the other hand, emaciated adult animals may have normal-sized popliteal lymph nodes that appear more prominent because of loss of fat and muscle mass.

Generalized lymphadenopathy usually indicates a systemic disease (e.g., immune-mediated disease, systemic infection, or more commonly neoplasia). Especially in the dog, the presence of markedly enlarged external lymph nodes that are firm and non-painful, is highly suggestive of lymphoma.[4]

1.2.2.7 Skin and subcutaneous tissue

The skin should be carefully inspected for areas of alopecia, inflammation, nodularity, and crustiness. Also, examination of the mucocutaneous junctions may reveal evidence for systemic immune-mediated diseases. Canine systemic lupus erythematous has occasionally been reported to cause megaesophagus, chronic small bowel diarrhea with PLE, and chronic hepatitis.[5–7]

Non-seasonal pruritus, erythema, and papules can be attributed to food hypersensitivity or "intolerance" in both dogs and cats. Concurrent presence of gastrointestinal and dermatological signs in dogs and cats is strongly suggestive of food hypersensitivity.[8–12]

Dramatic skin lesions (i.e., erythema, crusts, erosions, ulcers, alopecia, or shiny skin) can be seen in high-contact areas and on the ventral thorax and abdomen in patients with superficial necrolytic dermatitis, which can be caused by liver disease or glucagonoma. Also, pancreatic tumors have been reported as a cause of alopecia in dogs and cats.[13]

The integument should also be evaluated for changes in skin turgor, which is assessed in a consistent manner and location, usually on the lateral thorax. In evaluating skin turgor, the clinician should take into account the fact that skin turgor is dependent on the amount of subcutaneous fat and elastin, as well as on the interstitial volume. Thus, emaciated and older animals may appear more dehydrated than they actually are. On the other hand, obese animals may appear falsely well-hydrated based on their skin tenting.

1

Generalized soft tissue swelling or enlargement involving the four limbs, often associated with ascites, may be due to edema. Edema can be easily distinguished from other subcutaneous fluid accumulations or masses because pressure applied to an edematous area results in an indentation that stays for a short period of time. Subcutaneous edema can occasionally be seen in hypoalbuminemic dogs with PLE, PLN, or severe hepatic insufficiency.

1.2.2.8   Body temperature

At the time the temperature is taken, the clinician should also note if the rectal area is clean or soiled from diarrhea or matting, and whether the anal sacs are distended. The perineum is also observed for the presence of tapeworm proglottides. At the end of the examination, the thermometer should be examined for any blood, melena, or mucous. The appearance of blood in the feces can vary according to the site of bleeding, the transit time through the gastrointestinal tract, and the volume of blood lost.[14]

Hematochezia (i.e., fresh blood in the stool) is strongly suggestive of large bowel disease, in particular colitis. However, enterocolic and cecocolic intussusception, colorectal neoplasia and coagulopathies, especially platelet disorders, must also be considered, even though these are uncommon. Melena describes tar-, coal-, or asphalt-colored stools, resulting from digested blood and can be observed due to bleeding into the pharynx, esophagus, stomach, or upper small bowel. When melena is present, a complete physical examination should include careful inspection of the nares, oropharynx, and lungs for evidence of the source of bleeding. It is important to remember that a life-threatening volume of blood can accumulate within the gastrointestinal tract, with little or no visible signs of external blood loss. If gastrointestinal blood loss is associated with acute diarrhea, regardless of its cause, this signals a loss of normal intestinal mucosal integrity. With the loss of this barrier, the normal enteric flora can cross into the bloodstream, leading to septicemia. In this case, the clinician needs to address this life-threatening complication of diarrhea, while determining its cause.

There are many causes of fever in patients with gastrointestinal disease, ranging from infectious diseases (e.g., FeLV, FIV, FIP, canine distemper, feline panleukopenia, canine parvovirus, leptospirosis, salmonellosis, toxoplasmosis, leishmaniasis, histoplasmosis, blastomycosis, cryptococcosis, coccidiodomycosis, or rickettsial infections) to disorders involving the liver, exocrine pancreas, and the peritoneum, or neoplasia such as lymphoma or carcinoma.

In contrast, severely uremic patients, patients with sepsis and shock, or patients in the final stages of several severe systemic diseases can be hypothermic.

1.2.2.9   Pulse rate

The effects of many systemic and metabolic diseases on cardiac structure and function are well recognized. In some cases these may constitute the major clinical concern, while in others these effects may be subtle or of minimal importance. Common causes of tachycardia are excitement, fever, anemia, hemorrhage, shock, hypotension, significant alterations in the concentration of electrolytes or acid-base balance, congestive heart failure, and some infections.

Patients with GDV often show cardiac dysfunction, especially after surgical decompression. This is often associated with tachyarrhythmias or, less commonly, bradyarrhythmias.

Septic shock, often caused by gram-negative bacteria, can result in brick-red mucus membranes with a strong pulse during the initial stages, or pale mucus membranes and a weak pulse during the latter stages.

Electrolyte and acid-base abnormalities can produce significant alterations in cardiac function. These can often be documented during examination of the pulse; but are better recorded using an ECG. Severe hyperkalemia (usually >8 mEq/L) causes severe cardiac dysfunction. In addition to hypoadrenocorticism, hyperkalemia with hyponatremia (Na/K ratios <27:1) may also be found in dogs with gastrointestinal disease due to trichuriasis, salmonellosis, or a perforated duodenal ulcer and, although rare, in patients with peritoneal effusion.[15] Hyperkalemia without hyponatremia is almost always associated with impaired renal excretion due to oliguric or anuric renal failure.

Arrhythmias can also be observed in patients with hypokalemia. Hypokalemia is sometimes associated with alkalemia but more often is due to gastrointestinal loss of potassium or renal loss in patients with polyuric renal failure.

1.2.2.10   Respiratory rate

Respiratory rate and quality should be recorded before beginning the specific examination. It is important to differentiate between an increased respiratory rate that is due to a physiological response to exercise, hyperthermia, and anxiety, and one that is due to disease. Inspiratory dyspnea can be observed in patients with an elongated or edematous soft palate or feline patients with a pharyngeal polyp.

Animals with esophageal disease or vomiting can be presented to a veterinarian for respiratory distress due to aspiration pneumonia. Suspicion of megaesophagus or other esophageal diseases should be high if the owner reports that recurrent regurgitation or vomiting took place before the respiratory signs developed.

Severe and life-threatening dyspnea is often present in patients with pleural effusion and ascites associated with ascites due to hypoproteinemia or non-septic inflammation (i.e., FIP).

Rapid breathing can also be attributed to cranial displacement of the diaphragm by abdominal masses, fluid, or gas (e.g., gastric torsion) and/or acid-base imbalances. A compensatory hyperventilation is frequently seen in animals with metabolic acidosis caused by severe diarrhea, chronic renal disease, diabetic ketoacidosis, or hypoadrenocorticism.

1.2.3 Examination of the gastrointestinal tract

The examination of the gastrointestinal or digestive tract begins at the head (i.e., oral cavity), passes through the neck, down to the abdomen, and finishes with a rectal examination. Examination of the mouth and pharyngeal structures often provides important clues as to the pathogenesis of anorexia, vomiting, regurgitation, or drooling. In particular, drooling, which is best defined either as ptyalism (i.e., overproduction of saliva) or pseudoptyalism (i.e., dribbling or drooling of saliva that has accumulated in the oral cavity), occurs because animals are unable to swallow or are in too much pain to do so, as occurs during nausea, hepatic encephalopathy (especially in the cat), seizures, stomatitis, glossitis, gingivitis, pharyngitis, tonsillitis, and oral or pharyngeal dysphagia. Nasal discharge can also be associated with dysphagia, gagging and sometimes vomiting.

Swallowing and the gag reflex are assessed by placing an index finger at the base of the tongue or by observing the animal while it is drinking or eating. Tonsillitis or enlargement of the tonsils, mainly in the dog, can cause anorexia, vomiting, or dysphagia, and can occasionally be a sign of systemic disease (e.g., lymphoma). The tongue is examined for color and movement. The underside of the tongue is checked for masses, string foreign bodies (in the cat), or a laceration of the frenulum as a result of a string.

The **odor** of the breath can be indicative of dental or periodontal disease, but also of uremia or ketonemia.

The high frequency of **hyperthyroidism** in geriatric cats obliges the clinician to carefully palpate the paratracheal area, extending from the caudal larynx to the thoracic inlet, in order to detect nodular swelling suggestive of thyroid gland enlargement. The normal feline thyroid glands cannot be palpated.

Abdominal distension may be due to gas, fluid, organomegaly, or a poor abdominal muscle tone. Association with other clinical signs such as vomiting, diarrhea, abdominal pain, polydipsia, polyuria, polyphagia, or edema, may serve as a clue to the underlying etiology. In the dog, gastric tympany results in a flaring of the posterior rib cage and the hypochondrium. As gastric distension increases, the posterior abdomen also becomes visibly distended. If the enlarged abdomen is due to abdominal fluid, ballottement should be carefully performed to determine if a fluid wave is present. With experience, false positive results are infrequent.

Abdominal effusion is usually caused by hypoalbuminemia, portal hypertension, or peritoneal inflammation. Effusion due to gastrointestinal disease is primarily caused by PLE, hepatic failure, rupture of the alimentary tract, or leakage following anastomosis.[16,17] PLE in a young dog with chronic intermittent diarrhea, without hookworms, should prompt suspicion of a chronic intussusception and an abdominal ultrasound should be performed.[18]

Pyogranulomatous inflammation of the abdominal or thoracic cavity that is associated with a characteristic effusion is typical for the effusive form of FIP.

Malignant abdominal **tumors** may lead to obstruction of lymphatic flow, increased vascular permeability, accumulation of a modified transudate, or development of non-septic peritonitis. Modified transudates can also result from hepatic or cardiac disease. Hepatobiliary malignancies or other intra-abdominal malignant forms of neoplasia that have spread to the peritoneum can elicit an inflammatory reaction, with subsequent exudation of lymph, fibrin, and blood. This fluid may be serosanguinous, hemorrhagic, or pseudochylous in appearance.

Enlarged organs that most often account for increased abdominal size are the liver, spleen, and occasionally, the kidneys. Alternatively, single neoplastic masses of other organs also frequently lead to abdominal distension.

Abdominal palpation is the cornerstone of the physical examination in dogs and cats with clinical signs of gastrointestinal disease. This can be a most informative procedure for the cat, because of the ease with which most of the viscera can be palpated in this species.

If a gas-distended abdomen is suspected, digital abdominal percussion should be performed, listening for a tympanic sound. A sudden onset of a gas-distended abdomen, shock, and even death are often observed in dogs with intestinal volvulus.

Some animals tense their abdominal muscles in response to palpation. It is essential to determine whether this is caused by pain, anxiety, or the exertion of too much pressure during palpation. More significance is attributed to the pain response elicited in stoic animals and to pain that is localizable, repeatable, and evident after minimal manipulation. It is necessary to determine whether the painful area is superficial, located in the cranial or caudal abdomen, and whether it originates from a specific viscus. Cranial abdominal pain is commonly observed in dogs with pancreatitis, but less commonly observed in cats. Generalized abdominal pain with rigidity of the abdominal musculature suggests generalized peritonitis.

It is worth noting that if an animal arches its back during abdominal palpation the primary problem may be in the spinal cord. The empty stomach in cats and dogs is usually only palpable in thin patients, although if distended with food, it can be palpated in the upper left abdominal quadrant in most patients. The gallbladder and pancreas are not normally palpable. However, in patients with pancreatitis, pancreatic neoplasia, or a pancreatic pseudocyst, an abdominal mass and pain associated with palpation of the mass may be observed in the right cranial quadrant of the abdomen.

The **small intestine** is easily palpated as a thin-walled and smooth object that fills much of the mid-abdomen, and slides through the fingers. In the cat, the ileocecal area can often be palpated as a firm, knot-like structure in the mid-cranial abdomen, and should not be confused with an abdominal mass. The bowel should be carefully evaluated for thickness, rigidity, and irregular masses. A thickened intestinal wall may be felt in patients with intestinal infiltration by inflammatory or neoplastic cells and in patients with intestinal smooth muscle hypertrophy.[19]

Masses (e.g., lymph node enlargements, foreign bodies, omental steatitis, neoplasia, intussusception, or focal granulomatous lesions, such as those that can be seen in patients with a non-effusive form of FIP) can cause partial or total intestinal obstruction, but may go undetected during physical examination because of their small size.[20] Fluid-distended small bowel loops are often palpable in patients with acute enteritis. Aggregated or accordion-like small bowel loops are characteristic of a linear foreign body obstruction in cats. Palpable mesenteric lymph node enlargements are often associated with tumors, granulomas, or intestinal inflammation (with or without foreign body obstruction). A massive mesenteric lymphadenopathy is often typical of dogs and cats with alimentary tract lymphoma, but modest lymphadenopathy can also be found in patients with IBD or other chronic intestinal diseases.

A sick animal that vomits shortly after abdominal palpation should be suspected of having a GI obstruction, severe GI tract inflammation, or pancreatitis.

The **transverse and descending colon** are often full of fecal material and can easily be identified by palpation of the mid-posterior abdomen, just ventral to the spine. An impacted colon (the colon must be at least twice its normal diameter before megacolon can be considered), is caused by intestinal obstruction or dysmotilities.

The **liver** can be palpated routinely just caudal to the costal arch along the ventral body wall in both canine and feline patients, but may not be palpable in some cases. If the liver is not palpable, it does not automatically mean that it is abnormally small. Microhepatia is mainly seen in patients with a congenital portosystemic shunt or those with chronic hepatic disease with progressive loss of hepatocytes. However, hepatic size is better evaluated by radiography. In lean cats, it is possible to palpate the diaphragmatic surface of the liver. In animals with pleural effusion or other diseases that expand the thoracic volume, the liver may appear enlarged due to caudal displacement. The pattern of hepatic enlargement may be generalized or focal depending on its cause. Infiltrative and congestive diseases tend to result in smooth, firm, and diffuse hepatomegaly. Primary or metastatic neoplasia, nodular hyperplasia, and some chronic hepatic diseases associated with nodular regeneration can cause focal or asymmetric hepatic enlargement.

In icteric dogs and cats, hepatosplenomegaly may be attributable to mononuclear-phagocytic cell hyperplasia and extramedullary hematopoiesis secondary to immune-mediated hemolytic anemia or to infiltrative processes such as systemic mast cell disease, lymphoma, or myeloid leukemia.

Palpation of the spleen is not always possible, but sometimes the free distal portion is palpable on the floor of the mid-abdomen. The spleen is palpated for identification of an increase in size and for nodules or larger masses. In patients with severe splenomegaly, the spleen may occupy the entire ventral abdominal floor.[21] When the enlarged spleen is folded over, it may be mistaken for a mass. With experience, the clinican can sometimes unfold the spleen with his or her thumb, and thus the "real" shape of the organ can be evaluated.

The **kidneys** can only be easily palpated in cats because they are more loosely attached than they are in dogs. The kidneys are normally located in the retroperitoneal area, and the right kidney lies slightly more cranial than the left. The kidneys are evaluated for size, shape, location, firmness, pain, and surface irregularities. The left kidney (the only one that can be palpated in some dogs) is especially movable and can easily be mistaken for an abdominal mass. Enlarged, abnormally-shaped kidneys may be caused by acute renal failure, renal neoplasia, renal cysts, abscesses, granulomatous nephritis due to FIP, hydronephrosis, or hematoma. In contrast, small renal size is often associated with chronic renal disease.

During abdominal palpation of **intact female animals**, the normal non-gravid uterus is usually non-palpable. Massive uteromegaly caused by pregnancy, pyometra, mucometra, or hydrometra can sometimes give the mistaken impression of ascites and must be carefully differentiated.

Lastly, abdominal auscultation may sometimes be helpful. Failure to detect intestinal sounds after two or three minutes of auscultation is suggestive of ileus.

The **perineal area** should be examined for evidence of diarrhea caked in the hair coat, masses, or herniations. **Rectal examination** must always be performed and the clinician should be able to identify and evaluate the colonic mucosa, anal sphincter, anal sacs, pelvic canal bones, urogenital tract, and luminal contents. Mucosal polyps can easily be misinterpreted as mucosal folds, and it is possible to miss partial strictures that are large enough to allow a single finger to pass through.

Pelvic canal obstruction due to congenital and acquired causes can lead to constipation and megacolon, especially in cats.

Rectal discomfort, hematochezia, and mucous can be found in patients with colitis, proctitis, or large bowel neoplasia as described previously.

During the rectal examination, the prostate of all mature male dogs must be evaluated for size, symmetry, surface structure, and pain. If enlarged, the prostate may extend slightly over the brim of the pelvis or fall into the abdomen. In this latter situation, the prostate can be palpated in the caudal abdomen ventral to the colon and caudal to the urinary bladder. To assist in rectal palpation, the other hand of the examiner should be used to gently push the prostate into a more dorsal and caudal position via abdominal palpation.

Also, in order to complete the physical examination, the clinician should observe the act of defecation whenever possible, especially if there is a history of dyschezia or tenesmus.

Whether tenesmus occurs before or after defecation can also aid in differentiation of the underlying disease process. Obstructive disorders are more commonly associated with tenesmus before evacuation of feces, whereas inflammatory disorders are often associated with persistent tenesmus after the evacuation of feces.

🔑 Key Facts

- A life-threatening volume of blood can accumulate within the gastrointestinal tract, with little or no visible signs of external blood loss.
- Abdominal distension may be due to gas, fluid, organomegaly, or poor abdominal muscle tone.
- PLE in a young dog with chronic intermittent diarrhea, without hookworms, should prompt a suspicion of chronic intussusception.
- Aggregated (accordion-like) small bowel loops on abdominal palpation are characteristic of a linear foreign body obstruction in cats.
- A sick animal that vomits shortly after abdominal palpation should be suspected of having a GI obstruction, severe GI tract inflammation, or pancreatitis.
- Rectal examination should be performed in every patient presenting for evaluation of gastrointestinal disease.

References

1. Messieri A, Moretti B. *Semiologia e diagnostica medica veterinaria* [Veterinary clinical examination and diagnosis], *6th ed.* Tinarelli (ed.), Bologna, 1982; 1–1150.
2. Hostutler RA, Luria BJ, Johnson SE et al. Antibiotic-responsive histiocytic ulcerative colitis in 9 dogs. *J Vet Intern Med* 2004; 18: 499–504.
3. Franks JN, Howe LM. Evaluating and managing acute abdomen. *Vet Med* 2000; 1: 56–69.
4. Vail DM, MacEwen EG, Young KM. Canine lymphoma and lymphoid leukemias. In: Withrow SJ, MacEwen EG (eds.), *Small animal clinical oncology, 3rd ed.*, Philadelphia, WB Saunders, 2001; 558–590.
5. Guilford WG, Strombeck DR. Diseases of swallowing. *In*: Guilford WG, Center SA, Strombeck DR, Williams DA, Meyer DJ (eds.), *Strombeck's Small animal gastroenterology, 3rd ed.* Philadelphia, WB Saunders, 1996; 211–238.
6. Williams DA. Malabsorption, small intestinal bacterial overgrowth, and protein-losing enteropathy. *In*: Guilford WG, Center SA, Strombeck DR, Williams DA, Meyer DJ (eds.), *Strombeck's Small animal gastroenterology, 3rd ed.* Philadelphia, WB Saunders, 1996; 367–380.
7. Center SA. Chronic hepatitis, cirrhosis, breed-specific hepatopathies, copper storage hepatopathy, suppurative hepatitis, granulomatous hepatitis, and idiopathic hepatic fibrosis. *In*: Guilford WG, Center SA, Strombeck DR, Williams DA, Meyer DJ (eds.), *Strombeck's Small animal gastroenterology, 3rd ed.* Philadelphia, WB Saunders, 1996; 705–765.
8. White SD. Food hypersensitivity in 30 dogs. *J Am Vet Med Assoc* 1986; 188: 695–698.
9. White SD, Sequoia D. Food hypersensitivity in cats: 14 cases (1982–1987). *J Am Vet Med Assoc* 1989; 194: 692–695.

1

10. Guilford WG, Markwell PJ, Jones BR et al. Prevalence and causes of food sensitivity in cats with chronic pruritus, vomiting or diarrhea. *J Nutr* 1998; 128: 2790S–2791S.
11. Guilford WG, Boyd RJ, Markwell PJ et al. Food sensitivity in cats with chronic idiopathic gastrointestinal problems. *J Vet Intern Med* 2001; 15: 7–13.
12. Paterson S. Food sensitivity in 20 dogs with skin and gastrointestinal signs. *J Small Anim Pract* 1995; 36: 529–534.
13. Byrne KP. Metabolic epidermal necrosis-hepatocutaneous syndrome. *Vet Clin North Am (Small Anim Pract)* 1999; 29: 1337–1355.
14. Guilford WG. Approach to clinical problems in gastroenterology. *In*: Guilford WG, Center SA, Strombeck DR, Williams DA, Meyer DJ (eds.), *Strombeck's Small animal gastroenterology, 3rd ed.* Philadelphia, WB Saunders, 1996; 50–76.
15. Bissett SA, Lamb M, Ward CR. Hyponatremia and hyperkalemia associated with peritoneal effusion in four cats. *J Am Vet Med Assoc* 2001; 218: 1590–1592.

16. Hinton LE, McLoughlin MA, Johnson SE et al. Spontaneous gastroduodenal perforation in 16 dogs and 7 cats (1982–1999). *J Am Anim Hosp Assoc* 2000, 38: 176–187.
17. Ralphs SC, Jessen CR, Lipowitz AJ. Risk factors for leakage following intestinal anastomosis in dogs and cats: 115 cases (1991–2000). *J Am Vet Med Assoc* 2003; 223: 73–77.
18. Peterson PB, Willard MD. Protein-losing enteropathies. *Vet Clin North Am (Small Anim Pract)* 2003; 33: 1061–1082.
19. Diana A, Pietra M, Guglielmini C et al. Ultrasonographic and pathologic features of intestinal smooth muscle hypertrophy in four cats. *Vet Radiol Ultrasound* 2003; 44: 566–569.
20. Harvey CJ, Lopez JW, Hendrick MJ. An uncommon intestinal manifestation of feline infectious peritonitis: 26 cases (1986–1993). *J Am Vet Med Assoc* 1996; 209: 1117–1120.
21. de Morais HA, O'Brien T. Non-neoplastic disorders of the spleen. In: Ettinger SJ, Feldman EC (eds.), *Textbook of Veterinary Internal Medicine, 6th ed.* Philadelphia, Elsevier Saunders, 2005; 1944–1951.

1.3   Diagnostic Imaging

LORRIE GASCHEN

1.3.1   Introduction

The variety of diagnostic imaging modalities that have become available to veterinarians has led to the need for expanded expertise in ultrasound, computed tomography (CT), nuclear scintigraphy, and magnetic resonance imaging (MRI). However, conventional radiography and ultrasonography remain essential, cost-effective, and readily available methods for diagnosing many gastrointestinal disorders in dogs and cats. In the past 10 years, ultrasonography has become an invaluable diagnostic tool, which has virtually replaced the need for barium contrast studies in animals presenting for vomiting and/ or diarrhea. Historically, the combination of plain and contrast radiography was considered the gold standard for the examination of the gastrointestinal tract. Currently, however, the combination of sonography and endoscopy has become a more frequently used approach.

Radiography and ultrasonography of the abdomen should be performed together since they can each provide complementary information. Survey radiographs provide a global view of the abdomen that cannot be obtained with sectional imaging such as ultrasonography. Survey radiographs may also allow an immediate diagnosis to be made, as is the case in patients with an intestinal obstruction. Indications for plain **radiography** may include dysphagia, regurgitation, vomiting, acute abdomen, constipation, abdominal pain, abdominal distension, or a palpable mass. In animals with chronic diarrhea or marked abdominal effusion, abdominal radiographs are less beneficial.

The spectrum of gastrointestinal diseases that can be detected by **ultrasonography** include intussusceptions, pancreatitis, peritoneal infiltrative disease, gastrointestinal wall infiltrations, abdominal neoplasia, and hepatobiliary disease. Ultrasonography may also provide functional information in intestinal motility and hemodynamic disorders. Furthermore, ultrasound-guided, percutaneous tissue biopsy can be performed to collect samples for cytological or histological examination. However, the clinical usefulness of ultrasonography is highly operator-dependent and the detection and interpretation of changes relies heavily on the ultrasonographer's expertise.

Barium contrast studies of the gastrointestinal tract are generally only indicated when the combination of clinical information, survey radiography, and ultrasonography do not lead to a diagnosis.[1] Contraindications to performing barium contrast studies include survey radiographic evidence of obstructive disease or free peritoneal gas or liquid. Although iodinated contrast agents may be used, they should be avoided in debilitated or dehydrated patients since they can worsen the condition of the patient or lead to a hypovolemic state.[2]

Endoscopic ultrasound is commonly used in human gastroenterology to examine the gastrointestinal tract and for performing guided transluminal biopsies. Although this technique has been underutilized in veterinary medicine, it can be applied in both canine and feline patients.[3] A high frequency transducer mounted on the tip of a conventional video endoscope (Figure 1.8) allows the acquisition of high resolution images of the esophageal wall, stomach, liver, pancreas, lymph nodes, adrenal glands, intra-abdominal vasculature, kidneys, spleen, duodenum, jejunum, and proximal colon.

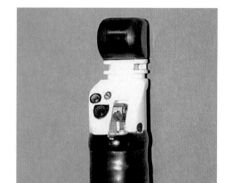

Figure 1.8:
Echoendoscope. This figure shows the tip of an Olympus GF-UC140-AL5 video gastroendoscope (Olympus Optical, Hamburg, Germany). The ultrasound transducer is mounted at the tip, while the optics and working channel are mounted at an angle on the side. The transducer is a multi-frequency (5–10 MHz) curved (180°) linear array transducer designed for guided tissue aspirations.

1

Contrast-enhanced ultrasonography is being used with increasing frequency in veterinary medicine. Modern ultrasound contrast agents are gas-containing stabilized microbubbles that remain intact in the vascular space for several minutes after intravenous injection and increase the intensity of the backscattered ultrasound.[4] In human medicine, contrast-enhanced ultrasound has been most widely used for the differentiation of malignant versus benign focal liver lesions.[5] It has recently been shown that contrast harmonic ultrasound of the liver can be used to detect portosystemic shunting in dogs.[6]

CT, MRI, and **nuclear scintigraphy** are alternative methods for the investigation of the abdomen in cats and dogs.[7,8,9] However, there are only a few reports about the use of these modalities in small animal gastroenterology and these methods have not yet attained common usage for investigating gastrointestinal disorders. CT may be performed for the detection of abdominal neoplasia, pancreatic imaging, or for the detection of portosystemic shunts.[10,11] Only a few reports concerning the use of MRI for the examination of the abdomen in dogs and cats are available and more work is clearly needed in this field.[12] Nuclear scintigraphy provides functional information about the gastrointestinal tract and has been well established in veterinary medicine. In the hands of an experienced user, rectal scintigraphy has significantly improved the rapid diagnosis of portosystemic shunts and allows for the quantification of the shunting fraction both pre- and postoperatively.[13,14] Nuclear scintigraphy has also been used for the diagnosis of hepatobiliary disease and the quantification of gastric emptying time.[7,15]

This chapter provides guidelines for a diagnostic imaging approach in dogs and cats with gastrointestinal disorders. Each section discusses the imaging of different anatomic regions according to specific clinical signs. Imaging for the evaluation of hepatobiliary and pancreatic disorders is described in a separate section. Although radiography and ultrasonography are emphasized, indications for alternative imaging modalities are also described.

1.3.2   Oropharynx

Patients with dysphagia and regurgitation on the one side or vomiting on the other are approached differently depending on which sign predominates. Dysphagia and regurgitation can often be differentiated from vomiting by a thorough history and physical examination. Regurgitation can occur with both oropharyngeal and esophageal disorders. Patients with exaggerated swallowing attempts, gagging, or pain when drinking or swallowing food, however, often have oropharyngeal dysphagia. Regurgitation is characterized by the passive retrograde expulsion of undigested food, whereas animals with vomiting show a forceful ejection of partially digested food with a marked abdominal effort.

Survey radiographs should always be performed to rule out structural abnormalities, such as fractures of the hyoid apparatus or radiopaque foreign bodies in the oropharyngeal region. The pharyngeal and laryngeal regions and the entire esophagus should be included in both lateral and ventrodorsal views. Thoracic radiographs in two planes are strongly recommended in animals with dysphagia to rule out the presence of aspiration pneumonia.

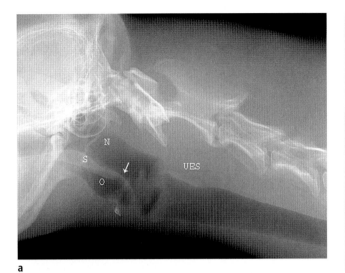

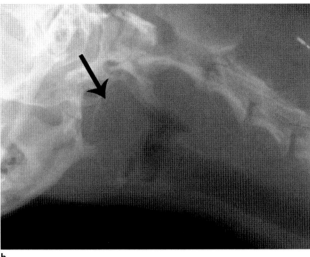

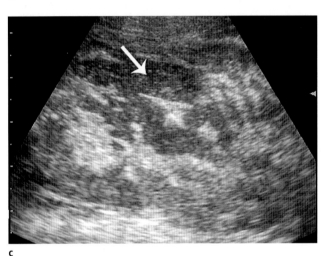

Figure 1.9a–c:
Imaging of the pharyngeal region.
(a) Normal pharynx. N=nasopharynx, O=oropharynx, S=soft palate, UES=upper esophageal sphincter, arrow=epiglottis
(b) Oblique lateral radiograph of the pharyngeal region in an 11-year-old Coton de Tuléar that presented in respiratory distress. In this dog, the nasopharynx is compressed and the pharynx is displaced dorsally (arrow) due to an opaque soft tissue space-occupying lesion.
(c) Ultrasonographic image of the soft tissue lesion from the patient shown in Figure 9b. A complex cavitary mass with fluid-filled pockets (arrow) in the center was identified. The mass was surgically removed and diagnosed as an abscess.

1.3.2.1 Structural abnormalities

Survey radiographs should be inspected for increased soft tissue opacities in the pharyngeal, retropharyngeal, or cervical region, which may impinge upon or displace the airways of the oropharynx, nasopharynx, larynx, or trachea (Figure 1.9). Soft tissue space-occupying lesions may be due to lymphadenomegaly, abscesses, polyps, neoplasias, or foreign body granulomas. Radiopaque foreign bodies may be immediately evident; however, radiolucent ones may only appear as space-occupying lesions of soft tissue opacities. The presence of gas within soft tissues can be seen with abscesses or percutaneous foreign body penetration.

Ultrasonography can be used to determine the origin of soft tissue swellings of the neck and retropharyngeal region. High frequency linear array transducers are best for the examination of the cervical region since most structures are very superficial. However, curved-linear array transducers are also adequate.[16] The thyroids and salivary glands and the retropharyngeal or mandibular lymph nodes can all be enlarged due to inflammation, abscessation, or primary or metastatic neoplasia. Perforating foreign bodies can be recognized as hyperechogenic structures of varying size with acoustic shadowing (Figure 1.10).[17] Pinpoint hyperechogenic structures with reverberation echoes signal the presence of air and should not be mistaken for foreign material. Lingual foreign bodies and abscesses can also be diagnosed with ultrasound using a ventral, inter-mandibular approach (Figure 1.11).[18]

MRI and CT are excellent alternative modalities for examining the cervical region, screening for foreign bodies, and for determining the origin of complex masses.

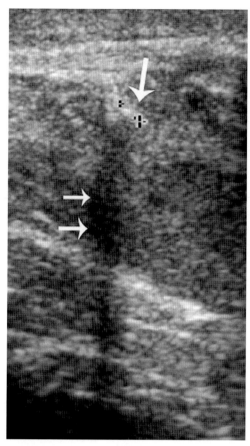

Figure 1.10:
Foreign body in the cervical region. Ultrasound image of the cervical region of a dog with a chronic draining fistula. A 3-mm long, hyperechoic, linear structure (arrow) with distinct acoustic shadowing (two smaller arrows) was detected in the soft tissue. Diagnosis: wood splinter with abscess.

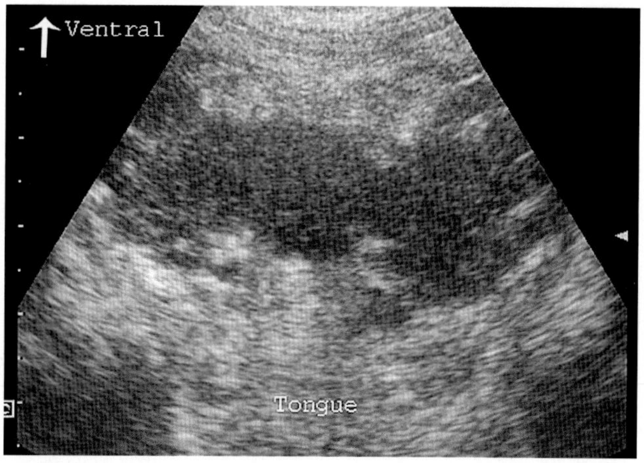

Figure 1.11:
Lingual foreign body. Ventral transverse ultrasound image of the caudal oral cavity at the level of the angular processes of the mandible in a dog with acute dyspnea, cyanosis, and pharyngeal swelling. A space-occupying lesion with a complex echotexture at the base of the tongue was identified. The mandibular rami can be seen as the anechoic structures on either side of the tongue. The lesion was explored surgically and found to be an abscess most likely to be due to a perforated foreign body.

1.3.2.2 Functional Disorders

Survey radiographs of animals with neuromuscular causes of oral, pharyngeal, and cricopharyngeal dysphagia are generally unremarkable. Thoracic radiographs are strongly recommended to rule out the presence of aspiration pneumonia, which can occur with cricopharyngeal dysphagia. Lateral radiographs of the oropharyngeal and cervical region are required to rule out structural abnormalities. Focal accumulations of gas may be detected in the proximal esophagus due to either esophagitis or functional disorders. The presence of an open, air-filled upper esophageal sphincter and an air-filled esophagus can be seen with cricopharyngeal chalasia since the sphincter cannot maintain a positive resting pressure (Figure 1.12). However, the finding of air in the esophagus in sedated or anesthetized animals is not uncommon and should be interpreted with caution.

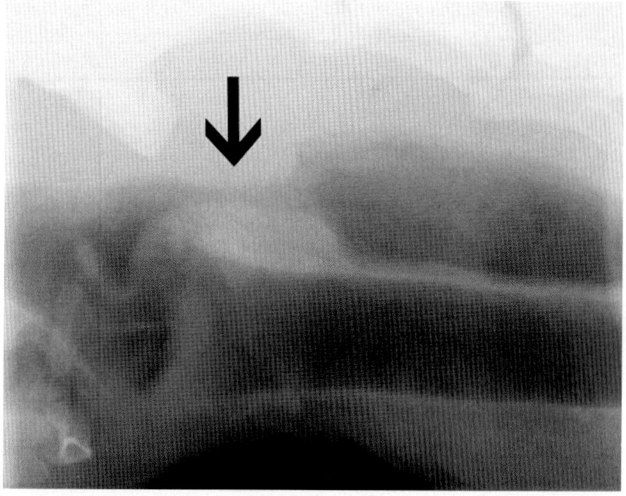

Figure 1.12:
Megaesophagus. Lateral radiograph of the pharynx in a 4-year-old German Shepherd with regurgitation due to megaesophagus. The upper esophageal sphincter is open and air-filled (arrow). The cervical esophagus is also dilated and air-filled. The presence of air in these structures signals the possibility of either a functional or structural disorder. The diagnosis in this dog was chalasia due to myasthenia gravis. (Image courtesy of Dr. Johann Lang, Division of Radiology, Faculty of Veterinary Medicine, University of Bern, Switzerland.)

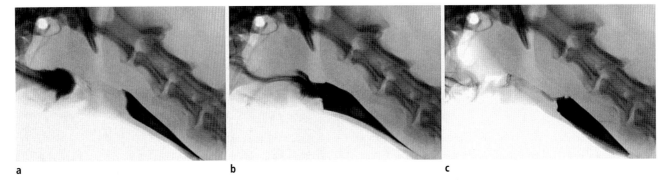

a   b   c

Figure 1.13a–c:
Barium swallow in a normal dog. Static digital fluoroscopic images of a barium swallow in a normal dog. The pharyngeal **(a)**, cricopharyngeal **(b)**, and esophageal **(c)** phases are shown. (Images courtesy of Dr. Johann Lang, Division of Radiology, Faculty of Veterinary Medicine, University of Bern, Switzerland.)

When survey radiographic examination is unremarkable, a contrast study performed with either fluoroscopy, serial radiographic exposures, or static radiographic images is indicated. However, without the possibility of fluoroscopy and dynamic acquisition of images, the details of bolus formation and passage can usually not be observed with static radiographic images alone.

Swallowing studies are generally performed in conscious animals since sedation may inhibit swallowing or increase the risk of aspiration. Initially, a liquid contrast agent should be administered into the oral cavity. Liquid barium sulfate suspensions (45–85% w/w) are preferred for barium swallows and 5–20 ml of the suspension is administered depending on the size of the animal. If the animal has a history of having difficulty swallowing food but not liquids, the study should be repeated using barium-coated food. With the animal in lateral recumbency, the act of swallowing should be observed immediately with fluoroscopy and recorded on video tape or using rapid serial radiography (Figure 1.13).

Retention of contrast medium in the oral cavity and its absence in the pharynx and esophagus can be observed in animals with oral dysphagia. When direct damage to the tongue is ruled out, a brain stem lesion (hypoglossal nerve) may be suspected as the underlying cause. Retention of substantial amounts of contrast medium in the pharynx following swallowing of the bolus is observed in pharyngeal phase dysphagia. Laryngeal aspiration may also be observed. When mechanical obstruction can be ruled out, idiopathic neuromuscular dysfunction is usually the cause.

Cricopharyngeal dysphagia is characterized by retention of contrast medium in the pharynx with reflux of the contrast medium into the oro- or nasopharynx, aspiration into the larynx, retention in the cervical esophagus, and hypertrophy or distortion of the upper esophageal sphincter. Often, very small amounts of contrast medium are observed to pass through the hypertrophied sphincter. This disease is often seen in young dogs and is called cricopharyngeal achalasia (Figure 1.14). In contrast, in patients with cricopharyngeal chalasia, the upper esophageal sphincter remains open and contrast can be observed moving freely between the esophagus and pharynx through an open sphincter (Figure 1.15). This should alert the clinician to a neuromuscular disorder such as myasthenia gravis.

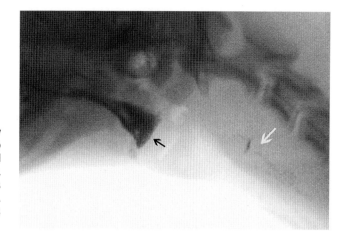

Figure 1.14:
Cricopharyngeal achalasia. Static digital fluoroscopic image of a barium swallow in a 5-month-old American Staffordshire Terrier with dysphagia and failure to thrive. The puppy showed clinical signs of cricopharyngeal dysphagia and could only swallow food intermittently. There is retention of contrast in the pharynx. Fluoroscopically, pharyngeal contractions were evident and the contrast bolus was repeatedly advanced towards a closed upper esophageal sphincter (black arrow). Occasionally, some contrast material could pass through the sphincter and was visible in the esophagus (white arrow). Diagnosis: cricopharyngeal achalasia.

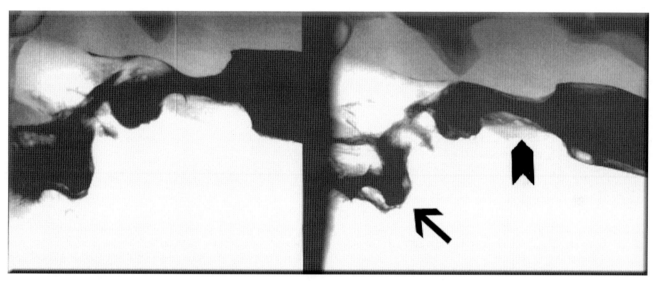

Figure 1.15:
Barium swallow in a dog with myasthenia gravis. This figure shows a barium swallow in the same dog as shown in Figure 1.12. Note that there is retention of contrast in the pharynx (arrow) and the upper esophageal sphincter remains open (arrow head) and filled with contrast. (Image courtesy of Dr. Johann Lang, Division of Radiology, Faculty of Veterinary Medicine, University of Bern, Switzerland.)

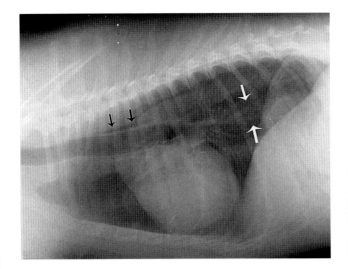

Figure 1.16:
Radiographic appearance of the esophagus in normal dogs. Lateral thoracic radiograph of a normal dog. Dogs and cats that are nervous and panting when radiographs are taken may have small amounts of air or fluid in the esophagus. Air is typically seen just cranial to the base of the heart (black arrows). The caudal esophagus may appear as a soft tissue opaque band (between white arrows) between the aorta and caudal vena cava.

1.3.3   Esophagus

The radiographic features that are associated with esophageal disease are listed in Table 1.7. Radiography is central to the diagnosis of megaesophagus. It allows rapid identification of the affected segments and also assessment of the degree of esophageal dilation. A small amount of air in the esophageal lumen can be expected in dogs that are panting or nervous during the radiographic procedure or those under sedation or general anesthesia (Figure 1.16). The presence of ventral pulmonary consolidations and pleural fluid on thoracic radiographs should raise the suspicion of mediastinitis and/or aspiration pneumonia (Figure 1.17).

Esophagography with barium sulfate creams or suspensions is indicated when esophageal disease is suspected and survey thoracic radiographs are unremarkable. In the presence of a pneumomediastinum or mediastinitis, aqueous iodine agents may be used orally, but if aspirated they may induce pulmonary edema due to their hypertonic nature. The goal of the esophagram should be to determine the location and type of esophageal abnormality. The esophagram may, however, only provide limited information since it can only differentiate intraluminal lesions from intramural or peri-esophageal ones. If the liquid barium suspension does not show a stricture, a barium-coated food bolus should be fed.

Peri-esophageal or intramural lesions that do not alter the esophageal mucosa may go unnoticed during conventional endoscopy of the esophagus. In contrast, echoendoscopy allows the detection of intramural neoplasms and extramural space-occupying lesions of the mediastinum that may compress the esophagus. The author has diagnosed both esophageal tumors and periesophageal lesions using echoendoscopy in both dogs and cats (Figure 1.19).

1.3.3.1   Generalized esophageal dilation

Generalized megaesophagus can be visualized by the presence of a dilated, gas-filled lumen along the entire length of the esophagus on survey radiographs. The tracheal stripe sign is present due to superimposition of the esophageal and tracheal walls and the longus colli muscle ventral to the 5th and 6th thoracic vertebrae (Figure 1.18). The caudodorsal thorax may also appear hyperlucent due to the presence of air in the esophagus. Differential diagnoses for generalized dilation of the esophagus are numerous. In young animals megaesophagus is most commonly idiopathic. In adults, central nervous system and neuromuscular disorders, such as myasthenia gravis, feline dysautonomia, polyneuritis, or polymyositis are more likely to be the cause. Endocrinopathies such as hypothyroidism or hypoadrenocorticism and toxicities, trauma, tetanus, and thymoma are additional differential diagnoses. Dilation can also be seen with hiatal hernias and gastric volvulus. Furthermore, an air-filled megaesophagus can be seen in cats with lower airway disease causing dyspnea and aerophagia. Mechanical causes of generalized dilation can be due to foreign bodies and strictures located either intraluminally, murally, or peri-esophageally.

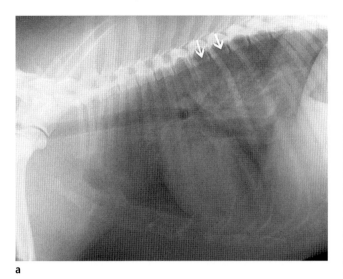

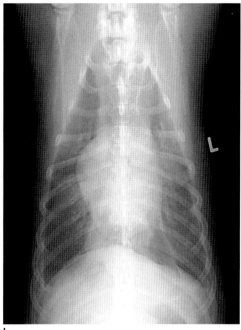

a

b

Figure 1.17a, b:
Perforated esophageal foreign body. Lateral **(a)** and ventrodorsal **(b)** thoracic digital radiographs of a 2-year-old American Staffordshire Terrier that presented in lateral recumbency and shock with severe abdominal pain. A mixed radiopacity in the region of the caudal esophagus is seen. Additional findings include the presence of pleural fluid and pneumothorax. Note the retracted border of the caudal lung lobe (arrows) with free air surrounding it dorsally. Differential diagnoses include trauma, pulmonary disease, and mediastinitis. A piece of rawhide was removed surgically from the esophagus, which was perforated.

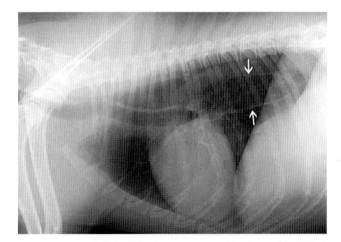

Figure 1.18:
Megaesophagus. Lateral thoracic radiograph showing generalized megaesophagus. The esophagus is air-filled, the dorsal thorax appears hyperlucent, and the thin walls of the esophagus can be identified (arrows).

Table 1.7: Radiographic signs of esophageal disease

- Increased visibility
- Tracheal stripe sign
- Dilation with air, fluid, or food
- Pneumomediastinum
- Mediastinal space-occupying lesion

- Ventral displacement of the trachea and heart
- Increased lucency of the dorsal thoracic region
- Ill-defined pulmonary consolidations located ventrally
- Pleural fluid

1

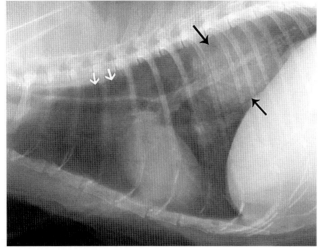

a

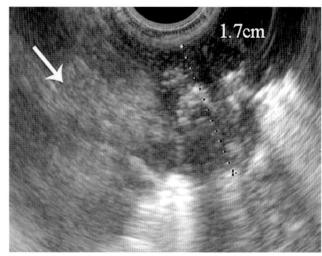

c

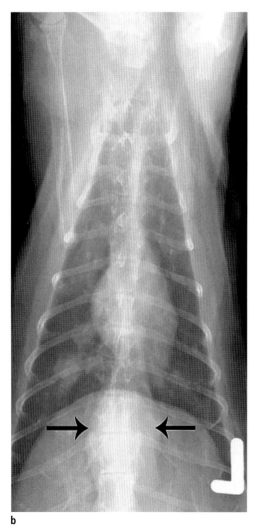

b

Figure 1.19a–c:
Esophageal mass.
(a+b) Lateral and ventrodorsal thoracic radiographs of a 16-year-old European Short Hair cat that presented with chronic dyspnea, anorexia, and weight loss. A round soft tissue opacity in the region of the caudal mediastinum can be seen (black arrows). Note the segmental dilation of the esophagus cranial to the lesion (white arrows). Additional pulmonary nodules are seen in the right caudal lung lobe. Possible origins of the mass are esophageal intraluminal, mural, or periesophageal as well as pulmonary. Differential diagnoses include neoplasia, granuloma, abscess, and esophageal foreign body.
(c) Esophageal echoendoscopy showed a nodular infiltration with disruption of the esophageal wall layering of 1.7 cm in diameter (distance shown: dotted line). The lesion has a complex echostructure that includes hyperechoic foci with reverberation echoes (gas bubbles in the mass). A separate portion of the lesion (arrow) was 2 cm in diameter, homogenous, and had broken through the esophageal wall to invade the periesophageal region. Multiple intralesional vessels with arterial flow could be shown by Doppler ultrasound. Histological diagnosis: esophageal carcinoma.

1.3.3.2 Segmental esophageal dilation

Localized or segmental esophageal dilations may be located anywhere along the esophagus. (Figure 1.19). Potential causes include foreign bodies, segmental hypomotility, esophagitis, diverticuli, hernias, foreign bodies, acquired strictures, and mural or extramural lesions due to inflammation or neoplasia. Foreign bodies and strictures may also present radiographically as mediastinal soft tissue opacities rather than focal dilations. Common sites of esophageal strictures are the thoracic inlet, the base of the heart, and at the gastroesophageal junction. In young dogs and cats, esophageal strictures are often due to vascular ring anomalies such as a persistent right aortic arch. These are recognized by a ventral displacement of the trachea in the cranial thorax and varying degrees of esophageal dilation cranial to the base of the heart. Barium esophagrams are contraindicated in the presence of large fluid- or food-filled esophageal dilations. Angiography should be performed to definitively rule out a vascular ring anomaly in any puppy or kitten with suspected vascular ring anomaly.

1.3.4 Stomach

Following the clinical history, physical examination, and laboratory data base, survey radiographs and ultrasound are important diagnostic tools in dogs and cats with vomiting. Radiography is a rapid method for assessment of extra-abdominal structures, the abdominal wall, diaphragm, vertebrae, and also the detection of obstructive lesions and radiopaque foreign bodies. The significance of the presence of radiopaque material in the gastrointestinal tract must be correlated to the type of foreign body, its size, and the clinical signs of the animal. Regardless of inherent diagnostic limitations, lateral and ventrodorsal survey radiographs should always be performed prior to contrast studies, ultrasonography, or endoscopy.

Prior to both radiography and ultrasonography, animals should be fasted for a minimum of 12 hours, though this may not be possible in emergency situations. Dependent upon the radiographic findings, a combination of ultrasonography and endoscopy may be deemed necessary. Ultrasonography should always be performed prior to endoscopy or barium studies since the presence of excessive intestinal gas or barium sulfate will create ultrasound artefacts that prohibit examination of the abdomen.

For the ultrasonographic evaluation of the gastrointestinal tract, high frequency curved linear array or sector transducers are recommended. High frequency transducers have the best resolution for evaluation of gastrointestinal wall layers. Moreover, linear transducers allow the best resolution of small intestinal layering and echogenicity (Figure 1.20). A 5- to 7.5-MHz transducer is adequate for large dogs whereas frequencies of

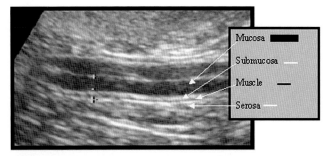

Figure 1.20:
Intestinal wall layering. Ultrasound image using a 7.5-MHz linear array transducer of a normal jejunal segment in a dog showing the normal wall layering.

>7.5 MHz are best for smaller animals. The ultrasound examination of the stomach and small bowel should include an assessment of the peritoneum, mesentery, and lymph nodes.

Gastrointestinal contents, especially air or barium, may hinder the ultrasonographic examination. Even under ideal conditions, it is difficult to examine the entire stomach during abdominal ultrasound, especially in large dogs or when the stomach is greatly dilated. In order to improve imaging of the stomach, it can be filled with small amounts of water by either allowing the animal to drink or by administering it by stomach tube. This may facilitate the examination of the gastric wall, which may be difficult when the stomach is contracted.

Ultrasonographic evaluation of the gastrointestinal tract should include assessment of the wall thickness, layering, and symmetry, localization and distribution of thickening, motility, and luminal content.

1.3.4.1 Gastric dilation and volvulus

Severe gastric distension may be caused by excess quantities of gas, food, and fluid in the stomach. If the stomach is dilated and food-filled but positioned normally, dilation is probably the most likely diagnosis (Figure 1.21a). Severe dilation together with displacement of the stomach is a sign of gastric volvulus. In gastric volvulus, the stomach appears compartmentalized or segmented with band-like soft tissue opacities apparent between the gas-filled segments (Figures 1.21b, c and d). The radiographic localization of the pylorus is the key to the diagnosis. The pylorus is usually displaced dorsally and to the left. A right lateral radiograph is usually sufficient to make the diagnosis of gastric volvulus, and the pylorus will be air-filled and located dorsally. The spleen is also often enlarged due to circulatory compromise and may also be displaced. The esophagus and small intestines may often appear dilated and air-filled. Gastric volvulus without severe distension may also

1

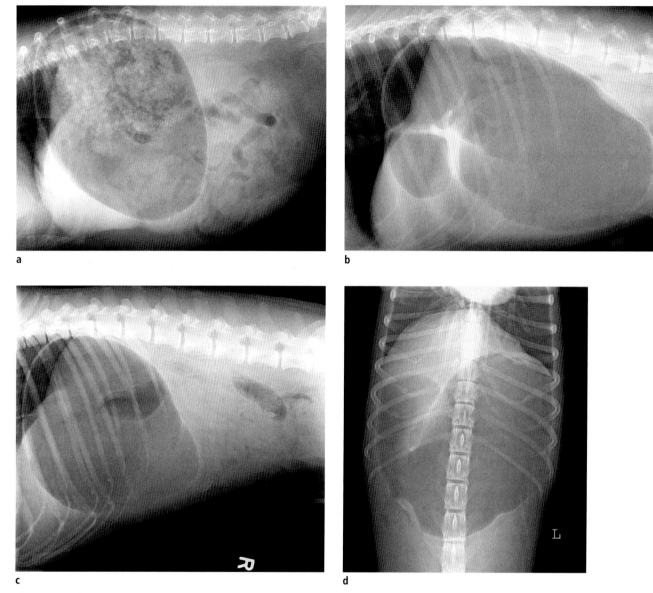

a

b

c

d

Figure 1.21a–d:
Gastric dilation, and gastric dilation and volvulus.
(a) Gastric dilation without volvulus. The gastric fundus is still located craniodorsally.
(b) Gastric dilation and volvulus. The gastric fundus is located caudoventrally, the pylorus craniodorsally. Folds in the stomach create the appearance of compartmentalization.
(c+d) 360° gastric torsion. The fundus appears to be in its normal position. Note the soft tissue band between the body and pylorus in the ventrodorsal image. A stomach tube could not be passed in this dog and the 360° nature of the torsion was confirmed surgically.

occur. Therefore, it is always important to interpret the radiographic findings in the light of the clinical findings. Dogs with previous gastropexy that present with recurrent vomiting may have some degree of gastric distension and displacement radiographically.

1.3.4.2 Gastric causes of chronic vomiting

Primary gastric causes of chronic vomiting include diffuse inflammatory infiltration, neoplasia, foreign body, polyps, ulcers, pyloric hypertrophy, and delayed gastric emptying. Their diagnosis can be challenging and often requires a combination of radiography, ultrasound, and endoscopy. Thickening of the stomach wall is commonly associated with chronic vomiting and is probably one of the most commonly over-interpreted findings on survey radiographs. Superimposition of fluid with the stomach wall may lead to the impression that the wall is thickened. The same is true for fluid within the small intestines. Thickening of the rugal folds in chronic gastritis is difficult to appreciate on survey radiographs for the same reason. Liquid barium contrast studies or preferably, ultrasonography, is required to confirm a radiographic suspicion of wall thickening. Negative contrast studies can be obtained by filling the stomach with air and performing radiographs in various positions.[1] This technique may allow detection of focal wall infiltrations. However, because both negative and positive contrast radiographic studies of the stomach are very time consuming and can be difficult to interpret, ultrasound is generally the method of choice for imaging the stomach wall.

Ultrasonographically, thickening of the stomach wall can be characterized as focal or diffuse, concentric or asymmetric. Attention to technique is necessary since oblique scanning of the stomach wall may lead to an artificially increased thickness and disruption of wall layering.[19] Therefore, scanning in multiple planes perpendicular to the stomach wall is necessary to avoid this error. Focal thickening with disrupted wall layering may be caused by neoplasia, granulomas, and ulcers. Generalized thickening is more commonly seen with inflammatory disease but can also occur with diffuse neoplastic infiltration. Thickening of the gastric wall is considered to be present when the wall thickness is greater than 5 mm in dogs and 3 mm in cats.

Radiopaque gastric foreign bodies such as ingested bone fragments are the most frequent incidental findings. If the object is still located in the stomach 1–2 days after the initial examination, its presence should be further investigated. Radiolucent foreign bodies can be identified by endoscopy, ultrasound, or contrast studies. Only a small amount of barium should be administered, or a double-contrast gastrogram should be performed since large volumes of barium can obscure both wall infiltrates and foreign material. Alternatively, a negative contrast gastrogram can be performed.

Chronic pyloric obstruction can occur either due to narrowing of the lumen because of wall infiltration or mechanical blockage of the orifice. Survey radiographs usually show some degree of gastric distension. Barium studies may help to identify pyloric obstructive disease. However, differentiating hypertrophic pyloric stenosis from inflammatory infiltrates or neoplasia is often difficult since they all lead to a narrowing of the pyloric orifice due to annular thickening, and they all have a similar appearance radiographically. Detecting intraluminal filling defects in the area of the pylorus is also possible. These may be due to foreign bodies, polyps, or severe inflammatory infiltrates and neoplasms.

The gastroduodenal junction can be examined ultrasonographically in dogs. Congenital hypertrophic pyloric stenosis and chronic hypertrophic gastropathy have a similar ultrasonographic appearance. Circumferential thickening (>3 mm) of the muscularis layer can be recognized by a hypoechoic layer that appears like a ring in cross-section. In chronic hypertrophic gastritis the mucosa can also be thickened. The strong peristaltic contractions against the thickened pylorus can also be observed. These contractions fail to propel food through the pylorus and a reflux movement of the gastric contents can be seen and recorded on video tape.

Gastric ulcers will lead to a disruption of the mucosal surface and they usually cannot be diagnosed using survey radiographs alone. Their diagnosis requires a contrast study, ultrasound, or endoscopy. It is important to remember that ulceration of the stomach wall has various causes and that the stomach wall should be thoroughly investigated, preferably with ultrasound, for evidence of underlying disease. Ultrasonographically, benign ulcers appear as a localized wall thickening. Mucosal craters with an irregular surface and the adherence of gas bubbles may also be detected.[20] Unfortunately, the presence of air, food, or lack of ultrasound beam penetration in large or obese dogs may make their detection difficult. Benign ulcers may appear similar to those associated with neoplasms. When the thickened stomach wall shows a loss of wall layering, gastric neoplasia should be suspected.

Gastric neoplasia is generally only diagnosed on survey radiographs when it is large enough and when the proliferative tissue is projected into the air-filled lumen. Lack of air in the stomach may cause mural lesions to be overlooked. Diffuse stomach wall infiltrations are even more difficult to diagnose radiographically. Generalized wall thickening may be seen with a number of conditions including chronic hypertrophic gastritis, eosinophilic gastritis, fungal infiltrations, and malignant histiocytosis. Both diffuse and localized gastric wall infiltrations may be detected with ultrasound, which often eliminates the need for contrast studies. Neoplasms can be recognized during abdominal ultrasound by observing thickening of the wall and the disruption of the normal wall layering, which is usually of decreased echogenicity and may create the appearance of pseudolayering.[21] Also, regional lymph nodes are often enlarged. Gastric lymphoma occurs in both dogs and cats and causes a generalized, hypoechoic thickening of the stomach wall with loss of wall layering.[22]

Tumors with increased vascularity can be diagnosed by Doppler ultrasound. However, no larger studies have been performed in dogs and cats describing the vascular patterns of neoplastic versus inflammatory gastric wall infiltrations. Contrast-enhanced ultrasound may have future potential in the characterization of gastric tumors but further studies are needed.

Ultrasound-guided percutaneous fine-needle aspiration or biopsy of the gastric wall can be performed in order to differentiate neoplastic and inflammatory infiltrates. The author performs percutaneous tissue sampling when the gastric wall lesion is located submucosally, rendering endoscopic biopsy collection largely unsuccessful. Fine-needle aspiration can be performed with a 20-gauge needle or biopsies can be taken with an 18-gauge spring-loaded biopsy device. When the gastric wall is thicker than 2 cm, a true-cut spring-loaded biopsy is feasible.

Endoscopic ultrasound represents a new and alternative imaging modality for gastric lesions. High-quality video endoscopes provide both optical and sonographic imaging of the gastrointestinal wall and of the perigastric organs. The author believes that echoendoscopic imaging of the stomach allows a more thorough examination than transabdominal ultrasound alone (Figure 1.22). However, more work needs to be performed in cats and dogs in order to establish the role of echoendoscopy in veterinary gastroenterology.

1.3.4.3   Diagnosis of delayed gastric emptying

Mechanical obstruction due to pyloric foreign body, gastric neoplasia, pyloric hypertrophy, antral mucosal hypertrophy, and antral polyps can generally be ruled out with a combination of radiography, ultrasound, and endoscopy. The diagnosis of other causes of delayed gastric emptying can be more difficult. Sequential radiographic imaging methods are often required. These can be time consuming and require restraint or sedation, both of which can potentially affect the results. Radiographic methods employ either indigestible radiopaque markers, barium meals, or liquid contrast agents (barium or iodine-containing).[15,23,24,25] However, radioscintigraphy is now considered the method of choice for detection of delayed gastric emptying.[15,23]

It has been shown that water intake, meal size, food type (dry vs. canned), and kibble shape can influence the rate of gastric emptying in cats.[26,27] The rate of gastric emptying in normal animals depends mainly on the state of filling of the stomach and the type of contrast medium used as well as stress and sedation in the patient. Animals should be kept in a quiet environment during the study and should not be sedated if possible. Iodine-containing contrast media have a much more rapid passage time than barium sulfate. Furthermore, a low dose of contrast medium may lead to longer emptying times. The dose of barium suspensions is 6 ml/kg in dogs and 10 ml/kg in cats and should be administered when the stomach is empty. Barium sulfate should be present in the duodenum by 15 minutes in the dog and by 5 minutes in the cat. The stomach should be free of barium after 1 to 4 hours in the dog and after 20 minutes in the cat. The presence of food in the stomach prior to the examination will delay gastric emptying for up to 15 hours or even more (longer for dry than moist food).

1.3.5   Small intestine

1.3.5.1   Ileus

Ileus is a failure of the intestinal contents to be transported and is recognized radiographically by the presence of dilated bowel segments. Survey abdominal radiographs should always be performed in animals suspected of having ileus. Ultrasound alone in such instances does not allow a global view of the abdomen, is much more time-consuming, and non-gastrointestinal causes of the patient's clinical signs as well as any secondary abnormalities may be overlooked. The radiographic appearance of ileus is dependent on its duration, location, and type. Acute or very proximal obstructions may show little intestinal dilation radiographically, whereas chronic or more distally located obstructions will show more severely dilated bowel segments. The two major types of ileus are obstructive (mechanical) and functional. Obstructive ileus may be partial or complete, and can be due to foreign bodies, torsion, volvulus, herniation, intussusception, adhesions, granulomas, and neoplasms.

Barium passage through the small intestines can be used to identify intraluminal, mural, or extramural obstructive as well as non-obstructive or partially obstructive lesions. However, it is a lengthy procedure and depending on the technique and experience of the clinician, may be difficult to interpret. Barium is also contraindicated prior to endoscopy or ultrasound, as it causes significant attenuation of sound and acoustic shadowing.

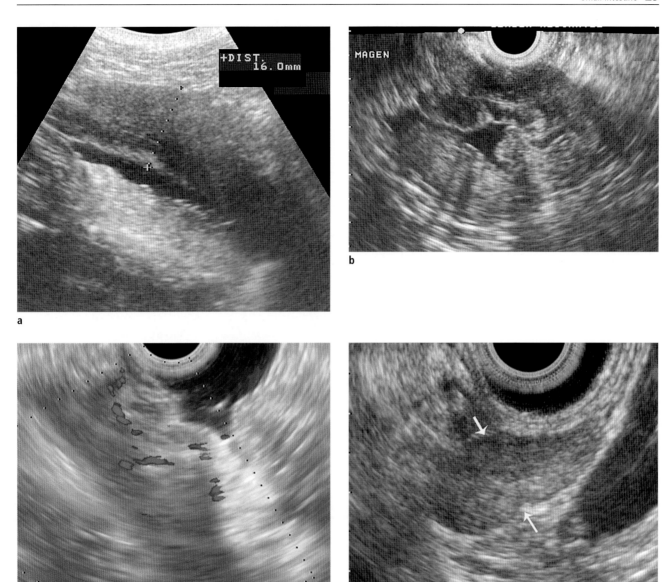

Figure 1.22a–d:
Gastric carcinoma.
(a) Transabdominal ultrasound image using a 7.5-MHz curved array transducer in a 45-kg Leonberger dog with chronic vomiting and weight loss. Localized thickening (1.6 cm) of the gastric wall with disruption of wall layering was identified.
(b) The dog underwent anesthesia for gastroscopy and an endoscopic ultrasound examination of the stomach was performed. The infiltration could be better localized to the lesser curvature of the stomach.
(c) In addition, Doppler showed the lesion to be well vascularized.
(d) The gastric lymph nodes were found to be enlarged and rounded (between arrows). Intraoperatively, the mass was non-resectable. Diagnosis: gastric carcinoma.

1.3.5.2 Partial obstructions

Fasted (>12 hours) or anorectic animals should not have small bowel segments containing granular material resembling that of food. Granular or more opaque small bowel contents may be detected in patients with a partial obstruction. The intestines in such cases may be mildly dilated (1–1.5 times the width of the second lumbar vertebral body [L2]) proximal to the obstruction or may be of normal diameter (Figure 1.23). Because fluid passes through the narrowed lumen, the contents remaining proximal to the partial obstruction become more dense and, therefore, radiographically more opaque (Figure 1.24).

1

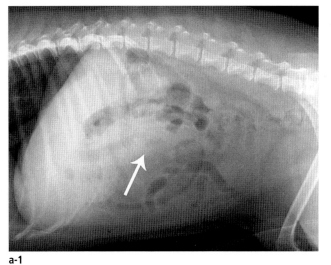

a-1

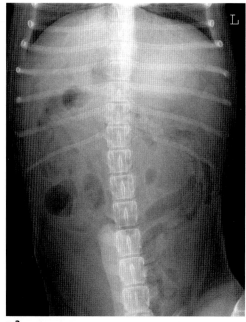

a-2

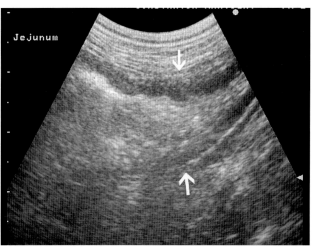

b-1

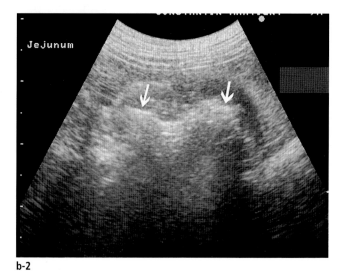

b-2

Figure 1.23a, b:
Small intestinal foreign body. Radiographic and ultrasonographic investigation of a 6-year-old West Highland White Terrier with a 1-month history of vomiting and weight loss. Upon clinical examination the dog's abdomen was painful.
(a) Lateral and ventrodorsal abdominal digital radiographs. There is a loss of mid-abdominal detail (white arrow) with mildly dilated small intestines. Although the dog was fasted over 12 hours, some of the small intestines have a granular content, which is difficult to differentiate from feces in the colon in this dog.
(b) An ultrasound examination showed dilated and fluid-filled jejunal segments proximal to an intraluminal structure with a hyperechoic wavy surface and acoustic shadowing. An unidentifiable foreign body was removed from the site surgically.

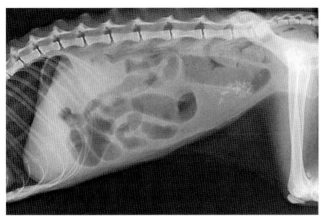

a-1

Figure 1.24a–c:

Small intestinal neoplasia.

(a) Lateral (left) and ventrodorsal (right) abdominal digital radiographs of the abdomen of a 9-year-old, castrated male European short-haired cat with a 5-month history of anorexia and weight loss. The cat's condition worsened 3 days prior to admission. The radiographs show cachexia with loss of abdominal detail. The majority of the small intestinal segments are severely dilated and air-filled. In the caudoventral abdomen there are multiple mineral opaque structures clumped together. Note that the descending colon is visible and filled with feces.

(b) Dilated and fluid-filled distal jejunal segment (between arrows). The wall is thickened (x–x) with disrupted wall layering. The irregular hyperechoic structures with clean distal shadowing are the stones that have collected proximal to the long-standing obstruction.

(c) The site of stenosis shows that the wall is thickened with an outer hypoechoic and inner hyperechoic wall layering. The regional lymph nodes (not shown) were enlarged and inhomogeneous. Histological diagnosis: adenocarcinoma.

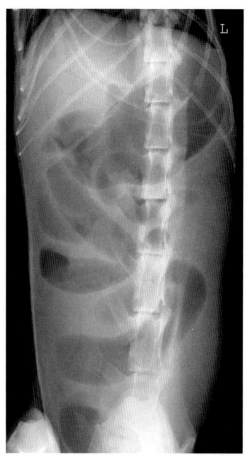

a-2

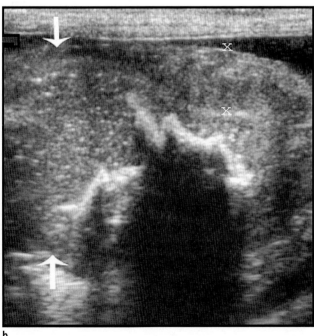

b

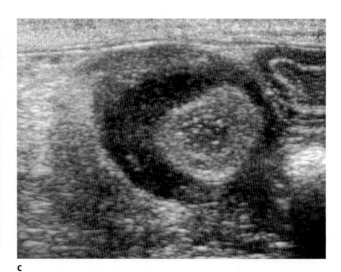

c

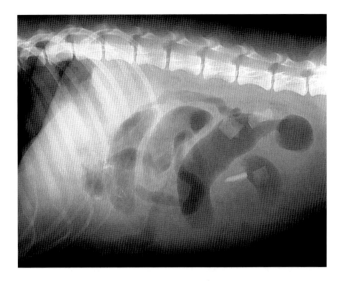
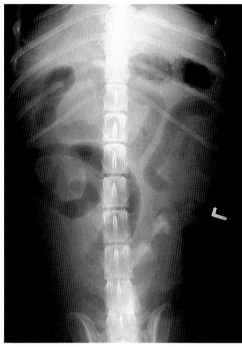

Figure 1.25:
Intestinal obstruction. Lateral and ventrodorsal abdominal radiographs in a dog with vomiting. Note that a few segments of small intestine are severely dilated and gas-filled while others are only mildly dilated. Foreign material with mineral opacity within the jejunal segments is also seen but was not the cause of obstruction. Diagnosis: mid-jejunal mechanical ileus due to radiolucent foreign body.

1.3.5.3 Complete obstructions

More severe dilation, usually with air, is seen in patients with complete obstructions (Figure 1.25). Dilation (1.5–2 times the width of the body of L2) is seen proximal to the site of obstruction and the segments distal to it usually appear empty and contracted. Due to this, the jejunal segments appear to have highly variable diameters. This is due to the continued peristaltic activity in the distal segments. Feces may still be present in the colon depending on the duration of the obstruction. Proximal duodenal or pyloric obstructions may show no radiographic abnormalities. Distal jejunal obstructions may cause generalized dilation and resemble a functional ileus radiographically.

1.3.5.4 Functional ileus

Another form of ileus that can be detected is a generalized and uniform mild intestinal dilation due to lack of peristaltic activity (Figure 1.26). This is known as adynamic, functional, or paralytic ileus. Functional ileus results in obstruction since the intestinal contents pool in the dependent areas of the gastrointestinal tract. It may affect the stomach, small and large intestines. Radiographically, the bowels may have a homogeneous soft tissue opacity when they are fluid-filled or a mixed pattern of air and fluid may also be present. Such an adynamic intestinal pattern can be due to the administration of pharmaceutical agents such as parasympatholytics or sedatives. Other causes are peritonitis, blunt abdominal trauma, electrolyte imbalance, or enteritis of various causes. Dysautonomia is a disorder of the autonomic nervous system that can also lead to generalized dilation of the gastrointestinal tract in both dogs and cats.[28] A complete obstruction in the distal jejunum or at the ileocecal level may also lead to the same radiographic appearance. Decreased peristalsis may be limited to the duodenum in patients with pancreatitis.

1.3.5.5 Detecting ileus with ultrasound

Generally, the clinical state of the animal in conjunction with radiographic findings provides adequate information to make a determination as to whether there is obstructive disease requiring surgery or not. However, when abdominal radiographic findings are unclear, an obstruction cannot be ruled out, or the radiographic findings do not explain the severity of the clinical signs, further diagnostic procedures are warranted.

Ultrasonography has the advantage that it does not require ionizing radiation and can be used to inspect the small intestines for wall layering, thickness, dilation, and peristalsis as well as for intraluminal, intramural, and extraluminal causes of obstruction. Lack of peristalsis occurring together with generalized dilation of the small intestines can be seen with functional ileus.[29] Contractions can be observed in two-dimensional real time imaging and approximately 5 contractions per minute are considered normal for the stomach and 1–3 are considered normal for the small intestine.

Radiolucent intestinal foreign bodies may be detected by ultrasound, especially when they cause mechanical obstruction. Solid material generally appears as a hyperechoic interface, which casts an acoustic shadow from the intestinal lumen.[30] Balls will have a round or curvilinear surface, peach pits are irregular, and bones generally have a smooth regular surface. Linear foreign bodies can sometimes be identified in plicated segments of small bowel. Foreign bodies tend to remain fixed in the same position and a repeat examination a short time later shows that they have not moved. The finding of severe dilation of one or more segments of the jejunum and the stomach together with empty, contracted bowel segments distally may indicate complete or partial obstruction. Care should be taken not to misinterpret a gas-liquid interface in dilated bowel segments as an obstruction. These appear as linear, hyperechoic intraluminal structures with acoustic shadowing. However, the bowel will often have a similar diameter proximally and distally to this artefact. This is usually not the case with intraluminal foreign bodies causing obstruction.

Localized mural infiltrations due to inflammation or neoplasia can slowly narrow the intestinal lumen. Some degree of intestinal dilation is present and solid foreign material such as small stones can collect proximal to the stricture. Ultrasonographically, neoplastic infiltrates produce intestinal wall thickening often with a loss of wall layering.[31] Lymphoma is the most common intestinal tumor in cats but also occurs frequently in dogs. It commonly leads to either a symmetrical or asymmetrical, transmural, circumferential thickening. The wall layers are difficult to identify and the entire wall appears hypo- to anechoic. The infiltration of the intestinal wall may be solitary, diffuse, or multifocal and regional lymph nodes may be enlarged. Complete intestinal obstructions often do not occur. Intestinal carcinoma often produces a solitary intestinal mass

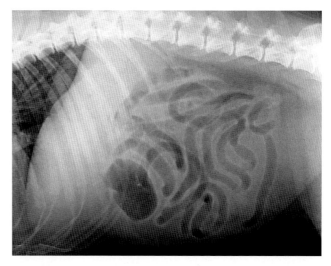

Figure 1.26:
Functional ileus. Lateral abdominal digital radiograph of a dog with vomiting and diarrhea for 2 days. The small intestines are moderately dilated, of uniform diameter, and air-filled. Diagnosis: functional ileus.

as can polyps, leiomyomas, or leiomyosarcomas. Carcinomas tend to be annular, irregular infiltrations that invade the lumen and cause obstructions.[32] Regional lymphadenopathy can also commonly be identified. Granulomatous infiltrations due to fungal infections may also cause diffuse or focal infiltration of the bowel wall and are difficult to distinguish from neoplasia ultrasonographically.[33] Histoplasmosis, for example, can produce localized and severe wall infiltrations that resemble lymphoma. Jejunal smooth muscle hypertrophy has been described in the cat and can also cause focal wall thickening but the wall layering is maintained.[34] Because the ultrasonographic appearance of the bowel wall alone is not sufficient for a definitive diagnosis, either full thickness biopsies, ultrasound-guided percutaneous biopsies, or fine-needle aspirates of the bowel wall are required for a definitive diagnosis of fungal disease.

1.3.5.6 Complicated ileus

Complicated forms of ileus include bowel perforation with peritonitis, free air in the abdominal cavity, and bowel ischemia due to thromboembolism, intussusception, or volvulus at the root of the mesentery. Linear foreign bodies can also lead to a complicated form of ileus. The presence of pneumoperitoneum together with abdominal effusion on an abdominal radiograph should alert the clinician to the fact that bowel perforation has occurred. The detection of free intra-abdominal air may require the use of ventrodorsal horizontal beam radiography with the patient in left lateral recumbency. Free air

1

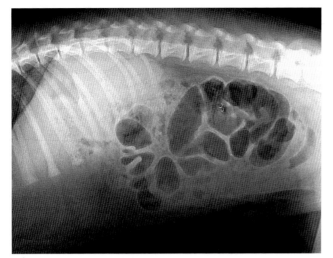

a-1

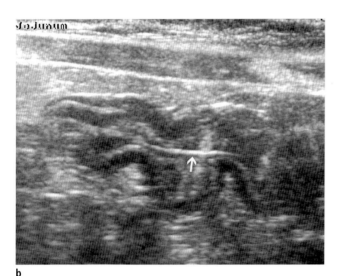

b

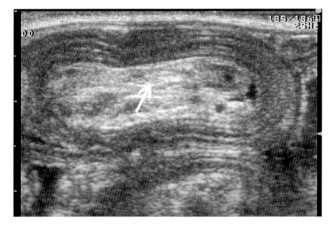

a-2

Figure 1.27a, b:
Linear foreign body.
(a) Lateral and ventrodorsal abdominal radiographs of a dog presented for vomiting. Note the "ribbon candy" appearance of the dilated and air-filled small intestinal segments. Irregularly shaped gas opacities can be seen in adjacent intestinal segments.
(b) Ultrasound image of a linear foreign body. The intestines appear plicated and pulled together. Although not always visible, in this case a string was identified sonographically (arrow).

Figure 1.28:
Intussusception. Ultrasound image of a jejunal intussusception in a young dog with diarrhea. Note the concentric intestinal layers. The hyperechoic center represents invaginated fat.

can be detected just under the right abdominal wall and lateral to the duodenum. Volvulus or mesenteric thromboembolism are recognized by the presence of generalized, severely dilated and air-filled jejunal segments. Linear foreign bodies produce characteristic changes on abdominal radiographs in both dogs and cats (Figure 1.27). The small intestinal loops appear convoluted and gathered or clumped together at one site (usually in the mid-right abdomen) and intraluminal gas bubbles appear asymmetrical and irregularly shaped. Ultrasonographically, the small intestinal segments will appear gathered up with the linear foreign material binding them together. The surrounding mesenterium should be examined for increased echogenicity and free fluid, which could be indicative of rupture.

Intestinal intussusception can usually be quickly diagnosed with ultrasound. Multilayered, concentric rings of bowel can be identified (Figure 1.28). The outer bowel segment is often thickened, edematous, and hypoechoic. More normal appearing inner segments can also be identified. Hyperechoic tissue representing invaginated mesenteric fat may also be detected. In older animals, careful examination of the affected bowel for nodular infiltrations of the bowel wall and regional lymphadenomegaly is important since underlying neoplastic disease may be responsible for the intussusception.

1.3.5.7 Chronic diarrhea

Chronic diarrhea due to small intestinal disease is common in dogs and cats. Survey radiographs are often nonspecific and gastrointestinal contrast studies are often unrewarding in patients with chronic diarrhea without vomiting. For detecting intestinal wall infiltrates, ultrasound is superior to survey and contrast radiography. Abdominal ultrasound allows for an assessment of wall thickness and layering, localization of lesions, motility, and potential involvement of regional lymph nodes. Recently, investigators have tried to correlate intestinal wall thickness in healthy dogs with body weight.[35] In that report the authors suggested normal values for jejunal wall thickness of ≤4.1 mm for dogs up to 20 kg, ≤4.4 mm for dogs between 20 and 39.9 kg, and ≤4.7 mm for dogs over 40 kg. Normal duodenal wall thickness was reported to be ≤5.1 mm for dogs up to 20 kg, ≤5.3 kg for dogs between 20 and 29.9 kg, and ≤6.0 mm for dogs over 30 kg.

1.3.5.8 Diffuse bowel wall infiltration

A number of gastrointestinal diseases lead to diffuse infiltration of the small intestinal wall. There are no known specific sonographic features that allow differentiation of the different infiltrative diseases. However, ultrasonography is important for localizing lesions within the gastrointestinal tract and allowing further characterization of the degree of infiltration inferred by wall thickness and the appearance of wall layering. The

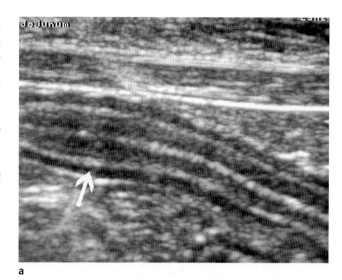

a

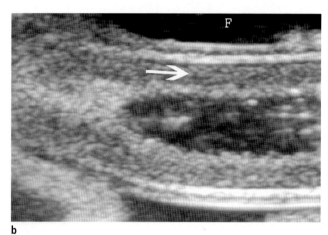

b

Figure 1.29a, b:
Eosinophilic enteritis and protein-losing enteropathy.
(a) Ultrasound image of a jejunal segment of a cat with an eosinophilic inflammatory infiltrate of the small intestine. The muscularis layer (arrow) was found to be very prominent.
(b) Ultrasound image of a jejunal segment of a dog with protein-losing enteropathy due to lymphangiectasia. The wall thickness is normal (3.8 mm), but the mucosa is hyperechoic and there is free fluid in the abdomen. The entire jejunum was affected. These sonographic findings are common in dogs with this syndrome.

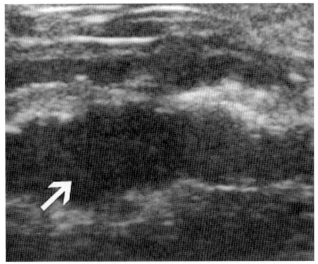

a

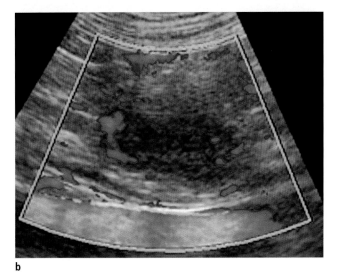

b

Figure 1.30a, b:
Intestinal lymphoma.
(a) Ultrasound images of a 9-year-old mixed-breed dog with chronic diarrhea, anemia, and weakness. Multifocal, hypoechoic, 1.2 cm diameter intestinal wall infiltrations were identified throughout much of the jejunum.
(b) Although Doppler examination initially showed no vascularity, following intravenous injection of 1 ml of Sonovue® ultrasound contrast medium, numerous perilesional and intralesional vessels were seen. Percutaneous, ultrasound-guided fine-needle aspiration of the intestinal wall was performed. Diagnosis: Lymphoma.

mucosal, submucosal, and muscularis layers are most commonly affected (Figure 1.29). The mucosa may also exhibit alterations in echogenicity varying in severity from diffuse pinpoint hyperechogenic foci to generalized hyperechogenicity. Severe mucosal thickening with increased echogenicity may be seen in animals with PLE and lymphangiectasia. In addition, the small intestine generally shows some dilation with fluid and gas and may have a decreased motility or a rigid appearance.

Thickening of the intestinal wall or a single layer due to inflammatory disease is difficult to differentiate from neoplastic infiltration. For example, a thickened muscularis layer alone can occur with either inflammatory or neoplastic infiltrates or can be due to smooth muscle hypertrophy. Lymph nodes may appear rounded, heterogenous, and possibly show target lesions in patients with either disease. Mycotic diseases such as histoplasmosis, pythiosis, and cryptococcosis can produce localized infiltrative disease that is sonographically similar to that of localized neoplasia.[33] However, neoplasia is considered to produce more disruption of the wall layering compared to inflammatory disease.[36] Sonographic changes in patients with alimentary lymphosarcoma may include thickening of the stomach or intestinal wall, loss of normal layering, a hypoechoic mass associated with the intestinal wall (Figure 1.30), and abdominal lymphadenomegaly.[37,38]

1.3.5.9 Gastrointestinal hemodynamic assessment with Doppler ultrasound

Dogs presenting with chronic diarrhea may be examined with Doppler ultrasound. Spectral Doppler waveforms of the celiac and cranial mesenteric arteries are generated at fasting and at 20, 40, 60, and 90 minutes postprandially.[39] Resistive (RI) and pulsatility indices (PI) calculated from these waveforms infer the degree of resistance to blood flow in the distal vascular bed of the intestinal tract. In a colony of Soft-coated Wheaten Terriers with food allergy, a prolonged lowered resistance (lowered RI and PI values) to blood flow was identified in response to stimulation with mucosal allergens.[40] More work will need to be carried out in this field in order to judge the clinical utility of this method in the assessment of dogs with chronic gastrointestinal disease.

1.3.6 Large intestine

Lateral and ventrodorsal radiographs of the pelvic region can provide helpful information in dogs and cats with constipation, hematochezia, or painful defecation. Abnormalities of the colon such as obstruction, megacolon, and obstipation can usually be recognized radiographically. Since a large quantity of feces may be present in the colon prior to defecation in a normal animal, the finding of a radiographically distended co-

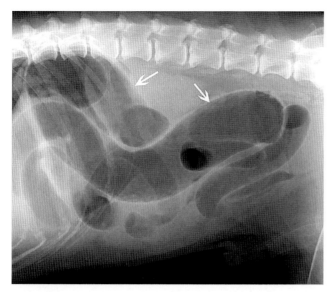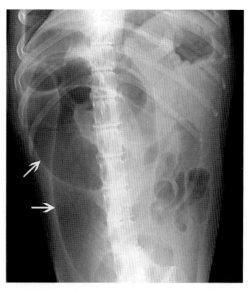

Figure 1.31:
Colonic torsion. Lateral and ventrodorsal abdominal digital radiographs of a 13-year-old German Shepherd dog with anorexia for 5 days and weakness in the hind limbs. Borborygmus and a tympanic abdomen were additional findings. Most of the gastrointestinal tract is dilated and air-filled. The entire colon (arrows) is severely dilated and air-filled. At the pelvic inlet, the gas pattern of the colon ends abruptly. Diagnosis: colonic torsion.

lon must be evaluated relative to the patient's clinical signs. Although not common, colonic torsion can occur causing severe dilation and displacement of the colon from its normal location (Figure 1.31). Mechanical obstruction due to previous pelvic trauma or space-occupying lesions can be ruled out radiographically. Sublumbar lymph node enlargement, extension of retroperitoneal masses, prostatomegaly in male dogs and uterine masses in females, and the presence of perineal herniation can also be detected radiographically. Dilation of the colon (greater than the length of a lumbar vertebra) with impaction of feces with increased radiopacity can be due to constipation, obstipation, or megacolon. Increased soft tissue opacities or displacement or compression of the colon within the pelvic canal indicate the need for further imaging procedures such as ultrasonography.

Ultrasonographically, the ileum, ileocecal junction, cecum, and ascending, transverse, and descending colon can be identified. When distended, the wall should have the appearance of having three layers and a thickness of 1–2 mm. The empty colon will appear contracted and many layers can be appreciated. This should not be misinterpreted as colonic wall thickening. Due to the presence of air and feces, it is often difficult to examine the entire colon by ultrasound. The bony pelvis also limits examination of the colon, but the rectum as well as the perirectal and perineal regions can be examined via a perineal approach. However, a certain length of rectum within the

pelvic canal cannot be examined in both dogs and cats. If the region of interest within the pelvic canal cannot be assessed due to overlying bone, radiographic contrast studies can be helpful in determining the origin of soft tissue masses causing displacement or compression of the colon. Negative and positive contrast studies of the colon may be performed, but they may be difficult to interpret due to the presence of intestinal contents or lack of experience with the procedure. Barium enemas can be useful in the diagnosis of ileocolic intussusceptions, cecal inversions, strictures, or wall infiltrations.

In dogs with diarrhea due to colitis, the colon may appear normal or irregular in form and may be air or fluid filled. Colitis due to diffuse, mild to moderate inflammatory infiltration will often show no radiographic or ultrasonographic changes and colonoscopy is the diagnostic method of choice in both dogs and cats. Soft tissue lesions such as neoplasia of the colon can be recognized radiographically as localized increased soft tissue opacities. However, they are not always evident on survey radiographs, and either a positive or negative contrast study of the colon may be required. Sonographically, focal infiltrations or intramural masses of the colonic wall may be detected and are associated with either neoplasms or granulomas (Figure 1.32). Both MRI and CT are alternative methods for examining the pelvic region or determining the involvement of the colon and surrounding tissues, especially when space-occupying lesions are present in that region.

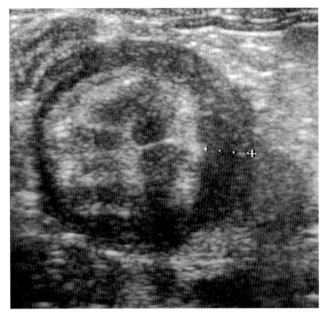

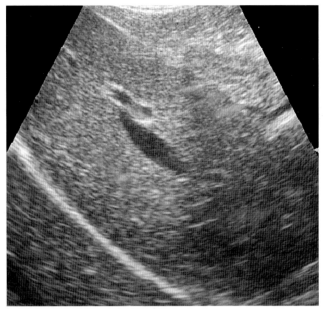

Figure 1.32:
Colonic neoplasia. Ultrasound image of the descending colon of a 12-year-old European short-haired cat with a history of tenesmus and hematochezia. Ultrasonographically, an irregular localized infiltration (4 mm) of the wall of the colon just cranial to the pelvis can be identified. The wall layering is disrupted and the echotexture is complex. The regional lymph nodes were found to be enlarged and rounded. Histological diagnosis: mucinous carcinoma.

Figure 1.33:
Normal canine liver. The liver has a medium echogenicity. Both portal (hyperechoic walls) and hepatic (no walls) veins are visible.

1.3.7 Liver and biliary tract

Clinical signs of hepatobiliary disease can be nonspecific and include anorexia, apathy, vomiting, diarrhea, polyuria, polydipsia, and icterus. The presence of icterus in the absence of anemia indicates hepatobiliary disease in both dogs and cats. Abdominal ultrasonography is the most useful non-invasive diagnostic tool for differentiating hepatic vs. post-hepatic causes of icterus. In cats, hepatic causes of icterus such as hepatic lipidosis are more common than pre- or post-hepatic disease. The liver, gallbladder, biliary tract, duodenal papilla, and pancreas should be examined with a high frequency transducer. Generally, curved array transducers with a small foot print are advantageous for examining these structures due to their location just behind and underneath the curvature of the ribs. Ultrasonographically, hepatic size can be estimated and its internal architecture, including its portal, venous, arterial, and biliary vasculature in addition to its echogenicity and echotexture can be evaluated (Figure 1.33). The wall thickness and contents of the gall bladder as well as the size of the cystic and the bile duct can also be assessed. In addition, the proximal duodenal papilla can be assessed for signs of obstruction. Finally, involvement of the pancreas in the disease process can also be assessed.

1.3.7.1 Hepatic parenchymal disease

Ultrasonographic changes in patients with hepatic parenchymal disorders are generally either focal or diffuse. Diffuse processes are more difficult to recognize than focal or multifocal ones and a change in the echogenicity of the liver is the main ultrasonographic finding. The liver may appear normal or have an increased, decreased, or mixed echogenicity.

In patients with **acute liver disease**, the liver may appear normal or enlarged with a generalized decrease in echogenicity. When the echogenicity is decreased, the portal veins appear much more visible, i.e. more hyperechoic than usual (Figure 1.34). This finding is nonspecific and the differential diagnoses may include toxic injury, infectious hepatitis, metabolic disease, trauma, vascular compromise, cholangiohepatitis, amyloidosis, lymphoma, or passive congestion.

Increased echogenicity of the liver can be detected in a number of conditions including fatty infiltration, steroid hepatopathy, and chronic hepatic diseases, such as hepatitis, cirrhosis, malignant histiocytosis, or lymphosarcoma.[41,42,43]

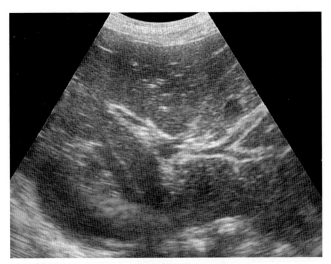

Figure 1.34:
Cholangiohepatitis. Ultrasound image of a hypoechoic liver in a 2.5-year-old male Cairn Terrier with icterus and vomiting. The liver is enlarged, hypoechoic, and the portal veins are very prominent and hyperechoic throughout the entire liver. Histopathologic diagnosis: cholangiohepatitis.

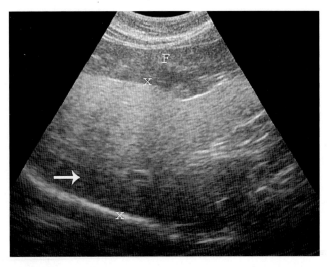

Figure 1.35:
Hepatic lipidosis. Ultrasound image of a hyperechoic liver in a 16-year-old, male European short-haired cat that presented with anorexia. The hyperechoic liver (between x–x) is homogenous and few vessels are visible. The echogenicity is equal to or greater than that of the spleen and surrounding mesentery and falciform fat (F). Note the hypoechoic appearance of the liver dorsally (arrow) due to beam attenuation. Differential diagnoses include hepatic lipidosis, diabetes mellitus, and neoplasia. Cytologic diagnosis: hepatic lipidosis.

Feline hepatic lipidosis is a common source of intrahepatic cholestasis that can be recognized ultrasonographically (Figure 1.35). The liver of affected cats is enlarged, rounded, shows an increased echogenicity equal to or greater than that of the spleen. In addition, the liver may appear isoechoic or hyperechoic compared to omental fat and hyperechoic to falciform fat.[44] Beam attenuation may also occur and the dorsal region of the liver may be difficult to visualize. The appearance of vascular structures is also diminished. Cytologic examination of a fine-needle aspirate is usually adequate for diagnosis of hepatic lipidosis.

Cirrhosis and **end-stage chronic inflammatory disease** is rare in cats compared to dogs, but hepatic fibrosis may be seen in cats. Hepatic cirrhosis and chronic hepatitis are difficult to diagnose by ultrasound. Furthermore, they can have a similar appearance as neoplastic disease. The liver may be small or normal in size and may contain nodules. Ascites may or may not be present. The nodules tend to be round and distinct and the surrounding liver may be of normal or increased echogenicity. Ultimately, a biopsy or fine needle aspiration is needed to make a more definitive diagnosis.

In the **presence of ascites** without venous hepatic congestion, spectral Doppler evaluation of the portal vein can be used to rule out portal hypertension. The velocity of the portal venous flow in patients with cirrhosis is generally reduced.[45] In the presence of portal hypertension and ascites, secondary portosystemic shunts may be detected. Secondary shunts can be recognized by the presence of many tortuous vessels in the abdomen. Doppler ultrasound will show the flow within these vessels to be monophasic and of low velocity, identifying them as portal in origin. In such instances, a surgical mesenteric portogram or a scintigraphic portogram is indicated (Figure 1.36).[46] Helical CT is a new alternative approach in veterinary patients with suspected portosystemic shunts.[47] Also, contrast harmonic ultrasound has been investigated in dogs for the detection of congenital portosystemic shunts.[6]

Diffuse hepatic changes with mixed echogenicity may also be seen in some patients. Neoplasia is the most common cause when the hepatic parenchyma appears diffusely complex or disrupted with poorly circumscribed areas of both increased and decreased echogenicity. Other possible causes of a complex echostructure in the liver are inflammation, toxicity, or necrosis.

1

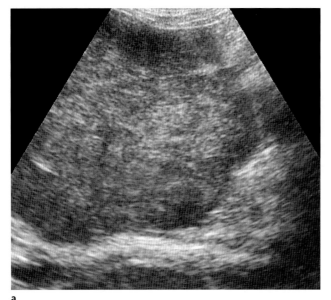

a

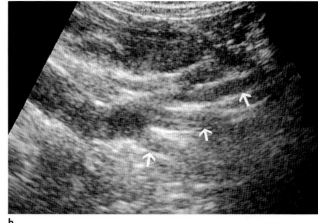

b

c

Figure 1.36a–c:

Extrahepatic portosystemic shunts. A 2-year-old female mixed-breed dog weighing 10 kg was presented with apathy and intermittent diarrhea. The serum chemistry profile showed hypoglycemia, hypoalbuminemia, and elevated pre- and postprandial bile acids concentrations.

(a) Ultrasound image of the liver. The liver was rounded, inhomogeneous, and had an irregular surface.

(b) Numerous aberrant vessels (arrows) with low velocity monophasic flow were identified caudal to the stomach and there was free fluid in the abdomen. Portal venous flow was greatly reduced at only 5 cm/sec. In addition, uroliths were identified in the urinary bladder.

(c) Intraoperative mesenteric venous portogram. Multiple, tortuous shunting vessels (arrows) are shown. A normal portal vasculature could not be demonstrated in this liver. Diagnosis: secondary extrahepatic portosystemic shunts due to chronic liver disease.

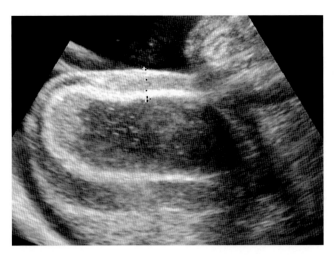

Figure 1.37:
Gall bladder wall edema. Ultrasound image of the gall bladder in a 5-month-old mixed-breed dog that presented with weight loss and inappetence of 3 weeks' duration. Serum hepatic enzyme activities and bilirubin concentration were elevated and there was a clinical suspicion of hepatitis. Ultrasonographically, the liver was hypoechoic with prominent portal vein walls. The gall bladder showed a "double-walled appearance". The gall bladder wall was 8 mm thick and hypoechoic with an inner and outer hyperechoic rim. Ascites was also detected. Note that the double-walled appearance in this instance is not due to the presence of ascites since the thickened wall itself can be visualized. Diagnosis: gall bladder wall edema.

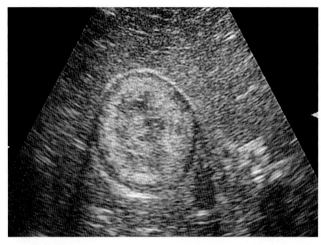

Figure 1.38:
Biliary mucocele. Ultrasound image of the gall bladder in an 8-month-old, male Rhodesian Ridgeback that was presented for vomiting of 2 days' duration and a painful abdomen. Radiographs of the abdomen showed signs of obstructive ileus and an ultrasound examination was performed. An invagination was diagnosed. In addition the liver and kidneys were enlarged and the gall bladder contents showed a complex echostructure with a thickened wall. The dog was diagnosed with leptospirosis, cholangiohepatitis, and a biliary mucocele. (Image courtesy of Dr. Johann Lang, Division of Radiology, Faculty of Veterinary Medicine, University of Bern, Switzerland.)

Contrast-enhanced ultrasonography has been found to be very useful for differentiating benign from malignant hepatic disease in human beings.[5,48] However, there are few reports describing its use in the assessment of dogs and cats with hepatic disease.

1.3.7.2 Non-obstructive biliary tract disease

Cholecystitis is a form of non-obstructive biliary disease and is usually seen with inflammation due to bacterial infection. The infection may spread to the liver causing cholangiohepatitis. If the cholecystitis is necrotizing, the infection may eventually lead to gall bladder rupture and bile peritonitis.

Thickening of the gall bladder wall is a common ultrasonographic finding in patients with cholecystitis and cholangiohepatitis.[49] Varying amounts of gall bladder sediment may be identified but this finding is nonspecific. Choleliths and mineralization of the gall bladder wall may also be seen but their significance is dependant on the clinical findings. The thickened wall is generally hyperechoic, possibly with an irregular inner surface. Polyps may occur in patients with chronic cholecystitis and appear as focal or multifocal wall infiltrations or nodules. Neoplasia could have a similar appearance, but gall bladder tumors are rare.

The gall bladder may also appear to have two echogenic double rims with a hypoechoic space in between (Figure 1.37). This double-walled appearance of the gall bladder can be seen with hypoalbuminemia, ascites, sepsis, acute inflammatory disease, or neoplasia. The presence of even small amounts of peritoneal fluid can create the appearance of a thickened gall bladder wall. Therefore, caution should be used in the interpretation of the gall bladder wall in patients with ascites.

Emphysematous cholecystitis may be detected radiographically as a zone of hyperlucency in the right cranioventral region of the liver. Ultrasonographically, reverberation echoes either within the gall bladder lumen or the wall may be recognized. This type of "dirty" shadowing can be differentiated from the "clean" shadowing that is seen with calculi in the gall bladder.

Gall bladder mucoceles are important findings in patients with hepatobiliary disease and icterus and various sonographic patterns have been described (Figure 1.38).[50] Gall bladder mucoceles have the potential to rupture and may cause bile peritonitis. In general, the gallbladder wall is thickened and contents with a complex echostructure and echogenicity can be observed. Ultrasonographic evidence of ascites can indicate the presence of rupture and bile peritonitis.

1

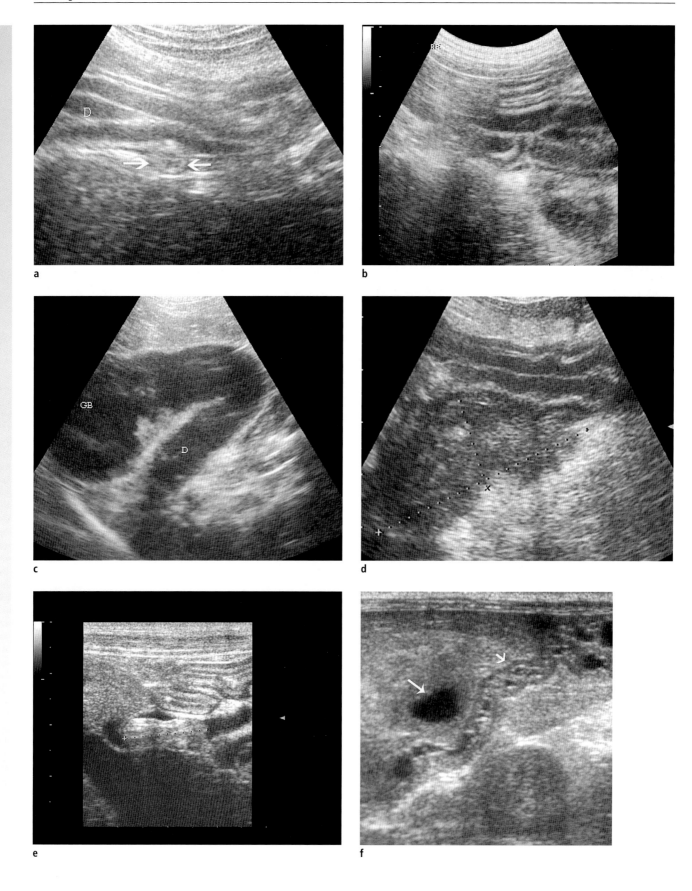

a

b

c

d

e

f

1.3.7.3 Obstructive disease

Ultrasound can be used to detect dilated and tortuous common and hepatic bile ducts, choleliths, or biliary and peri-biliary obstruction. Biliary calculi, pancreatitis, neoplasia, granulomas, or abscesses are possible causes of obstruction.[51] Liver flukes in cats are another cause in tropical and subtropical climates. If the patient is anorectic or has been fasted prior to examination, the gall bladder can be very large, which should not be misinterpreted as biliary obstruction. If obstructed, the gall bladder enlarges prior to the intrahepatic bile ducts, which may take days to weeks to dilate. Also, the common bile duct may take days to dilate following obstruction.

The porta hepatis and cranial duodenum can be challenging regions to examine with ultrasound. The presence of food and gas in the gastrointestinal tract is one of the main barriers. With the use of high frequency transducers, however, the duodenal papilla and bile duct can even be seen in normal dogs and cats (Figures 1.39 a and b). Therefore, visualization of the bile duct should not be considered the sole criterion for biliary obstruction. The normal bile duct diameter should not be more than 4 mm in dogs and 3–4 mm in cats.[52]

Extrahepatic cholestasis can be recognized by a distended gall bladder and bile duct (Figure 1.39 c). The pancreas and duodenal papilla can be sources of obstruction that can be evaluated ultrasonographically (Figure 1.39 d). Pancreatic abscesses, cysts, neoplasia, and choleliths as well as pancreatitis may cause mechanical obstruction of the bile duct (Figure 1.39 e). Bile duct carcinoma, pancreatic carcinoma, or lymphosarcoma in cats are additional causes. Long-standing obstructions may lead to intrahepatic bile duct dilation (Figure 1.39 f). Ultrasonographically, "too many vessels" can be visualized in the liver that do not show any blood flow when examined with color Doppler. Differential diagnoses for tubular fluid-filled structures in the liver are obstruction, biliary cysts, pseudocysts, biliary cystadenomas, and bile duct carcinoma.

Nuclear scintigraphy and contrast radiography are not commonly performed for the diagnosis of hepatobiliary disease in dogs and cats, but quantitative cholescintigraphy can be used to diagnose extrahepatic biliary obstruction.[53] Moreover, nuclear scintigraphy using Tc-99m-mebrofenin shows promise in dogs for the quantification of hepatic function.[54] Endoscopic retrograde cholangio-pancreatography (ERCP) uses a combination of endoscopy and fluoroscopy for radiographic contrast imaging of the biliary and pancreatic ducts. Investigators experienced with this method were able to identify an enlarged common bile duct, intraductal filling defects, a deviated course of the common bile duct, and a stenosis of the major duodenal papilla in some affected canine patients. This imaging modality requires specialized equipment and training, but may be promising for the diagnosis of biliary and pancreatic diseases in dogs in the future. [55, 56]

1.3.7.4 Interventional procedures of the liver and biliary system

Interventional procedures such as fine-needle aspiration or biopsy of the liver and pancreas can be performed using a 16- to 18-gauge biopsy needle depending on the size of the animal. Both manual and spring-loaded instruments may be used. Recently, the sensitivity and specificity of cytology and histology of tissue samples collected by fine-needle aspiration has come under criticism.[57] A coagulation profile should be performed prior to percutaneous true-cut biopsy, but it is not necessary prior to fine-needle aspiration unless there is a clinical suspicion of a coagulopathy. Complications following liver biopsy are extremely rare. Percutaneous ultrasound-guided cholecystocentesis can be performed for cytologic and bacteriologic analysis with a high degree of safety in dogs and cats. A 22-gauge, 1.5-inch (3.81-cm) needle with an attached 12-mL syringe is used via a right-sided transhepatic approach. Alternatively, a right ventral abdominal approach into the fundus of the gallbladder can be used.[58]

Figure 1.39a–f:
Ultrasonographic assessment of the bile duct.
(a) Normal duodenal papilla in a cat.
(b) Normal common bile duct entering the duodenal papilla in a dog.
(c) Enlarged gall bladder and cystic duct in a dog with extrahepatic bile duct obstruction.
(d) Pancreatitis in a dog that caused obstruction of the bile duct at the duodenal papilla resulting in cholestasis and icterus.
(e) Intraluminal bile concrements obstructing the bile duct in a dog with chronic cholecystitis and choleliths.
(f) Cystic dilation of the intrahepatic bile ducts in a cat with chronic cholestasis due to obstruction of the extrahepatic bile duct.

1

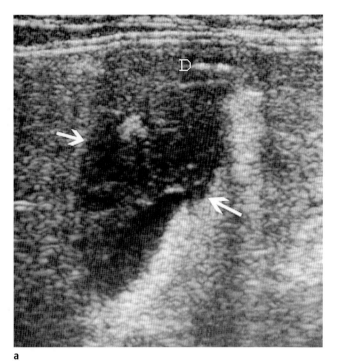

a

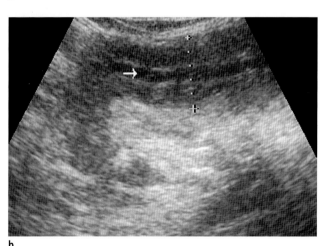

b

Figure 1.40a, b:
Acute pancreatitis in a cat.
(a) The right pancreatic limb is enlarged (arrows) and very hypoechoic. The surrounding mesenterium is hyperechoic, which is a sign of peripancreatic fat necrosis. D = duodenum.
(b) The left pancreatic limb in the same cat was smaller but hypoechoic. The pancreatic duct (arrow) is mildly dilated.

1.3.8 Pancreas

The ultrasonographic examination of the pancreas is highly operator dependent and an excellent knowledge of anatomy, including vascular anatomy as well as experience with ultrasonography is required to locate the pancreas and interpret its appearance. High resolution transducers are required to image the pancreas in normal animals. Excessive gas in the gastrointestinal tract as well as deep thoracic conformation may inhibit visualization of the entire pancreas. Obese animals pose an additional barrier, even for experienced ultrasonographers. Furthermore, animals with pancreatic disease often have abdominal pain and resent transducer pressure in the region of the pancreas, and analgesia may be necessary in order to perform a thorough examination. Another ultrasound tool for examination of the pancreas in either obese or painful animals is echoendoscopy. Using an echoendoscope, a high frequency transducer can be inserted into the stomach and the pancreas is imaged transgastrically.[59] Obesity and air pose fewer problems for echoendoscopic imaging compared to conventional transabdominal ultrasound. The author has been able to consistently examine the pancreas using this technique in both dogs and cats.

1.3.8.1 Pancreatitis

While ultrasound is generally considered a valuable tool for the diagnosis of canine pancreatitis, its sensitivity in cats with pancreatitis is variable.[60] In patients with acute pancreatitis the pancreatic parenchyma becomes hypoechoic and enlarged. The surrounding mesentery of the pancreas is often diffusely hyperechoic and poorly circumscribed. However, these changes may be subtle in cats. When the mesenterium is inflamed and the bowel loops are distended with gas, the pancreatic tissue itself may be difficult to identify ultrasonographically (Figure 1.40). Mild to moderate accumulations of free fluid may be detected in the cranial abdomen. Together with a hyperechogenic mesentery this may indicate the presence of focal peritonitis. In such cases, the small intestinal loops and especially the duodenum may be dilated due to functional ileus. This may contribute to lack of visualization of the pancreas due to fluid and gas accumulation. In cats, multiple hypoechoic round foci of a few millimeters in diameter may be recognized if high frequency (greater than 7.5 MHz) transducers are used. These findings may present either nodular hyperplasia or dilated pancreatic ducts.[61]

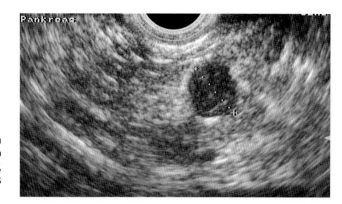

Figure 1.41:
Canine insulinoma. Echoendoscopic image of the body of the pancreas in a 7-year-old, female Bearded Collie with hypoglycemia. The pancreas was found to be normal in the transabdominal ultrasound examination. An 8.6-mm diameter, round, and hypoechoic nodule was identified echoendoscopically. The nodule was removed surgically and was diagnosed histologically as an insulinoma.

The ultrasonographic appearance of chronic pancreatitis in dogs and cats has not been well described. Recurrent episodes of pancreatitis may lead to chronic changes that can be identified ultrasonographically and are mainly due to fibrosis. The pancreas may be of normal size or enlarged with a heterogenous appearance. Mineralizations may be present and may lead to acoustic shadowing.

Cavities in the pancreatic parenchyma are typically either due to abscesses or pseudocysts and appear as anechoic or hypoechoic cavities, possibly with a thickened wall. Fine-needle aspiration for cytological analysis may be useful to differentiate them.

1.3.8.2 Pancreatic neoplasia

Pancreatic neoplasia is much less common than pancreatitis in both dogs and cats.[62] Neuroendocrine tumors are the most common pancreatic neoplasia, followed by adenocarcinoma and metastatic tumors. Differentiation of pancreatitis and pancreatic neoplasias with ultrasound is not always easy due to the overlapping nature of their appearance.[62] Lymphadenomegaly can occur with both and surrounding tissues are often similarly altered. Fine-needle aspiration or true-cut, laparoscopic, or surgical biopsy is often needed for conclusive differentia-

tion. Involvement of multiple organs can occur in both severe suppurative pancreatitis or primary liver, pancreatic, or bile duct neoplasia.[62] Neoplasia of any one of these structures may invade adjacent organs and simulate inflammatory or granulomatous disease. In such cases, biopsy of both the liver and pancreas is warranted. Diffuse infiltrative disease of the pancreas, liver, and other organs such as the stomach, duodenum, spleen, and lymph nodes may be seen in suppurative, granulomatous, as well as neoplastic disorders.

Depending on the size of a pancreatic nodule, the amount of gastrointestinal gas, and thoracic conformation of the patient, pancreatic neoplasms such as insulinomas and adenocarcinomas may be difficult to detect ultrasonographically. Endosonography of the pancreas via a transgastric approach may allow better assessment of the entire pancreas in dogs (Figure 1.41).[59] The author has been able to diagnose a number of insulinomas echoendoscopically that could not be visualized with conventional transabdominal ultrasound. Recently, CT and nuclear scintigraphy using radiolabeled leucocytes has been evaluated for assessing the canine and feline pancreas.[11,63] The MRI appearance of the normal feline pancreas has also been reported, but reports of its clinical use are lacking.[64] Such modalities may have future potential for diagnosing pancreatic disease but more clinical data is needed.

1

⚷ Key Facts

- Radiography and ultrasonography are two of the most valuable diagnostic tools for diagnosing gastrointestinal disease in dogs and cats.
- Thoracic radiography should be performed in every patient with regurgitation in order to assess the esophagus and rule out aspiration pneumonia. However, dynamic contrast studies are often necessary to diagnose the cause of dysphagia.
- High quality radiographs of the abdomen in two orthogonal planes should be performed in patients presented for vomiting and are important for ruling out obstructive ileus. Abdominal ultrasound and/or barium studies may be indicated when radiography does not allow definitive ruling out of an obstructive lesion.
- Ultrasound is indicated in dogs and cats presenting with icterus. Hepatic vs. post-hepatic causes can be investigated and ultrasound-guided biopsies of the liver or pancreas can be performed.
- Abdominal ultrasound is clinically useful for the diagnosis of pancreatitis in both dogs and cats. The examination should include assessment of the liver, gall bladder, mesentery, and regional lymph nodes in order to rule out multi-organ involvement.

References

1. Mahaffey E, Barber D. The Stomach. In: Textbook of Veterinary Diagnostic Radiology; ed. Thrall DE. WB Saunders, Philadelphia, 2002, *4th ed.*, 615–638.
2. Williams J, Biller DS, Myer CW et al. Use of iohexol as a gastrointestinal contrast agent in three dogs, five cats, and one bird. *J Am Vet Med Assoc* 1993; 202 (4): 624–627.
3. Gaschen L, Kircher P, Lang J. Endoscopic ultrasound instrumentation, applications in humans, and potential veterinary applications. *Vet Radiol Ultrasound* 2003; 44 (6): 665–680.
4. Correas JM, Bridal L, Lesavre A et al. Ultrasound contrast agents: properties, principles of action, tolerance, and artifacts. *Eur Radiol* 2001; 11 (8): 1316–1328.
5. Solbiati L, Tonolini M, Cova L et al. The role of contrast-enhanced ultrasound in the detection of focal liver lesions. *Eur Radiol* 2001; 11 Suppl 3: E15–E26.
6. Salwei RM, O'Brien RT, Matheson JS. Use of contrast harmonic ultrasound for the diagnosis of congenital portosystemic shunts in three dogs. *Vet Radiol Ultrasound* 2003; 44 (3): 301–305.
7. Newell SM, Graham JP, Roberts GD et al. Quantitative hepatobiliary scintigraphy in normal cats and in cats with experimental cholangiohepatitis. *Vet Radiol Ultrasound* 2001; 42 (1): 70–76.
8. Samii VF, Biller DS, Koblik PD. Normal cross-sectional anatomy of the feline thorax and abdomen: comparison of computed tomography and cadaver anatomy. *Vet Radiol Ultrasound* 1998; 39 (6): 504–511.
9. Samii VF, Biller DS, Koblik PD. Magnetic resonance imaging of the normal feline abdomen: an anatomic reference. *Vet Radiol Ultrasound* 1999; 40 (5): 486–490.
10. Frank P, Mahaffey M, Egger C et al. Helical computed tomographic portography in ten normal dogs and ten dogs with a portosystemic shunt. *Vet Radiol Ultrasound* 2003; 44 (4): 392–400.
11. Jaeger JQ, Mattoon JS, Bateman SW et al. Combined use of ultrasonography and contrast enhanced computed tomography to evaluate acute necrotizing pancreatitis in two dogs. *Vet Radiol Ultrasound* 2003; 44 (1): 72–79.
12. Muleya JS, Taura Y, Nakaichi M et al. Appearance of canine abdominal tumors with magnetic resonance imaging using a low field permanent magnet. *Vet Radiol Ultrasound* 1997; 38 (6): 444–447.
13. Forster-van Hijfte MA, McEvoy FJ, White RN et al. Per rectal portal scintigraphy in the diagnosis and management of feline congenital portosystemic shunts. *J Small Anim Pract* 1996; 37 (1): 7–11.
14. Daniel GB, Bright R, Ollis P et al. Per rectal portal scintigraphy using 99m-technetium pertechnetate to diagnose portosystemic shunts in dogs and cats. *J Vet Intern Med* 1991; 5 (1): 23–27.
15. Wyse CA, McLellan J, Dickie AM et al. A review of methods for assessment of the rate of gastric emptying in the dog and cat: 1898–2002. *J Vet Intern Med* 2003; 17 (5): 609–621.
16. Wisner ER, Mattoon JS, Nyland TG. Neck. In: Small animal diagnostic ultrasound, *2nd ed.* Philadelphia, WB Saunders, 2002; 285–304.
17. Armbrust LJ, Biller DS, Radlinsky MG et al. Ultrasonographic diagnosis of foreign bodies associated with chronic draining tracts and abscesses in dogs. *Vet Radiol Ultrasound* 2003; 44 (1): 66–70.
18. Rudorf H. Ultrasonographic imaging of the tongue and larynx in normal dogs. *J Small Anim Pract* 1997; 38 (10): 439–444.
19. Easton S. A retrospective study into the effects of operator experience on the accuracy of ultrasound in the diagnosis of gastric neoplasia in dogs. *Vet Radiol Ultrasound* 2001; 42 (1): 47–50.
20. Penninck D, Matz M, Tidwell A. Ultrasonography of gastric ulceration in the dog. *Vet Radiol Ultrasound* 1997; 38 (4): 308–312.
21. Penninck DG, Moore AS, Gliatto J. Ultrasonography of canine gastric epithelial neoplasia. *Vet Radiol Ultrasound* 1998; 39 (4): 342–348.
22. Richter KP. Feline gastrointestinal lymphoma. *Vet Clin North Am (Small Anim Pract)* 2003; 33 (5): 1083–98.
23. Goggin JM, Hoskinson JJ, Kirk CA et al. Comparison of gastric emptying times in healthy cats simultaneously evaluated with radiopaque markers and nuclear scintigraphy. *Vet Radiol Ultrasound* 1999; 40 (1): 89–95.
24. Agut A, Sanchezvalverde MA, Torrecillas FE et al. Iohexol as a gastrointestinal contrast-medium in the cat. *Vet Radiol Ultrasound* 1994; 35 (3): 164–168.
25. Lester NV, Roberts GD, Newell SM et al. Assessment of barium impregnated polyethylene spheres (BIPS (R)) as a measure of solid-phase gastric emptying in normal dogs-comparison to scintigraphy. *Vet Radiol Ultrasound* 1999; 40 (5): 465–471.
26. Armbrust LJ, Hoskinson JJ, Lora-Michiels M et al. Gastric emptying in cats using foods varying in fiber content and kibble shapes. *Vet Radiol Ultrasound* 2003; 44 (3): 339–343.
27. Goggin JM, Hoskinson JJ, Butine MD et al. Scintigraphic assessment of gastric emptying of canned and dry diets in healthy cats. *Am J Vet Res* 1998; 59 (4): 388–392.
28. Detweiler DA, Biller DS, Hoskinson JJ et al. Radiographic findings of canine dysautonomia in twenty-four dogs. *Vet Radiol Ultrasound* 2001; 42 (2): 108–112.
29. An YJ, Lee H, Chang D et al. Application of pulsed Doppler ultrasound for the evaluation of small intestinal motility in dogs. *J Vet Sci* 2001; 2 (1): 71–74.

30. Penninck D, Mitchell SL. Ultrasonographic detection of ingested and perforating wooden foreign bodies in four dogs. *J Am Vet Med Assoc* 2003; 223 (2): 206–209.

31. Penninck D, Smyers B, Webster CR et al. Diagnostic value of ultrasonography in differentiating enteritis from intestinal neoplasia in dogs. *Vet Radiol Ultrasound* 2003; 44 (5): 570–575.

32. Paoloni MC, Penninck DG, Moore AS. Ultrasonographic and clinicopathologic findings in 21 dogs with intestinal adenocarcinoma. *Vet Radiol Ultrasound* 2002; 43 (6): 562–567.

33. Graham JP, Newell SM, Roberts GD et al. Ultrasonographic features of canine gastrointestinal pythiosis. *Vet Radiol Ultrasound* 2000; 41 (3): 273–277.

34. Diana A, Pietra M, Guglielmini C et al. Ultrasonographic and pathologic features of intestinal smooth muscle hypertrophy in four cats. *Vet Radiol Ultrasound* 2003; 44 (5): 566–569.

35. Delaney F, O'Brien RT, Waller K. Ultrasound evaluation of small bowel thickness compared to weight in normal dogs. *Vet Radiol Ultrasound* 2003; 44 (5): 577–580.

36. Penninck D, Smyers B, Webster CR et al. Diagnostic value of ultrasonography in differentiating enteritis from intestinal neoplasia in dogs. *Vet Radiol Ultrasound* 2003; 44 (5): 570–575.

37. Penninck DG. Characterization of gastrointestinal tumors. *Vet Clin North Am (Small Anim Pract)* 1998; 28 (4): 777–797.

38. Grooters AM, Biller DS, Ward H et al. Ultrasonographic appearance of feline alimentary lymphoma. *Vet Radiol Ultrasound* 1994; 35: 468–473.

39. Kircher P, Lang J, Blum J et al. Influence of food composition on splanchnic blood flow during digestion in unsedated normal dogs: a Doppler study. *Vet J* 2003; 166 (3): 265–272.

40. Kircher P, Spaulding KA, Vaden S et al. Doppler investigations of gastrointestinal blood flow in a canine model of food allergy. *J Vet Intern Med* 2004; 18:605–611.

41. Newell SM, Selcer BA, Girard E et al. Correlations between ultrasonographic findings and specific hepatic diseases in cats: 72 cases (1985–1997). *J Am Vet Med Assoc* 1998; 213 (1): 94–98.

42. Ramirez S, Douglass JP, Robertson ID. Ultrasonographic features of canine abdominal malignant histiocytosis. *Vet Radiol Ultrasound* 2002; 43 (2): 167–170.

43. Biller DS, Kantrowitz B, Miyabayashi T. Ultrasonography of diffuse liver disease. A review. *J Vet Intern Med* 1992; 6 (2): 71–76.

44. Yeager AE, Mohammed H. Accuracy of ultrasonography in the detection of severe hepatic lipidosis in cats. *Am J Vet Res* 1992; 53 (4): 597–599.

45. Szatmari V, van Sluijs FJ, Rothuizen J et al. Ultrasonographic assessment of hemodynamic changes in the portal vein during surgical attenuation of congenital extrahepatic portosystemic shunts in dogs. *J Am Vet Med Assoc* 2004; 224 (3): 395–402.

46. White RN, Macdonald NJ, Burton CA. Use of intraoperative mesenteric portovenography in congenital portosystemic shunt surgery. *Vet Radiol Ultrasound* 2003; 44 (5): 514–521.

47. Thompson MS, Graham JP, Mariani CL. Diagnosis of a portoazygous shunt using helical computed tomography angiography. *Vet Radiol Ultrasound* 2003; 44 (3): 287–291.

48. Leen E. The role of contrast-enhanced ultrasound in the characterisation of focal liver lesions. *Eur Radiol* 2001; 11 Suppl 3: E27–E34.

49. Hittmair KM, Vielgrader HD, Loupal G. Ultrasonographic evaluation of gallbladder wall thickness in cats. *Vet Radiol Ultrasound* 2001; 42 (2): 149–155.

50. Besso JG, Wrigley RH, Gliatto JM et al. Ultrasonographic appearance and clinical findings in 14 dogs with gallbladder mucocele. *Vet Radiol Ultrasound* 2000; 41 (3): 261–271.

51. Fahie MA, Martin RA. Extrahepatic biliary-tract obstruction – A retrospective study of 45 cases (1983–1993). *J Am Anim Hosp Assoc* 1995; 31 (6): 478–482.

52. Leveille R, Biller DS, Shiroma JT. Sonographic evaluation of the common bile duct in cats. *J Vet Intern Med* 1996; 10 (5): 296–299.

53. Boothe HW, Boothe DM, Komkov A et al. Use of hepatobiliary scintigraphy in the diagnosis of extrahepatic biliary obstruction in dogs and cats – 25 cases (1982–1989). *J Am Vet Med Assoc* 1992; 201 (1): 134–141.

54. Matwichuk CL, Daniel GB, Denovo RC et al. Evaluation of plasma time-activity curves of technetium-99m-mebrofenin for measurement of hepatic function in dogs. *Vet Radiol Ultrasound* 2000; 41 (1): 78–84.

55. Spillmann T, Schnell-Kretschmer H, Dick M et al. Endoscopic retrograde cholangio-pancreatography in dogs with chronic gastrointestinal problems. *Vet Radiol Ultrasound* 2005; 46 (4): 293–299.

56. Spillmann T, Happonen I, Kahkonen T, Fyhr T, Westermarck E. Endoscopic retrograde cholangio-pancreatography in healthy Beagles. *Vet Radiol Ultrasound* 2005; 46 (2): 97–104.

57. Cole TL, Center SA, Flood SN et al. Diagnostic comparison of needle and wedge biopsy specimens of the liver in dogs and cats. *J Am Vet Med Assoc* 2002; 220 (10): 1483–1490.

58. Savary-Bataille KCM, Bunch SE, Spaulding KA et al. Percutaneous ultrasound-guided cholecystocentesis in healthy cats. *J Vet Intern Med* 2003; 17 (3): 298–303.

59. Morita Y, Takiguchi M, Yasuda et al. Endoscopic ultrasonography of the pancreas in the dog. *Vet Radiol Ultrasound* 1998; 39 (6): 552–556.

60. Saunders HM, VanWinkle TJ, Drobatz K et al. Ultrasonographic findings in cats with clinical, gross pathologic, and histologic evidence of acute pancreatic necrosis: 20 cases (1994–2001). *J Am Vet Med Assoc* 2002; 221 (12): 1724–1730.

61. Wall M, Biller DS, Schoning P et al. Pancreatitis in a cat demonstrating pancreatic duct dilatation ultrasonographically. *J Am Anim Hosp Assoc* 2001; 37 (1): 49–53.

62. Bennett PF, Hahn KA, Toal RL et al. Ultrasonographic and cytopathological diagnosis of exocrine pancreatic carcinoma in the dog and cat. *J Am Anim Hosp Assoc* 2001; 37 (5): 466–473.

63. Head LL, Daniel GB, Tobias K et al. Evaluation of the feline pancreas using computed tomography and radiolabeled leukocytes. *Vet Radiol Ultrasound* 2003; 44 (4): 420–428.

64. Newell SM, Graham JP, Roberts GD et al. Quantitative magnetic resonance imaging of the normal feline cranial abdomen. *Vet Radiol Ultrasound* 2000; 41: 27–34.

1

1.4 Laboratory Tests

1.4.1 Laboratory assessment of gastric disease

JAN S. SUCHODOLSKI

1.4.1.1 Introduction

While routine laboratory tests are nonspecific for gastric disease, they should always be performed in a patient with clinical signs consistent with gastric disease in order to rule out conditions that can lead to similar clinical signs or systemic disorders that can affect the stomach (e.g., renal failure). Determination of packed cell volume and total protein allow for evaluation of blood and protein loss in patients with gastric ulcers and also allow evaluation of the hydration status in patients that vomit. Animals with gastric ulcers may show a regenerative anemia and decreased total protein concentration. Chronic vomiting may lead to loss of electrolytes (mainly sodium and potassium) and acid-base disturbances (metabolic alkalosis or acidosis). Anemia, hypoglycemia, and increased liver enzymes may be observed in animals with gastric tumors.

Gastroscopy is currently the gold standard for diagnosis of gastric disease (see 1.5). In recent years, several new diagnostic tests for gastric disease have been developed. However, at the current time most of these new tests are employed predominantly in a research setting.

1.4.1.2 Evaluation for parasitic infestation

The feline stomach worm (*Ollulanus tricuspis*) can be detected during microscopic examination of vomitus. Eggs of the feline and canine stomach worm (*Physaloptera rara*) can be detected in fecal smears or by fecal sedimentation.[1]

Diagnosis of Helicobacter spp. infection

Bacterial culture for isolation of *Helicobacter* spp. only has a limited yield. Gastroscopy allows direct visualization of gastric lesions and also enables the collection of samples for indirect detection of these organisms. *Helicobacter* spp. can be detected in biopsy specimens obtained during gastroscopy by means of histopathology (Warthin-Starry or modified-Steiner stain), immunohistochemistry, polymerase chain reaction, or rapid-urease tests.[2] Alternatively, an impression smear can be taken from the gastric mucosa using a cytology brush. The brush is then rolled across a microscope slide and the slide is stained either with May-Grünwald-Giemsa, Gram, or Diff-Quick stain.[2] Many animals show a patchy distribution of *Helicobacter* spp. infestation and it is crucial that biopsy specimens or impression smears are obtained from several areas of the stomach.[3]

Minimally-invasive detection methods for *Helicobacter* spp. infection are easy to perform but have the limitation that they do not allow for identification of the presence of gastric disease. Detection of antibodies directed against *Helicobacter spp.* in serum has a relatively low sensitivity. In addition, antibodies circulate for up to 6 months after eradication of the organism and thus these antibody tests can not be used for the monitoring of therapeutic success.[4] The ^{13}C-urea breath or blood test is based on the detection of metabolic activity of *Helicobacter* spp.[5] The organisms produce the enzyme urease, which catalyzes the metabolism of orally administered ^{13}C-urea. The ^{13}C is released from the urea, incorporated into ^{13}CO$_2$, and can be quantified in either breath or blood samples.[5] This test can be used for both diagnosis and monitoring of therapy, but is not offered commercially at this time.

1.4.1.3 Sucrose permeability testing

Increased gastric permeability has been observed in human beings with gastric ulcers and NSAID- or *Helicobacter-pylori*-associated gastritis. Gastric permeability has traditionally been evaluated using radioactive markers (^{51}Cr-EDTA). Alternatively, the disaccharide sucrose can be used as a specific non-radioactive marker for gastric permeability.[6] Orally administered sucrose is too large to permeate the intact gastric mucosa and an increase in the urine (validated for dogs and cats) or serum (validated for dogs only) concentration of sucrose is indicative of an increased gastric permeability and is highly suggestive of gastric mucosal damage.

1.4.1.4 Minimally-invasive markers for gastric disease

Serum concentration of gastrin can be measured in both dogs and cats using an assay developed for measurement of gastrin in human serum. Gastrin is very labile and the serum must immediately be separated from the blood cells, frozen, and shipped on ice. It has been suggested that a 24-hour fasting serum gastrin concentration that is increased above 10-fold of the upper limit of the reference range is suggestive for a gastrinoma in dogs. However, this recommendation is based on human beings where atrophic gastritis is a common cause of moderate increases in serum gastrin concentrations. In contrast, atrophic gastritis has only been reported in the Norwegian Lundehund and other diseases that are associated with an increased serum gastrin concentration can easily be ruled out in the dog. However, if any uncertainty remains, a secretin stimulation test should be performed (see 9.4).

C-reactive protein, a highly sensitive but nonspecific marker of inflammation, correlates well with the degree of experimentally induced damage of the gastric mucosa.[7] Also, an increased plasma lactate concentration (>6.0 mmol/L) has been shown to be a negative prognostic marker for post-operative survival time in dogs following gastric dilation/volvulus.[8] Further studies evaluating the correlation of plasma lactate concentrations with long-term survival are warranted. Measurement of immunoreactive pepsinogen has been useful as a research tool for the diagnosis of gastritis in dogs, but has no diagnostic value in individual patients with spontaneous disease.[9]

1.4.1.5   Analysis of gastric juice

Analysis of gastric juice is performed rarely in veterinary medicine. This is due to the technical complexity and limited standardization. Also, analysis of gastric juice shows poor correlation with endoscopic and histopathological findings. The pH of gastric juice and concentrations of hydrochloric acid and pepsin can be evaluated either at baseline or after stimulation with pentagastrin. Gastroduodenal reflux can be demonstrated by use of a radioactive marker that is excreted in bile.[10]

1.4.1.6   Evaluation of gastric emptying time

Scintigraphy is currently the gold standard for evaluation of gastric emptying but requires the use of a radioactive marker. Alternatively, a radiopaque marker, such as barium-impregnated polyethylene spheres (BIPS), can be used. These markers have the disadvantage that, depending on their size, they only mimic emptying of either solid or liquid food.[11] Recently, ^{13}C-octanoic acid breath tests have been introduced to assess gastric emptying time in dogs and cats.[12] These tests allow labeling of a complex meal with ^{13}C-octanoic acid, a medium-chain fatty acid that is absorbed in the duodenum and oxidized in the liver, where the ^{13}C is released. A rise in $^{13}CO_2$ in the expiratory air indicates that gastric emptying has occurred.

Key Facts

- Routine laboratory tests are nonspecific for gastric disease but should be performed to rule out other diseases that are associated with clinical signs consistent with gastric disease or systemic diseases that affect the stomach.
- Currently, no laboratory tests are available that are specific for gastric disease.
- Gastroscopy is currently the gold standard for a definitive diagnosis of gastric disease.

References

1. Hasslinger MA. Der Magenwurm der Katze, *Ollulanus tricuspis* (Leuckart, 1865) – zum gegenwärtigen Stand der Kenntnis. *Tierärztl Prax* 1985; 13: 205–215.
2. Happonen I, Saari S, Castren L et al. Comparison of diagnostic methods for detecting gastric *Helicobacter*-like organisms in dogs and cats. *J Comp Pathol* 1996; 115: 117–127.
3. Neiger R, Simpson KW. *Helicobacter* infection in dogs and cats: Facts and fiction. *J Vet Intern Med* 2000; 14: 125–133.
4. Strauss-Ayali D, Simpson KW, Schein AH et al. Serological discrimination of dogs infected with gastric *Helicobacter* spp. and uninfected dogs. *J Clin Microbiol* 1999; 37: 1280–1287.
5. Cornetta AM, Simpson KW, Strauss-Ayali D et al. Use of a ^{13}C-urea breath test for detection of gastric infection with *Helicobacter* spp. in dogs. *Am J Vet Res* 1998; 59: 1364–1369.
6. Meddings JB, Kirk D, Olson ME. Non-invasive detection of canine NSAID-gastropathy. *Am J Vet Res* 1995; 56: 977–981.
7. Otabe K, Ito T, Sugimoto T et al. C-reactive protein (CRP) measurement in canine serum following experimentally-induced acute gastric mucosal injury. *Lab Anim* 2000; 34: 434–438.
8. dePapp E, Drobatz KJ, Hughe, D. Plasma lactate concentration as a predictor of gastric necrosis and survival among dogs with gastric dilatation-volvulus: 102 cases (1995–1998). *J Am Vet Med Assoc* 1999; 215(1): 49–52.
9. Suchodolski JS, Steiner JM, Ruaux CG et al. Concentrations of serum pepsinogen A (cPG A) in dogs with gastric lesions. *J Vet Intern Med* 2002; 16: 384 (abstract).
10. Happé RP, Van den Brom WE, Van der Gaag I. Duodenogastric reflux in the dog, a clinicopathological study. *Res Vet Sci* 1982; 33: 280–286.
11. Lester NV, Roberts GD, Newell SM et al. Assessment of barium impregnated polyethylene spheres (BIPS) as a measure of solid-phase gastric emptying in normal dogs – comparison to scintigraphy. *Vet Radiol Ultrasound* 1999; 40:465–471.
12. Wyse CA, Preston T, Love S et al. Use of the ^{13}C-octanoic acid breath test for assessment of solid-phase gastric emptying in dogs. *Am J Vet Res* 2001; 62: 1939–1944.

1

1.4.2 Laboratory tests for the diagnosis of intestinal disorders

CRAIG G. RUAUX

1.4.2.1 Introduction

The clinical investigation and definitive diagnosis of intestinal disorders is complicated by the inaccessibility of much of the intestinal tract to direct examination. While endoscopic examination of the intestinal tract can yield information on discrete lesions and gross alterations in mucosal appearance or architecture, endoscopy requires expensive equipment, a high level of expertise, and general anesthesia of the patient. Histological assessment of the intestinal tract is usually considered the gold standard for diagnosis of intestinal disease, yet no consistent system for the interpretation of intestinal histopathology sections has been described. In a recent study, there was a high degree of variability in histopathological interpretation between different observers and the reliability and consistency of diagnoses based on intestinal histopathology has been questioned.[1]

Laboratory assessment of the intestinal tract is less expensive and invasive than endoscopy or exploratory laparotomy with histopathology. Most clinicians, therefore, will use some form of laboratory assessment of the intestinal tract before proceeding to more invasive procedures.

As described in chapter 5.1, the intestinal tract as a whole has five major functions: secretion, digestion, absorption, motility, and barrier function. Secretion of fluid, ions, and enzymes, nutrient digestion and absorption occur primarily in the small intestine. The large intestine is a major site of absorption of water and ions. Clinical signs of intestinal disease result from alterations or disturbances in one or more of these major functions. Decreased digestion or absorption, or increased fluid secretion, will lead to diarrhea, one of the hallmark signs of intestinal disease.

Normal function of the intestine relies upon the presence of a healthy epithelium. Much of the function of the intestinal epithelium is dependant on subcellular structural elements such as the microvillar brush border and intercellular tight junctions, which can not be assessed by routine histopathological techniques.

Techniques for the functional assessment of the intestinal mucosa have only been developed and described relatively recently. Typically, the mucosal barrier function and absorptive capacity are the only functions assessed. Intestinal absorptive capacity can be assessed by the measurement of serum cobalamin and folate concentrations and by intestinal function testing using sugar probes. Intestinal barrier function can be assessed by fecal α_1-proteinase inhibitor concentration and permeability testing using sugar probes. Intestinal motility can be assessed using radiographic or ultrasonographic techniques but secretion and digestion are not readily measured in a non-invasive manner.

1.4.2.2 Assessment of serum cobalamin and folate concentrations

Cobalamin (Vitamin B12) and folate are water-soluble vitamins whose specific mechanisms and sites of absorption can provide information about the small intestinal mucosa and the bacterial flora present in the small intestine.

Cobalamin is a cobalt-containing vitamin that is synthesized exclusively by bacteria. No eukaryotic organisms are capable of synthesizing this compound, hence the essentiality of this vitamin. While cobalamin is exclusively bacterial in origin, the main dietary source of cobalamin for companion animal species is in complex with animal-sourced proteins. Dietary deficiency of cobalamin is highly unlikely in pets consuming commercial diets as they are fortified with cobalamin. Even homemade diets for companion animals are usually based on some form of animal protein, and thus provide sufficient cobalamin in most cases. As dietary deficiency of cobalamin is unlikely, alterations in the serum concentration of cobalamin most likely represent changes in the ability of the animal's gastrointestinal tract to absorb cobalamin. Thus, serum cobalamin concentrations can be used as a marker for gastrointestinal disease.

Cobalamin is absorbed through a complex, receptor-mediated mechanism (Figure 1.42). Dietary cobalamin, initially complexed to protein in the diet, is liberated in the stomach by the action of pepsinogen and gastric acid. The cobalamin is immediately bound to gastric and salivary R-protein, which carries the cobalamin into the duodenum. In the duodenum, the R-protein-cobalamin complex is broken down by pancreatic proteases, and the newly liberated cobalamin is complexed with another carrier protein, intrinsic factor. The site of intrinsic factor synthesis and secretion varies from species to species. In human beings, the gastric mucosa is the major source of intrinsic factor, while dogs produce intrinsic factor in both the stomach and the pancreas.[2] The domestic cat exclusively synthesizes intrinsic factor in the exocrine pancreas.[3,4]

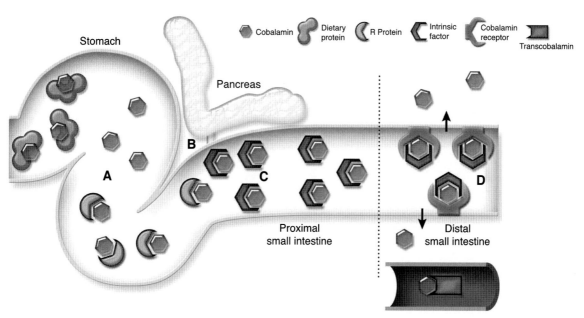

Figure 1.42:
Cobalamin absorption. Dietary cobalamin is bound to dietary protein. In the stomach, pepsin and hydrochloric acid degrade the dietary protein, releasing the cobalamin **(A)**. The cobalamin is immediately bound by R-protein, which is produced in the gastric mucosa. In the duodenum, pancreatic proteinases digest the R-protein, releasing the cobalamin. Free cobalamin in the duodenum is bound by intrinsic factor **(B)**. In dogs and human beings, intrinsic factor is produced by both the stomach and the pancreas, but in the cat 99% of intrinsic factor is synthesized by the exocrine pancreas. Cobalamin remains bound to intrinsic factor during its passage through the cranial small intestine **(C)**. In the distal small intestine, the cobalamin/intrinsic factor complexes are taken up by specific receptors found only on enterocytes in the ileum **(D)**. These enterocytes process the cobalamin/intrinsic factor complex and release cobalamin into the circulation, where a final set of binding proteins (transcobalamins) complex the vitamin and carry it to the cells. Reprinted from *Clinical Techniques in Small Animal Practice*, 18(4): Suchodolski and Steiner, "Laboratory assessment of gastrointestinal function" page 207, © 2003, with permission from Elsevier.

The final site of cobalamin absorption, in all species studied to date, is the ileum. Highly specialized cobalamin-intrinsic factor complex receptors are expressed on ileal mucosal enterocytes. Cobalamin that is not in complex with intrinsic factor is not readily absorbed, even if given orally in high doses.

As the exocrine pancreas is the only source of intrinsic factor in cats and an important source for intrinsic factor in dogs, exocrine pancreatic insufficiency is commonly associated with cobalamin deficiency in dogs and especially cats, and should be ruled out in patients with gastrointestinal signs and a decreased serum cobalamin concentration (see 1.4.4).[5]

Two other major mechanisms can reduce cobalamin availability from the small intestine, decreased mucosal absorptive capacity or excess utilization of cobalamin by the intestinal microflora. Some bacterial species commonly present in the intestinal tract, particularly some members of the *Clostridium* and *Bacteroides* genera, are able to absorb and utilize cobalamin after it has been complexed with intrinsic factor. In the normal individual with a healthy intestinal microflora, there is

sufficient cobalamin in the diet to supply the needs of both the host organism and the intestinal microflora. If the numbers of bacteria present in the intestine are increased, and particularly if *Clostridium* and *Bacteroides* spp. numbers are increased in the cranial part of the small intestine, the intestinal flora can effectively compete with the host for the available cobalamin, ultimately leading to a reduced serum cobalamin concentration in the host.

Mucosal disease in the ileum reduces expression of the cobalamin-intrinsic-factor complex receptor. With reduced expression of this receptor, mucosal uptake of cobalamin in the ileum is reduced, leading to cobalamin malabsorption, depletion of body stores of cobalamin, and ultimately a reduced serum cobalamin concentration. The same is true for diffuse intestinal disease as long as the ileum is involved in the disease process. Cobalamin normally undergoes enterohepatic circulation. In gastrointestinal disease the ability of the intestine to reabsorb cobalamin secreted in the bile is reduced, which can lead to dramatic shortening of the half-life of cobalamin in circulation, particularly in cats.[6]

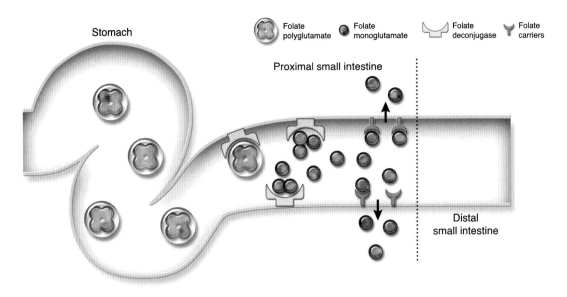

Figure 1.43:
Folate absorption. Dietary folate enters the gastrointestinal tract predominantly in the polyglutamate form. Folate deconjugase, a brush border enzyme in the cranial small intestine, deconjugates the folate polyglutamate to folate monoglutamate. Specific folate carriers present on enterocytes located in the cranial small intestine subsequently absorb folate monoglutamate. Both the deconjugase and folate carrier molecules are restricted to the cranial small intestine. There is no appreciable absorption of folate in the distal small intestine or the colon. Reprinted from *Clinical Techniques in Small Animal Practice*, 18(4): Suchodolski and Steiner, "Laboratory assessment of gastrointestinal function" page 208, © 2003, with permission from Elsevier.

Serum cobalamin concentration is not only of diagnostic importance. Cobalamin is essential for many cell functions and cobalamin deficiency can lead to gastrointestinal abnormalities, such as inflammatory infiltration of the mucosa, villous atrophy, and cobalamin malabsorption, as well as systemic abnormalities, such as peripheral and central neuropathies, or immunodeficiencies. Thus, patients with cobalamin deficiency may not respond to therapy of the primary disease process unless supplemented with cobalamin, and measurement of serum cobalamin is crucial in planning a rational therapy for these patients.

The normal mechanism of folate absorption is illustrated in Figure 1.43. Most folate in the diet is present in a poorly absorbable, polyglutamate form. Folate deconjugase in the jejunum removes most of the glutamate residues, leaving folate monoglutamate. Specific folate carriers in the upper small intestine then absorb folate monoglutamate.

Gastrointestinal disease may either increase or decrease serum folate concentrations, depending upon the type of pathology present. Mucosal disease in the upper small intestine or diffuse intestinal disease involving the upper small intestine may reduce folate absorption either by interfering with folate poly-glutamate deconjugation or reducing the presence of folate carrier proteins. Also, many intestinal bacteria, particularly those present in the lower bowel, are able to synthesize folate. These organisms release excess folate into the intestine. Thus, overgrowth of bacteria in the small intestine can lead to increased serum folate concentrations.[7]

Measurement of serum concentrations of cobalamin and folate is clinically indicated during the assessment of any patient with chronic diarrhea, particularly in those with clinical signs and history suggestive of small intestinal disease. Differential diagnoses to be considered with altered serum cobalamin and folate concentrations are summarized in Table 1.8. In order to rule out exocrine pancreatic insufficiency, concurrent measurement of serum trypsin-like immunoreactivity concentration is strongly recommended. Red blood cells have very high intracellular concentrations of folate, thus it is important to avoid hemolysis of samples for serum folate determination to reduce the chance of falsely elevated results.

Table 1.8: Interpretation of serum concentrations of cobalamin and folate in companion animals with gastrointestinal diseas

		Serum Cobalamin		
		Elevated	Normal	Subnormal
Serum Folate	Elevated	■ Increased bacterial numbers in cranial small intestine ■ Consider small intestinal bacterial overgrowth	■ Increased bacterial numbers in cranial small intestine ■ Consider small intestinal bacterial overgrowth	■ Small intestinal bacterial overgrowth or ileal mucosal disease ■ Measure serum TLI concentration to rule out EPI
	Normal	■ Elevated serum cobalamin with normal serum folate has no known significance	■ Normal serum cobalamin and folate does not rule out small intestinal disease	■ Ileal mucosal disease ■ Measure serum TLI concentration to rule out EPI
	Subnormal	■ Disease affecting the cranial small intestine ■ Consider IBD, lymphoma, or fungal disease	■ Disease affecting the cranial small intestine ■ Consider IBD, lymphoma, or fungal disease	■ Diffuse mucosal disease ■ Consider IBD, lymphoma, or fungal disease

1.4.2.3 Assessment of gastrointestinal protein loss

Many small intestinal diseases can lead to loss of protein into the gastrointestinal tract. Examples include inflammatory bowel disease, infiltrative diseases of the mucosa/submucosa, such as lymphoma, and lymphatic drainage abnormalities (lymphangiectasia). Protein loss into the intestine is a significant metabolic drain on the patient, and may alter bacterial numbers in the intestine by increasing available substrates for bacterial growth. Excess protein loss into the small intestine can lead to loss of plasma oncotic pressure and systemic pathology such as ascites, thoracic effusion, and edema.

Assessment of protein loss into the small intestine is complicated by the digestive function of the intestine and the presence of bacterial proteolytic enzymes. It is important to be able to quantify the loss of albumin into the GI tract, as albumin is a major contributor to the colloid oncotic pressure of the plasma. Unfortunately, albumin present in the gastrointestinal tract is rapidly degraded by the animal's own digestive proteases as well as bacterial proteases; therefore, it is not possible to accurately measure albumin in feces or intestinal fluid.

The traditional, gold-standard method for assessing gastrointestinal albumin loss is the ^{51}Cr-EDTA test.[8] Radioactive chromium bound to EDTA is administered parenterally to the patient, and subsequently binds to circulating plasma proteins, predominantly albumin. By collection of all fecal matter passed over 72 hours, and measurement of the accumulated radioactivity passed in the feces, the total intestinal protein loss can be measured. This technique is methodologically complex, requires consideration of radiation safety and the handling of radioactive waste, and is expensive. Consequently, this test is usually only used in institutional or research settings.

Alpha$_1$-proteinase inhibitor (α_1-PI) is a serum protein that is similar in molecular mass and size to albumin, and thus is lost into the intestine at a similar rate to albumin. As it is a proteinase inhibitor, it is able to resist proteolytic degradation in the intestine and is passed undamaged in the feces.[9] Following extraction from fecal samples, α_1-PI can be measured by use of an enzyme-linked immunosorbent assay. Species-specific assays for the measurement of α_1-PI are avaible for both dogs and cats (www.cvm.tamu.edu/gilab).

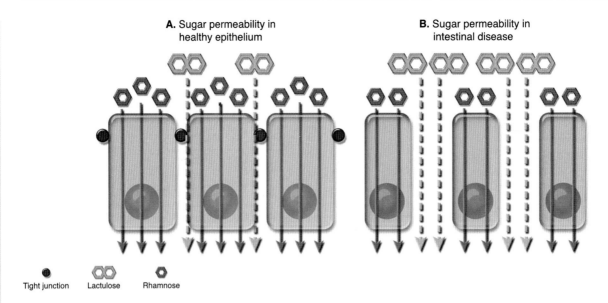

A. Sugar permeability in healthy epithelium

B. Sugar permeability in intestinal disease

Tight junction   Lactulose   Rhamnose

Figure 1.44:
Lactulose / rhamnose permeability testing. (A) Normal gastrointestinal mucosa has limited permeability to lactulose through tight-junction-associated paracellular channels, while rhamnose is taken up via a transcellular route. With gastrointestinal disease (B), the surface area of the mucosa available for rhamnose permeability is reduced and the integrity of the paracellular tight junctions is altered. The result is increased permeability to lactulose with a decreased permeability to rhamnose, leading to an increase in the L/R ratio in serum or urine. Reprinted from *Clinical Techniques in Small Animal Practice*, 18(4): Suchodolski and Steiner, "Laboratory assessment of gastrointestinal function" page 204, © 2003, with permission from Elsevier.

Ideally the loss of α_1-PI should be measured over 24 hours by collection of all feces, followed by thorough homogenization and extraction. However, this is not feasible under practice conditions. Thus the current recommendation is to collect three samples of 1 g each from three different bowel movements. It is important to keep the samples frozen from the time of collection until they are delivered to the laboratory. The average and maximum concentrations of fecal α_1-PI measured from the three samples are determined. At the time of writing, the presence of an average α_1-PI concentration $\geq 9.4\ \mu g/g$ feces, or in any one sample $\geq 15\ \mu g/g$ is considered suggestive of a protein-losing gastroenteropathy in the dog. The fecal α_1-PI test can detect significant protein loss before serum / plasma proteins are markedly reduced and before the onset of severe clinical signs related to hypoproteinemia. For example, Soft-coated Wheaten Terriers that have a familial PLE / PLN have increased fecal α_1-PI concentrations long before any clinical signs are present. Also, some patients with PLE may not show signs of gastrointestinal disease and measurement of fecal α_1-PI concentrations may help to diagnose the presence of gastrointestinal disease in these patients.

1.4.2.4 Assessment of intestinal absorptive capacity and barrier function

Recently, the use of sugar probes to measure intestinal mucosal permeability and absorptive capacity has been described in dogs and cats. The most common probes used for this type of study are mixtures of simple sugars, with quantification of either urinary or serum recoveries of these sugar probes.[10–12]

Measurement of the relative recoveries of the sugars lactulose and rhamnose can be used to assess the permeability of the small intestine. This technique has been described in both the dog and the cat.[10–12] Rhamnose is believed to be absorbed across the intestinal epithelium via a transcellular route, entering via small pores on the mucosal cell surface (Figure 1.44). Lactulose, a larger molecule, is unable to penetrate these small transcellular pores. Small quantities of lactulose are absorbed through paracellular pores that are apparently located in the area of the intercellular tight junctions (Figure 1.44). Absorption and recovery of lactulose and rhamnose can be expressed as a lactulose / rhamnose (L/R) ratio. When the mucosa is diseased, there is usually a reduction in the surface area of the mucosa (thus less transcellular pores are available) and an increase in the permeability of the tight junctions (Figure 1.44). Thus, with diseases of the gastrointestinal mucosa, the L/R ratio is increased.

Mucosal absorptive function can be measured by measuring the uptake of sugars that are absorbed through carrier-mediated mechanisms. Xylose and 3-O-methylglucose have been used to evaluate the intestinal absorptive capacity for fructose and glucose, respectively.[12] Absorptive capacity can be assessed for xylose and 3-O-methylglucose separately or can be expressed as the X/M ratio.

Currently, gastrointestinal permeability and mucosal function testing ideally requires the collection of all the urine produced over a 6-hour period in order to determine the urinary recovery of each sugar marker. Alternatively, a spot urine sample 4 to 6 hours after sugar administration can be utilized to calculate urinary sugar recovery ratios. A serum test, utilizing the ratios of serum sugar concentrations at a single time point is currently under development.

⚷ Key Facts

- Non-invasive serum and urine tests often yield clinically useful information for assessment of the small intestine.
- Functional assessment of the intestine may reveal disease when histopathology is normal.
- Serum concentrations of cobalamin and folate can aid in localization of intestinal disease, and may indicate the presence of an altered intestinal flora.
- Fecal concentrations of alpha$_1$-proteinase inhibitor (α_1-PI) are often elevated in animals with protein-losing enteropathy before hypoproteinemia develops.

References

1. Willard MD, Jergens AE, Duncan RB et al. Interobserver variation among histopathologic evaluations of intestinal tissues from dogs and cats. *J Am Vet Med Assoc* 2002; 220: 1177–1182.
2. Batt RM, Horadagoda NU, McLean L et al. Identification and characterization of a pancreatic intrinsic factor in the dog. *Amer J Physiol* 1989; 256: G517–G523.
3. Fyfe JC. Feline intrinsic factor (IF) is pancreatic in origin and mediates ileal cobalamin (CBL) absorption. *J Vet Intern Med* 1993; 7: 133 (abstract).
4. Ruaux CG, Steiner JM, Williams DA. Metabolism of amino acids in cats with severe cobalamin deficiency. *Amer J Vet Res* 2001; 62: 1852–1858.
5. Steiner JM, Williams DA. Feline exocrine pancreatic disorders. *Vet Clin North Amer* 1999; 29: 551–575.
6. Simpson KW, Fyfe J, Cornetta A et al. Subnormal concentrations of serum cobalamin (Vitamin B12) in cats with gastrointestinal disease. *J Vet Intern Med* 2001; 15: 26–32.
7. Batt RM, Needham JR, Carter MW. Bacterial overgrowth associated with a naturally occurring enteropathy in the German Shepherd dog. *Res Vet Sci* 1983; 35: 42–46.
8. Hall EJ, Batt RM, Brown A. Assessment of canine intestinal permeability, using ^{51}Cr-labeled ethylenediaminetetraacetate. *Amer J Vet Res* 1989; 50: 2069–2074.
9. Melgarejo T, Williams DA, Asem EK. Enzyme-linked immunosorbent assay for canine α_1-protease inhibitor. *Amer J Vet Res* 1998; 59: 127–130.
10. Rutgers HC, Batt RM, Proud FJ et al. Intestinal permeability and function in dogs with small intestinal bacterial overgrowth. *J Small Anim Pract* 1996; 37: 428–434.
11. Papasouliotis K, Gruffydd-Jones TJ, Sparkes AH et al. Lactulose and mannitol as probe markers for in vivo assessment of passive intestinal permeability in healthy cats. *Amer J Vet Res* 1993; 54: 840–844.
12. Steiner JM, Williams DA, Moeller EM. Kinetics of urinary recovery of five sugars after orogastric administration in healthy dogs. *Amer J Vet Res* 2002; 63: 845–848.

1.4.3 Laboratory tests for the diagnosis of liver disease

David A. Williams, Jan Rothuizen

1.4.3.1 Introduction

Definitive diagnosis of liver disease is often problematic. Many diseases lead to secondary hepatic changes (Table 1.9) and routine biochemical tests may reveal evidence of liver disease in animals that appear clinically normal. The clinician must determine whether or not abnormal test results reflect clinically significant liver disease. Careful consideration of the history, findings on physical examination, diagnostic imaging, and clinicopathological evaluation, when taken together generally guide the clinician in making this decision.[1–3]

Once primary hepatic disease is suspected, it is extremely important that clinical suspicion is directed by the overall clinical picture and all available data, not just the results of selected laboratory tests in isolation. It is often informative to monitor changes in observed abnormalities at 2 to 4 week intervals, particularly when test results are equivocal. Over such a time interval nonspecific changes may abate, secondary changes often remain fairly consistent depending on the primary disease process, and abnormalities associated with primary liver disease will often become more apparent. If the test results are initially equivocal and the clinical signs are vague, sequential evaluation may be necessary to allow time for the disease to be fully expressed.

Definitive diagnosis may ultimately require hepatic biopsy, but even histopathology may not provide a clear diagnosis since histological abnormalities may be patchy, diagnostic criteria are not well standardized between pathologists, and the size and quality of biopsy samples is often sub-optimal. It should be noted that a manual on the standardization of hepatic diseases in small animals has recently become available.[4] This manual also describes standards for histopathological evaluation of hepatic biopsies and is the result of the efforts of the WSAVA standardization group for hepatic diseases. The final diagnosis often involves integration of information based not only on laboratory findings but also those of diagnostic imaging (radiology, ultrasonography, and scintigraphy) taken together with histological changes.

Table 1.9: Diseases associated with secondary hepatic abnormalities

- Hyperadrenocorticism (dogs)
- Adrenal overproduction of sex hormones (dogs)
- Drugs
  - phenobarbital (dogs)
  - corticosteroids (dogs)
- Hyperthyroidism (cats)
- Hypoxia
  - autoimmune hemolytic anemia
  - shock
- Chronic small intestinal disease
- Acute pancreatitis
- Diabetes mellitus
- Periodontal disease
- Sepsis

1.4.3.2 Routine hematological testing, urinalysis, and fecal examination

There are few alterations in blood cells that suggest hepatobiliary disease. Most are changes in erythrocytes associated with fragmentation or changes in cell size or membrane composition. Microcytosis with normochromia or slight hypochromia is a rather common finding in dogs with congenital portosystemic shunts ($\geq 60\%$); it is less common in cats with congenital portosystemic shunts ($\geq 30\%$). Most of these animals are not anemic. The cause of microcytosis is poorly understood. Regardless of the mechanism, delay in attaining the full complement of hemoglobin causes erythrocytes to undergo an extra cell division, resulting in smaller than normal mature cells. The erythrocyte indices normalize after successful surgery to correct the portosystemic shunt. If there is also non-regenerative anemia, microcytosis must be distinguished from anemia of chronic disease (which may also include liver disease) causing microcytosis and relative iron deficiency, or from iron deficiency caused by chronic gastrointestinal blood loss.

Strongly regenerative anemia, with low hematocrit ($<20\%$), macrocytosis, high reticulocyte count, and normal to slightly increased serum protein concentration in a jaundiced dog, especially if spherocytes are also identified, indicates hemolytic anemia with the increased bilirubin formation being the cause of jaundice. Cats and dogs with hemolytic anemia typically also have high serum liver enzyme activities and bile acids concentrations, pointing to hepatic consequences developing secondary to the effects of marked hemolysis, such as hypoxia and thromboembolism which cause intrahepatic cholestasis.[1]

Few changes in the leukogram are expected in cats or dogs with hepatobiliary disease except when an infectious agent is the initiating cause of the disease (e.g., histoplasmosis, bacterial cholangitis, or leptospirosis in dogs) or when infection has complicated a primary hepatobiliary disorder (e.g., gramnegative sepsis in a dog with cirrhosis or septic bile peritonitis). Neutrophilic leukocytosis would be likely in such cases, whereas pancytopenia is typical of disseminated histoplasmosis and severe toxoplasmosis in cats and of early infectious canine hepatitis. In dogs and cats with portosystemic shunting (congenital or acquired), endotoxins and bacteria from the intestinal tract are not filtered out by the liver and may reach the systemic circulation, so that neutrophilic leukocytosis may occur in these diseases. However, a neutrophilia is not a consistent finding in dogs and cats with portosystemic vascular anomalies.

Platelet numbers may be normal or mildly decreased, but severe thrombocytopenia is rare in patients with liver disease.

The results of urine and fecal examinations are generally unhelpful in patients with liver disease. Dilute urine (specific gravity as low as 1.005) due to polyuria/polydipsia occurs frequently in dogs with chronic hepatobiliary diseases or dogs with portosystemic shunting. Other common findings on urinalysis consistent with hepatobiliary disease include excessive bilirubinuria in a non-anemic dog ($\geq$2+ bilirubin in urine of specific gravity $\leq$1.025), presence of bilirubin in the urine of cats, and ammonium biurate crystalluria. In dogs, excessive bilirubinuria may precede the onset of hyperbilirubinemia and jaundice. Kidneys of male dogs contain all enzymes needed to produce and conjugate bilirubin, so that 1–2+ bilirubin in a urine sample from a male dog is not abnormal, and small numbers of bilirubin crystals may be found in concentrated urine specimens from normal male dogs. However, ammonium biurate crystals in a freshly voided urine sample are not normal. These crystals occur when hyperammonemia combined with excess uric acidemia from diminished hepatic conversion to allantoin exceeds the renal threshold, and precipitation of ammonium biurate results. Their presence in the urine may fluctuate, but alkalinizing the urine specimen with a few drops of sodium hydroxide may precipitate ammonium biurate crystals and make them visible during sediment examination. About half of the dogs with congenital portosystemic shunts have these urine crystals. However, some breeds of dog, including Dalmatians, have an inherent inadequate conversion of uric acid to allantoin and display ammonium biurate crystalluria in the absence of portosystemic shunting.

Measurement of urinary urobilinogen has traditionally been used to assess the presence of extrahepatic bile duct obstruction. However, there are so many confounding factors (e.g., influences by the intestinal flora, renal function, urine pH and specific gravity, and the exposure of the urine sample to light) that the test is now considered without diagnostic value and obsolete.

Acholic feces characterized by absence of stercobilins (fecal pigments) and steatorrhea are very rarely seen in patients with severe, usually extrahepatic, cholestasis. Severe hemolysis causing increased bilirubin production and excretion may cause orange-colored feces.

1.4.3.3 Analysis of ascites fluid

If abdominal fluid is detected, a sample should be collected for laboratory analysis. In dogs with chronic liver disease causing intrahepatic portal hypertension, the ascitic fluid is a clear and colorless pure transudate. It contains very few cells (<2500/ml) and a low protein concentration (<2.5 g/dl). Consequently the specific gravity is below 1.016. In contrast, in dogs with post-sinusoidal hypertension due to right-sided heart failure, the fluid is nearly always slightly red. This typical modified transudate contains more protein ($\geq$2.5 g/dl), and has a specific gravity ranging from 1.010 to 1.033. Exudate (as seen with abdominal tumors or peritonitis) has a high cell and protein content. Blood (e.g., due to rupture of a hemangiosarcoma), and bile (i.e., due to gall bladder or bile duct rupture) have a typical but distinctly different character compared with the pure transudate associated with chronic liver disease and portal hypertension. In case of acute portal vein obstruction (thrombosis), the fluid is similar to that seen in right-sided heart failure. Urine in the abdominal cavity secondary to urinary tract rupture may resemble a yellow-colored modified transudate, but is associated with azotemia and hyperkalemia.

1.4.3.4 Classical serum parameters

While numerous serum markers for hepatic disease exist, the following section will focus primarily on bilirubin, alkaline phosphatase (ALP), alanine aminotransferase (ALT), and serum bile acids (SBA), four classical markers that are widely available and most consistently useful in the evaluation of patients with suspected liver disease.

1

Serum bilirubin concentration

Bilirubin is derived from the metabolism of heme proteins by the reticuloendothelial system. Hemoglobin is the source of most of the bilirubin present in serum, with smaller amounts originating from the degradation of other heme sources such as myoglobin. The product of heme metabolism is non-conjugated bilirubin, which travels to the liver bound to albumin where it is conjugated and excreted into the biliary system. Hyperbilirubinemia reflects failure of the normal mechanisms involved in metabolism and/or excretion of bilirubin, and can be categorized as prehepatic, hepatic, or posthepatic in origin (Table 1.10).[1] The liver has tremendous reserve capacity for metabolizing and excreting heme proteins and hemolysis alone does not necessarily result in elevated bilirubin levels. Failure to excrete bilirubin only occurs when hepatic hypoxia secondary to anemia leads to hepatocyte dysfunction. Evaluation of a CBC should determine if elevated bilirubin concentrations are prehepatic in origin. Causes of posthepatic hyperbilirubinemia resulting from biliary obstruction or leakage from the biliary tree can often be identified by abdominal ultrasonographic evaluation. Measurement of bilirubin concentration in abdominal fluid and comparison with serum concentrations can also be diagnostically useful, with higher bilirubin concentrations in abdominal fluid being consistent with leakage from the biliary system.

Although certain conditions may be associated with a relative increase in either the non-conjugated or the conjugated forms of bilirubin (usually determined using van den Bergh's test), sufficient overlap exists to make distinctions based on the relative proportion of these two forms diagnostically unreliable, so that their determination is not clinically useful.[1] This lack of benefit in using the van den Bergh's test relates to the fact that hemolytic diseases associated with hyperbilirubinemia lead to hepatic hypoxia, affecting the liver secondarily. Centrizonal liver cell necrosis then causes leakage of bile into the hepatic lymph so that conjugated bile pigments (and bile acids) are increased in the blood. Thus, only in the very early stages of hemolytic jaundice is the serum bilirubin concentration primarily determined by the increased production of unconjugated bilirubin. Hyperbilirubinemia caused by primary liver/cholestatic disease on the other hand, is naturally characterized by presence of conjugated pigment in the circulation. However, there is also increased erythrolysis and decreased clearance of unconjugated bilirubin in such diseases, so that there is again a mixture of conjugated and unconjugated pigment.

Erythrocyte membrane changes are often a component of many primary hepatobiliary disorders, and thus accelerated red blood cell (RBC) destruction often contributes to high serum bilirubin concentrations. These cases have strong clinicopathological evidence of cholestasis (i.e., high ALP activity with moderate to high ALT activity). If they are associated with anemia, it is mild and often poorly regenerative. Hyper-

Table 1.10: Causes of prehepatic, hepatic, and posthepatic hyperbilirubinemia

Prehepatic
- Immune-mediated
- Parasite-associated or toxin-induced hemolytic anemia
- Blood transfusion reaction
- Congenital erythrocyte defects

Hepatic
- Acute and chronic hepatitis, cholangitis, or cholangiohepatitis
- Hepatic necrosis
- Hepatic fibrosis or cirrhosis
- Hepatic lipidosis (cats)
- Hepatic neoplasia
- Bacterial and fungal infections

Posthepatic
- Bile duct obstruction (e.g., due to pancreatitis, neoplasia, or foreign body)
- Biliary tree rupture (e.g., due to trauma or necrotizing cholangitis)

bilirubinemia can be attributed to hemolysis when there is moderate to marked anemia (the hematocrit is usually <15%) with strong evidence of regeneration. Such dogs can have secondary cholestasis with clinicopathological evidence.

Serum alanine aminotransferase activity

Alanine aminotransferase (ALT) is the most specific enzyme of hepatic origin. However, it is not completely liver-specific and may also be elevated in patients with severe muscle necrosis. It is located in the cytosol of hepatic cells and readily leaks into the bloodstream when hepatocytes are damaged. Unfortunately, the degree of elevation does not always correlate well with the degree or severity of hepatic damage. Activities not only increase when there is active hepatocellular damage, but also when hepatocytes regenerate during the recovery phase following hepatic injury. Conversely, serum ALT may be normal in end-stage liver disease as a result of hepatocyte depletion in the face of severe hepatic failure.

Both the chronicity of increased activities and the degree of elevation, as well as the overall clinical picture, should be taken into consideration when evaluating the significance of abnormal serum ALT activities. It is important to note that severe hepatic disease can be present in patients with a normal or minimally increased serum enzyme activity. Therefore, finding such values should not preclude further investigation, especially if there are clinical signs or other laboratory evidence that suggest hepatobiliary disease. Especially with chronic liver diseases, when there is less hepatocellular damage per time unit, serum ALT activities may not be severely increased, yet the disease ultimately causes severe loss of hepatic functional capacity. On the other hand, acute diseases, during which many cells are affected and release enzymes in a short time period, usually are associated with very high elevations of liver enzyme activities in serum. Owing to the large functional reserve of the liver, hepatic functional capacity is usually not severely affected in such cases. The above considerations explain why it is important to assess both liver enzyme activities and liver function tests for screening purposes. A good combination to confirm or exclude liver diseases is serum ALT activity with SBA concentrations (see below). If both are within the reference range, the chance that there is clinically significant liver disease is very low (<0.5%). Conversely, elevation of one or both parameters indicates the presence of liver disease and serves as an indication to perform further diagnostic tests (e.g., ultrasonography or liver biopsy).

Other enzyme activities can also be used as markers of hepatocellular injury, including arginase, sorbitol dehydrogenase, glutamate dehydrogenase, and lactate dehydrogenase, but have no diagnostic advantage over ALT and are usually less sensitive and less specific. Methods to measure these enzyme activities are not routinely available commercially, and given their lower diagnostic utility their use is not recommended.

Serum alkaline phosphatase activity

Alkaline phosphatase (ALP) is an enzyme that is induced in the biliary tract whenever there is intrahepatic or extrahepatic obstruction to the flow of bile, or in dogs when there are increased concentrations of certain adrenal steroid hormones or other drugs in the blood. Thus increased activities are commonly and classically seen when there is posthepatic obstructive disease or in dogs with hyperadrenocorticism or iatrogenic steroid administration. Idiopathic overproduction of other steroid hormones in older dogs that do not have glucocorticoid overproduction is another more recently recognized cause of increased ALP activity.[5]

ALP activity is also present in non-hepatobiliary tissues such as osteoblasts, intestinal mucosa, renal cortex, and placenta. These tissues, however, produce ALP with a very short half life. Thus, these isoenzymes disappear quickly from the blood and do not contribute significantly to the ALP activity measured in serum. Only the bone isoenzyme has a long half life comparable with the isoenzyme from liver and biliary epithelium, so that there is some contribution by the bone isoenzyme in young, growing puppies and kittens. Dogs with aggressive osteolytic bone neoplasms may also show increased serum ALP activities. In such cases, the source of enzyme is usually readily apparent.

A high serum ALP activity of bone origin was reported in a group of healthy Siberian Husky puppies.[6] This change is believed to be benign and familial, and should be considered when Huskies are evaluated for the presence of liver disease.

Anticonvulsants (e.g., phenytoin, phenobarbital, and primidone) and corticosteroids can induce production of ALP, reflected by increased serum activities (up to 100-fold for ALP). This occurs only in dogs, but not in cats. Anticonvulsant drugs stimulate production of the hepatic ALP isoenzyme. In contrast, pharmacological doses of corticosteroids administered orally, by injection, or topically, or increased endogenous steroid production as in patients with spontaneous hyperadrenocorticism, stimulate the production of a unique ALP isoenzyme in dogs. The steroid-induced isoenzyme can be identified by electrophoresis and by specific immunoassays. It is also stable during heating at 65 °C, whereas the normal hepatic ALP isoenzyme is quickly inactivated at this temperature. Heating of the sample for two minutes inactivates hepatic ALP completely, while the steroid-induced isoenzyme is practically unaffected. The corticosteroid-induced ALP isoenzyme assay (determined by electrophoresis or heat inactivation) has become routine in several laboratories. Serum γ-glutamyl transferase (GGT) activity may also rise in response to corticosteroids, but not as much as ALP does, and its measurement confers no advantage over that of ALP alone.

Feline hepatic ALP has a shorter half life than canine hepatobiliary ALP. Serum activity of this enzyme is, therefore, lower in cats than it is in dogs with a similar degree of cholestasis, and ALP is an insensitive enzyme marker for the diagnosis of liver and biliary disease in cats. Conversely, any increase in feline serum ALP activity should be considered significant.

Serum bile acids concentration

Serum bile acids (SBA) analysis is one of the most useful and specific liver function tests in dogs and cats. The concentration of bile acids in serum is normally low as a result of efficient hepatic extraction of bile acids from the portal blood following reabsorption of conjugated bile acids from the ileum. Postprandial gall bladder contractions cause a large increase in intestinal bile acids concentrations, but due to the extremely efficient removal of the absorbed bile acids by hepatocytes, there is only a mild (approximately 2–3 fold) and transient increase in SBA concentrations as compared with those seen in the unfed state. However, when there is significant hepatic dysfunction or biliary obstruction, impaired clearance of bile acids leads to spillover from the portal circulation, with resultant increases in SBA concentrations, which is particularly pronounced in the postprandial state. Pre- and postprandial SBA concentrations are sensitive tests for the diagnosis of hepatobiliary disease, but it must be noted that biliary obstruction as well as hepatic dysfunction can lead to increased concentrations.[7,8] Thus, there is no clinical utility in determining SBA concentrations if biliary obstruction has been documented. Indeed, if the total serum bilirubin concentration is elevated due to either hepatocellular dysfunction or biliary obstruction; there is no need to analyze SBA concentrations, since the elevation of bilirubin alone indicates either severe hepatic dysfunction or biliary obstruction; and in either case measurement of SBA concentrations will not provide any additional useful information. However, dogs with hemolytic anemia may have an elevated serum bilirubin concentration in the face of normal SBA concentrations. Such cases can most often be easily diagnosed by assessment of a PCV. The advantage of measuring SBA concentrations over bilirubin concentration is that they are very sensitive markers of hepatic function, much more sensitive than serum bilirubin concentration.

Bile acids can be measured in both serum and heparinized plasma, with identical results, but most studies have reported concentrations in serum. Cholic and chenodeoxycholic acid (the primary bile acids) are exclusively synthesized and conjugated (primarily with taurine) in the liver. Bile is in part stored in the gallbladder, where it is concentrated tenfold. Cholecystokinin, released from the small intestine after a meal, is the main trigger for gall bladder contraction, which is a slow and gradual process. Conjugated bile acids in the small intestine facilitate fat absorption by emulsifying the fat. They are very efficiently reabsorbed in the distal small intestine and reach the portal vein. Bile acids are cleared by the liver and re-excreted into the bile (i.e., enterohepatic cycle). Healthy animals have 10–15 cycles per day and lose very little bile acids. A small percentage escapes resorption and is converted by intestinal bacteria to secondary bile acids, deoxycholic and lithocholic acid, of which the minority is also resorbed into the enterohepatic cycle. Especially lithocholic acid is very toxic to cells and when bile acids accumulate in case of cholestasis, lithocholic acid may exert hepatotoxic effects. Fasting animals have low concentrations of SBA in the systemic circulation (the fraction, which has escaped hepatic clearance from the portal vein; total <5 mmol/L by enzymatic assay). After a meal, a larger load of bile acids is delivered to the intestines so that postprandial concentrations (after 1–2 hours) are higher than fasting concentrations. Postprandial SBA concentrations may increase up to three- to fourfold over fasting values (15–20 mmol/L). There are no age-related effects on SBA concentration.

Abnormally high fasting and/or postprandial SBA concentrations reflect either portosystemic shunting (congenital or acquired) causing impaired hepatic clearance, or cholestasis (intra- or extrahepatic) causing reflux of bile via the hepatic lymph into the systemic circulation. Intrahepatic cholestasis is common in most liver diseases, so that SBA concentrations may be increased in nearly all liver diseases of dogs and cats.

The standard way to assess SBA concentrations is to collect a blood sample after food has been withheld from the animal for 12 hours. Subsequently, gallbladder contraction is stimulated by feeding a small amount of food. Two hours after the meal, another blood sample is collected. There is minimal risk of precipitating an episode of hepatic encephalopathy during this test, even in predisposed animals. After the serum is collected, the samples may be refrigerated for several days or frozen almost indefinitely without loss of SBA concentration.

The fasting SBA concentration is a sensitive test to detect liver disease. However, postprandial SBA concentrations are more frequently and often more abnormally increased than fasting concentrations, and so it is recommended that both determinations be made. If only one determination can be made and the animal will either eat or tolerate force-feeding, the postprandial value is most useful to determine the presence or absence of clinically relevant hepatobiliary disease in most cats and dogs. The authors recommend that for animals suspected of having acquired hepatobiliary disease, a biopsy should be considered when enzymatically assayed postprandial SBA concentrations exceed 20 mmol/L in cats and 25 mmol/L in dogs. No pattern of pre-prandial and postprandial values is pathognomonic for any particular hepatic disorder, but patterns may help direct the further diagnostic workup of the patient.

For the diagnosis of congenital portosystemic shunting in particular, both fasting and postprandial SBA determinations are recommended in order to enhance the sensitivity of the SBA testing procedure. It is not uncommon for both dogs and cats with congenital vascular anomalies to have fasting SBA concentrations within or barely above the reference range, but postprandial concentrations are often markedly increased. This incremental increase in SBA following feeding is often far greater in patients with portosystemic vascular anomalies than in those with cholestatic parenchymal or biliary diseases.

Because enzymatic assays for SBA are now routinely available, determination of total SBA has become a convenient, practical test of hepatobiliary function in both cats and dogs. However, it should be noted that the postprandial rise of SBA is quite variable between different animals. This may reflect in part that the ideal quantity and composition of the test meal have not been determined or standardized, and that not all patients will consume all the food offered. These factors may affect gastric emptying and intestinal transit. In some patients, the presence of intestinal disease (especially in the ileum) and changes in the intestinal microflora are additional unknown variables. Another variable is gallbladder contraction in response to the meal, which is known not to be an instantaneous or complete process. The gallbladder shows an increased tone for several hours, causing gradual release of bile into the duodenum. Therefore, the bile acids do not reach the small intestine in a sharp peak, but as a blunt and extended, irregular peak. Even with a very well specified stimulus in the form of intravenously injected cholecystokinin, the degree and duration of the gall bladder contraction and emptying is highly variable between different dogs. Finally, expulsion of bile during periodic physiological gallbladder contractions between meals may complicate interpretation of the fasted sample result. In summary, there are numerous explanations for the observed variations in both pre- and postprandial SBA concentrations. Despite these limitations, evaluation of both parameters usually gives a strong indication regarding the likely presence or absence of significant hepatobiliary disease and abnormal SBA concentrations should always be followed by additional diagnostic testing to identify the specific cause of the disease.

Bile acids can also be assayed in urine, and abnormally high values have recently been reported in both dogs and cats with liver disease.[9,10] While the measurement of urinary bile acids may be helpful in screening very small patients for which blood collection is difficult, this approach offers no advantage over measurement of SBA concentrations and may give less information than can be obtained by evaluation of pre- and postprandial SBA concentrations.

Recent studies have indicated that bile acids can be increased in the absence of liver disease in dogs with an altered intestinal microflora that can be associated with small intestinal disease or EPI.[11] In these patients, the abnormal intestinal microflora generates large amounts of unconjugated bile acids that are readily absorbed from the intestinal lumen but that are cleared relatively inefficiently from the portal blood. When SBA are increased in circumstances where other evidence supporting the presence of liver disease is not present, the possibility of underlying small intestinal disease should be further investigated.

1.4.3.5 Other serum markers

Many additional markers that may be of value in the evaluation of patients with suspected liver disease have been described, but they generally offer few advantages over those tests mentioned above, although there may be certain circumstances when they can be useful. Most notably, patients with severe liver disease associated with hepatic failure may also exhibit hypoalbuminemia, hypoglycemia, hyperglobulinemia, hypokalemia, hypocholesterolemia, low blood urea nitrogen concentration, and hyperammonemia. Since the liver is important in the synthesis and / or metabolism of many of these analytes, their concentration in blood changes when hepatic dysfunction is marked.

Blood ammonia and blood urea nitrogen (BUN)

Formation of urea as a means of detoxifying ammonia is a function unique to the liver. However, BUN concentration may be reduced by several non-hepatic factors. Most frequent causes of non-hepatic causes of decreased serum BUN are restricted protein intake (e.g., due to anorexia, intentional reduction with low protein diet) and renal medullary washout due to sustained polydipsia and polyuria. A low BUN concentration in the absence of reduced protein intake or polyuria / polydipsia may therefore indicate liver dysfunction.

Plasma ammonia concentration is a very sensitive and specific indicator of ammonia detoxification by the liver. As for many other hepatic functions, the liver has a huge reserve capacity for this function, so that increased ammonia or decreased BUN concentrations are rarely due to parenchymal liver dysfunction, but more commonly caused by portosystemic shunting. Virtually all ammonia is formed in the intestinal tract and reaches the liver through the portal blood supply. If portal blood bypasses the liver (i.e., due to congenital or acquired portosystemic shunting), it reaches the systemic circulation and becomes increased. The effect of shunting on BUN is much smaller, as the decreased portal blood supply of the liver induces an increased hepatic arterial blood flow. Much of the systemic ammonia-rich blood reaches the liver via the arterial route and is converted into urea. Blood ammonia concentration is, therefore, preferentially increased in patients with congenital and acquired portosystemic shunts, particularly after feeding, or after oral or rectal administration of ammonium sulfate (i.e., for the purpose of an ammonia tolerance test). Blood ammonia is also increased in patients with hepatic encephalopathy from other causes, and its assay can thus be useful to diagnose hepatic encephalopathy as a cause of neurological signs.

Plasma ammonia was formerly only available through specialized veterinary or human hospital laboratories. However, today there is reliable and affordable equipment for analysis of ammonia that is suitable for use in veterinary practice (e.g., Menarini Diagnostics, Blood Ammonia Checker II).[12] Fasting plasma ammonia values for normal dogs are ≤ 100 mg/dl (45 µmol/L) and ≤ 90 mg/dl (40 µmol/L) for normal cats. Food should be withheld for at least 6 hours before sample collection. Blood must be collected into EDTA-coated tubes, which are immediately put into melting ice. Blood or plasma samples cannot be stored because ammonia is spontaneously liberated from amino groups (e.g., proteins and urea) in the sample, causing artefactually high concentrations.

If the sample is not analyzed immediately but is transported to a specialized off-site laboratory, the blood should be spun immediately in a refrigerated centrifuge, and the plasma should be put in a new pre-cooled tube and stored on ice. Cooled plasma can be stored for only 45 minutes prior to analysis, so that transport is only possible to a nearby facility. Hemolysis should be avoided because erythrocytes contain about three times the ammonia concentration of plasma. It is also important to avoid the possibility of contact of the blood sample with ammonia-containing contaminants such as cigarette smoke and body fluids such as sweat or saliva that may contain more ammonia than the sample. The use of vacuum tubes with a rubber stopper may help in preventing such contamination.

If ammonia is increased above 150 mg/dl (75 µmol/L), this confirms that neurological signs are caused by hepatic encephalopathy, or that portosystemic shunting is present. How-

1

ever, in rare cases, and especially when there is only a low shunting fraction (e.g., due to mild congenital portal vein hypoplasia), basal fasting ammonia may be within normal limits. In such cases, an ammonia tolerance test can be performed, and will confirm or exclude the presence of portosystemic shunting with certainty.

Oral administration of ammonium compounds can induce vomiting. A rectal test, in which 2 ml/kg of a 5% ammonium sulfate or chloride solution is given by enema and deposited as proximally into the colon as possible, is better tolerated. Blood ammonia is measured before and 30 min after administration of the ammonium salt. Plasma values after ammonium chloride administration in normal animals or animals with parenchymal or cholestatic liver diseases without portosystemic shunting do not exceed a twofold increase over baseline concentrations. An exaggerated response indicates congenital or acquired portosystemic shunting. Possible rare exceptions include rare inborn errors of ammonia metabolism, cats with hepatic lipidosis, and animals with fulminant liver necrosis. Clinical experience has revealed little risk of aggravating hepatic encephalopathy during a rectal ammonia tolerance test.

Serum cholesterol concentration

Serum cholesterol concentration is often routinely included in serum biochemistry profiles by commercial laboratories but affords little useful information in the diagnosis of hepatobiliary diseases. Increased cholesterol can be found in practically all cholestatic and parenchymal liver diseases, whereas low cholesterol may be present in dogs and cats with portosystemic vascular anomalies, which is, however, not diagnostic.

Serum glucose concentration

Hypoglycemia is an unusual finding in patients with liver disease and reflects very severe loss of hepatic function. It may be seen in patients with chronic liver disease with less than 20% functional hepatocytes left, or in acute fulminant hepatitis, associated with severe necrosis of the liver. Dogs with congenital portosystemic shunting may also show hypoglycemia, which is usually not very severe, but may become important when the patient is fasted before surgery. Also, some hepatic neoplasms may produce insulin-like proteins that can lead to hypoglycemia.

Serum electrolyte concentrations

Serum electrolyte abnormalities may occur in anorectic and hypoalbuminemic dogs and cats with congenital or acquired portosystemic shunting. Hypocalcemia is usually mild and an incidental finding associated with hypoalbuminemia.

Hypokalemia may be a risk factor for the development of hepatic encephalopathy and can be caused by renal and gastrointestinal loss, reduced intake, and secondary hyperaldosteronism. Hypokalemia may induce hypokalemic alkalosis, which is an important factor facilitating hepatic encephalopathy by promoting a shift of ammonia to non-ionized NH_3, which can readily diffuse membranes.

1.4.3.6 Abnormalities of coagulation parameters

The impaired synthesis of coagulation factors may lead to prolonged clotting times or even bleeding episodes in rare instances. Coagulation abnormalities may occur in patients with liver disease because of either vitamin K malabsorption, reduced hepatic synthesis of coagulation factors, or DIC as a consequence of the underlying primary disorder. It is perhaps most common to find a subtle prolongation of aPTT (1.5 times normal), abnormal fibrin degradation products (10–40 µg/ml or >40 µg/ml), and variable fibrinogen concentrations (<100 to 200 mg/dl) in cats and dogs with severe parenchymal hepatic disease. Some animals with severe hepatic disease and relatively unremarkable routine coagulation test results have a high serum concentration of proteins induced by vitamin K antagonism (PIVKA) that could impart bleeding tendencies. Frank bleeding is rare, but can be severe and life threatening. Also, and more importantly, severe blood loss into the GI tract can precipitate hepatic encephalopathy. Parenteral vitamin K1 administration can correct coagulation abnormalities in some patients. Plasma or clotting factor administration may help arrest acute bleeding episodes in those that are not responsive to vitamin K or have evidence of more severe underlying problems. Finally, plasma activity of protein C, an anticoagulant protein, has recently been reported to be decreased in dogs with hepatic diseases, and may help differentiate subgroups of various hepatic diseases.[13]

1.4.3.7 Other hepatic function tests

Other function tests used to evaluate hepatic function in the past include evaluation of plasma clearance of intravenously administered synthetic dyes, most notably bromosulphthalein or indocyanine green, excreted by the liver. These tests were neither sensitive nor practical to perform in most clinical settings, and they never gained widespread application. In future, testing based on the clearance of stable isotope-labeled test substrates, such as aminopyrine, that are metabolized by hepatocytes may prove to be more sensitive, specific, and practical methods by which to quantify hepatic function.

1.4.3.8   Species differences

There are notable differences between cats and dogs regarding numerous aspects of hepatic structure and function, as well as the types and frequency of different diseases encountered in each species. Specific differences with regard to the evaluation of marker test results also exist. For example, in cats, serum ALP is not induced by adrenal steroids or other drugs, which is a common cause of increases in serum activities of this enzyme in dogs. Also, both the hepatic concentration and half life of ALP in cats are low, such that increases should always be considered significant in this species. GGT is similar in its origins to ALP and generally behaves similarly to ALP when there is hepatobiliary disease, although it may be less affected by cholestasis and drugs than ALP in dogs and more affected by cholestasis than ALP in cats. One notable observation is that cats with hepatic lipidosis, but not those with other hepatopathies, classically have very high serum ALP activities but normal GGT activities. As mentioned above, bilirubinuria may be an indicator of hepatic disease. However, it is not uncommon for normal dogs to have mildly to moderately elevated urine bilirubin concentrations. In contrast, this is not true in cats, and therefore bilirubinuria in this species should always be considered indicative of hepatic disease and investigated further.

🔑 Key Facts

- Serum alanine aminotransferase activity reflects hepatocellular damage but not hepatic function.
- Increased serum alkaline phosphatase activities in cats nearly always indicate significant hepatic disease, but in dogs numerous extrahepatic diseases, such as hyperadrenocorticism or bone disease can cause abnormalities.
- A pre- and postprandial serum bile acids concentration is the most clinically useful test to assess liver function in both dogs and cats.
- Blood ammonia concentration can help identify patients with hepatic encephalopathy.
- Results of hepatic laboratory testing must be evaluated in the light of the clinical picture and cannot be used in isolation to assess patients with suspected liver disease.

References

1. Bunch SE. Jaundice. In: Hall EJ, Simpson JW, Williams DA (eds.), *BSAVA manual of canine and feline gastroenterology*. Quedgeley, British Small Animal Veterinary Association, 2005; 103–108.
2. Watson P. Diseases of the liver. In: Hall EJ, Simpson JW, Williams DA (eds.), *BSAVA Manual of canine and feline gastroenterology* Quedgeley,. British Small Animal Veterinary Association, 2005; 240–268.
3. Rothuizen J. Diseases of the biliary system. In: Hall EJ, Simpson JW, Williams DA (eds.), *BSAVA Manual of canine and feline gastroenterology*. Quedgeley, British Small Animal Veterinary Association, 2005; 269–278.
4. Rothuizen J, Bunch SE, Charles JA, et al. WSAVA Standards for clinical and histological diagnosis of canine and feline liver disease. *1st ed.* Philadelphia, Saunders Elsevier, 2006; 1–130.
5. Hill KE, Scott-Moncrieff JC, Koshko MA et al. Secretion of sex hormones in dogs with adrenal dysfunction. *J Am Vet Med Assoc* 2005; 226: 556–561.
6. Lawler DF, Keltner DG, Hoffman WE et al. Benign familial hyperphosphatasemia in Siberian huskies. *Am J Vet Res* 1996; 57: 612–617.
7. Center SA, Baldwin BH, Erb HN et al. Bile acid concentrations in the diagnosis of hepatobiliary disease in the dog. *J Am Vet Med Assoc* 1985; 187: 935–940.
8. Center SA, Baldwin BH, Erb H et al. Bile acid concentrations in the diagnosis of hepatobiliary disease in the cat. *J Am Vet Med Assoc* 1986; 189 (8): 891–896.
9. Balkman CE, Center SA, Randolph JF et al. Evaluation of urine sulfated and nonsulfated bile acids as a diagnostic test for liver disease in dogs. *J Am Vet Med Assoc* 2003; 222: 1368–1375.
10. Trainor D, Center SA, Randolph F et al. Urine sulfated and nonsulfated bile acids as a diagnostic test for liver disease in cats. *J Vet Intern Med* 2003; 17: 145–153.
11. Williams DA, Ruaux CG, Steiner JM. Serum bile acid concentrations in dogs with exocrine pancreatic insufficiency. *Proc 14th ECVIM-CA Congress, Barcelona, Spain* 2005; 200 (abstract).
12. Gerritzen-Bruning MJ, van den Ingh TS, Rothuizen J. Diagnostic value of fasting plasma ammonia and bile acid concentrations in the identification of portosystemic shunting in dogs. *J Vet Intern Med* 2006; 20: 13–19.
13. Toulza O, Center SA, Brooks MB, et al. Evaluation of plasma protein C activity for detection of hepatobiliary disease and portosystemic shunting in dogs. *J Am Vet Med Assoc* 2006; 229: 1761–1771.

1

1.4.4 Laboratory tests for the diagnosis of exocrine pancreatic disorders

Jörg M. Steiner

1.4.4.1 Introduction

Exocrine pancreatic disease is common in both dogs and cats. In a study of necropsy findings, 1.5% of 9,342 canine pancreata and 1.3% of 6,504 feline pancreata examined at necropsy showed significant pathological lesions.[1] Pancreatitis is the most common exocrine pancreatic disorder in both species, followed by exocrine pancreatic insufficiency, exocrine pancreatic neoplasia, and rare conditions of the exocrine pancreas. Pancreatitis is also common in human beings. A recent study reported that 300,000 patients are discharged from the hospital each year with a diagnosis of pancreatitis in the USA alone.[2] This number does not include patients that only have mild forms of pancreatitis and are not admitted to a hospital or those that have severe disease leading to death. In addition, it has been estimated that approximately 90% of all cases of pancreatitis in human beings remain undiagnosed. It is likely that the number of undiagnosed cases in dogs and cats is at least as high as in human beings. Reasons for the difficulty of diagnosing exocrine pancreatic disease are the nonspecific clinical picture, the lack of specific changes on routine blood work, the low yield of diagnostic imaging in making a definitive diagnosis, and until recently, the lack of sensitive and specific markers for pancreatic function and pathology.

1.4.4.2 Pancreatitis

Serum amylase and lipase activities

Serum amylase and lipase activities have been used for several decades to diagnose pancreatitis in both human beings and dogs. Unfortunately, neither one of these diagnostic tests is both sensitive and specific for pancreatitis. After total pancreatectomy in dogs significant serum amylase and lipase activities remain, clearly indicating that there are other sources of serum amylase and lipase activity than the exocrine pancreas.[3] This lack of specificity is also reflected by clinical studies that showed a specificity of serum amylase and lipase activities for pancreatitis of only approximately 50%.[4] Many non-pancreatic diseases, such as renal, hepatic, intestinal, and neoplastic disease can lead to increases in serum amylase and lipase activities.[5] Steroid administration can also lead to an increase in serum lipase activity and a variable response in serum amylase activity.[6,7] Thus, in dogs, serum amylase and lipase activities are only of limited clinical usefulness for the diagnosis of pancreatitis and should only be used until a more definitive diagnostic test, such as abdominal ultrasound, serum canine pancreatic lipase immunoreactivity (cPLI) concentra-

tion, or even exploratory laparotomy can be performed. Serum amylase and/or lipase activities that are 3–5 times the upper limit of the reference range in patients with clinical signs consistent with pancreatitis, are suggestive of pancreatitis. However, it is important to note that approximately 50% of dogs with an elevated serum lipase and/or amylase activity do not have pancreatitis. In cats, serum amylase and lipase activities appear to be of no clinical value for the diagnosis of pancreatitis.[8] While cats with experimental pancreatitis showed an increase in serum lipase activity and a decrease in serum amylase activity, these changes were not seen in cats with spontaneous disease.[8,9]

Serum trypsin-like immunoreactivity (TLI)

TLI concentration is a specific marker for exocrine pancreatic function. Serum TLI mainly measures trypsinogen, the only form of trypsin that circulates in the vascular space in healthy individuals. In addition, if present in serum, the TLI assay also measures trypsin and a portion of trypsin bound to some proteinase inhibitors. In healthy animals, serum TLI concentration is low as most of the trypsinogen synthesized by pancreatic acinar cells is released into the pancreatic duct and does not reach the vascular space (Figure 1.45). During pancreatitis an increased amount of trypsinogen leaks into the vascular space, which leads to an increase in serum TLI concentration.[10] Trypsin, which is prematurely activated during pancreatitis, may also contribute to this increase in serum TLI concentration. However, both trypsinogen and trypsin are small molecules that are quickly cleared by the kidney. In addition, any prematurely activated trypsin is quickly removed by proteinase inhibitors, such as α_1-proteinase inhibitor (α_1-PI) and α_2-macroglobulin. In turn, α_2-macroglobulin-trypsin complexes are removed by the reticuloendothelial system, mainly in the spleen and the liver. Therefore, the serum half life for TLI is short and a significant degree of active inflammation is required in order to have an increased serum TLI concentration. Also, some patients with peracute severe disease may have normal serum TLI concentrations. One possible explanation for this phenomenon is that not enough trypsinogen remains in the acinar cells to leak into the vascular space. In dogs, serum canine TLI (cTLI) concentration is of limited clinical usefulness for the diagnosis of pancreatitis. While it is more specific than serum amylase and lipase activity, its sensitivity is lower and for most veterinarians the turnaround time for this test is longer than that for serum lipase and amylase activities, thus making the measurement of serum cTLI less desirable as a diagnostic test for pancreatitis.[4] The sensitivity and specificity of serum TLI concentration in dogs and cats is similar with a specificity of approximately 90% and a sensitivity of 30–40%. While these performance indices are less than ideal, until recently, serum feline TLI (fTLI) concentration was the most sensitive and specific diagnostic test for feline pancreatitis available.[10] Abdominal ultrasound is also highly specific for pancreatitis if stringent criteria are applied, but the sensitivity of abdominal ultrasound is only between 10% and 35% in cats, and was lower than the sensitivity for serum fTLI concentration in every study in which both diagnostic parameters were evaluated.[10,11]

Pancreatic lipase immunoreactivity (PLI)

Serum PLI specifically measures the mass concentration of classical pancreatic lipase in serum, rather than its kinetic activity. Assays for the measurement of PLI in dog and cat serum have recently been developed and validated.[12,13] Serum PLI concentration has been shown to be highly specific for exocrine pancreatic function in both species.[14] Serum cPLI concentration has also been shown to be far more sensitive for the diagnosis of pancreatitis than any other diagnostic tool available.[15] Sensitivity for serum PLI concentration has been reported at 82% in the dog and at 67% to 100% in the cat.[15,16] Currently, measurement of serum fPLI concentration is only available through the Gastrointestinal Laboratory at Texas A&M University. However, a commercial assay for the measurement of cPLI concentration (Spec cPL®; Idexx Laboratories) has recently been introduced and performs the same as the original cPLI ELISA. Also, in-clinic assay kits for measurement of cPLI and fPLI, respectively, should be available in the near future. The current control range for serum cPLI concentration as measured by the Spec cPL assay is ≥200 µg/L, with a diagnostic cut-off value for canine pancreatitis of 400 µg/L. The current control range for fPLI concentration as measured by radioimmunoassay (RIA) is 1.2 to 6.8 µg/L with a diagnostic cut-off value for feline pancreatitis of 12 µg/L. Serum PLI concentrations between 200 and 399 µg/L in dogs and 6.9 to 11.9 µg/L in cats are considered in the questionable range, requiring repeat analysis and/or further diagnostic tests. Chronic renal failure has been shown to have no clinically significant effect on serum cPLI concentration.[17] Therefore, the assay can be used to diagnose pancreatitis in dogs with renal failure, underscoring the high specificity of this new diagnostic test. While this has not been confirmed in cats, there is little reason to believe that this would be different in this species. Also, oral administration of long-term high-dose prednisone (2.2 mg/kg daily for 4 weeks) did not alter serum cPLI concentration.

Other tests for the diagnosis of pancreatitis in dogs and cats have been evaluated. However, plasma trypsinogen activation peptide (TAP) concentration, urine TAP concentration, urine TAP/creatinine ratio, serum α_1-PI/trypsin complex concentration, and serum α_2-macroglobulin concentration have all been shown to be of little clinical usefulness for the diagnosis of spontaneous pancreatitis in dogs or cats.[4]

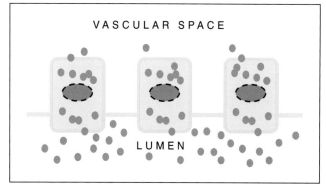

Figure 1.45:
Physiology of pancreatic enzyme secretion. Acinar cells secrete zymogens (e. g., trypsinogen) and pancreatic enzymes (e. g., pancreatic lipase) into the duct system of the exocrine pancreas, ultimately reaching the duodenum. However, a small amount of zymogens and enzymes is also secreted into the vascular space and can be measured by species-specific immunoassays.

1.4.4.3 Exocrine pancreatic insufficiency (EPI)

In the past, several fecal tests have been used to diagnose EPI. Microscopic fecal examination for fat and/or undigested starch or muscle fibers may suggest maldigestion, at best. In light of the wide-spread availability of tests with high accuracy for the diagnosis of EPI, microscopic fecal examination can no longer be clinically justified. Fecal proteolytic activity had been used for several decades to diagnose EPI in small animals. Several variations of the test have been described, the most simple involving digestion of the gelatin emulsion on a piece of radiographic film. Most of these methodologies, particularly the radiographic film clearance test, are completely unreliable.[18] One method, which utilizes pre-made tablets that can be used to pour a gelatin agar, has been found to be most useful.[18] However, false positive as well as false negative results have been reported and the clinical use of fecal proteolytic activity should be limited to species for which more specific assays to estimate pancreatic function are not available.

Serum trypsin-like immunoreactivity (TLI)

Serum TLI is the diagnostic test of choice for EPI in both dogs and cats.[19,20] Assays for TLI measure trypsinogen, the zymogen of trypsin, circulating in the vascular space. In healthy individuals only a small amount of trypsinogen is present in serum (Figure 1.45). In dogs and cats with EPI, serum TLI concentration decreases significantly and may even be undetectable (Figure 1.46). The reference range for serum canine TLI (cTLI) concentration is 5–35 µg/L with a cut-off value for EPI of ≤2.5 µg/L. Similarly, the reference range for serum

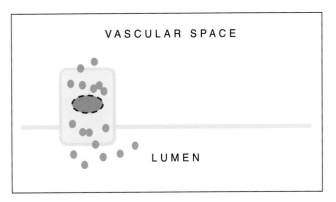

Figure 1.46:
Serum TLI in dogs and cats with EPI. Dogs and cats with EPI have a severely decreased functional mass of the exocrine pancreas. As a result, the secretion of digestive enzymes may be decreased to a point that maldigestion ensues and clinical signs of EPI become apparent. At the same time, leakage of trypsinogen into the vascular space is reduced and serum TLI concentration is decreased below the cut-off value for EPI.

feline TLI (fTLI) concentration is 12–82 µg/L with a cut-off value for EPI of ≤8.0 µg/L. Rarely, animals with a serum TLI concentration below the cut-off value are encountered that do not have clinical signs of EPI. This is probably due to the large functional reserve of the gastrointestinal tract. On the other hand, there are many dogs and cats with chronic diarrhea and weight loss that have a mild decrease in serum TLI concentration (2.6 to 4.9 µg/L in dogs, 8.1 to 11.9 µg/L in cats). Most of these animals have chronic small intestinal disease and should be worked-up accordingly. A small number of these dogs and cats may have EPI and if small intestinal disease can-

not be diagnosed, the serum TLI concentration should be reevaluated after a couple of months in these patients.

Serum pancreatic lipase immunoreactivity (PLI)

Similarly to serum TLI concentration, serum PLI concentration is highly specific for exocrine pancreatic function and could be used for the diagnosis of EPI.[14] However, there is a small degree of overlap for serum cPLI between normal dogs and dogs with EPI, making the measurement for PLI slightly inferior to TLI for a definitive diagnosis of EPI. The only exception to this is the rare patient with an isolated pancreatic lipase deficiency. Since pancreatic lipase is essential for fat digestion, clinical signs of maldigestion may ensue in these rare cases. The clinical utility of serum fPLI concentration for diagnosis of feline EPI has not been evaluated to date.

Fecal elastase

Recently, an assay for measurement of fecal elastase has been developed and validated. Fecal elastase concentration has a lower specificity than measurement of serum cTLI concentration.[21] Since the prevalence of EPI in dogs with chronic diarrhea and weight loss is only approximately 10%, the number of false positive test results for fecal elastase concentration is unacceptably high (23.1% in a recent study). Also, measurement of fecal elastase concentration is more cumbersome and more expensive than the measurement of serum cTLI concentration. The only scenario in which fecal elastase concentration may be clinically useful is a patient with EPI due to obstruction of the pancreatic duct. However, this condition has not been described in dogs or cats to date.

☞ Key Facts

- Serum amylase and lipase activity are not useful for the diagnosis of feline pancreatitis
- Serum amylase and lipase activities have limited clinical value for the diagnosis of canine pancreatitis and the diagnosis must be verified by other means.
- Serum PLI concentration is the most sensitive and specific diagnostic test for pancreatitis in both dogs and cats.
- Serum TLI concentration remains the test of choice for EPI in dogs and cats.

References

1. Hänichen T, Minkus G. Retrospektive Studie zur Pathologie der Erkrankungen des exokrinen Pankreas bei Hund und Katze. *Tierärztl Umschau* 1990; 45: 363–368.
2. Lowenfels AB. Epidemiology of diseases of the pancreas: clues to understanding and preventing pancreatic disease. In: Grendell JH, Forsmark CE (eds.), *Controversies and clinical challenges in pancreatic diseases*. Bethesda, American Gastroenterological Society, 1998; 9–13.
3. Simpson KW, Simpson JW, Lake S et al. Effect of pancreatectomy on plasma activities of amylase, isoamylase, lipase and trypsin-like immunoreactivity in dogs. *Res Vet Sci* 1991; 51: 78–82.
4. Mansfield CS, Jones BR. Trypsinogen activation peptide in the diagnosis of canine pancreatitis. *J Vet Intern Med* 2000; 14: 346 (abstract).
5. Strombeck DR, Farver T, Kaneko JJ. Serum amylase and lipase activities in the diagnosis of pancreatitis in dogs. *Am J Vet Res* 1981; 42: 1966–1970.
6. Parent J. Effects of dexamethasone on pancreatic tissue and on serum amylase and lipase activities in dogs. *J Am Vet Med Assoc* 1982 180: 743–746.
7. Fittschen C, Bellamy JE. Prednisone treatment alters the serum amylase and lipase activities in normal dogs without causing pancreatitis. *Can J Comp Med* 1984; 48: 136–140.
8. Parent C, Washabau RJ, Williams DA et al. Serum trypsin-like immunoreactivity, amylase and lipase in the diagnosis of feline acute pancreatitis. *J Vet Intern Med* 1995; 9: 194 (abstract).
9. Kitchell BE, Strombeck DR, Cullen J et al. Clinical and pathologic changes in experimentally induced acute pancreatitis in cats. *Am J Vet Res* 1986; 47: 1170–1173.
10. Gerhardt A, Steiner JM, Williams DA et al. Comparison of the sensitivity of different diagnostic tests for pancreatitis in cats. *J Vet Intern Med* 2001; 15: 329–333.
11. Swift NC, Marks SL, MacLachlan NJ et al. Evaluation of serum feline trypsin-like immunoreactivity for the diagnosis of pancreatitis in cats. *J Am Vet Med Assoc* 2000; 217: 37–42.
12. Steiner JM, Gumminger SR, Williams DA. Development and validation of an enzyme-linked immunosorbent assay (ELISA) for the measurement of canine pancreatic lipase immunoreactivity (cPLI) in serum. *J Vet Intern Med* 2001; 15: 311 (abstract).
13. Steiner JM, Wilson BG, Williams DA. Development and analytical validation of a radioimmunoassay for the measurement of feline pancreatic lipase immunoreactivity in serum. *Can J Vet Res* 2004; 68: 309–314.
14. Steiner JM, Rutz GM, Williams DA. Serum lipase activities and pancreatic lipase immunoreactivity concentrations in dogs with exocrine pancreatitic insufficiency. *Am J Vet Res* 2006; 67: 84–87.
15. Steiner JM, Broussard J, Mansfield CS et al. Serum canine pancreatic lipase immunoreactivity (cPLI) concentrations in dogs with spontaneous pancreatitis. *J Vet Intern Med* 2001; 15: 274 (abstract).
16. Forman MA, Marks SL, De Cock HEV et al. Evaluation of serum feline pancreatic lipase immunoreactivity and helical computed tomography versus conventional testing for the diagnosis of feline pancreatitis. *J Vet Intern Med* 2004; 18: 807–815.
17. Steiner JM, Finco DR, Gumminger SR et al. Serum canine pancreatic lipase immunoreactivity (cPLI) in dogs with experimentally induced chronic renal failure. *J Vet Intern Med* 2001; 15: 311 (abstract).
18. Williams DA, Reed SD. Comparison of methods for assay of fecal proteolytic activity. *Vet Clin Pathol* 1990; 19: 20–24.
19. Steiner JM, Williams DA. Serum feline trypsin-like immunoreactivity in cats with exocrine pancreatic insufficiency. *J Vet Intern Med* 2000; 14: 627–629.
20. Williams DA, Batt RM. Sensitivity and specificity of radioimmunoassay of serum trypsin-like immunoreactivity for the diagnosis of canine exocrine pancreatic insufficiency. *J Am Vet Med Assoc* 1988; 192: 195–201.
21. Spillmann T, Wittker A, Teigelkamp S et al. An immunoassay for canine pancreatic elastase 1 as an indicator for exocrine pancreatic insufficiency in dogs. *J Vet Diag Invest* 2001; 13: 468–474.

1.4.5 Molecular-genetics-based laboratory tests

Roger M. Batt, H. Carolien Rutgers

1.4.5.1 Introduction

Molecular-genetics-based tests have already been developed for some diseases in small animals, providing an early flavor of these powerful tools that add a new dimension to diagnosis in veterinary medicine. These tests are based on the detection of inherited mutations in DNA that typically have an adverse effect on structure, function, or quantity of specific proteins, resulting in disease or susceptibility to disease. These new tests are powerful tools because they facilitate accurate diagnosis of clinical disease, allow for selective breeding, and can also identify susceptible animals so that onset of disease can be delayed or prevented by prophylactic intervention.

Selective breeding for appearance has reduced the genetic diversity within breeds of pedigree dogs, and in some breeds it has unintentionally increased the likelihood of inheriting gene mutations that cause disease or disease susceptibility. Over 400 inherited disorders have already been identified in dogs, and it seems certain that many more will be characterized.[1,2] Sequencing and mapping the entire canine genome is well advanced, providing the tools to identify genomic markers for inherited diseases in dogs.[3,4] The situation in the cat is different as the majority of cats are domestic shorthair cats. As a consequence, there has been little selective breeding and there are few known inherited disorders in cats.[5]

There is considerable potential for the application of molecular-genetics-based tests for gastrointestinal disorders in dogs, underlined by emerging knowledge of inheritance and pathogenesis of the many breed-associated conditions already described (Table 1.11). Currently, the mode of inheritance has been identified in a few, and the genetic abnormality in only one instance.[6] The barriers to progress include the complex nature of many gastrointestinal disorders, for some of which there may be environmental factors operating with genetic drivers of disease.

1.4.5.2 Test Development

Molecular-genetics-based tests are typically dependent on the identification of DNA markers or mutations within or close to key genes that drive specific traits or diseases. These tests are performed on genomic DNA extracted from cheek swabs or whole blood. Identification of mutations in the gene or genes involved could be considered to provide the ultimate reliable test. This can be achieved by a candidate gene approach, based on genes that have been identified in similar conditions in other species or by knowledge of the pathophysiology of the disease. Alternatively, DNA markers within or in close proximity may be used to detect abnormal genes. Informative microsatellite markers may be identified by linkage analysis, which relates a specific allele of a particular microsatellite marker with disease. This approach is used when candidate genes are either unknown or uncertain. Alternatively, informative SNPs (single nucleotide polymorphisms) can be identified by association studies.

There are many practical considerations in the development of molecular-genetics-based tests for gastrointestinal diseases in dogs. The most important is accurate characterization and identification of the target phenotype that should be distinct (for example, EPI or hepatic copper toxicosis). A distinct phenotype facilitates accumulation of data from extended families to determine inheritance and for linkage analysis. Clearly, development of genetic tests is much more difficult for conditions that are less distinct or that are multifactorial, such as IBD. However, provided there is an inherited component, other types of molecular-genetic studies can be done in large numbers of unrelated dogs; for example, using disequilibrium linkage analysis of microsatellite data, SNPs, or sequencing of candidate gene(s). Results from these studies may in fact help to redefine the phenotype.

Complexity of inheritance is also important. Tests for single gene disorders are easiest to develop and most likely to be used not only to identify but also to eliminate a condition by selective breeding. Complex genetic diseases are at the other end of the spectrum, where multiple genes drive disease susceptibility and disease expression may depend on an environmental component, such as an allergen or pathogen. Selective breeding with the goal of elimination is not a practical option for complex genetic diseases, but genetic tests may direct treatment and preventative strategies.

Table 1.11: Putative and/or proven inherited gastrointestinal diseases of dogs

Disease	Breeds	Inheritance
Intestinal		
■ Basenji enteropathy	Basenji	Not known
■ Gluten-sensitive enteropathy	Irish Setter	Autosomal recessive
■ Histiocytic ulcerative colitis	Boxer dogs	Not known
■ Idiopathic small intestinal bacterial overgrowth	Beagle German Shepherd	Not known
■ Lymphangiectasia	Norwegian Lundehund	Not known
■ Protein-losing enteropathy	Soft-coated Wheaten Terrier	Not known
■ Selective cobalamin malabsorption	Beagle Border Collie Giant Schnauzer Shar Pei	Autosomal recessive
Pancreatic		
■ Exocrine pancreatic insufficiency	German Shepherd	Autosomal recessive
Hepatic		
■ Copper hepatotoxicosis	Bedlington Terrier	Autosomal recessive
	Dalmatian	Not known
	Labrador Retriever	Not known
	Skye Terrier	Not Known
	West Highland White Terrier	Not Known
■ Portovascular anomalies:		
– Intrahepatic shunt	Irish Wolfhound	Autosomal recessive (single gene)
– Extrahepatic shunt	Cairn Terrier	Autosomal recessive
	Yorkshire Terrier	Not known
■ Microvascular dysplasia	Terrier breeds	Not known

1.4.5.3 Diseases of the esophagus and stomach

Little is known about the genetics of these diseases in dogs. Breed predispositions for gastric dilation/volvulus are most likely related to anatomical features (large, deep-chested dogs). Antral gastric hypertrophy has been described as a congenital disorder in small brachycephalic dogs, but there is not enough information to describe this condition as an inherited trait.

1.4.5.4 Intestinal diseases

Selective cobalamin malabsorption

Selective intestinal malabsorption of cobalamin (vitamin B12) accompanied by proteinuria is inherited as a simple autosomal recessive trait in Giant Schnauzers, and has also been described in Beagles, Border Collies, and Shar Peis.[7,8,9] Affected puppies show chronic inappetence and failure to thrive, and have low serum cobalamin concentrations, megaloblastic anemia, and methylmalonic aciduria. Clinical signs can be reversed with parenteral, but not oral, cobalamin supplementation. These patients have a defective expression of the intrinsic factor-cobalamin receptor (IFCR) in the ileal brush border membrane, which has been attributed to mutations affecting either of the two proteins (cubilin, amnionless) that mediate endocytosis of the IF-cobalamin complex.[10]

Gluten-sensitive enteropathy (GSE)

GSE is a well-characterized small intestinal disease in Irish Setters, and potentially other breeds of dogs, which can cause weight loss with or without diarrhea.[11,12] GSE has several similarities with human celiac disease, which involves immune-mediated damage of the small intestine, but differs because it does not correlate with MHC II haplotypes.[11] GSE in Irish Setters has been shown to be inherited at a single autosomal recessive locus, but currently there is no DNA test available.[12]

Lymphangiectasia

This disease has an increased prevalence in Yorkshire Terriers, Soft-coated Wheaten Terriers, and Norwegian Lundehunds, but can also occur in many other breeds. Familial occurrence has been demonstrated in the Norwegian Lundehund,[13] but the mode of inheritance is unknown.

Protein-losing enteropathy (PLE)

PLE can occur in many breeds and in many disease processes, but a distinctive familial predisposition for both PLE and/or PLN has been recognized in Soft-coated Wheaten Terriers.[14]

Pedigree analysis suggests a common male ancestor, but the mode of inheritance is as yet unknown.

Basenji enteropathy

Basenji enteropathy is a severe form of IBD in Basenji dogs, which closely resembles the non-secretory form of human immunoproliferative small intestinal disease.[15] Asymptomatic Basenji dogs can have abnormal intestinal function and gastrointestinal lesions on biopsy. This disease is likely to have a hereditary basis, although the mode of inheritance is unclear.

Small intestinal bacterial overgrowth (SIBO)

SIBO is characterized by relatively high numbers of bacteria in the lumen of the upper small intestine. It is frequently associated with a change from an aerobic to a predominantly anaerobic flora.[16] SIBO has recently been named "antibiotic-responsive diarrhea" by some authors.[17] SIBO may occur as an idiopathic abnormality, secondary to other gastrointestinal diseases, or as a subclinical finding in apparently healthy Beagle and German Shepherd dogs.[16] While German Shepherds appear to have a predisposition to SIBO, its inheritance has not been established. Development of molecular marker(s) for predisposition may be facilitated by identification of a key driver of disease, such as defective intestinal protection due to deficiency or dysregulation of secretory IgA.[18]

Histiocytic ulcerative colitis

This disease is a form of inflammatory large bowel disease that occurs predominantly in Boxer dogs, although it also has been reported in a few Bulldogs and other breeds. Inheritance has not been established, but a genetic predisposition is suggested by its strong breed predisposition. Pathologically, it is characterized by colonic mucosal ulceration and a mixed inflammatory infiltrate typically including PAS-positive macrophages. The immunohistochemical changes are similar to those reported in human ulcerative colitis. Recent studies suggest that an infectious agent responsive to antibiotics plays an integral role in the clinical manifestation of this disease.[19]

Inflammatory bowel disease (IBD)

There are many potential causes of this disease phenotype, which is likely to involve a complex interaction of genetic predisposition and environmental factors, such as intestinal microflora and dietary antigens. The genetic background in dogs is obscure but there is emerging evidence of susceptibility due to gene mutations in human beings.[20]

1

1.4.5.5 Pancreatic disease

Pancreatic acinar atrophy (PAA)

PAA is the most common cause of EPI in the dog, and is mainly seen in German Shepherd dogs and Rough-coated Collies. Recent studies suggest that PAA may occur as the end stage of lymphocytic pancreatitis.[21] PAA has been shown to be a hereditary disease in German Shepherd dogs, most likely due to an autosomal recessive gene.[22]

Pancreatitis

Hereditary pancreatitis has been described in human beings and several mutations have been associated with an increased risk for pancreatitis. Chronic pancreatitis is also commonly seen in the Miniature Schnauzer, which may be due to the increased incidence of fasting lipidemia and hypertriglyceridemia in this breed. However, screening for mutations of the anionic and cationic trypsinogen genes has not revealed any associations.

1.4.5.6 Liver disease

Hepatic copper toxicosis

Hepatic copper toxicosis can result either from a primary defect in hepatic copper metabolism or from an altered biliary excretion of copper. An inherited copper storage hepatopathy has been documented in Bedlington Terriers, and there is evidence for familial copper storage liver disease in West Highland White Terriers, Skye Terriers, Dalmatians, Labrador Retrievers, and possibly Doberman Pinschers. Secondary copper accumulation, due to long-standing cholestatic liver disease (copper-associated hepatopathy), may occur in many dog breeds but does not lead to levels high enough to be hepatotoxic. Copper accumulation has been reported in a large number of breeds with cholestatic liver disease in which it is a secondary event. Copper hepatotoxicosis in the Bedlington Terrier is the best-described example of a primary abnormality in hepatic copper metabolism. Accumulation of toxic levels of copper in the liver results in hepatocellular necrosis, hepatitis, and ultimately cirrhosis. This disease has been shown to be autosomal recessive, and has a high prevalence in the breed. Diagnosis used to be by histological assessment and measurement of copper content in liver biopsies. More recently, a microsatellite marker, CO4107, closely linked with the copper toxicosis gene has been used to screen Bedlington Terriers, but this test has been controversial.[23] Recently, the copper toxicosis locus has been mapped to canine chromosome 10 at locus CFA 10q28, and the disease has been sugges-

ted to be due to a deletion in the MURR1 gene, paving the way for the development of an accurate DNA test.[6] The microsatellite C04107 lying in an intron of the MURR1 gene is highly associated with the disease but shows haplotype diversity.[24] The only solid molecular test for the disease is thought to be by showing the deletion in exon-2 in cDNA in liver tissue; this test is not robust on RNA from peripheral leukocytes because of their low MURR1 expression level. A quantitative PCR (Q-PCR) test on genomic DNA was shown to correlate well with the microsatellite marker and with RT-PCR data from blood samples, buccal swabs, and liver biopsies.[25]

A familial copper-associated liver disease that has recently been described in Dalmatians also may involve a primary metabolic defect in copper metabolism, but the mechanism and genetic basis for the disease have not been assessed. There is, furthermore, evidence for different forms of familial copper-associated liver disease in West Highland White and Skye Terriers, but in these dogs inflammatory changes precede copper accumulation, suggesting a different pathogenesis than in Bedlington Terriers and Dalmatians.

Portovascular anomalies

Congenital portosystemic shunts are characterized by a single anomalous connection between the portal vein and the systemic circulation, bypassing the hepatic sinusoids. Single intrahepatic shunts are found primarily in large breed dogs, and they are thought to be inherited as a single gene autosomal recessive trait.[26] Irish Wolfhounds also may have inherited transient hyperammonemia due to a defect in the urea cycle enzyme arginine succinate synthetase, which should not be mistaken for portovascular anomalies.[27,28] Single extrahepatic shunts occur primarily in small dog breeds, especially those having a Terrier heritage. In Cairn Terriers, test matings have shown extrahepatic shunts to be inherited as an autosomal recessive trait, which is most likely polygenic or monogenic with variable expression.[29] Portosystemic shunts are also thought to be inherited in Yorkshire Terriers.[30]

Hepatic microvascular dysplasia (MVD)

MVD is a congenital and probably inherited disorder of the microscopic architecture of the liver, which occurs mostly in small breed dogs, especially Terrier breeds (e.g., Yorkshire, Cairn, and Maltese Terriers). The genetic relationship between MVD and portovascular anomalies is uncertain but considered possible because of their association in certain breeds, similar histological features, and evidence that they may occur together.

🔑 Key Facts

- A breed predilection is commonly observed for gastrointestinal disorders in dogs, but less commonly in cats, suggesting a hereditary nature or effect in the pathogenesis of these diseases.
- To date the only molecular-based diagnostic test available for the diagnosis of inherited gastrointestinal disorders in dogs or cats is for copper hepatotoxicosis in the Bedlington Terrier.
- Major advances are to be expected in this field and new diagnostic tests for hereditary gastrointestinal diseases should be available in the near future.

References

1. Aguirre, GD. DNA testing for inherited canine diseases. In: Bonagura, JD (ed.), *Current Veterinary Therapy XIII.* Philadelphia, WB Saunders, 2000; 909–913.
2. Meyers-Wallen VN. Ethics and genetic selection in purebred dogs. *Reprod Domest Anim* 2003; 38: 73–76.
3. Guyon R, Lorenten TD, Hutte C et al. A 1-MB resolution radiation hybrid map of the canine genome. *Proc Natl Acad Sci USA* 2003; 100: 5296–5301.
4. Dukes-McEwan J, Jackson IJ. The problems and promise of linkage analysis by using the current canine genome map. *Mamm Genome* 2002; 13: 667–672.
5. Malik R. Genetic diseases in the cat. *J Feline Med Surg* 2001; 3: 109–113.
6. Klomp AE, van de Sluis B, Klomp LW et al. The ubiquitously expressed MURR1 protein is absent in canine copper toxicosis. *J Hepatol* 2003; 39: 703–709.
7. Fyfe JC, Ramanujam KS, Ramaswamy K et al. Defective brush-border expression of intrinsic factor-cobalamin receptor in canine inherited intestinal cobalamin malabsorption. *J Biol Chem* 1991; 266: 4489–4494.
8. Fordyce HH, Callan MB, Giger U. Persistent cobalamin deficiency causing failure to thrive in a juvenile beagle. *J Small Anim Pract* 2000; 41: 407–410.
9. Morgan LW, McConnell J. Cobalamin deficiency associated with erythroblastic anemia and methylmalonic aciduria in a Border Collie. *J Am Anim Hosp Assoc* 1999; 35: 392–395.
10. Fyfe JC, Madsen M, Hojrup P et al. The functional cobalamin (vitamin B12)-intrinsic factor receptor is a novel complex of cubilin and amnionless. *Blood* 2004; 103: 1573–9.
11. Polvi A, Garden OA, Houlston RS et al. Genetic susceptibility to gluten sensitive enteropathy in Irish setter dogs is not linked to the major histocompatibility complex. *Tissue Antigens* 1998; 52: 543–549.
12. Garden OA, Pidduck H, Lakhani KH et al. Inheritance of gluten-sensitive enteropathy in Irish Setters. *Am J Vet Res* 2000; 61: 462–468.
13. Flesja K, Yri T. Protein-losing enteropathy in the Lundehund. *J Small Anim Pract* 1977; 18: 11–23.
14. Littman MP, Dambach DM, Vaden SL et al. Familial protein-losing enteropathy and protein-losing nephropathy in Soft-Coated Wheaten Terriers. *J Vet Intern Med* 2000; 14: 68–80.
15. De Buysscher EV, Breitschwerdt EB, MacLachlan NJ. Elevated serum IgA associated with immunoproliferative enteropathy of Basenji dogs: lack of evidence for alpha heavy-chain disease or enhanced intestinal IgA secretion. *Vet Immunol Immunopathol* 1988; 20: 41–52.
16. Rutgers HC, Batt RM, Elwood CM et al. Small intestinal bacterial overgrowth in dogs with chronic intestinal disease. *J Am Vet Med Assoc* 1995; 206: 187–192.
17. German AJ, Day MJ, Ruaux CG et al. Comparison of direct and indirect tests for small intestinal bacterial overgrowth and antibiotic-responsive diarrhea in dogs. *J Vet Intern Med* 2003; 17: 33–43.
18. German AJ, Hall EJ, Day MJ. Relative deficiency of IgA production by duodenal explants from German Shepherd dogs with small intestinal disease. *Vet Immunol Immunopathol* 2000; 76: 25–43.
19. Hostutler RA, Luria BJ, Johnson SE et al. Antibiotic-responsive histiocytic ulcerative colitis in 9 dogs. *J Vet Intern Med* 2004; 18: 499–504.
20. Mathew CG, Lewis CM. Genetics of inflammatory bowel disease: genetics and prospects. *Hum Mol Genet* 2004; 13: R161–R168.
21. Wiberg ME, Saari SA, Westermarck E. Exocrine pancreatic atrophy in German Shepherd Dogs and Rough-coated Collies: an end result of lymphocytic pancreatitis. *Vet Pathol* 1999; 36: 530–541.
22. Moeller ME, Steiner JM, Clark LA et al. Inheritance of pancreatic acinar atrophy in German Shepherd Dogs. *Am J Vet Res* 2002; 63: 1429–1434.
23. Haywood S, Fuentealba IC, Kemp SJ et al. Copper toxicosis in the Bedlington terrier: A diagnostic dilemma. *J Small Anim Pract* 2001; 42: 181–185.
24. van de Sluis B, Peter AT, Wijmenga C. Indirect molecular diagnosis of copper toxicosis in Bedlington Terriers is complicated by haplotype diversity. *J Hered* 2003; 94: 256–259.
25. Favier RP, Spee B, Penning LC et al. Quantitative PCR method to detect a 13-kb deletion in the MURR1 gene associated with copper toxicosis and HIV-1 replication. *Mamm Genome* 2005; 16: 460–463.
26. Ubbink GJ, van de Broek J, Meyer HP et al. Prediction of inherited portosystemic shunts in Irish Wolfhounds on the basis of pedigree analysis. *Am J Vet Res* 1998; 59: 1553–1556.
27. Meyer HP, Rothuizen J, Tiemessen I et al. Transient metabolic hyperammonaemia in young Irish wolfhounds. *Vet Rec* 1996; 138: 105–107.
28. Rothuizen J, Ubbink GJ, Meyer HP et al. Inherited liver diseases: New findings in portosystemic shunts, hyperammonemia syndromes, and copper toxicosis in Bedlington Terriers. *Proc 19th ACVIM Forum* 2001; 637–639.
29. van Straten G, Leegwater PA, de Vries M et al. Inherited congenital extrahepatic portosystemic shunts in Cairn terriers. *J Vet Intern Med* 2005; 19: 321–324.
30. Tobias KM. Determination of inheritance of single congenital portosystemic shunts in Yorkshire terriers. *J Am Anim Hosp Assoc* 2003; 39: 385–389.

1

1.5 Endoscopy

Michael D. Willard

1.5.1 Introduction

Endoscopy is the use of an instrument (i.e., the endoscope) to look into a cavity or orifice. Its main value to veterinary gastroenterology consists of allowing the collection of tissue samples without surgery, although observation of morphological changes of the mucosal surface or removal of foreign bodies is also useful. Gastroduodenoscopy is the most important flexible endoscopy technique, although colonoileoscopy can also be important.

1.5.2 Indications

Esophagogastroduodenoscopy is primarily indicated a) to biopsy the gastrointestinal mucosa in patients with clinical signs of gastrointestinal disease, such as vomiting, diarrhea, weight loss, anorexia, or hypoalbuminemia; b) to detect and remove foreign bodies; c) to detect a gastric outflow obstruction and determine the cause of such an outflow obstruction; d) to look for sites of upper GI bleeding; e) to inspect and/or biopsy the esophagus in patients suspected of having esophagitis or anatomic lesions of the esophagus; f) to dilate benign esophageal strictures; g) to help place gastrostomy tubes; and h) to remove polyps.[1–3] Colonoileoscopy is primarily indicated a) to biopsy the ileum in patients with small bowel disease; b) to biopsy the colon in patients with chronic colonic disease that is either non-responsive to therapeutic trials or that is characterized by concurrent hypoalbuminemia, weight loss, or systemic signs of illness; c) to determine the cause of persistent hematochezia or dyschezia; and d) to examine patients with known/suspected polyps or masses of the large bowel.[4] However, colonoscopy is done less frequently than gastroduodenoscopy as large bowel disease can often be effectively diagnosed and treated using less-invasive modalities.

Imaging is typically performed shortly before gastroduodenoscopy or colonoileoscopy. Radiographic imaging and especially abdominal ultrasonography may reveal evidence of infiltrative disease that is out of reach of the endoscope (e.g., mid-jejunum), free air or fluid (suggestive of a perforation), or widespread infiltrative disease (e.g., metastatic disease) that can be diagnosed by less invasive means (e.g., ultrasound-guided fine needle aspiration). Abdominal ultrasound is relatively specific but not as sensitive for diagnosing infiltrative disease. Thus, it can be appropriate to endoscopically biopsy the GI tract even if there is no ultrasonographic evidence of infiltrative disease, which is the case in many patients with IBD or intestinal lymphoma. Ultrasonography before colonoscopy is indicated if there is evidence for diffuse disease or systemic complications or if a tumor is suspected based upon rectal examination.

1.5.3 Basic principles of endoscopy

1.5.3.1 Choice of endoscopes

Entering and biopsying the duodenum is often the most important but also most difficult part of gastroduodenoscopy. An endoscope with a smaller outer diameter makes it easier to enter the duodenum. However, endoscopes with a smaller diameter also have a smaller biopsy channel (e.g., 2.0 to 2.2 mm). Larger diameter biopsy channels (i.e., 2.8 mm) facilitate obtaining good quality tissue samples as well as the removal of foreign bodies. For cats and most dogs, a one meter long insertion tube will allow visualization and biopsy of the duodenum and ileum, but some large dogs and those with long body conformations may require a 1.4 to 1.6 meter insertion tube. Unfortunately, the extra 0.4 to 0.6 meter in length can be very awkward when scoping cats and medium to small-sized dogs. Video endoscopes generally provide superior visualization compared to fiberoptic scopes, plus they allow two people to work together when removing some difficult to remove foreign bodies. However, fiberoptic scopes are less expensive and allow a competent endoscopist to accomplish almost everything that can be done with a video endoscope.

Having a selection of endoscopes is optimal (e.g., a pediatric gastroduodenoscope with a 7.9-mm outer diameter and a 1-meter-long insertion tube and a 2.2-mm biopsy channel; a standard gastroduodenoscope with a ≤9.0-mm outer diameter and a 1-meter-long insertion tube and a 2.8-mm biopsy channel; and a pediatric colonoscope with an outer diameter of 11 mm, a 1.4-meter-long insertion tube and a 2.8- to 3.0-mm biopsy channel). If only one scope is to be purchased, the dimensions should depend on the size of animals that most commonly undergo endoscopy (i.e., cats versus dogs) and the number of endoscopies anticipated to be performed on a weekly basis. If only 2–3 gastroduodenoscopies will be done per month, it is probably best to obtain a smaller diameter scope (e.g., 7.9-mm outer diameter) because it is doubtful that the endoscopist will achieve a high level of skill in passing the endoscope into the duodenum of cats and small dogs. If at least two endoscopies will be done weekly, then one is likely to become proficient enough to be able to maneuver slightly larger endoscopes (i.e., 8.6- to 9.0-mm outer diameter) with larger biopsy channels (i.e., 2.8 mm) into the duodenum of most adult cats.

1.5.4 Esophagogastroduodenoscopy

1.5.4.1 Preparation and anesthesia

Patients with GI disease and especially those that are vomiting sometimes have delayed gastric emptying. Therefore, food should be withheld for at least 24 hours prior to the procedure. One should not administer barium or sucralfate for at least 1 and preferably 2 days before the procedure. Various preanesthetic-anesthetic regimens may be used; glycopyrrolate plus either butorphanol or acetylpromazine is effective. However, narcotics (e.g., morphine, oxymorphone, or fentanyl) and prokinetic agents (e.g., metoclopramide) should be avoided.[5,6] Ketamine may relax the feline pylorus and may thus facilitate entry into the duodenum, although it also relaxes the lower esophageal sphincter, often making it necessary for someone to occlude the esophagus so that the stomach can be kept inflated during the procedure. Induction with propofol and maintenance with isoflurane is effective. Sevoflurane is also useful, especially in very ill animals, but it is important to assist respiration when using sevoflurane because the diminished tidal volume due to insufflation of the stomach with air may cause the patient to wake up in the middle of the procedure. The patient is placed in left lateral recumbency with the head slightly extended. A reliable mouth gag is always used, as a single bite on the endoscope may cause severe damage that requires expensive repairs.

1.5.4.2 Technique

The hollow viscus to be evaluated should be insufflated with enough air so that all of the mucosal surface can be inspected. Excessive insufflation of the stomach, which causes symptomatic gastric dilation, should be avoided. Also, panoramic views are often more effective than getting too close. This is especially true when a "red out" (i.e., the endoscope is too close to the mucosa and everything is out of focus) is experienced. The endoscope should only be advanced when the lumen can be visualized. Finally, while advancing the endoscope, it is often best to try to keep the tip of the scope aimed at the center of the lumen.

1.5.4.3 Gastroduodenoscopy[2,7]

The insertion tube is lightly lubricated and gently inserted into the mouth, much like an orogastric tube. As the larynx is approached and one can see the endotracheal tube entering the trachea, the tip of the endoscope is directed slightly dorsally and gently advanced towards the cricopharyngeal sphincter. Immediately upon entering the cricopharyngeal sphincter, the operator should begin to insufflate so that there is moderate distension of the esophagus allowing one to inspect the mucosa while advancing the endoscope towards the lower esophageal sphincter (LES) and the stomach. The LES usually appears as a "slit" although it sometimes is wide open. If the LES is closed, the operator should aim for the center of the sphincter and advance the endoscope gently rather than pushing hard and trying to force the tip into the stomach. The next step is determined by the size of the patient and the area(s) of interest. In small or medium-sized animals, one should first distend and examine the stomach (i.e., "typical gastroduodenoscopy"). In large or very long dogs in which examination and biopsy of the duodenum is important, it is often better to enter and examine the duodenum before examining the stomach (i.e., "modified gastroduodenoscopy" – see below).

Typical gastroduodenoscopy

It is critical to systematically examine all mucosal surfaces of the stomach because gastric lesions can be localized. After entering the stomach, the stomach is distended with air until the entire gastric mucosal surface can be examined. If the stomach cannot be distended because air escapes through an open LES, then an assistant should gently apply pressure on both sides of the cervical trachea in order to occlude the cervical esophagus and trap air in the upper GI tract. However, insufflation must be limited in order to avoid excessive gastric distension. Even moderate overdistension impedes ventilation with both oxygen and inhalant anesthetics, and it may even become necessary to deflate the stomach so that the patient can be maintained under anesthesia.

After the stomach is distended, a four-quadrant scan of the stomach should be performed. Starting with the tip of the scope near the LES, the tip is moved in a square pattern going from 10 o'clock to 2 o'clock to 5 o'clock to 7 o'clock. Second, the tip of the scope is advanced and then maximally retroflexed so that the LES and fundus can be examined (i.e., one can see the insertion tube of the endoscope entering the stomach through the LES). Insufficient examination of the fundic area is a common mistake of inexperienced operators, but this is the area where many foreign bodies as well as some infiltrative lesions can be found. After complete inspection of the gastric fundus, the tip of the endoscope is straightened and is advanced into the antrum by pushing the insertion tube into the patient. In this way, the tip of the scope will slide along the greater curvature, advancing into the antrum and towards the pylorus. The endoscopist may need to deflect the tip of the endoscope just a little bit upwards in order for it to enter the antrum without catching on a mucosal fold. Upon entering the antrum, one can see the pylorus at the back and to the left. The entire antral mucosa should be examined while advancing the tip of the endoscope towards the pylorus.

1

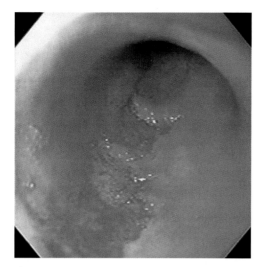

Figure 1.47:
Abrasions of the duodenal mucosa. Endoscopic view of duodenal mucosa with a linear abrasion caused by the endoscope. Such iatrogenic lesions must be distinguished from spontaneous ones.

To enter the duodenum, the pylorus should be kept in the middle of the viewing field while advancing the tip. It should be noted that the tip of the endoscope is larger than the field seen by the endoscopist because the viewing port at the tip of the endoscope generally comprises <20% of the scope diameter. Therefore, while the pylorus may appear as a "large hole" with plenty of room to admit the endoscope, it may really be smaller than the diameter of the scope. The endoscopist may advance the tip of the scope against the pylorus with modest pressure, as long as the pylorus can be seen in the middle of the viewing field. As the scope is advanced, the field of view often becomes blurred due to the scope being so close to the mucosa. Insufflating air while pushing against the pylorus can help the endoscopist see the opening. If the pylorus can not be kept in the center of the field of vision, even by rotating the endoscope, it sometimes helps to pass a biopsy forceps 5–10 mm into the pylorus and use it as a guide wire. This approach can cause erosions and hemorrhage, but is sometimes useful. With practice, the endoscopist should be able to routinely enter the duodenum with a 9.0 mm scope in cats and also dogs weighing more than 3 kg.

The mucosa just inside the pylorus can be difficult to examine, especially when disease causing mucosal swelling, such as an ulcer, is present. After entering the pylorus, the duodenum immediately turns to the right (from the perspective of the image on the screen). To find the duodenal lumen, it sometimes helps to back up the tip of the scope a millimeter or two while insufflating with air. Once the duodenal lumen is located, the operator should advance the scope as far as possible into the duodenum, keeping the lumen in the center of the field of vision. Due to the friable nature of the duodenum, it is especially important to visualize the entire circumference of the duodenal mucosa as the scope is being advanced. One should always remember that it is easy to create artifacts (i.e., linear erosions) by pushing the tip of the endoscope against the duodenal mucosa (Figure 1.47).

Modified gastroduodenoscopy procedure for very large and long-bodied dogs

As the stomach is distended with air, the distance the tip of the endoscope must travel as it slides along the greater curvature towards the pylorus becomes greater. In small or medium-sized dogs this is not a problem. However, in larger dogs (e.g., >30 kg) or in very long-bodied dogs (e.g., Greyhounds), insufflation may result in the insertion tube being too short to enter the duodenum. If this is a concern, one should start by insufflating as little air as possible into the esophagus. Once in the stomach, one should slightly deflect the tip of the endoscope up about 30 degrees and gently advance it (blindly at times) attempting to slide it into the antrum. This can be done in almost all cases, although a small amount of air must sometimes be insufflated so that one can see the direction to the antrum (i.e., rugal folds point towards the antrum). If this approach is taken, the stomach cannot be examined until after the duodenum has been examined and biopsied.

Patients in which it is difficult to enter the antrum

Occasionally it becomes impossible to direct the tip of the endoscope into the antrum. This can be caused by the configuration of the stomach or because of abdominal viscera (e.g., an enlarged spleen) pushing into the stomach and diverting the tip of the scope as it travels along the greater curvature of the stomach. This usually occurs when scoping larger dogs. Repositioning the dog into dorsal recumbency while the scope is still in the stomach will usually allow the endoscopist to direct the tip of the endoscope into the antrum. Then, with the tip of the endoscope in the antrum, the dog is repositioned into left lateral recumbency so that the pylorus can be entered.

Sometimes it is necessary to view the gastric mucosa during abdominal exploratory surgery to pinpoint lesions that cannot be identified from the serosal surface during laparotomy. For intraoperative endoscopy the patient is typically in dorsal recumbency, which sometimes makes it more difficult to enter the antrum and duodenum. However, the surgeon can help to direct the endoscope in such cases.

1.5.5 Colonoileoscopy

1.5.5.1 Preparation and anesthesia

Food should be withheld for at least 24 and preferably 36 hours before the procedure. The colon must be cleaned thoroughly, which can be achieved by use of gastrointestinal lavage solutions (e.g., Colyte®, Schwarz Pharma, Milwaukee, WI) and/or enemas.[8] Enemas are easier and less expensive, but it is crucial to perform several enemas before the procedure. Properly performed enemas consist of administering copious amounts of warm water (no soap) with the enema tube inserted as far into the colon as possible. At least one liter of warm water is administered per enema to dogs weighing more than 10 kg. For large breeds (e.g., >30 kg) 2 liters per enema can be used. Water often starts exiting the anus before the enema is finished, but the full amount should be administered. Three to four such enemas should be given the night before the procedure and 1–2 more the next morning, at least 2–3 hours before the procedure. Administering bisacodyl (5 mg) the night before the procedure also can be useful. The colon in cats is particularly hard to clean with enemas. Also, one must avoid over distension of the colon with the enema, which could result in vomiting. Cats usually receive 50–60 ml of warm water via a soft latex catheter and a syringe.

Lavage solutions are more effective for cleaning the colon than enemas alone.[4,9] These solutions are especially useful in large patients (i.e., >30 kg) or in patients with rectal pain. A volume of 25–30 ml/kg of the lavage solution is administered twice, at least 2 hours apart, the night before the procedure. Another dose of the solution is usually administered again the morning of the procedure. An enema will then be administered to wash out the lavage solution. Very rarely, gastric dilation and volvulus occurs after administering such large volumes of lavage solution.

Almost any anesthetic regime may be used for colonoscopy. Severely ill patients may only need sedation or manual restraint, unless ileoscopy is also planned. Ileal biopsies typically require anesthesia, and one should avoid drugs like oxymorphone and fentanyl.

1.5.5.2 Technique[4]

Flexible colonoscopy is simple to perform compared to gastroduodenoscopy, and rigid colonoscopy is very easy. A digital rectal examination should always be performed immediately before either endoscopy to detect potential problems (e.g., perineal hernia or a mass) and help straighten out the rectal canal so as to make entry into the colon easier. For rigid colonoscopy, the patient is positioned in right lateral recumbency so that any fluid present in the colon will pool in the ascending and transverse colon.[8] The tip of the colonoscope is inserted about 3 cm into the rectum with the obturator in place. Then, the obturator is removed, the glass window closed, and air is insufflated into the colon. As the colonic lumen opens up, the operator can follow the lumen orad until the entire length of the scope is inserted or the descending colon turns and becomes the transverse colon. Rigid colonic biopsy forceps provide tissue samples that are far superior to those that can be obtained by use of flexible biopsy forceps. However, rigid colonoscopy is limited to the descending colon. Fortunately, most, but not all, diffuse colonic lesions involve the descending colon.

If the entire colon is to be examined, flexible colonoscopy is required. The patient is positioned in left lateral recumbency, which prevents other abdominal organs from pushing down on the ileocolic valve area. The endoscope is advanced along the lumen until the ileocolic valve is seen. If the colon will not distend because air is escaping from the rectum, an assistant can hold the rectum tightly against the endoscope, thus trapping the air.

The ileocolic valve region is often not as a clean as the rest of the colon because of ingesta continually exiting the small bowel and entering the colon. In the dog, it is easy to bypass the ileocolic valve obscured with ingesta and inadvertently pass the endoscope tip into the cecum, thinking that the endoscope is still in the colonic lumen. If the colon appears to be making a spiral curve and the scope cannot be further advanced, the scope should be withdrawn as the operator carefully looks for the ileocolic valve that was previously missed.

The ileocolic valve is a dynamic structure in the dog. It can appear as a "mushroom" with a slit in the center (Figure 1.48), it can retract and look like an opening in the colonic wall, or it can appear anywhere in between these two extremes.[4] The feline ileocolic valve region is different. The cecum is simply a blind sac, and the ileocolic valve is usually a slit opening in the mucosa (Figure 1.49). This region is seen immediately after the tip of the scope negotiates the flexure between the descending colon and the ascending/transverse colon. In some cases, the tip of the scope will pass the ileocolic valve and the scope will have to be partially withdrawn in order to see the valve.

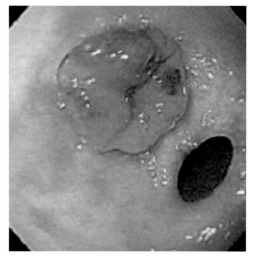

Figure 1.48:
Ileocolic valve of a dog. The ileocolic valve is the mushroom-shaped structure near the center of the photograph. The orifice below and to the right is the opening to the cecum.

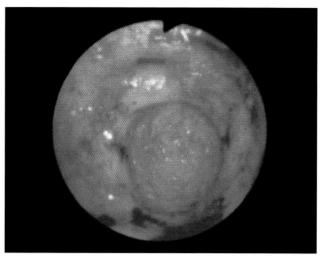

Figure 1.49:
Cecum and ileocolic valve in a cat. The cecum is the blind pouch and the ileocolic valve is the horizontal "slit" seen above the cecum.

In dogs weighing >7 kg, one can typically enter the ileum with an endoscope that has an outer diameter of <9.8 mm. The technique is similar to that used to enter the duodenum.[3] In small dogs or cats, the operator can blindly pass a biopsy forceps through the ileocolic valve and biopsy the ileum without visualizing the mucosa.

1.5.6 Proctoscopy

Proctoscopy is the best diagnostic modality to evaluate rectal lesions.[8] Proctoscopy does not require insufflation of air, is simple, easy, and quick. The distal rectum is cleaned out with one or two enemas about one hour before the procedure. The patient is sedated or anesthetized (depending upon the need). A digital rectal examination is performed and then the proctoscope is carefully inserted to its maximum depth in the rectum. The obturator is removed and the mucosa examined as the scope is slowly withdrawn.

1.5.7 Diagnostic procedures

1.5.7.1 Biopsy

Generally, during esophagogastroduodenoscopy the esophagus, stomach, and duodenum are carefully examined before starting to take biopsies. There are exceptions to this (e.g., see modified gastroduodenoscopy section above), but collecting biopsies produces bleeding, which can obscure nearby lesions.

It is relatively easy to obtain good quality gastric tissue samples by approaching the gastric mucosa at as near to a 90° angle as possible, pushing the jaws of the biopsy forceps into the mucosa with enough pressure to cause a slight indentation but without having the forceps sliding off the mucosal surface, closing the jaws firmly, and pulling the forceps back into the endoscope.[2] Better samples are obtained if the stomach is not overly distended. The antral and pyloric mucosa is tougher than that of the rest of the stomach, and one must close the forceps more tightly and sometimes vigorously pull the forceps back into the endoscope to obtain good quality tissue samples. It is important to biopsy the antrum, greater curvature, lesser curvature, and fundus because lesions are often localized. Two samples of each area are desirable. If an obvious lesion (e.g., ulcer, mass, erosion, or discolored area) is found, it should be biopsied first so that bleeding from other biopsy sites does not obscure the primary lesion. Biopsies from such lesions should be placed into a separate formalin container. If an ulcer is found, biopsies of both the center (one should take care not to

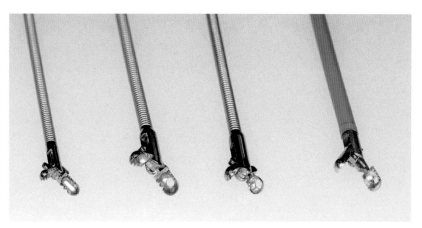

Figure 1.50:
Endoscopic biopsy forceps. Four flexible endoscopic biopsy forceps. The forceps on the far left is for a 2.0-mm biopsy channel. It obtains a sample substantially smaller than the next three forceps, which are all for a 2.8-mm channel. The second forceps from the left has an ellipsoidal jaw with fenestrated cups and serrated jaws; this is the more desirable forceps. The third forceps from the left has round jaws and obtains a relatively small tissue sample. The forceps on the far right is a disposable biopsy forceps that also takes a smaller sample than the one next to it.

push so hard as to perforate the stomach) as well as the periphery of the ulcer should be collected. Although the ulcer center can be necrotic, diagnostic samples often have been collected from that area. Ulcers caused by scirrhous tumors can be very tough, and one may not be able to obtain a diagnostic biopsy using flexible endoscopy forceps. For masses that are below the mucosa, a "well digging" technique may be employed by biopsying the same site repeatedly, each time placing the biopsy forceps into the hole that was made by the previous biopsy.[10]

The duodenal mucosa is the hardest tissue to collect consistently high quality biopsy samples from. The author prefers biopsy forceps that are ellipsoid (as opposed to round) with fenestrated cups, serrated jaws, and without a needle (Figure 1.50). However, there are numerous opinions as to which is the best biopsy instrument.[11–13] Poor biopsy quality is sometimes explained as being due to dull forceps. While this may be true for biopsies from the antral mucosa, it is not an acceptable excuse for poor duodenal, colonic, ileal, or gastric body biopsies. Disposable biopsy forceps typically have the sharpest edges, but in the author's experience these forceps routinely obtain tissue samples inferior to those retrieved with standard, reusable forceps.

An excellent sample of duodenal mucosa generally has the following characteristics: a) it tends to have a white or near white color as opposed to the reddish brown to very dark tan color of most poor quality samples, b) it is obviously an intact

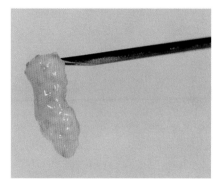

Figure 1.51:
Duodenal biopsy. An example of a good-quality duodenal biopsy sample. This section of mucosa is intact and can be held up much like a fillet of meat, as opposed to being a mass of villus tips with a more "gummy" or "jello-pudding"-like texture.

piece of tissue (as opposed to the non–distinct material that characterizes samples primarily composed of villus tips) that can be unfolded and handled (Figure 1.51), and c) it fills the cup of the biopsy instrument.[14] Pushing the biopsy forceps into the mucosa at as near to a 90° angle as possible (as opposed to a more acute angle) is desirable.[13] One technique, known as the "turn and suction" technique involves inserting the biopsy instrument until the jaws extend several millime-

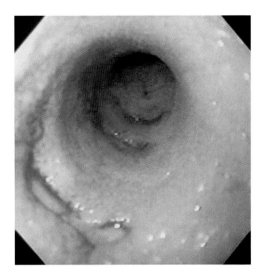

Figure 1.52:
Biopsy site. Endoscopic view of a site where a biopsy has been taken. Note the white submucosal tissue showing that a full thickness section of mucosa was obtained.

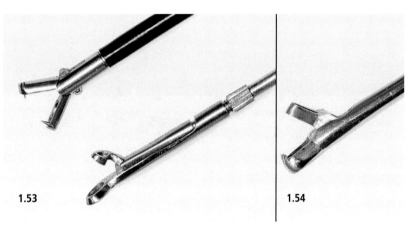

1.53   1.54

Figure 1.53:
Biopsy forceps. The top one is a "double spoon" forceps, which is preferred for laparoscopic liver biopsies. The lower one has a smaller punch that fits into the lower cup much like a pair of scissors, which is preferred for biopsy of colonic mucosa.

Figure 1.54:
Biopsy forceps. Heavy duty rigid forceps that will be able to cut through very dense, infiltrative lesions.

ters in front of the scope tip.[10] Then the biopsy instrument jaws are opened and the forceps are gently withdrawn until the opened jaws are resting against the tip of the scope. Now, the tip of the scope is maximally deflected up or down, whichever makes the tip of the scope as near perpendicular to the mucosa as possible. This will produce a "red out" (i.e., the scope tip rests against the mucosa causing the endoscopist to see a red blur). Next, suction is applied and then the biopsy instrument is advanced into the mucosa for 2–4 mm. The biopsy instrument is closed when there is substantial resistance to advancing the tip. The scope is straightened in order to avoid damaging the biopsy channel, and the forceps are withdrawn. Sometimes one may look at the mucosa after performing an excellent biopsy and see obvious, whitish submucosa, which

indicates that a full-thickness mucosal biopsy was obtained (Figure 1.52). Another technique is the "push-off" technique, which is, however, not described here.[10] If the duodenum cannot be entered, one may blindly pass the biopsy forceps through the pylorus to biopsy duodenal mucosa. However, such biopsies typically yield non-diagnostic, artifact-riddled tissue samples. At least eight excellent tissue samples from the duodenum, should be collected in the hope that one or two of them will be oriented in an optimal fashion for evaluation by the pathologist.[15]

For flexible endoscopic biopsy of the colon and ileum, the same technique is employed. If a rigid scope is used, one can obtain a tissue sample superior to anything that a flexible scope can provide. A fold of colonic mucosa is created by gently moving the endoscope back and forth a little, and then the edge of this fold is cut off using rigid forceps.[8] The best biopsy forceps for collecting colonic mucosal biopsies are those where the small upper punch fits into a larger lower cup and cuts the tissue much like a pair of scissors rather than the "double spoon" type (Figure 1.53).

For rectal lesions with a dense submucosal infiltrate (e.g., scirrhous carcinomas), it is imperative to biopsy the underlying submucosa and not just the overlying mucosa. In order to collect these tissue samples, heavy, rigid forceps with the shearing action described above are necessary (Figure 1.54). It can be very difficult to sample a densely infiltrated submucosa and it sometimes works best if the scope is removed from the anus, and a gloved finger guides the forceps to the thickest part of the lesion. The opened jaws of the forceps are carefully placed over the thickest part, pushed firmly into the lesion, and forcefully closed. This often results in an audible "crack" as the dense underlying tissue is cut.[8] The tissue must be inspected after removal from the forceps. If the presence of submucosa is not obvious the biopsy must be repeated.

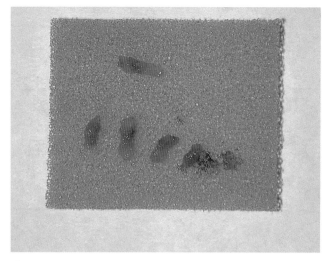

Figure 1.55:
Biopsy handling. Example of how tissue samples should be placed on a sponge or other media prior to fixation. Note how the biopsies have been gently unfolded after they were taken from the biopsy forceps.

1.5.7.2 Mounting and handling tissue samples

It is critical that the clinician consults with the pathologist to establish how the samples are to be submitted, and how the lab will process the samples. In particular, duodenal samples are very difficult to get embedded correctly, but are often the samples most likely to provide valuable information. The author places tissue samples on a non-absorbent, plastic sponge that fits into the histopath cassette.[14,15] Duodenal and ileal samples are oriented such that the submucosal side of the sample is on the sponge and the villi are pointing away from the sponge (Figure 1.55). It is crucial to not allow the tissue samples to dry out. The sponges with the attached tissue samples are placed upside down in formalin and submitted to the laboratory. The laboratory embeds these samples in paraffin by turning them 90 degrees so that they will be sectioned longitudinally. This should enable the pathologist to see a well-oriented section of mucosa from the villus tips to the junction of the mucosa and muscularis mucosa (Figure 1.56). For gastric and colonic mucosal samples, it does not matter which side is against the sponge. However, care must be taken not to stretch colonic or gastric mucosa when placing it on the sponge.

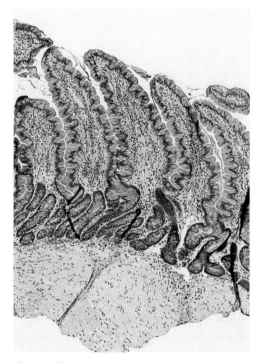

Figure 1.56:
Duodenal mucosa. A photomicrograph of a good-quality, well-oriented section of duodenal mucosa. Note that the entire thickness of the mucosa can be seen and that some submucosa is included. Not all endoscopic biopsies are as high-quality as the one shown, but it should be the aim of the clinician and pathologist that at least some samples from every case are oriented this well.

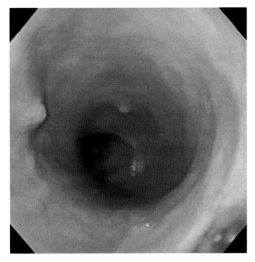

Figure 1.57:
Duodenal papilla. Endoscopic view of a duodenum showing the duodenal papilla at the 9-o'clock position. (From: Fossum T (ed.) *Small Animal Surgery, 2nd ed.* 2002, page 113; used with permission.)

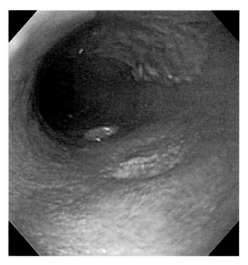

Figure 1.58:
Lymphoid follicle. Endoscopic view of a duodenum showing a crater-like depression at the 5-o'clock position, which represents a normal lymphoid follicle.

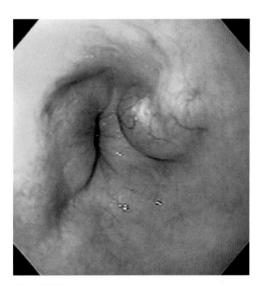

Figure 1.59:
Submucosal leiomyoma in a dog. (From: Nelson R, Couto G (eds.), *Small Animal Internal Medicine, 3rd ed.* 2003, page 416; used with permission.)

1.5.8 Appearance of the upper gastrointestinal tract

The normal esophagus has a smooth texture, except in the cat where the distal esophagus has a ribbed texture where the striated muscle is replaced with smooth muscle.[1,7] Black pigment is usually visible in Chow Chows or Shar Peis. The LES may have a reddened area protruding slightly into the esophageal lumen, which is normal. The stomach should have a smooth texture.[2] One may see numerous dots on the mucosa in some patients. The duodenum has a definite, fine texture due to the villi.[3] One can typically see the duodenal papilla (Figure 1.57) as well as depressions that represent lymphoid follicles (Figure 1.58). When using a video endoscope the examiner can often appreciate individual villi.

1.5.8.1 Abnormal findings

Esophagus

Although endoscopy may help to detect a grossly distended esophagus (i.e., megaesophagus), endoscopy is often a poor diagnostic tool for the diagnosis of esophageal weakness.[7] Only patients with marked esophageal dilation will be obvious during endoscopy; fluoroscopy is a much more sensitive (and less invasive) way to diagnose esophageal weakness. Also, some preanesthetics (e.g., ketamine or xylazine) can cause the esophagus, stomach, and intestines to become flaccid.[18]

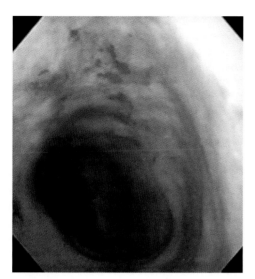

Figure 1.60:
Esophagitis. Note obvious areas of hyperemia.

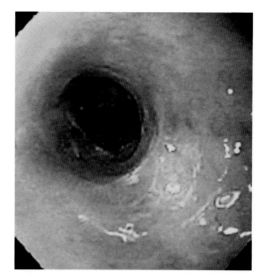

Figure 1.61:
Esophageal stricture. Note the narrowing of the lumen and the white tissue (scar tissue) at the 4-o'clock position.

Some esophageal tumors present as distinct masses while others cause strictures.[7,19] Sarcomas may be caused by *Spirocerca lupi*. *Spirocerca lupi* granulomas appear as nodules with some having a small "crater" or "nipple" from which a red worm may occasionally protrude. Sarcomas, carcinomas, and melanomas are all easily diagnosed by biopsy. Leiomyomas are typically submucosal and are covered with normal mucosa (Figure 1.59). It is often impossible to diagnose these tumors with flexible endoscopic forceps because such forceps cannot cut through the stratified esophageal mucosa. In some cases leiomyomas at the LES may only be visible through the retroflexed position from inside the stomach. Finally, esophageal polyps are rare, and if found may represent an underlying malignancy that has produced a benign, adenomatous growth over it. A deep biopsy (i.e., surgical or performed with a rigid biopsy forceps) that includes the submucosa is necessary for diagnosis.

Esophagitis is usually obvious; the operator can find a roughened, hyperemic, bleeding mucosa (Figure 1.60).[19,20] Care should be taken to not further damage the esophagus by excessive or rough endoscopic technique. The esophageal mucosa may be biopsied in order to confirm the diagnosis. Rare patients may have fungal infections. The clinician should always seek to identify the cause of esophagitis, and carefully examine the stomach and intestines in affected patients for concurrent lesions. Hiatal hernias are sometimes responsible and may be obvious or occult at endoscopy. Obvious hiatal hernias can have a wide opening at the LES with gastric mucosa protruding into the opening. However, not all patients with a hiatal hernia have esophagitis.

Strictures secondary to esophagitis are usually obvious (Figure 1.61).[21,22] They may occur anywhere, but are more common near the LES. Larger animals may have their esophageal lumen decreased by ≥75% and still allow the endoscope to easily pass through it. Strictures adjacent to the LES may be mistaken for the LES, especially if the endoscope readily passes through it.

Stomach

Many animals with moderate to severe gastritis have a grossly normal appearing gastric mucosa. Therefore, the gastric mucosa should be biopsied in any vomiting or anorexic patient undergoing gastroduodenoscopy. Most gastric lesions are not uniformly distributed throughout the entire gastric mucosa; therefore, one must carefully inspect and biopsy the entire gastric mucosal surface.[7] Any food or water in the stomach should be aspirated, and hairballs or other foreign material removed so that the entire mucosal surface can be examined. If blood is present, one should aspirate as much as possible so that all bleeding lesions may be identified and more closely examined. The operator can also infuse water into the stomach through the tip of the endoscope to help wash out the stomach. The inside of the pylorus is perhaps the hardest place to adequately visualize, but ulcers and *Physaloptera* organisms are sometimes found there.

1

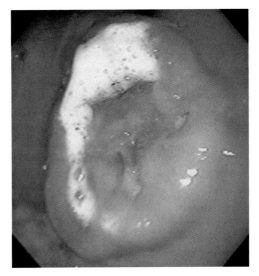

Figure 1.62:
Gastric tumor. This is a leiomyoma on the greater curvature of the stomach.

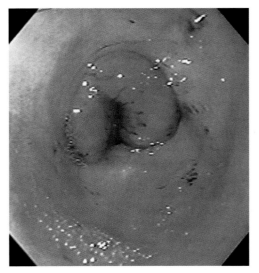

Figure 1.63:
Antral mucosal hypertrophy. Endoscopic view of a dog's pyloric area. The pylorus is obscured by a mass. This lesion is non-neoplastic and represents antral mucosal hypertrophy.

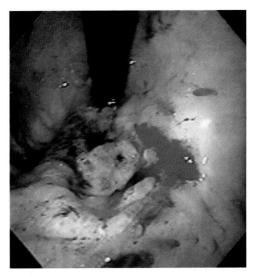

Figure 1.64:
Neoplastic ulcer. Endoscopic view of a large ulcer near the LES. This is a neoplastic ulcer caused by a scirrhous carcinoma. It was not possible to diagnose this tumor with an endoscopic biopsy because the tissue was too tough and dense to collect a biopsy from it.

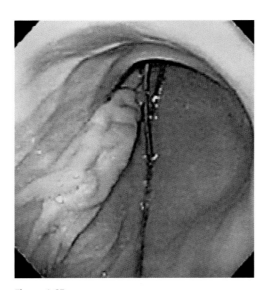

Figure 1.65:
Greater curvature and antrum. Endoscopic view of the greater curvature and entrance to the antrum with an incision line extending into the antrum. The incision line is raised and could be mistaken for an infiltrative lesion.

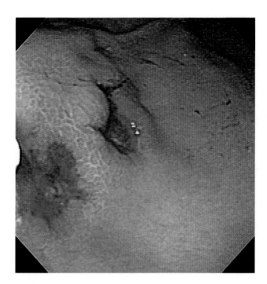

Figure 1.66:
Non-neoplastic ulcer. Note the obvious defect in the mucosa plus marked hyperemia at the site.

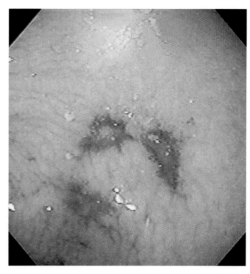

Figure 1.67:
Gastric erosions. There is marked hyperemia but a defect is not obvious.

Tumors can cause obvious proliferations (Figure 1.62). However, gastric antral mucosal hypertrophy (Figure 1.63) and benign gastric polyps can closely mimic their appearance.[23] Tumors can also cause mucosal ulcerations without any obvious proliferation (Figure 1.64). Lymphosarcoma is usually easily diagnosed by collection of biopsies with flexible biopsy forceps, but scirrhous tumors, leiomyomas, or pythiosis may be impossible to diagnose with flexible biopsy instruments. Prior gastric surgery can be seen as an elongated mucosal mass that could be mistaken for a tumor (Figure 1.65). Sometimes areas which have diffuse submucosal infiltrates are detected because they remain collapsed and cannot be distended by air insufflation – this may be more obvious in the gastric antrum.

Ulcers and erosions can be surprisingly easy to miss. Digested blood is dark brown-black and absorbs light, making it difficult for the operator to critically examine the mucosa. Also, debris often accumulates on top of erosions or ulcers, making the aspiration of debris necessary. Unless the stomach is adequately distended, erosions and ulcers can also be hidden in between rugal folds. Ulcers are deep mucosal defects that often are discolored (Figure 1.66), while erosions are hyperemic areas, which sometimes can be seen to have a minor mucosal defect (Figure 1.67).[2] Healed ulcers may cause a "stellate" appearance in which "rays" seem to radiate out from a central flat area. Submucosal hemorrhage (Figure 1.68) may be caused by coagulopathies or may signify areas of ulcer formation. Linear gastric lesions can be caused by over-inflating a diseased stomach or pushing an endoscope into the stomach wall with too much pressure.

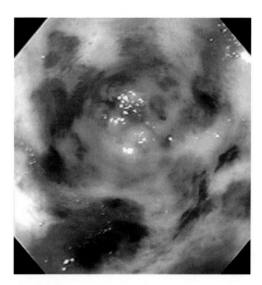

Figure 1.68:
Submucosal hemorrhage. Endoscopic view of submucosal hemorrhage. This lesion was caused by a coagulopathy, but could also represent a site that will soon ulcerate.

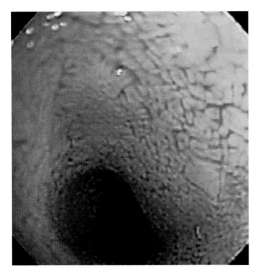

Figure 1.69:
Duodenal infiltrative disease. Endoscopic view of duodenal mucosa with a very coarse pattern consistent with marked infiltration. Instead of a fine-textured rug appearance, it looks more like cracks in drying mud. This cat had alimentary lymphoma. However, severe IBD could appear similar.

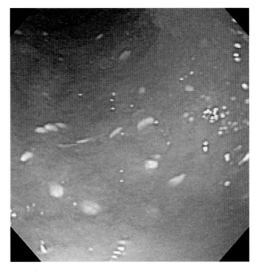

Figure 1.70:
Lymphangiectasia. Endoscopic view of a dog with numerous, large white villi that are not associated with lymphoid follicles. This is very suggestive of lymphangiectasia.

Rarely, a previously unsuspected, non-distended gastric torsion will be diagnosed when the endoscopist cannot find the entrance to the antrum.

Duodenum

The duodenal mucosa typically has a fine texture. Infiltration can cause the texture to be coarser, and severe infiltrates may cause the mucosa to resemble dried mud with cracks (Figure 1.69). Duodenal ulcers may have obvious craters or may appear as focal areas of exudate or spots of hemorrhage. Large, deep ulcers that occur near the pylorus may represent damage due to excessive gastric acid secretion. Extensive, eroded areas can have a smooth appearance, due to lack of villi. Areas of hyperemia may indicate infiltration, erosion, or coagulopathy. Masses and strictures may be obvious, although sometimes the only hint of a focal infiltrative lesion (e.g., tumor or fungal granuloma) is a roughened section of mucosa that does not smooth out when the rest of the bowel distends. However, the operator must ensure that such findings are not due to inadequate insufflation.

Finding large white dots scattered over the mucosa (Figure 1.70) is suggestive of lymphangiectasia.[24] The white dots represent dilated lacteals and are different from the generalized, delicate, fine textured white villi that can be seen in any normal animal that has recently had a fatty meal. Large white lacteals are often seen in the area of lymphoid follicles, but are not diagnostic of lymphangiectasia. Finding a substantial amount of white froth in the duodenum during and after biopsy also suggests lymphangiectasia because biopsying disrupts dilated lymphatics, allowing chyle to escape into the lumen.

Colon

Occasionally areas of obvious colonic inflammation (e.g., histoplasmosis, pythiosis) or ulceration are seen (e.g., histiocytic ulcerative colitis). However, most of the dramatic colonic lesions are seen near the anus, where tumors and polyps are most common (Figure 1.71).[4] Tumors are occasionally seen further up the colon. One cannot distinguish benign polyps from malignant tumors based upon gross appearance alone. Sometimes, polyps can be multiple and small, resembling inflammatory disease. Occasionally, unsuspected whipworm infestation is noted. Intussusception of the ileum or cecum into the colon can occasionally be found (Figure 1.72).

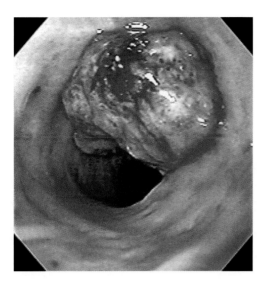

Figure 1.71:
Polypoid mass. Endoscopic view of the distal colon of a dog with a polypoid mass. Despite the polypoid appearance, this lesion turned out to be an adenocarcinoma.

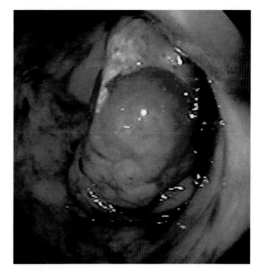

Figure 1.72:
Ileocolic valve area of a dog. The mass that is protruding is an intussuscepted cecum.

1.5.9 Interventional procedures

1.5.9.1 Foreign body removal

Esophagus

Esophageal foreign bodies (FB) can often be removed with flexible equipment.[19,25] However, the use of a rigid colonoscope and rigid forceps is superior to flexible endoscopy in many cases.[26] The length of the rigid scope is the major limiting factor. Fortunately, most dogs with esophageal FB are small to medium-sized. Plain radiographs are taken immediately before endoscopy to look for pneumothorax, pneumomediastinum, or pleural effusion, which may all be indicators for esophageal perforation (contrast procedures are rarely appropriate). The rigid endoscope is carefully advanced to the FB. Although not obvious, the edges of the FB will often have eroded into the mucosa. Thus, simply pulling on the FB can cause perforation. Instead, the operator must gently manipulate the FB so that the edges are no longer caught in the erosions before pulling with any force. In the case of bones (especially poultry bones), one can advance the scope until the tip of the scope is putting slight pressure against the bone. One may then use the rigid grasping forceps to grasp the bone, pull it snugly against the end of the rigid endoscope, and then tear off pieces or break it, thus facilitating removal. Once the FB is freed from the erosions, it may be pulled partially or completely inside the scope while being removed, thus protecting the rest of the

esophagus and making it easier for the remaining fragments to be pulled through the cricopharyngeal sphincter.

Fishhooks can often be removed, depending on the size of the barb and the location of the hook.[19,27] Small barbs can easily be torn out of the mucosa with a rigid scope, but hooks with large barbs often cannot. If the hook has passed completely through the esophagus, it can still be removed endoscopically by tearing it back out of the esophagus, as long as the hook is not in the vicinity of any important vessels. If the point of the hook is directed caudally, then the bend of the hook is tightly grasped with rigid forceps, and the hook is pulled cranially while keeping the hook as straight as possible. If the point of the hook is directed cranially, a rigid scope is passed until the edge of the scope is against the bend of the hook. The eye of the hook is grasped with the forceps so as to keep the shaft of the hook straight, and then the scope and forceps are pushed about 1 cm further into the esophagus. This action will push the hook out of the esophageal mucosa.

In some cases when a FB cannot be removed, it may be pushed into the stomach, where it can either be removed or, in the case of bones, allowed to dissolve.[19,26] This must only be done if one can be certain that there are no sharp edges on the FB, as pushing a FB with sharp edges may lead to esophageal perforation. In the case of a textured FB (e.g., racket ball), one may need to apply lubrication around the FB so that it can be pushed through the LES.

1

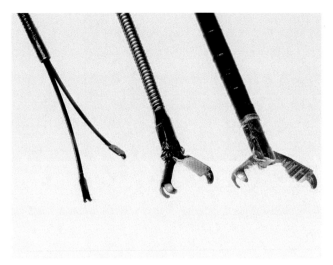

Figure 1.73:
Foreign body retrieval devices. The one on the left is a W-type coin forceps. In the middle is a "shark's tooth", and on the right an "alligator jaws" forceps. The one on the left can fit in a 2.0-mm biopsy channel, but the other two require a 2.8 mm-channel.

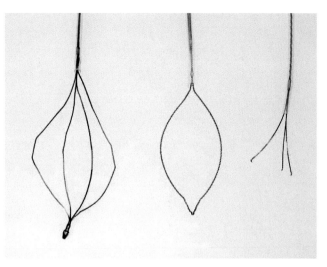

Figure 1.74:
Foreign body retrieval devices. A four-wire basket is shown on the left. Note how widely it opens. In the middle is a snare that can be used to retrieve foreign bodies or remove polyps with electrocautery. On the right is a three-prong wire snare, which does not have the grabbing power of any of the devices shown in Figure 1.73.

The operator should be extremely careful when insufflating air during endoscopic removal of an esophageal FB. If one causes gastric distension by insufflating air into the esophagus but one cannot enter the stomach with the scope, one may have to trocharize the stomach to relieve the pressure. Also, insufflating too much air may cause a severely ulcerated esophagus to rupture and produce a tension pneumothorax. In any case, a lateral thoracic radiograph should always be taken after removing an esophageal FB that has caused deep ulceration to look for evidence of pneumothorax as a sign for perforation. If the esophagus is severely diseased, endoscopic placement of a gastrotomy tube may also be valuable.

Stomach and intestines

It is important to have several good FB retrieval devices.[25] Some of the more useful devices require a 2.8-mm working channel (i.e., shark's tooth, alligator jaws; Figure 1.73), although some fit through a 2.2-mm channel (i.e., W-type coin forceps). A W-type coin forceps is useful for many objects besides coins. Objects that create a lot of resistance when being pulled across the mucosa require obtaining a substantial "grip" in order to remove them, and a "sharks tooth" and/or an "alligator jaws" forceps allows perhaps the most tenacious hold possible (Figure 1.73). A four-wire basket is very useful for balls and rocks. However, the wires should be very soft and pliable, and must open widely (i.e., at least 2 cm) in order to reliably snare most FB (Figure 1.74). A simple snare is also useful. Three wire graspers are often supplied with endo-

scopes, but are poor substitutes for the preferred instruments (Figure 1.74).

When a FB is located, it should first be studied in order to consider the best way to remove it. Pulling a FB through the LES is usually the most difficult task, and one must carefully decide which side should be grasped and pulled into the esophagus first. Objects with sharp points should be grasped so that sharp points or edges are oriented away from the mouth. It sometimes helps to a) partially deflate the stomach and b) gently rotate the scope as one is pulling the object through the LES.

An overtube can also be helpful for removing FBs.[25] The endoscope is passed through the larger diameter overtube. After snaring a sharp FB, one may pull the endoscope and the sharp FB into the overtube, thus protecting the esophagus. Additionally, because the overtube is larger than the endoscope, one may also use it to dilate the LES more than the endoscope alone would. By opening the LES those few additional millimeters, one may be able to pull a FB through the LES that would not otherwise pass. Also, administering ketamine or xylazine will relax the LES, which sometimes helps to pull a FB through the LES.

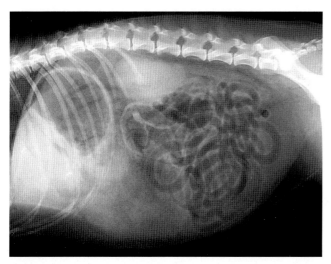

Figure 1.75:
Duodenal perforation. Lateral radiograph of a dog in which biopsy of a deep duodenal ulcer resulted in perforation. Free air is noted by the ability to see both the serosal and mucosal surfaces of the stomach.

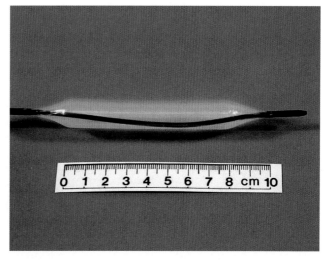

Figure 1.76:
Ballon catheter. This balloon catheter is used to dilate esophageal strictures. Note the length of the balloon. It is useful to keep the balloon in the center of the stricture when inflating it.

Linear foreign bodies

Linear FB, which have lodged at the pylorus and trail down the duodenum present a particular challenge. In the author's experience, about 20% of these linear FB can be removed via endoscopy. First, the duodenum should be entered. Then the endoscope tip should be carefully advanced to as near the end of the FB as possible. This can be very tedious, and may require the endoscope tip to repeatedly be advanced and pulled back. The goal is to grab the FB as near the distal (i.e., aborad) end as possible and then pull it out of the duodenum and into the stomach. In rare cases, one may be able to push the orad end of the linear FB (which has lodged at the pylorus) into the duodenum. Doing this often alleviates the problem because a linear FB only causes a problem if one end is lodged (usually at the base of the tongue or at the pylorus) and the rest is trailing off into the intestines. Because of the risk for perforation, one should perform a lateral abdominal radiograph after endoscopically removing a linear FB to look for free air as evidence for perforation (Figure 1.75).

1.5.9.2   Percutaneous gastrostomy tube

There are many techniques for placing percutaneous endoscopic gastrostomy tubes (PEG tubes), including devices that do not require endoscopy. Endoscopy is advantageous as PEG tubes can easily be placed incorrectly (i.e., too near the LES or too far caudally) or the mesentery or other organs can be damaged or impaled when using "blind" devices.

1.5.9.3   Dilation of esophageal strictures

Benign esophageal strictures can be dilated using either bougienage or balloon dilation.[19,20] It has been suggested that balloon dilation is associated with less shearing effects and therefore causes less unnecessary trauma, but studies in humans have shown that both bougienage and balloon dilation are effective if the operator is well trained. To date, balloon dilation is performed more commonly in small animals and will thus be discussed here. One needs to have balloon catheters specifically designed for this purpose. Round balloons as found on Foley catheters and endotracheal tubes do not work well for this purpose. Balloons of catheters designed for this purpose are long (Figure 1.76), making it easier to position the middle of the balloon at the stricture so that the balloon will not migrate as it is being inflated. First, a transfer wire is placed through the endoscope and the stricture. Then, the endoscope is removed while the wire is held in place by continually feeding it into the scope as the scope is removed. Next, the endoscope is replaced into the esophagus so that the stricture can be visualized with the transfer wire running alongside the scope. An over-the-wire balloon catheter is passed down over the wire and through the stricture, so that the stricture is at the middle of the balloon. First, a small diameter balloon is chosen and then the size is progressively increased for repeated ballooning. The balloon is maximally inflated for a few seconds. If the stricture is being torn, the patient typically shows increased heart or respiratory rates and some bleeding. How much to dilate the stricture is debatable and is a matter of personal choice. The goal is not necessarily to restore the esophagus to

1

its former size, but rather to make the patient able to consume regular or softened food. For most cats and small dogs, 15- to 20-mm balloons provide more than adequate dilation.

It is important to avoid causing excessive trauma in order to prevent restricturing. When aspirating blood and fluid from the esophageal lumen, one should be careful not to also aspirate strips of esophageal mucosa. The more esophageal mucosa that is damaged, the more likely is a reformation of a stricture. Some patients are permanently cured after one ballooning procedure. However some patients, especially those with concurrent esophagitis or with very dense, mature strictures, have recurrent strictures, and repeat ballooning procedures are necessary. Anywhere from 1 to 20 ballooning procedures may be needed, but most patients require <3–4.[21,22] In some patients with recurrent strictures, repeating the ballooning 2–3 times a week for 1–4 weeks will resolve the problem. Systemic steroids help prevent inflammation, but their efficacy in preventing restricturing is debatable. Endoscopic injection of steroids at the stricture site has been beneficial in humans, but there are no objective data to support or refute their routine application in dogs and cats.[21,28] If dilation can be done frequently enough, the majority of patients return to functionality (but may require softened food).

In some cases of very thick or very mature strictures, dilation is associated with severe, deep tearing that primarily occurs in one part of the stricture. Such deep tearing promotes reformation of the stricture. One technique that has been used is to make three or four equidistant cuts into the stricture with either an electrocautery snare (see below) or a papillotomy knife so that dilation causes a more uniform breaking of the stricture at three or four locations, as opposed to just one place.[19] Rarely there will be substantial bleeding after the dilation procedure. As during FB removal, one should take care to not overly insufflate air into the esophagus as this may lead to gastric dilation. Finally, if there is substantial damage to the esophagus, placement of a PEG tube might also be useful.

1.5.9.4 Electrocautery techniques

Briefly, while there are numerous endoscopic instruments that can be attached to an electrocautery unit (i.e., biopsy forceps, cutting snares, coagulation probes, or papillotomy knives), these techniques should only be done by individuals trained in their use. It is easy to cause substantial damage to the patient and/or destroy the endoscopic video processor if these tools are used incorrectly. The main indications for their use are a) removal of gastric or colonic polyps, b) performing three- or four-quadrant cuts of benign esophageal strictures prior to dilation, and c) stopping severe, potentially life-threatening hemorrhage while waiting to surgically remove a lesion.

⚷ Key Facts

- Not every dog and cat with signs of gastrointestinal disease needs gastrointestinal endoscopy. Cases for gastrointestinal endoscopy must be carefully selected.
- In general, the largest diameter endoscope with the largest diameter biopsy channel that can safely be used for a procedure is the best choice.
- Normal and abnormal tissue can often not be distinguished by gross appearance alone and a biopsy must be collected.
- Taking adequate endoscopic samples of gastrointestinal mucosa requires training.
- To be able to remove most foreign bodies requires a selection of 3–5 assorted baskets, snares, and forceps.

References

1. Sherding RG, Johnson SE, Tams TR. Esophagoscopy. In: Tams TR (ed.), *Small Animal Endoscopy, 2nd ed.* Philadelphia, Mosby, 1999; 39–96.
2. Tams T. Gastroscopy. In: Tams TR (ed.), *Small Animal Endoscopy, 2nd ed.* Philadelphia, Mosby, 1999; 97–172.
3. Tams TR. Endoscopic Examination of the Small Intestine. In: Tams TR (ed.), *Small Animal Endoscopy, 2nd ed.* Philadelphia, Mosby, 1999; 173–215.
4. Willard MD. Colonoscopy. In: Tams TR (ed.), *Small Animal Endoscopy, 2nd ed.* Philadelphia, Mosby, 1999; 217–245.
5. Donaldson LL, Leib MS, Boyd C et al. Effect of preanesthetic medication on ease of endoscopic intubation of the duodenum in anesthetized dogs. *Am J Vet Res* 1993; 54(9): 1489–1495.
6. Matz ME, Leib MS, Monroe WE et al. Evaluation of atropine, glucagon, and metoclopramide for facilitation of endoscopic intubation of the duodenum in dogs. *Am J Vet Res* 1991; 52 (12): 1948–1949.
7. Twedt DC. *Gastrointestinal Endoscopy in Dogs and Cats.* Wilmington, The Gloyd Group Inc, 2001; 1–71.
8. Willard MD. Colonoscopy, proctoscopy, and ileoscopy. *Vet Clin N Am* 2001; 31: 657–669.
9. Burrows CF. Evaluation of a colonic lavage solution to prepare the colon of the dog for colonoscopy. *J Am Vet Med Assoc* 1989; 195 (12): 1719–1731.
10. Golden DL. Gastrointestinal endoscopic biopsy techniques. *Sem Vet Med Surg* 1993; 8: 239–244.

11. Danesh BJZ, Burke M, Newman J et al. Comparison of weight, depth, and diagnostic adequacy of specimens obtained with 16 different biopsy forceps designed for upper gastrointestinal endoscopy. *Gut* 1985; 26: 227–231.

12. Woods KL, Anand BS, Cole RA et al. Influence of endoscopic biopsy forceps characteristics on tissue specimens: results of a prospective randomized study. *Gastrointest Endoscop* 1999; 49: 177–183.

13. Jergens AE, Moore FM. Endoscopic biopsy specimen collection and histopathologic considerations. In: Tams TR (ed.), *Small Animal Endoscopy, 2nd ed.* Philadelphia, Mosby, 1999; 323–340.

14. Mansell J, Willard MD. Biopsy of the gastrointestinal tract. *Vet Clin N Am* 2003; 33: 1099–1116.

15. Willard MD, Lovering SL, Cohen ND et al. Quality of tissue specimens obtained endoscopically from the duodenum of dogs and cats. *J Am Vet Med Assoc* 2001; 219: 474–479.

16. Wilcock B. Endoscopic biopsy interpretation in canine or feline enterocolitis. *Sem Vet Med Surg* 1992; 7 (2): 162–171.

17. Willard MD, Jergens AE, Duncan RB et al. Interobserver variation among histopathologic evaluations of intestinal tissues from dogs and cats. *J Am Vet Med Assoc* 2002; 220: 1177–1182.

18. Hall JA, Watrous BJ. Effect of pharmaceuticals on radiographic appearance of selected examinations of the abdomen and thorax. *Clin Rad* 2000; 30: 349–375.

19. Gualtieri M. Esophagoscopy. *Vet Clin N Am* 2001; 31: 605–630.

20. Sellon RK, Willard MD. Esophagitis and esophageal strictures. *Vet Clin N Am* 2003; 33: 945–967.

21. Melendez LD, Twedt DC, Weyrauch EA et al. Conservative therapy using balloon dilation for intramural, inflammatory esophageal strictures in dogs and cats: a retrospective study of 23 cases. *Eur J Com Gastroenterol* 1998; 3: 31–36.

22. Leib MS, Dinnel H, Ward DL et al. Endoscopic balloon dilation of benign esophageal strictures in dogs and cats. *J Vet Intern Med* 2001; 15: 547–552.

23. Leib MS, Saunders GK, Moon ML et al. Endoscopic diagnosis of chronic hypertrophic pyloric gastropathy in dogs. *J Vet Intern Med* 1993; 7: 335–341.

24. Peterson PB, Willard MD. Protein-losing enteropathies. *Vet Clin N Am* 2003; 33: 1061–1082.

25. Tams TR. Endoscopic removal of gastrointestinal foreign bodies. In: Tams TR (ed.), *Small Animal Endoscopy, 2nd ed.* Philadelphia, Mosby, 1999; 247–295.

26. Houlton JEF, Merrtage ME, Taylor PM et al. Thoracic oesophageal foreign bodies in the dog: a review of ninety cases. *J Small Anim Pract* 1985; 26: 521–536.

27. Michels GM, Jones BD, Huss BT et al. Endoscopic and surgical retrieval of fishhooks from the stomach and esophagus in dogs and cats 75 cases 1977–1993. *J Am Vet Med Assoc* 1995; 207 (9): 1194–1197.

28. Kochhar R, Makharia GK. Usefulness of intralesional triamcinolone in the treatment of benign esophageal strictures. *Gastrointest Endoscop* 2002; 56: 829–834.

1.6 Diagnostic Laparoscopy

DAVID C. TWEDT

1.6.1 Introduction

Diagnostic laparoscopy is a technique for viewing and for the biopsy of organs of the abdominal cavity. The technique involves distension of the abdominal cavity with gas followed by placement of a rigid telescope through a portal in the abdominal wall to examine the contents of the peritoneal cavity. Biopsy forceps or other instruments are then passed into the abdomen through adjacent portals to perform various diagnostic procedures.

As with the advent of newer laboratory tests and imaging techniques, laparoscopy has also become a valuable diagnostic tool for many gastroenterology cases when appropriately applied. The limited degree of invasiveness, diagnostic accuracy, and rapid patient recovery make laparoscopy an ideal technique for tissue biopsy or to perform selected ancillary procedures. Although an increasing number of diagnostic and surgical procedures are currently being performed using laparoscopy, this chapter will only concentrate on laparoscopic techniques associated with the gastrointestinal tract, including the liver and the pancreas.

1.6.2 Indications

Common indications for diagnostic laparoscopy in gastroenterology include the examination and biopsy of abdominal organs or masses (Table 1.12). Laparoscopy is frequently used as a method for obtaining liver, pancreas, kidney, splenic, and intestinal biopsies.[1,2] Laparoscopy is also used to diagnose and

Table 1.12: Laparoscopic procedures in small animal gastroenterology

Diagnostic Procedures	Surgical Procedures
■ Liver biopsy	■ Feeding tube placement
■ Cholecystocentesis	■ Gastropexy
■ Pancreatic biopsy	■ Gastric foreign body removal
■ Intestinal biopsy	

to stage the extent of neoplastic conditions of the abdominal cavity.[3] Laparoscopy may reveal small (0.5 cm or less) metastatic lesions, peritoneal metastases, or other organ involvement not easily observed by other techniques. An unexplained abdominal effusion is another indication for laparoscopy when other diagnostic modalities used to determine the cause are unsuccessful. Full-thickness intestinal biopsies can also be performed using laparoscopic assistance. Other ancillary diagnostic techniques using laparoscopic guidance include gallbladder aspiration (cholecystocentesis), and splenoportography.[1]

The advantages of laparoscopy over a conventional surgical laparotomy include improved patient recovery because of smaller surgical sites, lower postoperative morbidity, and decreased infection rate, postoperative pain, and hospitalization time. Other less obvious benefits of laparoscopy are related to fewer stress mediated factors than do occur with surgery.[4]

Due to the limited degree of invasiveness of this procedure there are few contraindications for laparoscopy. Often, the high-risk surgical patients are good candidates for a laparoscopic procedure. Abdominal effusion, abnormal clotting times, and poor patient condition are only relative contraindications. Fluid can be removed prior to or during a laparoscopic procedure and has little influence over the success rate of the procedure. Abnormal clotting times may also not definitively preclude the use of laparoscopy. Abnormal coagulation due to hepatic failure does not always correlate with excessive bleeding at the biopsy site.[2] Laparoscopy further makes it possible to visually select areas that appear to be less vascular and to monitor the extent of bleeding following the collection of a biopsy. If bleeding is considered to be excessive, various laparoscopic techniques can be used to control hemorrhage.

Absolute contraindications for laparoscopy include septic peritonitis or conditions for which surgical intervention is clearly indicated. Relative contraindications include the patient's condition, small body size, and obesity. The procedure becomes difficult in extremely small (<2 kg body weight) or obese patients.

1.6.3 Laparoscopic equipment and technique

1.6.3.1 Basic equipment

The basic equipment required for diagnostic laparoscopy includes the telescope, corresponding trocar cannula, light source, gas insufflator, Veress needle (for insufflation), and various forceps and ancillary instruments. Telescopes most frequently used in small animal laparoscopy generally range in diameters from 2.7 to 10 mm. The author recommends and uses a 5-mm diameter 0-degree field of view telescope for

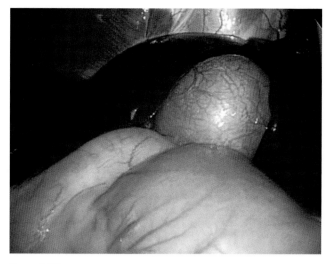

Figure 1.77:
Liver, gallbladder, and intestine. Laparoscopic view through a right lateral abdominal approach showing the liver, gallbladder, and intestines of a normal dog.

routine diagnostic laparoscopy.[1] The 0-degree designation means that the telescope views the visual field directly in front of the telescope in an 180° circumference. Angled viewing scopes enable the operator to look over the top of organs and see into small areas but the angulation also makes the orientation more difficult for the inexperienced operator.

The telescope is connected to a light source using a light guide cable. It is generally recommended that a high-intensity light source such as a xenon light source be used for laparoscopy.[1] Light sources used for gastrointestinal endoscopy are generally sufficient for laparoscopy. A video camera attached to the telescope allows the image to be viewed on a video screen. Video-assisted laparoscopy is imperative when performing surgical procedures.

A Veress needle is used for the initial insufflation of the abdominal cavity. The needle consists of an outer cutting tip and, contained within the needle, a spring-loaded obturator that retracts into the needle shaft as it traverses the abdominal wall. Once in the abdominal cavity, the obturator is once again advanced beyond the sharp tip and prevents needle injury to internal abdominal organs. The needle is then connected to the automatic gas insufflator. Most automatic insufflators are similar and function to dispense gas at a prescribed rate while maintaining a predetermined intra-abdominal pressure. Carbon dioxide is the gas most often used in order to prevent air emboli and spark ignition during cauterization.[1]

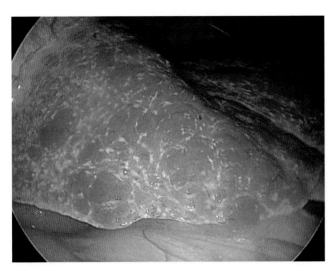

Figure 1.78:
Nodular liver. View of a nodular liver in a dog with hepatocutaneous syndrome.

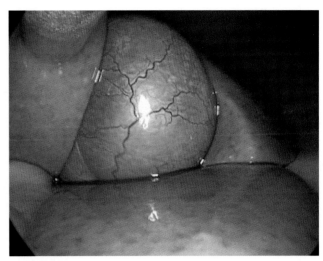

Figure 1.79:
Idiopathic hepatic lipidosis. View of the liver and gallbladder of a cat with idiopathic hepatic lipidosis.

The trocar cannula units are required to enter the abdominal cavity and are of a corresponding size to receive either the telescope or the biopsy instruments. There are a number of different types of cannula units available but the most common ones consist of a sharp trocar housed in an outer cannula. Together they are used to penetrate the abdominal wall. Once in the abdomen, the trocar is removed while the cannula remains in place traversing the abdominal wall and it becomes a portal for the introduction of the telescope or instruments into the abdominal cavity while maintaining the pneumoperitoneum.

Common accessory instruments include a palpation probe used to move and palpate abdominal organs and biopsy forceps. The author prefers a 5-mm diameter biopsy forceps with oval biopsy cups to obtain liver, spleen, abdominal mass, and lymph node biopsies. A variety of other biopsy forceps, tissue graspers, and aspiration needles are also available for diagnostic laparoscopy. A "true-cut" type or similar biopsy needle is required for both kidney and deep tissue biopsies. Biopsy needles are passed directly through the abdominal wall and guided to the area to be sampled without the need for a cannula.

1.6.3.2 Procedural considerations

The patient should be fasted for at least 12 hours before the procedure and the urinary bladder should be evacuated. Laparoscopy is commonly performed using general gas anesthesia and most patients tolerate the anesthesia and laparoscopy

well.[5,6] In some situations, the author will perform diagnostic laparoscopy using only heavy sedation in conjunction with local anesthesia at the entry sites.

In order to select the appropriate cannula portal placement sites, one must first determine the objectives of the laparoscopic procedure. The two most common approaches are a right lateral and a midline approach. The right lateral approach is recommended for diagnostic evaluation of the liver, gallbladder, right limb of the pancreas, duodenum, right kidney, and the right adrenal gland. A ventral approach is useful for many operative procedures, and offers good visualization of the liver, gallbladder, pancreas, stomach, intestines, reproductive system, urinary bladder, and spleen. With the ventral approach, visualization is sometimes hindered by the location of the falciform ligament. A complete description of a step-by-step technique of the laparoscopy procedure is beyond the scope of this chapter and has been previously described.[1]

1.6.4 Biopsy techniques

1.6.4.1 Liver biopsy

Laparoscopic liver biopsy is considered by many clinicians to be the preferred method of liver biopsy.[7] Often, other diagnostic modalities do not provide sufficient tissue or information on gross appearance of the liver and adjacent organs (Figures 1.77, 1.78, and 1.79). Generally, a right lateral approach is used for

1

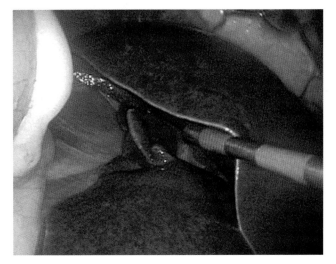

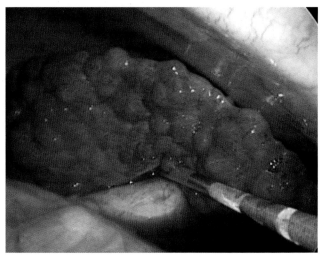

Figure 1.80:
Palpation probe. View of a palpation probe with centimeter markings used to elevate a liver lobe in a normal dog.

Figure 1.81:
Cirrhosis. View of a palpation probe elevating a liver lobe in a dog with cirrhosis and ascites.

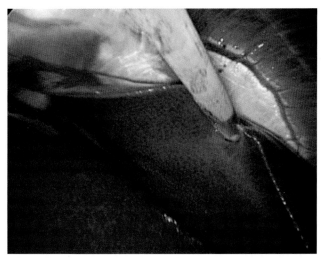

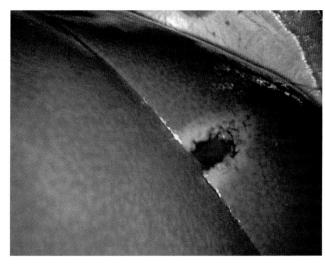

Figure 1.82:
Liver biopsy. View of a liver biopsy taken at the edge of a liver lobe using an oval biopsy cup forceps.

Figure 1.83:
Liver after biopsy. View of the liver following a biopsy taken with an oval biopsy cup in a normal dog.

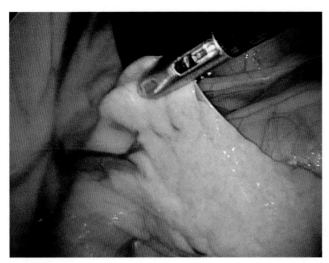

Figure 1.84:
Pancreatic biopsy. View of an oval cup biopsy forceps taking a pancreatic biopsy in a normal dog.

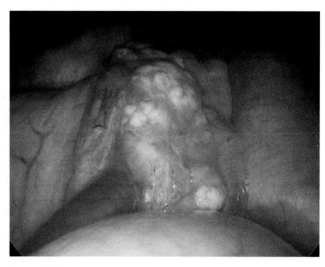

Figure 1.85:
Pancreatic atrophy. A laparoscopic view of pancreatic atrophy in a dog with clinical and laboratory evidence of exocrine pancreatic insufficiency.

evaluation of the liver, the extrahepatic biliary system, and the right limb of the pancreas. With this approach one is able to examine over 85% of the hepatic surface. Laparoscopic liver biopsies also provide enough tissue for culture, metal analysis, or other diagnostic uses.[8]

Prior to liver biopsy, coagulation parameters, including a buccal mucosal bleeding time, are evaluated. Mild coagulopathies are generally considered as a relative contraindication for hepatic biopsy because the coagulation status does not necessarily predict if the patient will bleed from a liver biopsy site. The author will frequently biopsy dogs or cats with slightly abnormal coagulation parameters or low platelet counts and rarely has identified problems from excessive bleeding.

Once the liver and extrahepatic biliary system have been examined, palpated, and the decision to obtain a liver biopsy has been made, the palpation probe is removed (Figures 1.80 and 1.81). For liver biopsies, the author recommends using a 5-mm oval cup biopsy forceps. A recent study emphasized the benefit of laparoscopic cup "wedge" biopsies as compared to 18-gauge needle biopsies finding that histopathology findings from evaluation of the smaller needle biopsies correlated only in approximately 50% of the cases with those from evaluation of the larger laparoscopic cup biopsies.[8] The author uses oval biopsy cups to biopsy either an edge of the liver or obtain samples over the flat surface of the liver. It is important to biopsy areas that appear normal as well as those that appear abnormal. Some authors suggest that biopsies taken at the edge of the liver often do not reflect deeper lesions and that the histopathology at the subcapsular edge of the liver is usually

more reactive. However, the author believes that the samples collected by laparoscopic cup biopsy are so large that this should not be considered a major concern. In rare instances when a deep hepatic lesion is suspected but not readily evident over the surface of the liver, a core biopsy needle can be directed into the lesion. Needles of 16 gauge or larger are required to obtain samples of adequate size.

Once the location of the biopsy site is selected, the biopsy cups are opened then closed around the sample area (Figure 1.82). The author generally holds the cups tightly closed for approximately 30 seconds before pulling the sample away from the liver. Generally, three to four biopsy samples from representative sites are taken from the liver. The biopsy site is then closely monitored for excessive bleeding (Figure 1.83). Usually little if any blood is lost at the biopsy site. If bleeding is considered to be excessive several steps can be taken. First, the palpation probe can be directed to the biopsy site in order to apply pressure over the site of bleeding. Alternatively, a small piece of saline soaked Gel-Foam® can be placed into the biopsy site using either laparoscopic grasping or biopsy forceps. In almost all cases this is sufficient for controlling bleeding. If continued excessive bleeding occurs, electrocoagulation, ligature clip, or loop ligature placement may be required.

1.6.4.2 Pancreatic Biopsy

Laparoscopic forceps are also used to biopsy the pancreas (Figures 1.84 and 1.85).[7] The author finds pancreatic biopsies to be generally free of complications and a study evaluating

1

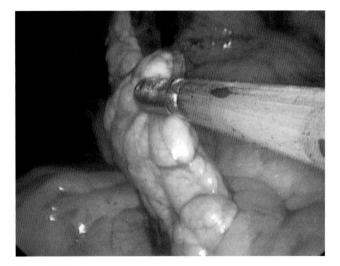

Figure 1.86:
Chronic fibrosing pancreatitis. View of an oval cup biopsy forceps taking a pancreatic biopsy from a cat having chronic fibrosing pancreatitis.

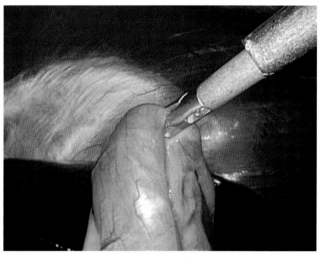

Figure 1.87:
Small intestinal biopsy. View of grasping forceps holding a portion of the small intestine to be exteriorized for a full-thickness biopsy.

laparoscopic pancreatic biopsies in normal dogs found no postoperative complications or evidence of secondary pancreatitis.[9] Indications for pancreatic biopsies include cases suspected of having either acute or chronic pancreatitis or pancreatic neoplasia. The author sometimes uses laparoscopy to confirm the presence of acute pancreatitis and to concurrently place a jejunostomy feeding tube. It is also possible to lavage the pancreatic area using laparoscopic guidance of a lavage and suction apparatus. Chronic pancreatitis is a common finding in the cat and is often associated with cholangiohepatitis and IBD (Figure 1.86). Laparoscopy is well suited for the diagnosis of these conditions and for the biopsy of all three organs.

Generally, "punch type" biopsy forceps work well for collection of a pancreatic biopsy. For evaluation of the pancreas, a right lateral approach is preferred. This approach gives an excellent view of the duodenum, the right limb of the pancreas, as well as the extrahepatic biliary system and the liver. The left limb of the pancreas is more difficult to examine from this approach and requires a ventral approach and retraction of the omentum. The suggested biopsy location is on the edge of the pancreas away from the pancreatic ducts that traverse the center of the gland and enter the duodenum. The author generally only takes one or two representative biopsy samples of the pancreas unless multiple lesions are present.

1.6.4.3　Intestinal biopsy

Full-thickness small intestinal biopsies can be obtained using laparoscopy by exteriorizing a piece of intestine through the abdominal wall and collecting the sample externally as would be done when performing a standard surgical biopsy.[1] An atraumatic forceps with multiple teeth is used to grasp the intestine at the site to be sampled. It may be necessary to "run" the bowel with two grasping forceps in order to select a section of the bowel for biopsy. The antimesenteric border is then firmly grasped with the forceps. The intestine is pulled to the cannula (Figure 1.87). Using a scalpel blade, the grasping forceps cannula incision is extended large enough to exteriorize the loop of bowel. One should see the scalpel blade enter internally parallel to the cannula shaft. The blade then cuts away from the cannula increasing the length of the abdominal incision. The cannula, forceps, and intestine together are then withdrawn through the incision. When a 3- to 4-cm loop of intestine is exteriorized, stay sutures are placed in the intestine to prevent it from falling back into the abdominal cavity. A small full-thickness biopsy is then obtained in the same manner as one would do when performing an exploratory laparotomy. Following the biopsy and closure of the intestine, the intestinal loop is returned into the abdominal cavity.

An intestinal biopsy should always be the last laparoscopic procedure to be performed as the pneumoperitoneum is lost during the procedure. If additional intestinal biopsies or other laparoscopic procedures are to be performed, the trocar cannula must be reintroduced through the abdominal incision, the incision sealed around the cannula, and a pneumoperitoneum reestablished. A technique for multiple biopsies of the intestine in conjunction with a serosal patch graft has also been described.[10] This involves retaining each segment of the bowel biopsied with stay sutures and then suturing together all of the biopsy sites in order to create a serosal patch graft.

1.6.4.4 Other biopsy techniques

A number of other biopsy techniques can also be performed using laparoscopic direction, including biopsy of mass lesions, lymph nodes, the spleen, and other organs. Splenic biopsies are generally safe to perform using the cup-type biopsy forceps. Technique, precautions, and coagulation control are similar to those of a liver biopsy. Laparoscopy may also be used to determine the cause of an unexplained abdominal effusion. The fluid is aspirated under laparoscopic guidance in order to enable examination of the abdominal contents.

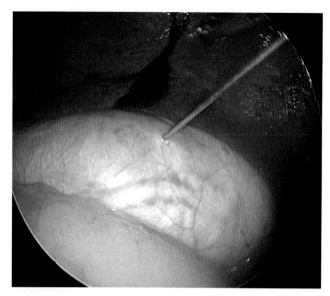

Figure 1.88:
Cholecystocentesis. View of a laparoscopy-guided cholecystocentesis using a 20-g needle.

1.6.5 Ancillary procedures

Additional diagnostic procedures that can also be performed using laparoscopic guidance include cholecystocentesis, cholecystography, and portography.

1.6.5.1 Cholecystocentesis and cholecystography

The gallbladder is best evaluated in a right lateral or ventral approach. The normal gallbladder should be soft and fluctuant and the ductal system should not be distended. Obstructive biliary tract disease is often associated with a hard firm gallbladder and a distended duct system. In these cases, the liver and biliary ducts are also often bile stained and the biliary lymphatics are generally distended.

When inflammatory or infectious biliary tract disease is suspected a laparoscopic-guided cholecystocentesis with a 22-gauge, 10-cm or longer needle is used to collect a sample for culture and cytology.[1] The needle is directed through the abdominal wall, the gallbladder is punctured, and the contents aspirated (Figure 1.88). It is important to remove as much bile as possible to empty the gallbladder and prevent leakage when the needle is removed. The bile should be submitted for both culture and cytology. It is also important to make sure the aspiration needle is placed through the abdominal wall caudal to the diaphragm. Piercing the diaphragm may produce a pneumothorax from abdominal gas passing into the thoracic cavity through the needle track in the diaphragm.

An alternative technique for gallbladder aspiration involves passing the needle through the right middle lobe of the liver and then into the gallbladder where it is attached to the liver surface. With this technique, bile leakage is minimal because bile drains back into the liver and not into the peritoneal cavity. Performing this technique, however, is difficult because the angle of the needle generally requires traversing the diaphragm.

If obstruction of the extrahepatic biliary system is suspected, an iodine contrast study can also be performed following cholecystocentesis. To perform cholecystography, a needle is placed into the gallbladder, bile is removed, and a radiopaque iodine contrast agent designed for IV use is injected into the gallbladder.[1] A volume of 5–15 ml is usually adequate to delineate abnormalities. Care should be taken not to overly distend the gallbladder in order to avoid leakage. Static radiographs or fluoroscopy are then used to evaluate the bile duct system for any blockages. The contrast agent should normally flow freely into the duodenum.

1.6.5.2 Portography

It is possible to evaluate the portal system using laparoscopic guidance.[11] Both congenital and acquired portal systemic shunts can be identified using this technique. This procedure should always be performed in conjunction with a liver biopsy. Splenoportography involves placement of iodine radiographic

1

contrast medium into the portal vascular system to outline portal blood flow downstream to where the splenic vein enters the portal vein. Laparoscopic splenoportography should be performed in the radiology suite, so that radiographs can be taken immediately following injection.

Splenoportography requires a left lateral approach. The spleen is located and an 18- to 20-gauge, 10-cm spinal needle with stylet is inserted through the ventrolateral abdominal wall near the area of the spleen. The needle is inserted into the body of the spleen parallel with the long axis of the spleen. The needle should be inserted 1–3 cm into the splenic parenchyma. Once the needle is firmly seated in the spleen, the telescope is withdrawn and the pneumoperitoneum is evacuated. The needle hub is then attached to extension tubing and gently flushed with several milliliters of heparinized saline. It is now also possible to measure splenic pulp pressure in centimeters of water by attaching the extension tubing to a standard water mano-

meter. The pressures in the splenic parenchyma are a reflection of portal blood pressure. Normal splenic pulp pressures range from 10–15 cm of water.[13] Animals with portal hypertension will have much higher pressures.

Following pressure measurements an iodine contrast agent intended for intravenous use is hand-injected at a dose of 0.25–0.5 ml/kg body weight over approximately 10 to 20 seconds. Radiographs are obtained halfway through the injection and immediately after completion of the injection. In almost all cases, one is able to delineate the portal blood flow to document congenital or acquired shunting. We find this procedure to be safe and associated with minimal complications.

An alternative method for portography involves exteriorizing a jejunal vein for direct catheter placement into that vein. The method for jejunal vein presentation is similar to that used for the intestinal biopsy technique.

1.6.5.3 Other procedures

A number of other laparoscopic procedures include gastrostomy or jejunostomy feeding tube placement and preventive gastropexy.[11,12] For these three techniques, the bowel is exteriorized through a trocar-cannula site. Feeding tubes are then placed or for the case of the preventive gastropexy the antral muscle is sutured to the abdominal wall.

1.6.6 Complications of laparoscopy

The complication rate of laparoscopy is low.[13] In a review by the author of a series of cases involving diagnostic laparoscopy, the complication rate was less than 2%.[1] Potential complications are listed in Table 1.13. Serious complications include anesthetic- or cardiovascular-related death, bleeding, or air embolism.[14] Minor complications are generally operative and are associated with inexperience or failure to understand the limitations and potential complications.

Table 1.13: Potential laparoscopic complications

Anesthesia related

Veress needle / trocar insertion
- Injury to abdominal wall vasculature
- Penetration of organs
- Perforation of hollow viscus

Insufflation
- Subcutaneous emphysema
- Peritoneal tenting
- Inappropriate insufflation
- Pneumothorax
- Gas embolism

Operative complications
- Bleeding
- Tissue injury

Technical problems
- Lack of experience
- Equipment-related problems

🗝 Key Facts

- Laparoscopy is a valuable diagnostic tool used in small animal gastroenterology.
- Laparoscopy is less invasive than exploratory laparotomy for obtaining biopsy samples from the organs of the abdominal cavity and is associated with a low complication rate.
- Laparoscopy is considered the best means for obtaining liver biopsies for histology, culture, and metal analysis.
- Laparoscopic pancreatic biopsies can confirm pancreatitis and/or pancreatic neoplasia and is rarely associated with complications.
- Full-thickness intestinal biopsies can be obtained using laparoscopy-assisted techniques.

References

1. Monnet E, Twedt DC. Laparoscopy. *Vet Clin North Am (Small Anim Pract)* 2003; 33: 1147–1163.

2. Richter KP. Laparoscopy in dogs and cats. *Vet Clin North Am (Small Anim Pract)* 2001; 4: 707–727.

3. Johnson GF, Twedt DC. Endoscopy and laparoscopy in the diagnosis and management of neoplasia in small animals. *Vet Clin North Am* 1977; 7: 77–92.

4. Bessler M, Whelan RL, Halverson A et al. Is immune function better preserved after laparoscopic versus open colon resection? *Surg Endosc* 1994; 8: 881–883.

5. Bufalari A, Short CE, Giannoni C et al. Evaluation of selected cardiopulmonary and cerebral responses during medetomidine, propofol, and halothane anesthesia for laparoscopy in dogs. *Am J Vet Res* 1997; 12: 1443–1450.

6. Duke T, Steinacher SL, Remedios AM. Cardiopulmonary effects of using carbon dioxide for laparoscopic surgery in dogs. *Vet Surg* 1996; 1: 77–82.

7. Twedt DC. Laparoscopy of the liver and pancreas. In: Tams TR (ed.), *Small Animal Endoscopy, 2nd ed.* St. Louis, Mosby 1999; 44–60.

8. Cole TC, Center SA et al. Diagnostic comparison of needle and wedge biopsy specimens of the liver in dogs and cats. *J Am Anim Hosp Assoc* 2002; 220: 1483–1490.

9. Harmoinen J, Saari S, Rinkinen M et al. Evaluation of pancreatic forceps biopsy by laparoscopy in healthy beagles. *Vet Ther* 2002; 3: 31–36.

10 Rawlings CA, Howerth EW, Bement S et al. Laparoscopic-assisted enterostomy tube placement and full-thickness biopsy of the jejunum with serosal patching in dogs. *Am J Vet Res* 2002; 63: 1313–1319.

11. Rawlings CA, Foutz TL, Mahaffey MB et al. A rapid and strong laparoscopic-assisted gastropexy in dogs. *Am J Vet Res* 2001; 6: 871–875.

12. Rawlings CA. Laparoscopic-assisted gastropexy. *J Am Anim Hosp Assoc* 2002; 38: 15–19.

13. Freeman LJ. Complications. In: Freeman LJ (ed.), *Veterinary Endosurgery*. St. Louis, Mosby 1999; 93–101.

14. Gilroy BA, Anson LW. Fatal air embolism during anesthesia for laparoscopy in a dog. *J Am Vet Med Assoc* 1987; 5: 552–554.

1.7   Cytology

Johannes Hirschberger

1.7.1   Introduction

Fine-needle aspiration (FNA) cytology is a minimally invasive technique. Fine-needle aspiration of the liver, pancreas, and intestine, even when performed without sedation and local anesthesia, is well tolerated in almost all small animal patients. Fine-needle aspiration cytology can be performed immediately after identification of an abnormal ultrasound finding. Despite some limitations (e.g., the differentiation of hepatic disease), this technique has great diagnostic utility. Fine-needle aspiration cytology shows high sensitivity and specificity for the diagnosis of certain diseases such as neoplasia and diffuse vacuolar hepatopathy.[1–5]

1.7.2   Technique

Fine-needle aspiration should be performed under sonographic guidance. In order to avoid excessive blood contamination of FNA specimens from organs with a rich blood supply (e.g., spleen or liver), the duration of aspiration should be kept as short as possible. The operator should only aspirate during brisk advancement of the needle into the liver for approximately one second. Alternatively, a needle can be advanced into the liver without subsequent aspiration. However, the first approach with a very short aspiration time is the preferred technique.

1.7.3   Liver

Hepatic cytology can be classified into normal, hyperplastic, neoplastic, inflammatory, degenerative / metabolic, and cholestatic abnormalities; extramedullary hematopoiesis; and mixed results.[4,6,7]

1.7.3.1   Normal liver cells

Normal liver cells show only slight anisocytosis. The cytoplasm often contains fine granules. The nuclear:cytoplasmic ratio ranges from 1:4 to 1:5. A nucleolus is clearly identifiable within the nucleus. Some normal liver cells may contain two nuclei. Bile duct epithelium and mesothelial cells can also be found in some liver FNA specimens. Leucocytes found on FNA cytology may originate from blood contamination and do not necessarily indicate infiltration of the liver with inflammatory cells. In unclear cases, the leucocyte:erythrocyte ratio should be compared between peripheral blood and the FNA cytology specimen. It should also be noted that FNA cytology can be contaminated with neutrophilic granulocytes originating from a purulent peritonitis, and leading to a false interpretation of liver cytology.

1

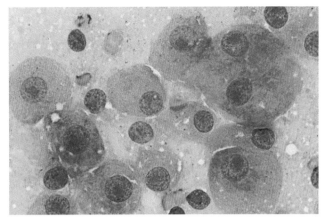

Figure 1.89:
Hepatoma. Cytologic preparation from an FNA of a 20-cm large liver tumor in a Collie. The liver cells show anisocytosis, slight anisokaryosis, a variable nuclear: cytoplasmic ratio, and slightly clumped chromatin. Occasionally, cell wall hyperchromasia can be observed.

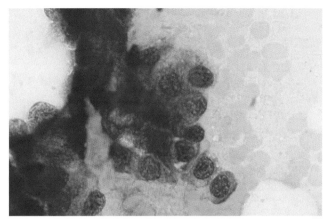

Figure 1.90:
Hepatocellular carcinoma. The hepatic FNA from a dog is highly cellular. The tumor cells show slight to moderate anisocytosis, anisokaryosis, and a variable nuclear: cytoplasmic ratio. The chromatin is irregular and clumped. Nucleoli are strikingly angular. The tumor cells are phenotypically recognizable as liver cells.

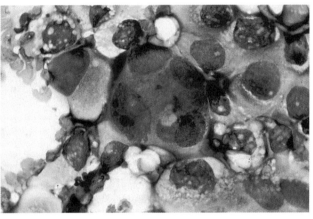

Figure 1.91:
Metastatic carcinoma in the liver. Epithelial cells with numerous criteria of malignancy are seen in this cytological preparation of a hepatic FNA from a Doberman. The primary tumor could not be determined in this patient.

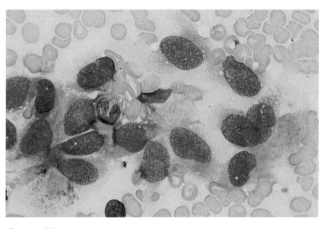

Figure 1.92:
Hepatic sarcoma. FNA cytology from a malignant spindle cell tumor in the liver of a Dachshund. The spindle cells with their plump, round nuclei show numerous criteria of malignancy.

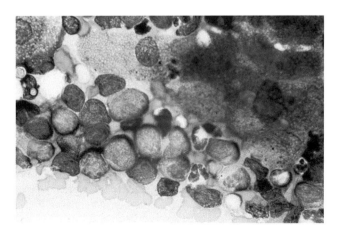

Figure 1.93:
Malignant lymphoma. A large number of large, immature lymphatic cells are present in a highly cellular hepatic aspirate from a cat. Normal hepatocytes can be observed between the lymphatic cells.

1

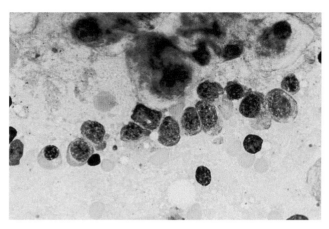

Figure 1.94:
Extramedullary hematopoiesis. This cytological preparation of an FNA from a mixed-breed dog with autoimmune hemolytic anemia shows erythropoetic cells. Glycogen incorporation into the cytoplasm of hepatocytes is due to glucocorticoid treatment.

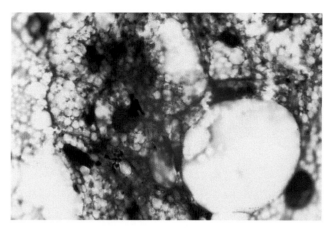

Figure 1.95:
Hepatic lipidosis. The hepatocytes in this cat are filled with vacuoles. Large fatty vacuoles or fat cells are observed in between. All liver aspirates obtained from this cat showed severe changes and severe hepatic lipidosis was diagnosed. Vacuoles can be characterized using Sudan-III stain.

1.7.3.2 Hyperplasia

Hyperplastic areas contain only few pleomorphic cells. It can be difficult to distinguish hyperplastic from normal liver cells or from cells from a well-differentiated hepatocellular carcinoma.

1.7.3.3 Inflammation

The different types of inflammation are classified based on the predominant leucocyte population. An increased number of neutrophilic granulocytes may be caused by suppurative hepatitis. Bacterial infection is a common cause and bacteria can be found on microscopic examination in some cases. Bacterial toxins will often cause degeneration of the neutrophil granulocytes. Also, in many cases bacteria can no longer be identified after treatment with antibiotics has been initiated. In these cases, fewer degenerated neutrophils are often observed.

Lymphoplasmacytic inflammation is characterized by the presence of small lymphocytes and plasma cells. Subtle indications for hepatitis are the presence of intra- or extracellular bile pigment, vacuolar degeneration, and hyperplasia or proliferation of the bile duct epithelium. Other indications for hepatitis include signs of fibrosis (presence of a pink, protein-rich substance that is infrequently infiltrated with fibrocytes), and signs of hepatocellular regeneration.

Eosinophilic granulocytes can be nonspecific and can be observed during inflammation with various other predominant cell types or they can represent primary eosinophilic inflammation as would occur during eosinophilic enteritis, systemic mast cell tumors, or liver fluke infestation in cats (*Amphimerus pseudofelineus*) in some states of the USA.

1.7.3.4 Neoplasia

Malignant tumors can be classified either as primary (hepatocellular carcinoma or bile duct carcinoma), or secondary (malignant lymphoma, metastasis of sarcoma or carcinoma, mast cell tumor, malignant histiocytosis, and myeloproliferative disease). The most common hepatic tumors in the dog are hepatocellular carcinomas, malignant lymphomas, sarcomas, and undifferentiated carcinomas. The most common hepatic tumors found in cats are bile duct carcinomas and malignant lymphomas (Figures 1.89–1.93).[4,6,7]

1.7.3.5 Other abnormalities of the liver

Extracellular hematopoiesis is characterized by the presence of precursor cells and various maturation stages of hematopoietic cells (Figure 1.94). Metabolic and degenerative abnormalities include hepatic lipidosis and steroid-induced hepatopathy. Hepatic lipidosis occurs mainly in cats and is characterized by round cytoplasmic vacuoles (Figure 1.95). Steroid-induced hepatopathy, which predominantly occurs in dogs, is characterized by a moth-eaten appearance, which starts at the cell edges and is due to glycogen incorporation (Figure 1.96).

1

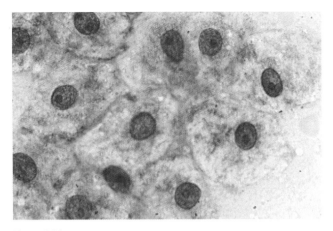

Figure 1.96:
Steroid-induced hepatopathy. Hepatocytes from this dog have a moth-eaten appearance, which is more severe at the cell edges but extends towards the nuclei. These abnormalities occur irregularly. In some areas of the smear, they occur frequently while in other areas they are absent. These changes in the cytoplasm are typically seen with steroid-induced glycogen incorporation, but can also be caused by ischemia or hepatic toxins. A specific characterization of glycogen storage could be achieved using PAS stain.

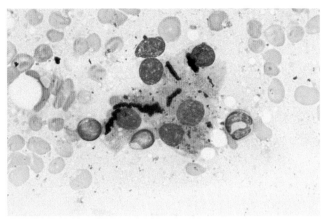

Figure 1.97:
Bile pigment cholestasis. Intra- and extracellular bile pigment can be seen as a black-green pigment in this cat with a cholestatic disorder.

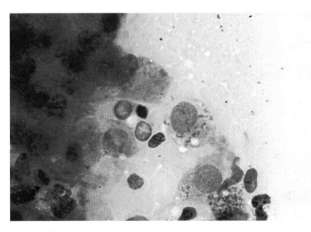

Figure 1.98:
Leishmaniasis. Macrophages in the liver of a dog, also known as Kupffer cells, have phagocytized parasites. Leishmania have a bright cytoplasm, an oval-shaped nucleus, and a small dark kinetoplast.

Necrosis is characterized by vacuolization of the cytoplasm and nuclear degeneration and fragmentation. Different types of pigments may also be seen, either dark green bile pigment (cholestasis, hepatitides), gold-brown hemosiderin, or light-green copper (mainly in Bedlington Terriers). Lipofuscin granules, a normal finding in hepatocytes of older cats, should not be confused with intra-cytoplasmic bile pigment (Figure 1.97). Differentiation of various cytoplasmic abnormalities may be achieved using a variety of different stains (Table 1.14).[4,8] Due to the fact that hepatic cirrhosis is characterized by structural changes (lobular structure, fibrosis, and areas of reconstruction and regeneration), this condition can not be diagnosed based on liver cytology.[9,10] Occasionally microorganisms can be observed on FNA cytology (Figure 1.98).

The diagnostic accuracy of hepatic cytology depends considerably on the experience of the observer. Table 1.15 lists different disorders that are easy to diagnose even for the less experienced observer. Considerable experience is necessary to diagnose and differentiate the various types of inflammation or a well-differentiated hepatocellular carcinoma.[1,2,4]

Table 1.14: Special stains used for differentiation of hepatic pigments[4,8]

Pigment	Stain
Copper	Rubeanic acid
Fat	Sudan-III stain
Glycogen	PAS stain
Hemosiderin	Prussian blue stain
Lipofuscin	Luxol blue stain

Table 1.15: Disorders that can easily be diagnosed based on FNA cytology[1,2,4,6,7]

Diagnosis	Cytologic features	Possible problems
Steroid-induced hepatopathy	Moth-eaten appearance of hepatocytes	
Hepatic lipidosis	Vacuolar cytoplasmic abnormalities	
Lymphoma of liver and pancreas; also in patients with circumscribed lesions of the intestinal wall	Frequently approximately 50% lymphoblasts; occasionally as few as 5% lymphoblasts	It can be difficult to distinguish lymphoma from lymphocytic cholangiohepatitis
Mast cell tumor	Mast cells	Presence of well differentiated mast cells may lead to formation of cell groups
Metastatic tumors	Epithelial or mesenchymal cells with criteria of malignancy surrounded by normal hepatocytes	Can be confused with mesothelial cells and bile duct epithelial cells
Suppurative hepatitis	Mostly degenerated neutrophils, in some cases with intra- and extracellular bacteria	

1.7.3.6 Bile

Bile can be obtained by FNA und subsequently evaluated under the microscope. Neutrophilic granulocytes or bacteria present in bile are evidence for an inflammatory or infectious condition, respectively.

1.7.4 Pancreas

Cytology of the pancreas, obtained either as FNA under sonographic guidance or intraoperatively using impression smears or scrapings, may yield a rapid diagnosis while the patient is still under anesthesia. The risk for complications is minimal with these procedures. However, FNA under sonographic guidance requires experience.

An indication for pancreatic FNA cytology is the evaluation of unexplained pancreatic enlargements observed during ultrasonographic examination. Neoplastic and cystic abnormalities need to be distinguished from an inflammatory process. Inflammation is characterized by the presence of numerous neutrophils, which frequently are degenerated, macrophages, and necrotic material. Inflammation also leads to slight dysplasia of pancreatic cells (Figure 1.99). However, it should be noted that pancreatitis is frequently localized, and a negative result of a single FNA does not rule out the presence of pancreatitis.

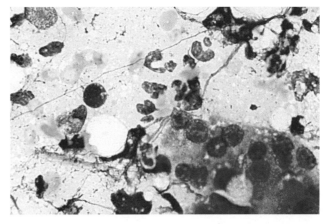

Figure 1.99:
Pancreatitis. This cytological preparation of an FNA from a pancreas of a Dachshund shows large numbers of mostly degenerated neutrophilic granulocytes, intermixed with some macrophages and lymphocytes. The pancreatic acinar cells exhibit mild dysplastic changes (slight anisocytosis, anisokaryosis, and vacuolization). Observed fatty vacuoles are due to steatitis and lipolysis. In some cases, lipophages can be seen (not on this slide).

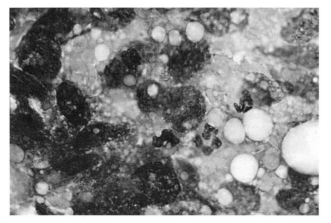

Figure 1.100:
Pancreatic adenocarcinoma. The FNA cytology of a pancreatic mass shows numerous epithelial cells with various criteria of malignancy (severe anisocytosis, anisokaryosis, macrocaryosis, variable nuclear:cytoplasmic ratio, and atypical nuclei and nucleoli). Only few inflammatory cells can be observed in the background.

Malignant neoplasia is characterized by the presence of so-called criteria of malignancy: anisokaryosis, pleomorphic cells, and excessive cellularity. A poorly differentiated pancreatic carcinoma is easy to diagnose (Figure 1.100). However, malignant tumors lead to extensive secondary inflammation, which makes the diagnostic differentiation of pancreatitis and pancreatic carcinoma by cytology extremely difficult, especially in cases where the pancreatic cells exhibit only a slight dysplasia with concurrent inflammation. In addition to primary tumors, metastatic tumors can also be diagnosed in the pancreas based on FNA cytology. Cysts und pseudocysts are characterized by the presence of encapsulated fluid that contains only few cells.[5]

1.7.5 Stomach and intestines

Rectal scrapings can lead to a diagnosis in some cases. Eosinophils can be observed in patients with eosinophilic colitis or gastroenterocolitis. Neutrophils can be observed in patients with other inflammatory disorders. In rare cases, neoplasia can be diagnosed based on a rectal scraping. Rectal scraping is considered most useful for the diagnosis of infectious organisms, such as *Histoplasma capsulatum*, *Cryptococcus neoformans*, *Prototheca*, *Pentatrichomonas hominis*, *Balantidium coli*, and *Entamoeba histolytica*.[11,12]

FNA cytology of masses of the gastrointestinal tract that are discovered during ultrasonographic examination and impression smears of endoscopically obtained biopsy specimens can be useful for the identification of infectious organisms or the diagnosis of neoplasia (Figures 1.101–1.104).

🔑 Key Facts

- Fine-needle aspiration rarely leads to complications.
- Tumors of the gastrointestinal tract can often be diagnosed based on cytology.
- Degenerative hepatic disease often displays characteristic cytological features.
- Hepatitis and hepatic cirrhosis cannot be accurately diagnosed based on cytology alone.
- In some cases microorganisms can be identified on cytology.

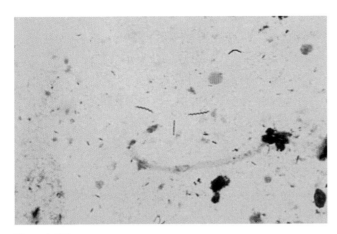

Figure 1.101:
Helicobacter infestation. Impression smear of a gastric biopsy specimen obtained from a cat. Large spiral-shaped organisms can be seen. Cytology is one of the most sensitive methods for detection of *Helicobacter*-like organisms.[13]

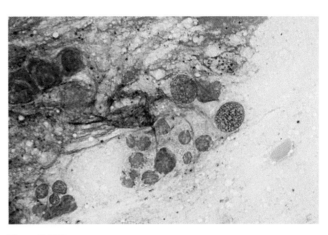

Figure 1.102:
Impression smear of an intestinal biopsy specimen in a cat. This cytology slide shows large quantities of eosinophilic granulocytes. Histopathology of this intestinal biopsy was indicative of lymphoplasmacytic enteritis. This is a good example that cytologic and histopathologic findings of gastrointestinal specimens do not always agree.

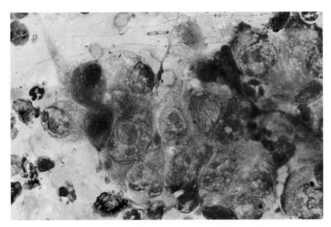

Figure 1.103:
Gastric carcinoma. Poorly differentiated epithelial cells with numerous criteria of malignancy are found on an impression smear of a gastric mucosal biopsy specimen. Neutrophilic granulocytes, few lymphocytes, and mast cells can be seen in the background.

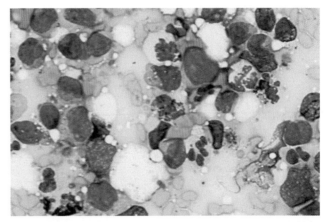

Figure 1.104:
Intestinal lymphoma. The FNA of an intestinal mass shows a homogenous population of large immature lymphocytes as well as a large number of inflammatory cells with mostly degenerated neutrophils with intra- and extracellular bacteria. Malignant lymphomas of the intestines are often contaminated with bacteria and often show large numbers of microorganisms and inflammatory cells on FNA cytology.

References

1. Hirschberger J. Organzytologie. In: Kraft W, Dürr UM (eds.), *Klinische Labordiagnostik in der Tiermedizin*. Stuttgart, Schattauer, 1997; 260–266.
2. Stockhaus C, Teske E. Klinische Anwendbarkeit der Leberzytologie bei Hund und Katze. *Kleintierpraxis*. 1997; 42: 687–701.
3. Stockhaus C, van den Ingh TS, Rothuizen J et al. A multistep approach in the cytologic evaluation of liver biopsies of dogs with hepatic diseases. *Vet Clin Pathol* 2002; (in press).
4. Weiss DJ, Moritz A. Liver cytology. *Vet Clin North Am (Small Anim Pract)* 2002; 32: 1267–1291.
5. Bjorneby JM, Kari S. Cytology of the Pancreas. *Vet Clin North Am (Small Anim Pract)* 2002; 32: 1293–1312.
6. Bolliger Provencher A. Cytology of the liver. *Proc of the 6th ESVIM Forum*. 1996; 66–67.
7. Blue JT, French TW, Meyer DJ. The liver. In: Cowell RL, Tyler RD, Meinkoth JH (eds.), *Diagnostic cytology and hematology of the dog and cat, 2nd ed.* St. Louis, Mosby, 1999; 183–194.
8. Teske E, Brinkhuis BG, Bode P et al. Cytological detection of copper toxicosis in Bedlington terriers. *Vet Rec* 1992; 131: 30–32.
9. Lundquis A, Akerman M. Fine needle aspiration biopsy in acute hepatitis and liver cirrhosis. *Ann Clin Res* 1970; 2: 197–203.
10. Perry MD, Johnston WW. Needle biopsy of the liver for diagnosis of nonneoplastic liver disease. *Acta Cytol* 1985; 29: 385–390.
11. Rakich PM, Latimer KS. Rectal mucosal scrapings. In: Cowell RL, Tyler RD, Meinkoth JH (eds.), *Diagnostic cytology and hematology of the dog and cat, 2nd ed.* St. Louis, Mosby, 1999; 249–253.
12. Baker R, Lumsden JH. The gastrointestinal tract – intestines, liver, pancreas. In Baker R, Lumsden JH (eds.), *Color Atlas of Cytology of the Dog and Cat, 1st ed.* St. Louis, Mosby, 2000; 177–197.
13. Kuffer-Frank M, Gerres A, Neuhaus B et al. Vergleich diagnostischer Methoden zum Nachweis von Gastric *Helicobacter*-like Organisms bei Hund und Katze. *9. Jahrestagung der Fachgruppe Innere Medizin und Klinische Laboratoriumsdiagnostik der Deutschen Veterinärmedizinischen Gesellschaft*, München, 6.–8. 3. 2000; 64–65.

1.8 Histopathology

THOMAS BILZER

1.8.1 Introduction

Modern histopathology emphasizes the definitive diagnosis in the live patient for a rational therapeutic regimen and – possibly – the prevention of disease. The accessibility of the gastrointestinal tract (GI tract) to direct visualization by endoscopy has generated a considerable increase in the number of biopsy samples, a trend that is expected to continue as a result of advancing technology and quality of care in small animal medicine. The clinician expects detailed, reliable, and relevant information from the mucosal biopsy specimens. This requires significant expertise of the histopathologist with the interpretation of gastrointestinal biopsies. But it also requires for the clinician to provide representative material as well as all relevant clinical data, as a lack of clinical information complicates the interpretation of biopsy specimens.

1.8.2 Types of gastrointestinal biopsies

Several biopsy techniques have been established to evaluate the GI tract.[1,2,3] Irrespective of the biopsy type collected, the tissue removed should be representative, sufficient, and well preserved.

1.8.2.1 Endoscopic biopsies

Specimens taken by endoscopic forceps are the most common type of GI tract biopsies. They allow accurate sampling of multiple sites and thus are a good compromise between minimal invasion on one hand and sufficient amount of tissue for evaluation on the other. The working channel of endoscopes commonly range in size from 2.2 to 2.8 mm and determine the size of the biopsy forceps that can be used to collect the samples. Biopsy samples should include samples from different areas of the stomach, i.e., cardia, fundus, corpus, antrum, and pylorus, as well as samples from duodenum and if indicated colon. This is not always possible or even indicated depending on the size of the patient or the clinical signs the patient was presented for.

1.8.2.2 Full-thickness biopsies

Surgical excisional and incisional biopsies vary considerably in size ranging from punch samples of a few millimeters in diameter to mass lesions measuring several centimeters in diameter. Ideally, samples should encompass the whole lesion or at least a representative portion of the lesion. In case of a disseminated process, more than one lesion should be sampled. Also, in order to allow for proper assessment of the disease process all layers of the gastrointestinal wall should be included.

1.8.2.3 Needle biopsies

Samples can also be collected by use of a needle when the lesion cannot be fully represented by endoscopic biopsies. Wide-bore cutting needle samples will be of higher diagnostic value than fine-needle biopsies.

1.8.2.4 Brushing and curettage samples

These samples comprise of exfoliations of individual cells and cell aggregates. Such samples should be investigated by cytology (see 1.7).

1.8.3 Advantages and disadvantages of different biopsy techniques

(Table 1.16)

The main advantage of endoscopic biopsies is the collection of biopsy samples under visualization.[4] Therefore, samples are representative of mucosal lesions observed during endoscopy of the stomach, duodenum, terminal ileum, or colon. The relatively small size (3-mm maximum diameter) of the samples is compensated for by the availability of multiple samples. The major disadvantages of endoscopic biopsies are crushing artefacts or the potential for insufficient depth, which can lead to separation within the mucosa. This is especially true for the duodenum, where the main problem is the distortion and disruption of villi, in particular when samples are collected blindly. Another disadvantage is the limited access to the jejunum and ileum. Furthermore, endoscopic biopsies are not deep enough to allow for evaluation of submucosal structures. Finally, the mucosa cannot be oriented prior to sectioning. However, in our own experience orientation within a good quality endoscopic biopsy is sufficient to identify structural alterations typical for many if not most intestinal diseases. The ideal endoscopic biopsy sample to enable histopathological diagnosis should include intact mucosa, with attached muscularis mucosae and parts of the submucosa, even if the relationship and size of villi and crypts cannot be determined accurately in comparison to full-thickness biopsies.

Advantages of full-thickness biopsies include the larger size compared to endoscopic biopsies leading to easier handling and orientation. Also, when abnormalities are located outside the mucosa, such as a leiomyoma or plexus lesions, or if endoscopic biopsies are inconclusive due to size, poor quality, or a non-representative sample, full-thickness biopsies can lead to a diagnosis. Also, crushing and disruption artefacts are rare with full-thickness biopsies. The disadvantages of full-thickness biopsies include the limited number of specimens that can be collected and the degree of invasiveness, which can be associated with an increased risk for complications.

The main advantage of fine-needle aspiration, brushing, or curettage is the ease and inexpensiveness of these procedures (see 1.7). However, they cannot reflect structural changes.

1.8.4 Tissue handling and processing

Most importantly, any sample should be protected from crushing, dehydration, and autolysis. Also, biopsy handling needs to be tailored to the investigations that are to be performed, such as histopathology, immunohistochemistry, or biochemistry. For morphologic assessment, tissue samples should be collected very carefully and handled with great delicacy in order to preserve tissue structure and to avoid artefacts. It also requires optimal condition of the cutting instruments, such as the biopsy forceps, needles, or others as well as proper placing of the specimens into containers with 7% buffered formalin enabling immediate fixation. Larger samples should be incised or dissected. Needle biopsies and endoscopic samples should be lifted from the instruments by use of a needle or flushed off with sterile saline. Any excessive or rough handling of the tissue

---

Table 1.16: Comparison of advantages and disadvantages of full- and partial-thickness gastrointestinal biopsies

Full-thickness biopsies collected by exploratory laparotomy or laparoscopy	Partial-thickness biopsies collected by endoscopy
■ Visualization/palpation of the GI tract, liver, pancreas, and lymph nodes	■ No macroscopic orientation; associated organs not visible
■ Blind and potentially inappropriate sampling (except of lesions that are apparent from the serosal surface)	■ Visualization of lesions of the GI tract mucosa
■ Sufficient sample size and appropriate orientation	■ Small sample size and potentially insufficient orientation
■ Limited number of samples	■ Numerous samples
■ Representative sample	■ Sample may not be representative
■ All layers of the gastrointestinal tube	■ Limited to mucosa and maybe submucosa
■ Biopsies from associated organs	■ No biopsies from associated organs
■ Increased risk	■ Minimal invasiveness
■ Requires experienced pathologist	■ Requires a very experienced pathologist

specimen will lead to artefacts and thus will limit their diagnostic value. The biopsy sample should also be accompanied by a detailed description of any relevant clinical data and a diagram of the sample collection site. Some authors have recommended placing small samples on lens paper, foam, thin cards, or even slices of cucumber in order to prevent distortion and to allow better tissue localization and orientation. However, this should be done with extreme caution as those efforts may result in additional artefacts rather than in their prevention. Some investigators allow the samples to adhere to the support surface for a short period of time. However, this may cause additional stress and is not recommended. In the author's experience it is sufficient to pool biopsies of the same region, but to keep different sites or specific lesions separate. It is not recommended to pool samples from different sites of the GI tract. Identification of the samples by included pencil-written labels and/or labeling the containers is of fundamental importance. Containers should be stable and adequate for storage and transport and should prevent accidental leakage. They should be shatter-proof with a twisted cap. Containers should be shipped in padded packaging materials.

Samples for electron microscopy should be immersed in 2.5% glutaraldehyde as a fixing solution. Biopsies for biochemical, immunological, and molecular biological purposes should be snap-frozen at $-135\,°C$ in isopentane, kept on liquid nitrogen, and then handled, transported, and further processed on dry ice. Under these conditions, samples for histopathological evaluation can also be sent unfixed as long as the tissue samples are protected against dehydration (<1-cm^3 container, no additives) and the transport to the pathologist within several hours can be assured.

Samples for bacteriology should be collected natively into small sterile containers and delivered to a bacteriology laboratory as soon as possible. Sample preparation for virology should be undertaken according to the guidelines of the virology laboratory.

For routine histopathological evaluation, formalin-fixed tissue specimens from one biopsy site are embedded into one paraffin block, then cut in series, and mounted on the same slide in order to have a representative set. Since orientation of small endoscopic samples is impossible prior to embedding it can be useful to re-orient or rotate microscopic slides during evaluation in order to improve orientation.

Although the majority of diagnoses can be made on the basis of the hematoxylin and eosin (H&E) stained slides alone, increasingly specific expectations by the clinician often require additional investigations. Special stains for connective tissue (e.g., van Gieson's Elastica, Masson's, or Goldner's Trichrome stain), mucopolysaccharide (e.g., periodic acid Schiff [PAS] stain), infective agents (e.g., Giemsa stain), reticulin fibers (e.g., Tibor Pap's silver stain), mast cells (e.g., Giemsa stain), as well

as immunohistochemical reactions for leucocyte typing, neuroendocrine markers, tumor markers, and the identification of infective agents are very helpful to arrive at a definitive diagnosis. The same is true for molecular genetics techniques; for example, in-situ-hybridization, polymerase chain reaction (PCR), and a combination of the two (in-situ-PCR). For many of these additional techniques, special handling of the specimen may be required and the pathologist should be consulted for guidelines in advance.

1.8.5 Interpretation and misinterpretation of GI tract biopsies

In order to correctly classify histopathological lesions, a systematic classification of histopathological lesions should be undertaken (Figure 1.105).

Macroscopic, endoscopic, and histologic appearance of the normal GI tract mucosa is highly variable.[1] This might be one reason for the failure to establish rigid guidelines to assess the limit between normal and abnormal.[5] Especially in the stomach and small intestine, evaluation of the significance of histopathological findings is only possible when considering the normal variation. Therefore, whenever possible, biopsy specimens should be collected from the entire GI tract. Also, sampling of evidently normal tissue can be very helpful. It is crucial that adequate clinical and laboratory information is provided to the histopathologist. Another frequent problem is the poor quality of samples. Inadequate tissue volume and crushing artefacts are the most common phenomena leading to reduction or even invalidation of the collection procedure. Especially in the small intestine, this is often accompanied by insufficient biopsy depth, i.e. the lack of full mucosal thickness, with collection of disrupted villi. Fixation artefacts in small biopsies are rare and mostly result from an inadequate fixative (e.g., alcohol, non-buffered formalin, and acetone).

Since the mucosal histology of the different stomach regions varies and gastric diseases can have a highly localized appearance, multiple small samples should be collected from several areas. Abnormalities in duodenal histology should be evaluated in the light of normal variations at this site and the susceptibility of biopsies from the small intestinal mucosa for artifacts, such as variable degrees of edema, fresh hemorrhage, vascular and/or lymphatic dilation, and epithelial flattening. A common problem of interpretation might be the underestimation of the variability of the normal spectrum of histological findings identified by the pathologist. This is especially true for features of inflammation, textural deformities, atrophy, epithelial metaplasia, and nuclear and cytoplasmic metachromasia. Thus, definitive identification of nonspecific inflammation can be very difficult. A grading system for IBD based mainly

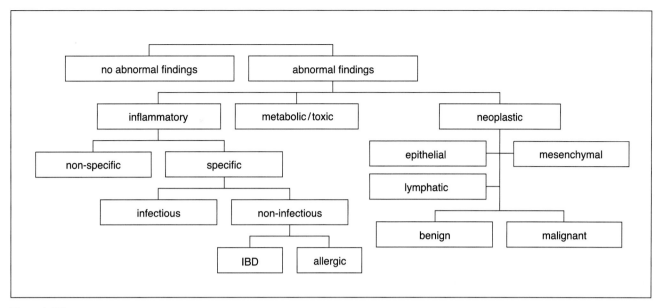

Figure 1.105:
Classification of lesions. This figure shows a systematic classification tree for histopathological samples collected from the gastrointestinal tract.

on the extent of mucosal textural damage and epithelial changes, and regardless of the number of infiltrating cells has been described:[5,6]

- mild IBD: cellular infiltrates, no textural damage, no glandular and epithelial necrosis, no signs of immaturity or fibrosis within the lamina propria
- severe IBD: cellular infiltrates, destruction of the mucosal architecture, extensive ulceration, necrosis, villus atrophy, glandular hyperplasia or loss, and fibrosis in the lamina propria
- moderate IBD: between mild and severe IBD

Further classification can be achieved according to the dominant cell type, for example, eosinophilic, suppurative, or granulomatous. However, clinical symptoms are often not reflected by the histopathological changes and vice versa.

Although it is usually easy to differentiate between an inflammatory and a neoplastic process, differential diagnosis of, for example, inflammatory bowel disease and alimentary tract lymphoma in older cats can be challenging and often requires

immunochemistry. In general, the expertise of histopathologists concerning feline GI tract disease is limited.[3,7,8] Interpretation of biopsies from the GI tract requires considerable expertise, an interest in this area, and continuous training. Close contact between the pathologist and the clinician is very important, since clinical information makes the search for and the interpretation of pathological findings much easier. This is especially true for endoscopic biopsies, where their small size hamper the identification of individual lesions or systemic disease. If the pathologist fails to identify any lesions, additional sections should be cut. The final diagnosis is often dependant on a discussion between the clinician and the histopathologist. Clinicians and pathologists must be cautious about correlating clinical signs and histopathology of intestinal biopsy specimens. Substantial interobserver variation in the evaluation of histopathological changes exists and urgently requires international standardization of pathologic descriptions of intestinal tissue.[9] It is, therefore, promising that an international gastrointestinal standardization group has been established by the WSAVA in 2004.

🔑 Key Facts

- Histological assessment of endoscopic biopsies allows a definitive diagnosis in many dogs and cats with gastrointestinal disease.
- Endoscopic biopsy handling is demanding and requires an experienced investigator.
- Communication between the clinician and the histopathologist is of paramount importance for meaningful biopsy interpretation.

References

1. Else RW. Biopsy collection, processing and interpretation. In: Thomas D, Simpson JW, Hall E. J. (eds.), *BSAVA Manual of canine and feline gastroenterology*. Shurdington, British Small Animal Veterinary Association, 1996; 37–56.
2. Mansell J, Willard MD. Biopsy of the gastrointestinal tract. *Vet Clin North Am (Small Anim Pract)* 2003; 33: 1099–1116.
3. Zoran DL. Gastroduodenoscopy in the dog and cat. *Vet Clin North Am (Small Anim Pract)* 2001; 31: 631–656.
4. Moore LE. The advantages and disadvantages of endoscopy. *Clin Tech Small Anim Pract* 2003; 18: 250–253.
5. Jergens AE, Schreiner CA, Frank DE et al. A scoring index for disease activity in canine inflammatory bowel disease. *J Vet Intern Med* 2003; 17: 291–297.
6. Jergens AE. Inflammatory bowel disease: Current perspectives. *Vet Clin N Am (Small Anim Pract)* 1999; 29: 501–521.
7. Willard MD. Feline inflammatory bowel disease: a review. *J Feline Med Surg* 1999; 1: 155–164.
8. Richter KP. Feline gastrointestinal lymphoma. *Vet Clin North Am (Small Anim Pract)* 2003; 33: 1083–1098.
9. Willard MD, Jergens AE, Duncan RB et al. Interobserver variation among histopathologic evaluations of intestinal tissues from dogs and cats. *J Am Vet Med Assoc* 2002; 220: 1177–1182.

1.9 Assessment of Gastrointestinal Motility

ROBERT J. WASHABAU

1.9.1 Disorders of gastrointestinal motility

Disorders of gastrointestinal motility represent a diagnostic and therapeutic challenge. Gastrointestinal motility disorders may result in delayed transit, accelerated transit, impaired relaxation, or inappropriate relaxation.[1] The delayed transit disorders are the most important motility disorders of companion animals and may involve the esophagus (e.g., idiopathic megaesophagus), stomach (e.g., delayed gastric emptying), small intestine (e.g., ileus or pseudo-obstruction), or colon (e.g., constipation) independently, or as a more generalized and diffuse gastrointestinal motility disorder (e.g., dysautonomia).[2]

Idiopathic megaesophagus. Idiopathic megaesophagus is the most common cause of regurgitation in the dog. The disorder is characterized by esophageal hypomotility and dilation, progressive regurgitation, and loss of body condition. Several forms of the syndrome have been characterized, including congenital, acquired secondary, and acquired idiopathic megaesophagus.[1,2]

Gastric emptying disorders. Gastric emptying disorders are fairly common in dogs and cats, and are an important cause of nausea and vomiting. Primary conditions that have been associated with delayed gastric emptying include infectious and inflammatory diseases (e.g., IBD), gastric ulceration, and post-surgical gastroparesis, while secondary causes include electrolyte disturbances, metabolic disorders, concurrent drug usage (e.g., cholinergic antagonists, adrenergic agonists, or opioid agonists), acute stress, and acute abdominal inflammation.[2] Recovery from gastric dilation/volvulus (GDV) is almost always associated with significant myoelectrical and motor abnormalities in the dog.[2]

Small intestinal transit disorders. Several small intestinal disorders that are associated with altered transit have been described in the dog and cat, including IBD, post-surgical pseudo-obstruction, nematode infection, intestinal sclerosis, and radiation enteritis.[2] Vomiting and diarrhea are the most important clinical signs associated with these disorders. Overgrowth of small intestinal bacteria, a common sequela to altered gastrointestinal motility, may also contribute to these clinical signs.

Colonic motility disorders. Constipation, obstipation, and megacolon are primarily disorders of the domestic cat.[2,3] An extensive list of differential diagnoses (e.g., neuromuscular, mechanical, inflammatory, metabolic, endocrine, pharmacologic, environmental, and behavioral causes) have been proposed, but most (>96%) cases are accounted for by idiopathic megacolon (62%), pelvic canal stenosis (23%), nerve injury (6%), or Manx sacral spinal cord deformity (5%).[1,3]

Dysautonomia. Dysautonomia is a generalized autonomic neuropathy that was originally reported in cats in Great Britain, which has now also been documented in dogs and cats throughout Western Europe and the United States. The clinical signs reflect a generalized autonomic dysfunction, leading to megaesophagus and esophageal hypomotility, gastric dilation and delayed gastric emptying, ileus and intestinal pseudo-obstruction, and megacolon and obstipation.

1.9.2 Methods for assessing gastrointestinal motility

Methods available for evaluation of gastrointestinal motility include 1) radiography – survey, barium contrast, and radiopaque indigestible solids (e.g., barium-impregnated polyethylene spheres or BIPS), 2) quantitative videofluoroscopy, 3) ultrasonography, 4) nuclear scintigraphy, 5) tracer studies, 6) manometry, and 7) functional MRI (Table 1.17).

1.9.2.1 Survey radiography

Survey abdominal radiography provides very little information about gastrointestinal motility, but is the imaging technique of choice in the initial assessment of any patient with a gastrointestinal disorder. Survey radiographs are useful in providing information about gastrointestinal tract position and content that may help to delineate mechanical obstruction from functional motility disorders. Survey radiographs are also helpful in determining the size and shape of other abdominal organs (e.g., spleen, liver, biliary tract, and urogenital tract) and their relationship to the gastrointestinal tract.

1.9.2.2 Contrast radiography – liquid barium

Barium contrast radiography is often used in clinical practice to detect gross abnormalities of esophageal peristalsis, gastric emptying (Table 1.18), intestinal transit (Table 1.19), and colonic motility, but the technique does have some distinct limitations.[4] In gastric emptying studies, for example, gastric emptying of a radionuclide-labeled solid meal was markedly delayed in a group of dogs with pyloric hypertrophy, although emptying of liquid barium was thought to be normal.[5] Also, the barium swallow technique that is currently used to assess esophageal peristalsis provides only a qualitative assessment unless it can be coupled with quantitative videofluoroscopy. The latter technique requires sophisticated equipment and computer software that are generally not available in a clinical practice setting. Barium enemas are now rarely performed in clinical practice, and this technique has been superseded by other imaging techniques. In general, liquid barium studies will be useful only in documenting gross abnormalities of gastrointestinal motility.

1.9.2.3 Contrast radiography – barium meal

Esophageal peristalsis, gastric emptying (Table 1.18), and intestinal transit (Table 1.19) are affected by the physical properties of the meal (solids vs. liquids), size of the ingested particles (large vs. small), and chemical composition (lipids vs. proteins vs. carbohydrates).[1,2] Barium mixed with food is thought to be a better contrast agent for the determination of gastrointestinal transit. Despite this, barium can dissociate from the food and re-distribute into the liquid phase of the ingested meal, which likely accounts for the wide variability in reported transit times when using this technique. For example, the gastric emptying time for ground kibble (8 g/kg) mixed with a barium sulfate suspension (5–7 ml/kg) was reported in the range of 5–10 hours in mature Beagle dogs, while total gastric emptying time ranged from 7–15 hours in other studies.[6,7] Also, as with liquid barium studies, gastrointestinal motility disorders can be diagnosed only if the transit/emptying times are markedly prolonged.

1.9.2.4 Contrast radiography – BIPS

Small, indigestible radiopaque markers such as barium-impregnated polyethylene spheres (BIPS) have been used to quantify gastric emptying (Table 1.18) and intestinal transit (Table 1.19) times in dogs and cats.[8] BIPS are administered in food as recommended by the manufacturer's package insert, and two to four abdominal radiographs are taken over the next 13–24 hours.[8] The percentage of BIPS that have been passed to the stomach and intestine is calculated and compared with standard emptying and transit curves (provided in the manufacturer's package insert). Unfortunately, interpretation of BIPS emptying and transit data has some of the same limitations as liquid barium and barium meal studies. However, because of the widespread availability of radiographic equipment and practitioner expertise, radiographic methods employing liquid barium, barium meal, or BIPS will continue to be the methods of choice for most practitioners.

1.9.2.5 Ultrasonography

Ultrasonographic equipment is now more widely available in veterinary practice, and recent studies suggest that ultrasound may be a useful non-invasive method for quantitative assessment of gastric emptying (Table 1.18) in dogs and cats.[9] In healthy dogs fed a solid meal labeled with ^{13}C-octanoic acid, there was a strong correlation between the rate of solid-phase gastric emptying assessed by use of gastric emptying ultrasonography and the ^{13}C-OBT (^{13}carbon-labeled octanoic acid breath test) in dogs.[9] Further research will be necessary to validate this method against nuclear scintigraphic imaging and to describe reference ranges for healthy and diseased animals.

1.9.2.6 Nuclear scintigraphy

Nuclear scintigraphic imaging is a very effective means of evaluating gastrointestinal motility and is now considered to be the standard method of assessment.[7,8,12] ^{99m}Technetium (bound to sulfur, albumin colloid, disofenin, or mebrofenin) and ^{111}indium (bound to diethylene triamine penta-acetic acid

[DPTA]) are the radioisotopes most widely used because they are safe, simple to use, and non-absorbable. Two radionuclide markers can be tracked simultaneously, which allows solid and liquid emptying to be assessed during the same test period. Animals are fasted for 12–24 hours after which a test meal is fed incorporating one or two radioisotopes. Left lateral, right lateral, and ventral images are acquired with a gamma-camera and integrated using a nuclear scintigraphy software package. Gastric, intestinal, and/or colonic regions of interest are identified, and the radioactive counts in these regions are recorded, usually at regular intervals for 6–9 hours (gastric emptying), 12–24 hours (intestinal transit), or 24–36 hours (colonic transit). The expense, limited availability, and radiation hazards (mostly for the staff rather than the patient) associated with this method have limited its widespread clinical application in dogs and cats.

1.9.2.7 Tracer studies

Several types of tracer studies, including gastric content, plasma, breath, and blood tracers, have been developed for the assessment of gastric emptying and/or intestinal transit (Tables 1.18 and 1.19).

Gastric tracer studies involve the serial aspiration of gastric contents after administration of a known concentration of a non-absorbable marker substance in food or by gastric intubation. Chromium oxide, polyethylene glycol, and phenol red have all been used to assess solid (chromium oxide) or liquid phase (polyethylene glycol or phenol red) gastric emptying. The invasive nature of this method precludes its use in anything other than the research setting.

Plasma tracer studies take advantage of the site-specific absorption of orally administered drugs following gastric emptying (acetaminophen) or orocecal transit (sulfasalazine). Acetaminophen is poorly absorbed in the stomach, but rapidly absorbed in the duodenum, and the appearance of acetaminophen in plasma therefore reflects gastric emptying time of acetaminophen. Sulfasalazine is a compound molecule of sulfapyridine and 5-aminosalicylate linked by an azochemical bond. After oral dosing, most of the sulfasalazine is transported unmetabolized to the distal GI tract, where cecal and colonic bacteria metabolize the drug to its component parts. Sulfapyridine is largely absorbed intact by the colonic mucosa but much of the 5-aminosalicylate remains in the colonic lumen, where it inhibits mucosal cyclooxygenase and the inflammatory cascade. The appearance of sulfapyridine in plasma therefore reflects the orocecal transit time of sulfasalazine. Acetaminophen and sulfasalazine plasma tracer studies have been validated in the dog, but there are no published studies comparing animals in health vs. disease.[11,12]

Breath tracer studies take advantage of the site-specific absorption of orally administered compounds following gastric emptying (^{13}C-octanoic acid), or of the site-specific fermentation (molecular hydrogen [H_2] generation) of orally ingested food or carbohydrate following orocecal transit. Both can be detected in expired breath, one reflecting gastric emptying time (^{13}C), the other representing orocecal transit time (H_2). The ^{13}C-OBT has been validated as a measure of solid phase gastric emptying in the dog, but there are no published studies comparing animals in health vs. disease.[9] The H_2 breath test has been validated as a measure of orocecal transit time in both dogs and cats.[12] Finally, gastric emptying can also be assessed by a ^{13}C-octanoid blood test. However, only limited data are available about the clinical utility of this test.

1.9.2.8 Manometry

Manometry has limited application in the diagnosis of cricoesophageal and gastroesophageal achalasia, gastroesophageal reflux, and aganglionic megacolon (Hirschsprung's disease), but this technique is currently only performed at major referral centers and university teaching hospitals.

1.9.2.9 Functional MRI

Functional MRI has been used to quantify gastric emptying in human beings, but this technique has not yet been validated in the dog or cat. Future MRI usage will likely be limited by expense and access to specialized equipment.

Table 1.17: Methods available for assessment of gastrointestinal transit in dogs and cats

	Esophagus	Stomach	Small Intestine	Colon
Survey radiography	+	+	+	+
Liquid barium contrast radiography	+	+	+	+*
Barium meal contrast radiography	+	+	+	–
BIPS contrast radiography	–	+	+	+
Ultrasonography	–	+	–	–
Nuclear scintigraphy	+	+	+	+
Tracer studies				
Gastric	–	+	–	–
Plasma	–	+	+	–
Breath	–	+	+	–
Blood	–	+	–	–
Manometry	+	–	–	–
Functional MRI	–	–	–	–

* rarely performed

Table 1.18: Gastric emptying times of solids and liquids in dogs and cats

50% GET (hours)	75% GET (hours)	95% GET (hours)	Substrate	Method	Species	n	Reference
Solids							
–	–	–	Hill's P/D + ^{99m}Tc	Nuclear scintigraphy	dog	6	13
2.5 ± 0.3	–	–	Dinty Moore + ^{99m}Tc	Nuclear scintigraphy	dog	6	14
1.1 ± 0.3	–	–	Eggs, starch, glucose	Nuclear scintigraphy	dog	27	15
1.3 ± 0.34	–	–	Mighty Dog + ^{99m}Tc	Nuclear scintigraphy	dog	6	10
2.5 ± 0.71	–	–	Purina + ^{99m}Tc	Nuclear scintigraphy	cat	10	16
1.9 ± 0.78	–	–	Bread, egg, milk	Ultrasound	dog	10	9
6.5 ± 1.2	–	–	Food + 1.5 mm BIPS	Radiography	dog	24	17
6.5 ± 3.2	–	–	Food + 1.5 mm BIPS	Radiography	dog	11	18
6.9 ± 1.3	–	–	Food + 1.5 mm BIPS	Radiography	dog	6	19
7.7 ± 0.7	–	–	Food + 1.5 mm BIPS	Radiography	dog	7	20
3.5	5	5	Hill's Sci. Diet + markers	Radiography	dog	26	21
–	–	7.0 ± 1.86	Ground kibble + barium	Radiography	dog	5	6
–	–	5.43 ± 1.0	Beef stew + barium	Radiography	dog	29	22
–	–	10.9 ±0.76	Purina + barium	Radiography	dog	9	7
7.7	–	12	Whiskas + 1.5 mm BIPS	Radiography	cat	12	23
8.1	–	10	Whiskas + 5 mm BIPS	Radiography	cat	12	23
5.36 ± 3.62	5.89 ± 4.06	6.54 ± 3.68	Hill's R/D + 1.5 mm BIPS	Radiography	cat	10	8
3.4 ± 0.50	–	–	Bread, egg, margarine	^{13}C breath test	dog	11	24
3.4 ± 0.48	–	–	Bread, egg, milk	^{13}C breath test	dog	10	9
Liquids							
0.2 ± 0.05	–	–	Saline + ^{99m}Tc	Nuclear scintigraphy	dog	4	25
–	–	0.66 ± 0.15	Saline	Ultrasound	dog	14	26
–	–	1.05 ± 0.29	12.5% Soup Solution	Ultrasound	dog	14	26
–	–	0.90	3% Phenol Red	Dye dilution	dog	6	27
0.16 ± 0.02	–	–	Saline	Duodenal recovery	dog	4	28
0.67 ± 0.12	–	–	3% Psyllium + Saline	Duodenal recovery	dog	4	28
0.57 ± 0.08	–	–	1.5% Guar + Saline	Duodenal recovery	dog	4	28
		1.27 ± 0.29	60% BaSO4	Radiography	dog	5	4
		3.5	Liquid barium	Radiography	dog	6	29

50% GET =   50% gastric emptying time, or the time it takes to empty 50% of the ingested/fed meal.
75% GET =   75% gastric emtying time;
95% GET =   95% gastric emtying time;
100% GET = 100% gastric emptying time
BIPS – Barium impregnated polyethylene spheres

Table 1.19: Orocecal transit times in dogs and cats

OCTT	Substrate	Method	Species	n	References
3.4 ± 0.75 hrs	Mashed potatoes	Sulfapyridine transit	dog	8	11
3.7 ± 0.9 hrs	Dog food	Sulfapyridine transit	dog	18	30
3.0 ± 0.9 hrs	Dog food	Sulfasalazine transit	dog	6	12
2.3 ± 0.8 hrs	Dog food	Breath H_2 excretion	dog	6	12
1.6 ± 0.4 hrs	Lactulose	Breath H_2 excretion	cat	10	31
2.8 ± 0.34 hrs	Cat food	1.5 mm BIPS	cat	10	8
3.0 ± 0.23 hrs	Cat food	1.5 mm BIPS	cat	10	32

OCTT – Orocecal transit time is the time taken from the oral administration of the test meal to the time when the first portion of the meal reaches the colon.
BIPS – Barium impregnated polyethylene spheres

🔑 Key Facts

- Gastrointestinal motility disorders are important causes of gastrointestinal signs (e. g., nausea, vomiting, diarrhea, abdominal discomfort, and constipation) in dogs and cats.
- Gastrointestinal motility disorders may involve the esophagus (e. g., idiopathic megaesophagus), stomach (e. g., delayed gastric emptying), intestine (e. g., ileus or pseudo-obstruction), or colon (e. g., constipation), independently, or as a more generalized and diffuse gastrointestinal motility disorder (e. g., dysautonomia).
- Gastrointestinal motility may be assessed by a number of different methods including survey and contrast radiography, ultrasonography, nuclear scintigraphy, tracer studies, manometry, and MRI (Table 1.17).

References

1. Washabau RJ, Holt DE. Pathophysiology of gastrointestinal disease. In: D. Slatter (ed.), *Textbook of Veterinary Surgery, 3rd ed.* Philadelphia, WB Saunders, 2003; 1142–1153.
2. Washabau RJ. Gastrointestinal motility disorders and gastrointestinal prokinetic therapy. *Vet Clin N Am* 2003; 33: 1007–1028.
3. Washabau RJ, Holt DE. Diseases of the large intestine. In: Ettinger SJ, Feldman EC (eds.), *Textbook of Veterinary Internal Medicine, 6th ed.* Philadelphia, WB Saunders, 2005; 1378–1408.
4. Miyabayashi T, Morgan JP, Atilola MAO et al. Small intestinal emptying time in normal beagle dogs: a contrast radiographic study. *Vet Radiol* 1986; 27: 164–168.
5. Hornof WJ, Koblik PD, Strombeck DR et al. Scintigraphic evaluation of solid-phase gastric emptying in the dog. *Vet Radiol* 1989; 30: 242–248.
6. Miyabayashi T, Morgan JP. Gastric emptying in the normal dog: a contrast radiographic technique. *Vet Radiol* 1984; 25: 187–193.
7. Burns J, Fox SM. The use of a barium meal to evaluate total gastric emptying time in the dog. *Vet Radiol* 1986; 27: 169–172.
8. Chandler ML, Guilford WG, Lawoko CR et al. Gastric emptying and intestinal transit times of radiopaque markers in cats fed a high fiber diet with and without low-dose intravenous diazepam. *Vet Radiol Ultrasound* 1999; 40: 3–8.
9. McLellan J, Wyse CA, Dickie A et al. Comparison of the carbon 13-labeled octanoic acid breath test and ultrasonography for assessment of gastric emptying of a semisolid meal in dogs. *Am J Vet Res* 2004; 65: 1557–1562.
10. Theodorakis MC. External scintigraphy in measuring rate of gastric emptying in beagles. *Am J Physiol* 1980; 239: 1285–1291.

11. Mizuta H, Kawazoe Y, Ogawa K. Effects of meals on gastric emptying and small intestinal transit times of a suspension in the beagle dog assessed using acetaminophen and salicylazosulfapyridine as markers. *Chem Pharm Bull* 1990; 38: 2224–2227.
12. Papasouliotis K, Gruffydd-Jones TJ, Sparkes AH et al. A comparison of orocaecal transit times assessed by the breath hydrogen test and sulphasalazine/sulphapyridine method in healthy Beagle dogs. *Res Vet Sci* 1995; 58: 263–267.
13. Orihata M, Sarna SK. Contractile mechanisms of action of gastroprokinetic agents: cisapride, metoclopramide, and domperidone. *Am J Physiol* 1994; 266: G665–G676.
14. Gullikson GW, Virina MA, Loeffler R et al. Alpha-2 adrenergic model of gastroparesis: validation with renzapride, a stimulator of motility. *Am J Physiol* 1991; 261: G426–G432.
15. van den Brom WE, Happe RP. Gastric emptying of a radionuclide-labelled test meal in healthy dogs: a new mathematical analysis and reference values. *Am J Vet Res* 1985; 47: 2170–2174.
16. Steyn PF, Twedt DF, Toombs W. The scintigraphic evaluation of solid phase gastric emptying in normal cats. *Vet Radiol Ultrasound* 1995; 36: 327–331.
17. Weber MP, Stambouli F, Martin LJ et al. Influence of age and body size on gastrointestinal transit time of radiopaque markers in healthy dogs. *Am J Vet Res* 2002; 63: 677–682.
18. Allan FJ, Guilford GW, Robertson ID et al. Gastric emptying of solid radiopaque markers in healthy dogs. *Vet Radiol Ultrasound* 1996; 37: 336–344.
19. Lester NV, Roberts GD, Newell SM et al. Assessment of barium-impregnated polyethylene spheres (BIPS) as a measure of solid phase

gastric emptying in normal dogs – comparison to scintigraphy. *Vet Radiol Ultrasound* 1999; 40: 465–471.

20. Nelson OL, Jergens AE, Miles KG et al. Gastric emptying as assessed by barium-impregnated polyethylene spheres in healthy dogs consuming a commercial kibble ration. *J Am Anim Hosp Assoc* 2001; 37: 444–452.

21. Hall JA, Willer RL, Seim HB et al. Gastric emptying of non-digestible radiopaque markers after circumcostal gastropexy in clinically normal dogs and dogs with gastric dilatation-volvulus. *Am J Vet Res* 1992; 53: 1961–1965.

22. Papageorges M, Breton L, Bonneau NH. Gastric drainage procedures: effects on normal dogs. II. Clinical observations and gastric emptying. *Vet Surg* 1987; 16: 332–340.

23. Sparkes AH, Papasouliotis K, Barr FJ et al. Reference ranges for gastrointestinal transit of barium-impregnated polyethylene spheres in healthy cats. *J Small Anim Pract* 1997; 38: 340–343.

24. Wyse CA, Preston T, Morrison DJ et al. The ^{13}C-octanoic acid breath test for assessment of solid phase gastric emptying in dogs. *Am J Vet Res* 2001; 62: 1939–1944.

25. Chaudhuri TK. Use of 99mTc-DTPA for measuring gastric emptying time. *J Nuc Med* 1974; 15: 391–395.

26. Choi M, Seo M, Jung J et al. Evaluation of canine gastric motility with ultrasonography. *J Vet Med Sci* 2002; 64: 17–21.

27. Leib MS, Wingfield WE, Twedt DC et al. Gastric emptying of liquids in the dog: serial test meal and modified emptying-time techniques. *Am J Vet Res* 1985; 46: 1876–1880.

28. Russell J, Bass P. Canine gastric emptying of fiber meals: influence of meal viscosity and antroduodenal motility. *Am J Physiol* 1985; 249: G662–G667.

29. Scrivani PV, Bednarski RM, Meyer CW. Effects of acepromazine and butorphanol on positive contrast upper gastrointestinal examination in dogs. *Am J Vet Res* 1998; 59: 1227–1233.

30. Weber MP, Martin LJ, Biourge VC et al. Influence of age and body size on orocecal transit time as assessed by use of the sulfasalazine method in healthy dogs. *Am J Vet Res* 2003; 64: 1105–1109.

31. Papasouliotis K, Muir P, Gruffydd-Jones TJ et al. Decreased orocecal transit time, as measured by the exhalation of hydrogen, in hyperthyroid cats. *Res Vet Sci* 1993; 55: 115–118.

32. Chandler ML, Guilford WG, Lawoko CRO. Radiopaque markers to evaluate gastric emptying and intestinal transit times in healthy cats. *J Vet Intern Med* 1997; 11: 361–364.

2 Clinical Evaluation of Dogs and Cats with Specific Clinical Signs

2.1 Clinical Evaluation of Patients with Acute Signs of Gastrointestinal Disease

KEITH P. RICHTER

2.1.1 Introduction

Acute gastrointestinal disease is a common reason for dogs and cats to be presented for veterinary care. Clinical signs can range from mild and self-limiting to severe and life-threatening. These signs can be divided into regurgitation, vomiting, diarrhea, or any combination there of. The initial clinical evaluation must take into account the severity of the animal's condition. This will help determine the extent of the diagnostic evaluation and guide initial treatment strategies. In cases with mild clinical signs, the diagnostic evaluation may be limited, and require only outpatient symptomatic care. In animals with severe clinical signs, a more thorough evaluation and inpatient care may be necessary. Complications of vomiting and diarrhea include dehydration, electrolyte imbalances, acid-base disturbances, aspiration pneumonia, and malnutrition and/or protein depletion. In most cases, it is helpful to establish a definitive diagnosis, but this is not always necessary or possible.

2.1.2 Diagnostic evaluation of vomiting

2.1.2.1 Vomiting versus regurgitation

It is critical to distinguish between vomiting, regurgitation, and gastroesophageal reflux when obtaining the initial history, because the diagnostic and treatment approaches are vastly different. Vomiting is a reflex act that includes prodromal signs followed by active abdominal contractions.[1] The prodromal signs may include behavioral changes, salivation, and repeated swallowing attempts.[1] It must be emphasized that these signs are variable. In contrast, regurgitation is a passive act that is often spontaneous or associated with changes in body position. There are no prodromal signs and there are no repetitive abdominal contractions. Regurgitation is typically associated with disorders of the esophagus (see 3.3). The best way to differentiate these two clinical signs is to imitate the two acts for the client, emphasizing the repetitive abdominal contractions seen in the vomiting patient as the most reliable distinguishing feature. The timing of the event with respect to eating, the

volume of material brought up, or the character of the contents (unless it contains bile, suggestive of vomiting) do not reliably distinguish vomiting from regurgitation.

2.1.2.2 The vomiting reflex

The vomiting reflex begins with afferent receptors located in visceral organs (including GI tract, pancreas, heart, liver, genitourinary tract, and peritoneum) and the pharynx.[1] The afferent impulses travel through the vagus and sympathetic nerves to the vomiting center located in the medulla. Vomiting can also be initiated by stimulation of the chemoreceptor trigger zone (CRTZ) located in the area postrema of the medulla.[1] The CRTZ is sensitive to blood-borne substances. The vomiting reflex can also be initiated by input from the cerebral cortex (rare in animals vs. human beings) and from the vestibular apparatus (i.e., motion sickness). Thus, vomiting can be initiated through a "humoral" pathway, caused by blood-borne substances stimulating the CRTZ, or a "neural" pathway, caused by stimulation of the vomiting center from vagosympathetic, CRTZ, vestibular, or cerebral neurons. Examples of vomiting caused by activation of the humoral pathway include chemotherapy drugs, digitalis, uremic toxins, and apomorphine. Examples of vomiting caused by activation of the neural pathway include gastroenteritis, pancreatitis, peritonitis, motion sickness, and emotions (cerebral input). It has also been suggested that vomiting can be initiated by both of these pathways simultaneously.[1] Knowledge of the cause of the vomiting will also aid the clinician in selecting the most appropriate antiemetic drug.

2.1.2.3 Etiology of vomiting

Acute vomiting can be caused by numerous disorders. These can be divided into gastrointestinal disorders and extra-gastrointestinal disorders (Table 2.1). It is beyond the scope of this chapter to discuss in detail the clinical findings and treatment of each disorder, however, many of these are discussed in other sections of this book.

2.1.2.4 History and physical examination

As mentioned above, it is critical to distinguish vomiting from regurgitation. In addition, there are several other historical features that help the clinician either determine the cause or direct the diagnostic workup. The client should be questioned for any

Table 2.1: Etiology of acute vomiting

Gastrointestinal Causes	Extra-Gastrointestinal Causes
Inflammatory ■ Inflammatory bowel disease (IBD) ■ Infectious (viral, bacterial, parasitic) ■ Hemorrhagic gastroenteritis (HGE) ■ Nonspecific ("garbage can intoxication") ■ Ulcer	**Hepatobiliary disorders** **Renal disorders** **Endocrine disorders** ■ Hypoadrenocorticism ■ Feline hyperthyroidism ■ Diabetic ketoacidosis
Drugs and toxins	**Exocrine pancreatic disease** ■ Acute pancreatitis
Mechanical ■ Foreign body ■ Gastric dilation-volvulus ■ Intestinal volvulus ■ Intussusception ■ Neoplasia ■ Pyloric stenosis	**Reproductive disorders** ■ Pyometra ■ Prostatitis ■ Testicular torsion ■ Orchitis
Functional ■ Primary motility disorders ■ Motility disorders secondary to GI inflammation or peritonitis	**Miscellaneous disorders** ■ CNS disorders ■ Drugs ■ Toxins

previous illness that could relate to the current problem. There should be a complete history including the current diet (or any dietary changes), vaccination and deworming status, onset of clinical signs, other systemic signs, exposure to drugs, toxins, or garbage, and exposure to foreign objects. The history should also help determine the severity of the clinical signs, and should therefore include the severity and frequency of vomiting, and the appearance of the vomitus. The presence of anorexia, profuse vomiting and hematemesis often warrant a more intense diagnostic and treatment plan. The physical examination should be thorough for all organ systems, and include careful abdominal palpation, an examination under the tongue for a possible string foreign body, and careful rectal palpation. The physical examination should also help determine the severity of the patient's illness. Features that suggest that more aggressive supportive care will be required include weakness, dehydration, severe depression, fever, abdominal distension, severe abdominal pain, an abdominal mass, and findings suggestive of shock. These findings also warrant laboratory and ancillary testing to determine a specific diagnosis if possible, and to assess metabolic consequences such as electrolyte and acid-base disturbances. It must be recognized early whether there are disorders that require immediate medical intervention (such as severe viral enteritis) or surgical intervention (such as gastric dilation / volvulus or a small intestinal obstruction).

2.1.2.5 Laboratory and ancillary testing

The thoroughness of laboratory and ancillary testing will depend on the severity of the problem, as determined by the factors described above. The minimum data base should include a complete blood count (CBC), serum biochemistry profile, and urinalysis. These data would screen for some of the extra-gastrointestinal causes of vomiting, help assess electrolyte abnormalities, and screen for an abnormal leukogram that may suggest a viral or inflammatory disorder. Endocrine testing may be warranted, including a serum total T4 concentration in cats, and possibly an ACTH stimulation test in dogs that are suspected of having hypoadrenocorticism. Abdominal radiographs are warranted to look for mechanical causes of vomiting, including gastric dilation / volvulus, gastrointestinal foreign body, and small intestinal obstruction. If these disorders are suspected based on plain radiographs, one could proceed directly to surgery. The features of an intestinal obstruction have been described elsewhere, and include most commonly dilated gas- and fluid-filled bowel loops.[2] In some instances, it cannot be determined whether a dilated gas-filled loop of bowel is small bowel (suggesting an obstruction) or large bowel (typically normal). An inexpensive easy test to distinguish large bowel gas from small bowel gas is a pneumocolonogram. This is performed by placing a Foley catheter (or large red rubber catheter) into the rectum and slowly infusing 20 ml/kg of room air. Lateral and ventrodorsal radiographs are obtained immediately. If the dilated loops of bowel in question are small intestinal in origin, they will remain separate from the dilated air-filled colon. If the dilated loops of bowel in question are large intestinal in origin, they will disappear and "blend" in with the dilated air-filled colon. In some instances, an upper gastrointestinal barium series is necessary to determine if an obstruction is present. It is important that the proper amount of barium is administered (10–12 ml/kg).[3] Iodinated contrast is given if there is suspected gastrointestinal perforation or if endoscopy may be performed with contrast material in the stomach. Endoscopy is generally only warranted in the evaluation of acute vomiting if there is a suspected gastric or duodenal foreign body, or possible ulceration in these regions. Abdominal ultrasonography may be helpful in certain instances, including screening of organs outside of the gastrointestinal tract. The liver, biliary system, kidney, reproductive tract, and pancreas can be examined by transabdominal ultrasonography. Gastrointestinal disorders that can be evaluated by ultrasonography include intussusception, small intestinal obstruction due to neoplasia or foreign body, peritonitis, and pancreatitis. Finally, specific laboratory testing for specific diseases may be warranted. Serum pancreatic lipase immunoreactivity is helpful in the diagnosis of pancreatitis (see 1.4.4.2). Infectious disease testing may include specific fecal cultures for *Salmonella* spp., *Campylobacter* spp., and *Yersinia* spp., testing for fecal enterotoxins from *Clostridium* spp., and specific fecal antigen testing for canine parvovirus, *Giardia* spp., or *Cryptosporidium parvum*.

2.1.3 Diagnostic evaluation of acute diarrhea

Acute diarrhea is a common clinical problem, and one that varies in severity depending on the underlying cause. Acute diarrhea is often self-limiting and may or may not require treatment. Often the etiology is unknown, either because diagnostic testing is not performed, the animal gets better prior to diagnostic testing, or diagnostic testing fails to reveal a definitive cause. In other instances, acute diarrhea can be severe and life threatening (as with acute parvoviral enteritis or hemorrhagic gastroenteritis). In these cases, there will be a need for a more intense diagnostic workup and treatment, with attempts to identify an underlying etiology and correct electrolyte, acid-base, and nutritional disturbances, potential sepsis, and other metabolic consequences. It is also important to keep in mind that chronic gastrointestinal disorders (such as IBD) can develop acute exacerbations.

2.1.3.1 Etiology of acute diarrhea

As with acute vomiting, the causes of acute diarrhea can be divided into gastrointestinal and extra-gastrointestinal causes (Table 2.2). Again, it is beyond the scope of this chapter to discuss in detail the clinical findings and treatment of each disorder; however, many of these are discussed in other sections of this book.

2.1.3.2 Pathophysiological changes with acute diarrhea

There are several mechanisms that can result in acute diarrhea. These include osmotic diarrhea, secretory diarrhea, exudative diarrhea, and abnormal motility.[4,5] Of these, osmotic diarrhea is the most common, and generally results from malassimilation of nutrients leading to an increase in osmotically active particles in the bowel lumen and therefore a net water and electrolyte loss. Examples of this include lactose intolerance, overeating, ingestion of food items that cannot be absorbed, and parvovirus enteritis. Excessive secretion leading to diarrhea can occur from bacterial enterotoxins, malabsorbed substances (such as non-absorbed bile acids), intestinal inflammation, and certain drugs.[5] Exudative diarrhea generally occurs with infectious causes, including viral enteritis and severe bacterial enteritis. Abnormal motility as a primary cause of acute diarrhea is uncommon. More commonly, motility disturbances are a consequence of the diarrhea. The most common motility derangement in the small intestine is a hypomotile gut with loss of rhythmic segmental contractions and thus decreased resistance to flow.[5] In this setting, very little peristalsis is required to propel intraluminal material through the relatively flaccid tube. The pathogenesis of abnormal motility in the large intestine also involves inflammation, thus stimulating the defecation reflex resulting in more frequent defecation. In many instances of diarrhea, multiple mechanisms occur simultaneously in the same patient.

Diarrhea usually results in loss of fluids that are isotonic to plasma, resulting in loss of sodium, chloride, organic anions, and potassium. This results in a body deficit of primarily sodium and water, thus leading to dehydration and potentially hypovolemic shock (as is the case with viral enteritis). Since there usually is isotonic fluid loss, serum electrolyte concentrations are often normal initially. Eventually, potassium depletion may also occur (through gastrointestinal and urinary losses). There may also be bicarbonate loss, in particular with distal small bowel disease (the site of bicarbonate secretion), resulting in metabolic acidosis. Thus, the patient with severe acute diarrhea may present with hypokalemia, and metabolic acidosis. If there is concurrent severe vomiting, this could further complicate these metabolic derangements. Additional consequences of severe mucosal disease relate to bacterial

2

Table 2.2: Etiology of acute diarrhea

Gastrointestinal Causes	Extra-Gastrointestinal Causes
Viral ■ Canine parvovirus ■ Feline panleukopenia virus ■ Canine coronavirus ■ Feline enteric corona virus ■ Canine distemper ■ FeLV or FIV related	**Hepatobiliary disorders** **Exocrine pancreatic disease** ■ Acute pancreatitis **Renal disorders**
Bacterial ■ *Salmonella* spp. ■ *Campylobacter* spp. ■ *Clostridium* spp. ■ *Yersinia* spp. ■ Enterotoxigenic *E. coli* ■ Bacterial peritonitis	**Endocrine disorders** ■ Hypoadrenocorticism ■ Feline hyperthyroidism **Miscellaneous disorders** ■ Drugs ■ Toxins
Helminth parasites ■ *Trichuris vulpis* ■ *Ancylostoma / Uncinaria* ■ *Strongyloides* ■ *Toxascaris / Toxocara*	
Protozoan parasites ■ *Giardia* spp. ■ *Cryptosporidium* spp. ■ Other coccidia ■ *Pentatrichomonas* (usually chronic) ■ *Balantidium coli* ■ *Entamoeba*	
Other infectious agents ■ *Neorickettsia* spp. (Salmon poisoning) ■ *Histoplasma* (usually chronic) ■ *Prototheca* (usually chronic)	
Miscellaneous causes ■ Hemorrhagic gastroenteritis (HGE) ■ Ingestion of garbage / foreign material ■ Diet change / overeating ■ Partial obstruction ■ Peritonitis	

translocation and the subsequent development of endotoxic shock. The presence of hemorrhagic diarrhea, leukopenia, vascular collapse, and hypoglycemia should alert the clinician to this possibility. Severe gastrointestinal protein loss can occur with severe exudative processes. This can lead to decreased plasma oncotic pressure and subsequent peripheral edema. Due to the complexities of the multiple pathophysiological derangements, it is important to be thorough in the evaluation of these potential changes.

2.1.3.3 History and physical examination

The initial history should help give the clinician clues as to the cause of acute diarrhea, but also help determine the severity of the illness in order to determine the aggressiveness of the diagnostic approach and treatment plan. The same historical information needed for patients with acute vomiting is also important for patients with acute diarrhea, including previous illness, current diet and diet changes, vaccination and deworming status, onset of clinical signs, presence of systemic signs, exposure to drugs, toxins, or garbage, and also the appearance of the diarrhea. Puppies and kittens are more likely to have parasitic diseases, viral enteritis, bacterial enteritis, intussusception, foreign body, garbage ingestion, or an adverse reaction to dietary changes. The character of the diarrhea will also help determine if there is primarily a large or small intestinal problem. This will help to allow the clinician to select appropriate diagnostic tests and medications. Small intestinal disorders typically result in a normal to increased frequency of defecation, lack of tenesmus and unproductive defecation attempts, and feces of large volume with a lack of fresh blood or mucus. Large intestinal disorders typically result in a marked increase in frequency of defecation, tenesmus, urgency, and unproductive defecation attempts. Each defecation episode is usually of small volume, with fresh blood and mucus frequently present in the feces. However, these characteristics are not absolute and patients with diffuse disease often present with mixed signs of small and large bowel disease.

The physical examination should be thorough and include a rectal examination. This should also allow the clinician to obtain a fresh fecal specimen for additional diagnostic testing. The patient should also be assessed for hydration status and the need for systemic volume replacement. The presence of profuse and/or bloody diarrhea, hypothermia, hyperthermia, severe depression, weakness, dehydration, or signs suggestive of shock require a more intense diagnostic approach and treatment plan.

2.1.3.4 Laboratory and ancillary testing

Since infectious and parasitic diseases are among the most common causes of acute diarrhea, fecal testing is imperative in the initial data base regardless of the severity. A direct fecal smear is easy to perform following collection of fresh feces from the rectal examination. A small amount is placed onto a slide, mixed with one to two drops of saline, and a cover slip is placed on top. The sample should be examined under X 100 magnification for motile trophozoites of protozoan parasites, including *Giardia* spp., *Entamoeba histolytica*, *Pentatrichomonas hominis*, and in cats *Tritrichomonas foetus*.[4,6,7] A fecal flotation should also be performed looking for ova, oocysts, and cysts. A centrifugation method using zinc sulfate gives the highest yield, especially for protozoan parasites such as *Giardia* spp., but it is also a good choice for diagnosis of a nematode infestation.[8] Centrifugation improves the yield of fecal flotation.[8] Though sugar centrifugation techniques are adequate for di-

agnosis of nematode infestation, *Giardia* spp. cysts are more difficult to detect.[4] Some parasites are shed intermittently, such as *Trichuris* spp. and *Giardia* spp. Therefore, multiple flotations may be required to detect infestation with these parasites (a minimum of three flotations over five to seven days is considered a good screen).[7] A stained rectal scraping or fecal smear is also helpful in some cases. This will allow detection of bacterial pathogens such as *Campylobacter* spp. and cysts of *Clostridium* spp. A sample is obtained by placing a moistened cotton swab in the rectum and gently rolling it a few times against the rectal mucosa. Alternatively, a gloved finger can be used to gently scrape the rectal mucosa.[7] The swab is then rolled onto a slide, air dried, and stained with an in-house stain, such as Diff-Quik. The slide should be examined for white blood cells, bacterial organisms, *Clostridium* spp. cysts, and fungal organisms. The presence of spores of *Clostridium* spp. has been suggested to implicate this organism as a cause of acute or chronic diarrhea,[9] but recent evidence suggests that the presence of spores is not specific for clostridial toxin-associated diarrhea.[10,11] Acid-fast staining of a fecal smear may detect the presence of *Cryptosporidium parvum*, appearing as a 4- to 6-μm diameter organism that will stain pink to red.[4] Fecal culture for specific pathogens, including *Salmonella* spp., *Campylobacter* spp., and *Yersinia* spp. may be warranted, especially in puppies or kittens, or when a rectal scraping reveals large numbers of neutrophils. In addition to these techniques, specific immunologic methods can be used to detect enteric pathogens. These tests include enzyme-linked immunosorbent assay (ELISA) testing for canine parvovirus, *Giardia* spp., *Cryptosporidium parvum*, and *Clostridium* spp. enterotoxins. Immunofluorescent assays are also available for detecting some of these pathogens. Although *Tritrichomonas foetus* usually causes a more chronic clinical picture, fecal culture or PCR testing for *Tritrichomonas foetus* may be warranted in some cats presenting for acute gastrointestinal signs.

For animals that are systemically ill, additional testing should include a CBC, serum biochemistry profile, urinalysis, and venous blood gas analysis. This will allow the clinician to look for extra-gastrointestinal causes of diarrhea, and to assess for metabolic, acid-base, and electrolyte abnormalities. Endocrine testing may be warranted, including a serum total T4 concentration in cats and an ACTH stimulation test in dogs that are suspected of having hypoadrenocorticism. Abdominal radiographs and ultrasound are low-yield test in dogs and cats with acute diarrhea. However, certain abnormalities may be detected such as peritonitis, intestinal intussusception, and partial obstruction. In these cases, vomiting usually accompanies the diarrhea.

2

🔑 Key Facts

- In cases with mild clinical signs, the diagnostic evaluation may be limited, and patients may require only outpatient symptomatic care.
- In animals with severe clinical signs, there may be severe electrolyte and acid-base disturbances, and a more thorough evaluation and in-patient care may be necessary.
- It is critical to distinguish vomiting versus regurgitation when obtaining the initial history, because the diagnostic and treatment approaches are vastly different.
- Acute vomiting and diarrhea can be caused by gastrointestinal and extra-gastrointestinal causes.
- Acute diarrhea is often self-limiting and may or may not require treatment. Often the etiology remains unknown.

References

1. Washabau RJ, Elie MS. Antiemetic therapy. In: Bonagura JD, Kirk RW (eds.), *Current Veterinary Therapy XII*. Philadelphia, WB Saunders, 1995; 679–684.
2. O'Brien TR, Biery DN, Park RD et al. *Radiographic diagnosis of abdominal disorders in the dog and cat*. Philadelphia, WB Saunders, 1978; 302–311.
3. Wallack ST. *The handbook of veterinary contrast radiography*. Solana Beach, California, 2003, 62–67.
4. Triolo A, Lappin MR. Acute medical diseases of the small intestine. In: Tams TR (ed.), *Handbook of small animal gastroenterology*. Philadelphia, WB Saunders, 2003; 195–210.
5. Guilford WG, Strombeck DR. Classification, pathophysiology, and symptomatic treatment of diarrheal disease. In: Guilford WG, Center SA, Strombeck DR et al (eds.), *Strombecks' Small Animal Gastroenterology, 3rd ed.* Philadelphia, WB Saunders, 1996; 351–366.
6. Lappin MR, Calpin JP. Laboratory diagnosis of protozoal infections. In: Greene CE (ed.), *Infectious diseases of the dog and cat, 2nd ed.* Philadelphia, WB Saunders, 1998; 437–441.
7. Matz ME, Guilford WG. Laboratory procedures for the diagnosis of gastrointestinal tract diseases of dogs and cats. *NZ Vet J* 2003; 51: 292–301.
8. Zajac AM, Johnson J, King SE. Evaluation of the importance of centrifugation as a component of zinc sulfate fecal flotation examinations. *J Am Anim Hosp Assoc* 2002; 38: 221–224.
9. Twedt DC. *Clostridium perfringens*-associated enterotoxicosis in dogs. In: Kirk RW, Bonagura JD (eds.), *Current Veterinary Therapy XI*. Philadelphia, WB Saunders, 1992; 602–604.
10. Marks SL, Melli A, Kass PH et al. Evaluation of methods to diagnose *Clostridium-perfringens*-associated diarrhea in dogs. *J Am Vet Med Assoc* 1999; 214: 357–360.
11. Cave NJ, Marks SL, Kass PH, et al. Evaluation of a routine diagnostic fecal panel for dogs with diarrhea. *J Am Vet Med Assoc* 2002; 221: 52–59.

2.2 Clinical Evaluation of Patients with Chronic Vomiting

JOHN V. DE BIASIO

2.2.1 Introduction

Vomiting is one of the most common problems for which dogs and cats are presented to their veterinarian. Vomiting is a complex physiological mechanism mediated by the emetic center located in the medulla. It is there that triggered input from abdominal viscera (e.g., secondary to inflammation, distension, chemical irritation, or osmolality shifts), CRTZ (e.g., secondary to toxins carried by the blood), semicircular canals of the vestibular apparatus, and cerebral cortex and limbic system (e.g., secondary to excitement, stress, fear, or increased intracranial pressure) are processed and ultimately result in a coordination of abdominal and visceral muscle contractions leading to the expulsion of material from the stomach and/or proximal small intestine.[1,2] Chronic vomiting is defined as persistent vomiting, either intermittent or continuous, of greater than ten days duration. The chronicity need not be the result of some insidious problem, but may be due to an acute problem unresponsive to initial therapy or for which therapy was never instituted. Chronic vomiting as a clinical sign can result from a multitude of different disease states and the clinical approach can be daunting as well as frustrating to both the veterinarian and the client alike (Table 2.3). Furthermore, the workup of this common problem can vary significantly based on the severity of the illness, availability of certain diagnostic modalities, and regional differences in disease prevalence. If vomiting has been occurring for months with no concurrent clinical signs, the diagnostic approach may be staged. If the patient has been vomiting frequently over a period of a few

2

Table 2.3: Causes of chronic vomiting

Drugs
- NSAIDs
- Antimicrobials (e.g., metronidazole)
- Many others (usually acute)

Gastrointestinal tract obstruction
- Gastric outflow obstruction
  - Benign pyloric stenosis
  - Foreign body
  - Gastric antral mucosal hypertrophy
  - Neoplasia
  - Chronic gastric malpositioning (GDV)
- Intestinal obstruction
  - Foreign body
  - Neoplasia
  - Cicatrix
  - Non-neoplastic infiltrative disease (e.g., pythiosis)
  - Intussusception
  - Adenomatous polyps (in cats)

Gastrointestinal Inflammation
- Inflammatory bowel disease
- Small intestinal bacterial overgrowth
- *Helicobacter* spp. infection
- Food hypersensitivity
- Food intolerance
- Chronic gastritis ± ulceration
- Bilious vomiting syndrome
- Parasitic – *Physaloptera* spp., *Ollulanus tricuspis,* Ascarids, *Giardia* spp., and *Aonchotheca putorii*
- Viral – FIV, FeLV, FIP virus
- Chronic colitis

Abdominal Inflammation
- Chronic peritonitis
- Chronic pancreatitis
- Cholecystitis

Endocrine Disorders
- Hypoadrenocortism
- Hyperthyroidism
- Diabetes mellitus

Metabolic Disorders
- Renal failure
- Hepatobiliary disease
- Hypercalcemia

Toxins
- Lead
- Zinc
- Plant toxins
- Grapes and raisins

Neurological
- Limbic epilepsy
- Neoplasia
- Meningitis / encephalitis
- Increased intracranial pressure
- Hydrocephalus
- Psychogenic
- Vestibular disease

Miscellaneous
- Abdominal steatitis
- Dysautonomia
- Feline heartworm disease
- Hiatal hernia
- Idiopathic delayed gastric emptying
- Idiopathic hypomotility
- Mast cell tumors
- Obstipation
- Overeating
- Sialoadenitis / sialoadenosis
- Others

weeks with concurrent weight loss, anorexia, and / or dehydration, a more aggressive approach is warranted so that a targeted treatment plan can be instituted as soon as possible. In the end, the workup of a patient with chronic vomiting requires the assimilation of data from the history, physical examination, and diagnostic testing to establish a diagnosis that permits a focused and specific management strategy. This chapter represents the view of the author on a rational systematic approach to the evaluation of a patient with chronic vomiting.

2.2.2   Initial evaluation

The first step in the investigation of virtually all clinical problems is a thorough history. With a patient presenting for chronic vomiting, it is essential to determine if the animal is in fact vomiting as opposed to regurgitating (Figure 2.1). Vomiting is usually preceded by nausea, which may be manifested by pacing, depression, lip licking, swallowing, salivation, and occasionally vocalization (cats). Retching, non-productive, rhythmic, abdominal contractions usually follow, culminating in the act of vomiting. In contrast, regurgitation occurs passively, with animals expelling tubular undigested food or foamy white liquid with little or no effort. Vomitus may contain bile pigment, while regurgitation should not. Both may look "digested" especially if regurgitated food has been retained in the

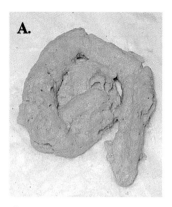
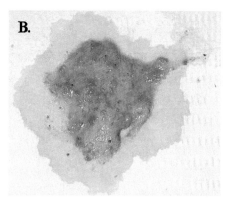

Figure 2.1:
Differentiation of vomiting and regurgitation. Panel **(A)** shows a classic example of regurgitated tubular undigested food. Panel **(B)** also shows an example of regurgitated material. However, in this case the food appears digested. Panel **(C)** shows bile-tinged vomitus. (Courtesy of Dr. Mike Willard, Texas A&M University, College Station, Texas.)

esophagus for a prolonged period of time, so this is not a reliable distinguishing characteristic.

Once it has been established that the animal has truly been vomiting, a more targeted historical investigation should be performed. First, a thorough dietary history should be obtained. It is especially important to question the owner for any evidence of dietary indiscretion, including ingestion of table scraps, garbage, foreign materials (including excessive amounts of hair), toxins, or plants (especially in cats). Questions concerning the consistency of the current diet or any dietary changes should also be asked. The content of the vomitus needs to be examined, looking for the presence of bile, undigested food, or clear liquid. Fresh or digested blood strongly suggests gastrointestinal ulceration; whereas, hair suggests the presence of trichobezoars or a motility disorder. Furthermore, the duration, frequency, and progression of the vomiting may also point to an underlying etiology. It is common for healthy cats to vomit occasionally up to once weekly; however, changes in the frequency or development of concurrent clinical signs such as anorexia warrant further investigation. It is also important to evaluate any temporal relationship between vomiting and eating. Although not pathognomonic, vomiting of undigested or partially digested food 8–10 hours after eating may indicate a gastric outflow obstruction or another gastric motility disorder.

It is also very important to determine what medications the animal is currently being given. Although most medications (e.g., antibiotics, chemotherapeutics, and digoxin) cause acute vomiting, they may play a role in chronic vomiting, especially if the connection between the two events is not made initially or the vomiting is mild and sporadic. Non-steroidal anti-inflammatory drugs (NSAIDs) and steroids, when used chron-

ically, can lead to chronic vomiting and hematemesis secondary to gastrointestinal ulceration, and thus, the potential use of these drugs should always be inquired of specifically.

Signalment and past history also can be extremely helpful. For example, a Miniature Schnauzer with previous bouts of pancreatitis may suggest another episode of pancreatitis. Finally, a thorough body systems review may also facilitate a diagnosis. The presence of concurrent clinical signs such as diarrhea, dyschezia, coughing, sneezing, polyuria, dysuria, anorexia, and lethargy all may provide important information, which not only may help to pinpoint the cause of the vomiting, but also to decide on how aggressive to pursue a diagnosis. Finally, inquiry into the patient's vaccination status, deworming schedule, and travel history may help in ruling out particular infectious diseases.

Also a "head to tail" physical examination building on the history can pick-up subtle abnormalities. The physical examination is essential for localizing the cause of the clinical signs and ascertaining the severity of disease. First, the body condition needs to be assessed, along with mentation and gait observed from a distance. Also, special attention should be paid to the presence of cranial abdominal pain or discomfort, a distended colon (especially in cats), linear foreign bodies caught around the base of the tongue (especially in cats), irregular or painful kidneys, organomegaly, thyroid nodules (in cats), abdominal masses, and other signs of systemic disease such as evidence of weight loss, dehydration, altered mentation, icterus, cardiac arrhythmias, mucous membrane pallor, pyrexia, or oral ulceration. Chronically vomiting dogs and cats are most often well hydrated; if the animal is vomiting frequently enough to become significantly dehydrated, the patient will usually present acutely. A digital rectal examination, especially to evaluate the

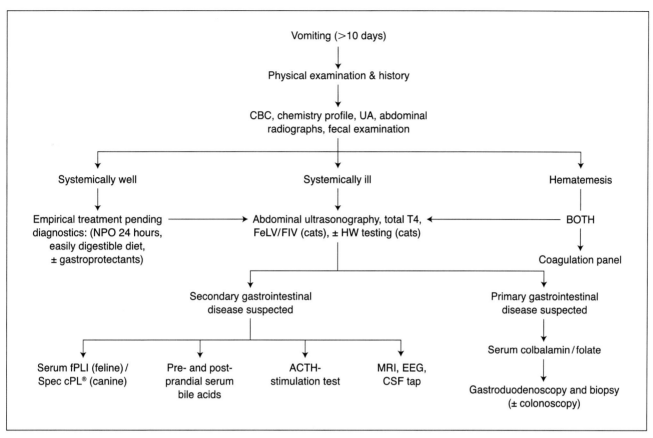

Figure 2.2:
Systematic diagnostic approach to patients with chronic vomiting. This figure shows a suggested systematic workup for dogs and cats with chronic vomiting. CBC = complete blood count; UA = urinalysis; FeLV = feline leukemia virus; FIV = feline immunodeficiency virus; HW = heartworm; NPO = nothing per os; MRI = magnetic resonance imaging; EEG = electroencephalogram; CSF = cerebrospinal fluid; ACTH = adrenocorticotrophic hormone; fPLI = feline pancreatic lipase immunoreactivity; Spec cPL® = canine pancreas-specific lipase.

feces for consistency and signs of occult bleeding, is also crucial. Neurological disease may lead to chronic vomiting and clinical signs of vestibular disease, such as a head tilt, ataxia, or nystagmus may be present. A complete neurological examination may be needed to detect more subtle central nervous system abnormalities. The combined findings from signalment, history, and physical examination allow the clinician to develop a complete clinical picture that will aid in formulating a list of differential diagnoses and necessary diagnostics.

2.2.3 Diagnostic approach (Figure 2.2)

The diagnostic approach to patients with chronic vomiting can vary greatly depending on the information obtained by signalment, history, and physical examination. If the animal has been receiving NSAIDs and now is vomiting blood, further

diagnostics may be indicated to simply aid in determining the severity of disease and guiding the therapeutic approach. Ideally, a minimum database should be obtained from all patients with chronic vomiting consisting of a CBC, serum biochemistry profile with electrolytes, urinalysis (UA), fecal analysis, and abdominal radiographs. In situations where results of these tests may not be readily available, a microhematocrit (PCV), total solids (TS), blood glucose, blood urea nitrogen, and if possible, a urine specific gravity can serve to guide the initial therapy. If the animal is systemically well with only mild intermittent vomiting, it is reasonable to stage the workup and treat empirically (e.g., NPO for 24 hours, easily digestible diet when food is reintroduced, ± gastroprotectants and antiemetics) pending the results of the initial diagnostic tests. Symptomatic therapy may lead to resolution of vomiting, especially if the underlying cause is transient or has been successfully removed (e.g., drugs or dietary indiscretion) and no further workup may be necessary.

A more aggressive approach is warranted in those patients in which vomiting has not resolved or that present systemically ill. All patients should have a basic screen for secondary causes of vomiting (e.g., endocrine, metabolic, infectious), as well as for complications of vomiting, such as alterations in acid–base and electrolyte status. This should consist of a CBC, serum biochemistry profile with electrolytes, UA, and FeLV/FIV testing in cats. Clinicopathological findings are often normal in animals with primary gastrointestinal disease. However, underlying renal, hepatic, or endocrine disease (e.g., hypoadrenocortism, diabetes mellitus) are often associated with specific changes. It is a common mistake not to obtain a baseline urinalysis prior to the initiation of therapy. As fluid therapy commonly plays a role in therapy, the utility of UA especially in the assessment of renal function will be greatly reduced if obtained after a significant amount of intravenous fluids have been administered. The serum total thyroxine (T4) concentration should also be measured in all cats older than 5 years of age. If possible, additional serum should be collected and frozen for future analysis. Finally, in animals presenting with hematemesis, a coagulation profile is warranted to screen for coagulation abnormalities, which may necessitate the administration of plasma.

A fecal examination, especially in patients with concurrent diarrhea, can also be useful in determining the presence of underlying gastrointestinal parasitism, particularly ascarids in young animals and giardia in cats. Both a direct fecal smear and flotation should be performed to look for evidence of eggs and protozoal cysts or organisms. However, it is important to note that standard flotation methods are rarely useful in identifying the presence of stomach worms (e.g., *Physaloptera* spp. and *Ollulanus tricuspis*). Diagnosis of these nematodes is most commonly accomplished using Baermann concentration of vomitus or gastroscopy.[3] Diagnosis of giardiasis can also be difficult with direct fecal microscopy or standard floatation alone. The gold standard in ruling out giardiasis is to obtain three negative zinc sulfate concentration centrifugations (ZSC) done on feces collected over a 3–5 day period. Commercial enzyme-linked immunosorbent assay kits to detect *Giardia* spp. antigen for use with dog and cat feces have a high specificity but lower sensitivity than the ZSC, and may serve as an alternative.[4]

Imaging studies can also be useful in the workup of a patient with chronic vomiting. Dogs and cats should first be screened by survey abdominal radiographs to look for signs of intestinal obstruction, constipation (especially in cats), foreign objects, masses, peritonitis, visceral displacement, and free abdominal fluid or gas.[5] A loop of small intestine dilated greater than twice the width of the central portion of the body of a lumbar vertebra or 3–4 times that of a rib in a dog suggests an obstructive or functional ileus.[6] Delayed gastric emptying may also be evident by detection of food retained in the stomach more than 12 hours after a meal.[5] In most patients with in-

flammatory diseases such as gastritis and IBD, routine abdominal radiographs are normal. Contrast radiography may reveal ulcers, subtle obstructions, or thickening of the gastric and/or enteric walls but has largely been replaced by the increasing use of ultrasonography and endoscopy. Abdominal ultrasound, alone or in combination with abdominal radiography, ideally should be performed in all cases where other diagnostics have failed to determine an underlying cause for the vomiting or for which a further investigation of abdominal viscera is indicated (e.g., abdominal mass visualized on radiographs, renal azotemia, increased liver enzymes, etc.). Ultrasonography may allow detection of hepatobiliary and pancreatic disease, evaluation of gastrointestinal wall thickness and peristaltic activity, characterization of obstructive lesions, and an investigation for abdominal masses. It may also facilitate fine needle aspiration to aid in the definitive diagnosis of abdominal masses, cystic lesions, and lymphadenopathy.

2.2.4 Secondary gastrointestinal disease

Many diseases can lead to secondary gastritis. Most secondary gastrointestinal diseases can be ruled in or out based on the aforementioned initial diagnostics. If a diagnosis still has not been made, further diagnostics may be needed for characterization of the cause of vomiting.

2.2.4.1 Hyperthyroidism

Approximately 40% of hyperthyroid cats may vomit chronically.[7] Hyperthyroidism in cats usually is ruled in or out after careful palpation of the neck, detection of concurrent clinical signs (e.g., weight loss, polyphagia, hyperactivity, and irritability), and determination of a serum total T4 concentration. An elevation in serum total T4 concentration is sensitive and almost 100% specific for hyperthyroidism.[7] In a small subset of cats, non-thyroidal illness may suppress the total T4 concentration into the high end of the normal range. Repeat testing after several weeks or measurement of a free T4 concentration (only reliable if measured by equilibrium dialysis) can help in patients still suspected of having hyperthyroidism.[8]

2.2.4.2 Hepatobiliary disease

Hepatobiliary diseases, such as hepatic failure and lipidosis, gall bladder mucoceles, cholangiohepatitis, cholecystitis, and portosystemic shunts, can also all cause chronic vomiting.[9,10,11] Dogs and cats with liver failure most commonly have additional clinical signs, such as anorexia, diarrhea, weight loss, and in cases of hepatic encephalopathy, neurological signs. A serum biochemistry profile may reveal increased serum hepatic enzyme activities and hyperbilirubinemia. With decreased functional liver capacity, serum urea nitrogen, cholesterol, or albumin concentrations may all be decreased. Hepatobiliary disease usually can be ruled out by the absence of these clinicopathological abnormalities. However, if a suspicion remains, other diagnostic tests, such as measurement of pre- and postprandial serum bile acids concentrations, abdominal radiographs and ultrasonography, and trans-colonic or splenic scintigraphy may be required. Ultimately, hepatic biopsy may be necessary to obtain a definitive diagnosis.

2.2.4.3　Renal failure

Renal failure, if resulting in uremic gastropathy, may lead to chronic vomiting in both dogs and cats. The most important parameters for ruling out renal failure are serum creatinine and urea nitrogen concentrations, and the specific gravity on UA. If suspected, renal ultrasound may provide further information about structural renal changes and help determine prognosis. In general, gastrointestinal signs from renal failure are present in the more severe and chronic cases.[12]

2.2.4.4　Hypoadrenocorticism

Hypoadrenocorticism is another potential cause of chronic vomiting in dogs (rarely in cats) and is commonly missed due to its ability to mimic other diseases. Dogs with hypoadrenocorticism may have intermittent anorexia, lethargy, vomiting, diarrhea, and/or weakness. Hyperkalemia and hyponatremia may be evident on a serum biochemistry profile with the sodium:potassium ratio usually less than 27:1. However, in dogs with a sole glucocorticoid deficiency, termed atypical Addison's disease, the serum electrolytes will be normal.[13] The lack of a stress leukogram in an ill animal or the less commonly found "reverse" stress leukogram (i.e., lymphocytosis and rarely eosinophilia) on a CBC should raise suspicion that glucocorticoid deficiency may be present. If there is any degree of suspicion of hypoadrenocorticism, an ACTH stimulation test should be performed.

2.2.4.5　Pancreatitis

Pancreatitis can also lead to chronic vomiting but most often is accompanied by other clinical signs (e.g., lethargy, anorexia, and/or diarrhea). Cats with pancreatitis are almost invariably anorexic, so other causes of vomiting should be suspected in cats that are still eating well.[14] If chronic pancreatitis is suspected, a combination of abdominal ultrasonography and species specific serum pancreatic lipase immunoreactivity concentration (Spec cPL® in dogs and fPLI in cats) should be evaluated.[15]

2.2.4.6　Heartworm disease

Finally, heartworm disease is an uncommon cause of chronic vomiting in cats. In one study of cats diagnosed with *Dirofilaria immitis* infections, 34% had a history of vomiting and 10% had vomiting as the main clinical sign without any concurrent signs of respiratory disease.[16] A combination of antibody and antigen testing is usually necessary to assess exposure and likelihood of heartworm infection given the overall low worm burden and the consequently low number of antigen-shedding females in cats.[17]

2.2.5　Primary gastrointestinal disease

Ruling out the vast majority of secondary gastrointestinal diseases with initial testing should greatly increase the suspicion of an underlying primary gastrointestinal disease process. When such a suspicion exists and abdominal imaging fails to reveal or fully characterize a cause of vomiting, additional investigation is indicated.

Gastric emptying disorders are fairly common causes of chronic vomiting and can be the result of either a mechanical obstruction (e.g., neoplasia, hyperplasia, or foreign bodies) or a functional disorder.[18] The latter may be associated with an underlying gastrointestinal disease process including infectious, inflammatory, or ulcerative disease. The diagnosis of a primary gastrointestinal motility disorder is one of exclusion. Accurate determination of abnormal gastric emptying is quite difficult and a number of techniques have been described (see 1.9). Radioscintigraphy is still considered the gold standard; however, ^{13}C-octanoic breath and blood tests have been described for the assessment of gastric emptying and may prove easier alternatives in the future.[19]

Ultimately, endoscopy is almost always indicated when a primary gastrointestinal cause of chronic vomiting is suspected (see 1.5). Endoscopy is one of the most reliable and cost-effective tools currently available for the evaluation of chronic vomiting, when secondary gastrointestinal diseases have been ruled out. Endoscopy is fast, safe, and minimally invasive. It allows visualization of mucosal lesions and acquisition of gastric and intestinal biopsies.[20] Endoscopy may reveal a cause of gastric outflow obstruction, such as antral pyloric mucosal hypertrophy, foreign bodies, or neoplasia. Erosive/ulcerative lesions, hemorrhage, lymphoid follicular hyperplasia, gastric fluid retention, and mucosal friability throughout the stomach may also be discovered. Gastric neoplasia (e.g., carcinoma, leiomyosarcoma, or lymphoma) or pythiosis may be associated with irregular masses or mucosal thickening, which can be biopsied for definitive diagnosis. However, scirrhous carcinoma may be difficult to biopsy as it leads to extreme thickening resulting in only superficial penetration of the biopsy forceps into the overlying mucosa. If unexplained gastric erosions, ulcers, large amounts of fluid, or mucosal hypertrophy are present, determining serum gastrin concentrations should be considered for the diagnosis of gastrinoma.

The role of *Helicobacter* spp. in gastritis and chronic vomiting is still uncertain in dogs and cats. However, if organisms are present in a chronically vomiting animal, where no other cause can be identified, specific therapy for eradication of *Helicobacter* spp. may be indicated. Gastric brush cytology is an effective way of looking for *Helicobacter* spp. and is more sensitive than the rapid urease test of biopsy samples. Ultimately, a diagnosis of spiral bacteria is best made by histological evaluation of gastric biopsy samples. Given the still unclear pathogenicity of the organism, no consensus exists on what treatment if any should be initiated if these organisms are identified.[21]

Finally, it is important to investigate the small intestine as well, even if vomiting is the only clinical sign. Inflammatory bowel disease is a common cause for vomiting in dogs and cats and may be missed if only gastric causes are explored. In some cats with inflammatory bowel disease, vomiting is the predominant clinical sign, with diarrhea being a minor disease component. If endoscopy is performed, biopsies should be obtained from the stomach and duodenum. Additionally, biopsies of the ileum and ascending colon may be useful as the primary disease process, such as gastrointestinal lymphoma, may be localized with mild to moderate inflammatory infiltration of the remainder of the gastrointestinal mucosa.

If a definitive diagnosis is still not made, an exploratory laparotomy should be considered; especially when serosal disease is suspected or when potentially surgically curable lesions are suspected.

🔑 Key Facts

- A thorough history and physical examination can be extremely helpful for the assessment of patients with chronic vomiting.
- Hyperthyroidism and heartworm disease can cause chronic vomiting in cats.
- Hypoadrenocortism can mimic many other diseases and should always be considered in cases of chronic vomiting, especially, but not exclusively, in patients with hyponatremia and hyperkalemia.
- Endoscopy is very useful and cost effective for the evaluation of chronic vomiting after secondary causes of vomiting have been ruled out.
- A common presenting clinical sign of dogs and cats with inflammatory bowel disease is chronic intermittent vomiting.

References

1. Ganong WF. Central regulation of visceral function. In: *Review of Medical Physiology*. New York, Magraw-Hill Co, 2005; 232–255.
2. Hall JA. Clinical approach to chronic vomiting. In: August JR (ed.), *Consultations in feline medicine, 3rd ed.* Philadelphia, WB Saunders, 1997; 61–67.
3. Broussard JD. Optimal fecal assessment. *Clin Tech Small Anim Pract* 2003; 18: 218–230.
4. Barr SC. Giardiasis. In: Greene CE (ed.), *Infectious diseases of the dog and cat.* St. Louis, Elsevier Inc, 2006; 736–742.
5. Kantrowitz B, Biller D. Using radiography to evaluate vomiting in dogs and cats. *Vet Med* 1992; 87: 806–813.
6. McNeel SV, Riedesel EA. The small bowel. In: Thrall DE (ed.), *Textbook of veterinary diagnostic radiology*. Philadelphia, WB Saunders, 1998; 540–560.
7. Feldman EC, Nelson RW. Feline hyperthyroidism (thyrotoxicosis). In: *Canine and feline endocrinology and reproduction*. Elsevier Science, St. Louis, 2004, 152–218.
8. Peterson ME. Diagnostic methods for hyperthyroidism. In: August JR (ed.) *Consultations in feline medicine, 5th ed.* St. Louis, Elsevier Inc, 2006; 191–198.
9. Center SA. Feline hepatic lipidosis, *Vet Clin North Am (Small Anim Pract)* 2005; 35: 225–269.
10. Pike FS, Berg J, King NW et al. Gallbladder mucocele in dogs: 30 cases (2000–2002). *J Am Vet Med Assoc* 2004; 224: 1615–1622.
11. Edwards M. Feline cholangiohepatitis. *Compend Contin Educ Pract Vet* 2004; 26: 855–862.
12. Peters RM, Goldstein RE, Erb HN et al. Histopathologic features of canine uremic gastropathy: A retrospective study. *J Vet Intern Med* 2005; 19: 315–320.
13. Feldman EC, Nelson RW. Hypoadrenocorticism (Addison's disease). In: *Canine and feline endocrinology and reproduction*. St. Louis, Elsevier Science, 2004; 394–439.
14. Washabau RJ. Feline acute pancreatitis: important species differences. *J Feline Med Surg* 2001; 3: 95–98.
15. Steiner JM. Is it pancreatitis? *Vet Med* 2006; 101: 158–167.
16. Atkins CE, DeFrancesco TC, Coats JR et al. Heartworm infection in cats: 50 cases (1985–1997). *J Am Vet Med Assoc* 2000; 217: 355–358.
17. Atkins CE, Litster AL. Heartworm disease. In: August JR (ed.), *Consultations in feline medicine, 5th ed.* St. Louis, Elsevier Inc, 2006; 323–330.
18. Washabau RJ. Gastrointestinal motility disorders and gastrointestinal prokinetic therapy. *Vet Clin North Am (Small Anim Pract)* 2003; 33: 1007–1028.
19. Wyse CA, McLellan J, Dickie AM et al. A review of methods for assessment of the rate of gastric emptying in the dog and cat: 1898–2002. *J Vet Intern Med* 2003; 17: 609–621.
20. Mansell J, Willard MD. Biopsy of the gastrointestinal tract. *Vet Clin North Am (Small Anim Pract)* 2003; 33: 1099–1116.
21. Leib MS, Duncan RB. Diagnosing gastric *Helicobacter* infections in dogs and cats. *Compend Contin Educ Pract Vet* 2005; 27: 221–228.

2.3　Clinical Evaluation of Patients with Chronic Diarrhea

Elias Westermarck

2.3.1　Introduction

Diarrhea is defined as the passage of feces containing an excess amount of water and is generally considered to be chronic or intermittent when it lasts for 2 or 3 weeks, at which time it is recommended that the problem be more thoroughly evaluated using specific diagnostic tests and in some cases therapeutic trials. Many clinicians rank the definitive diagnosis and management of chronic intermittent or chronic persistent diarrhea as one of the most challenging and frustrating aspects of their medical practice. There are no universally accepted recommendations on how to work up patients with chronic or intermittent diarrhea. Prevalences of different disorders vary in different countries, making it difficult to develop a common workup protocol for use throughout the world. However, general principles apply and should be used as a guideline for a systematic approach to patients with chronic diarrhea. As an example, the workup protocol used at the Faculty of Veterinary Medicine, University of Helsinki is represented in Figure 2.3. In patients with chronic diarrhea, every effort should be made to achieve a specific diagnosis in order to allow for specific therapy. Unfortunately, this can not always be achieved, in which case empirical therapeutic trials are employed. There are conflicting opinions on how long empirical therapy should be attempted. We recommend 10 days if dogs have chronic diarrhea or if the intervals between intermittent diarrheal episodes are only a few days. If signs of diarrhea disappear or are relieved during the empirical treatment period, the latter should be continued for at least 2–6 weeks. If the intervals between episodes in patients with intermittent diarrhea are long, for example more than one week, the length of the empirical treatment period should be prolonged.

The workup protocol for patients with chronic or intermittent diarrhea is applicable to most veterinary practices. Also, it is useful regardless of the presence of clinical signs that are typical for large- or small-intestinal disease. There is a high prevalence of diseases that can simultaneously affect the small and large intestines. Isolated colitis, which is a common condition in human beings, is uncommon in cats and rare in dogs.

2.3.2　General workup

2.3.2.1　Case history

It is essential to obtain a thorough case history in all patients (see 1.1). This is best accomplished by asking a series of broad-based questions. The most important questions cover the present condition as to the duration of clinical signs and their characterization. In addition, questions concerning the previous clinical history, including previous diagnoses and therapies, should always be asked. Finally, questions concerning travel and dietary history should be asked. Characterization of the stool may help to differentiate signs of small and large bowel diarrhea. Small bowel diarrhea is most often characterized by the presence of large quantities of soft-formed, bulky, or watery stools. Steatorrhea may also be evident. Chronic cases of small bowel diarrhea are also often accompanied by weight loss. In contrast, large bowel diarrhea most often is associated with a loose and stringy consistency due to increased mucus content. Streaks of fresh blood and tenesmus may also be present.

2.3.2.2　Physical examination

The physical examination should begin by observing the unrestrained patient on the floor. The animal's size, weight, mentation, posture, and behavior should be evaluated.

Abdominal palpation is an important part of the physical examination. Palpation must be systematic and the best sensitivity is afforded by alternating application and release of firm inward pressure on the abdomen by the fingers of both hands laid flat against the patient's abdomen. Raising the front end of the animal facilitates palpation of cranial abdominal organs. The intestines should feel soft, smooth, and should slide freely between the examiner's fingers.

A digital examination of the rectum is also important. The rectal examination also provides a stool sample, enabling evaluation of its consistency, color, and odor. Also, the fecal sample can be examined for any evidence of fresh blood, mucus, or melena.

2.3.2.3　Laboratory evaluation

Basic laboratory evaluation includes a CBC and a serum biochemistry profile comprising a minimum of blood urea nitrogen, creatinine, glucose, alanine aminotransferase (ALT), alkaline phosphatase (ALP), total protein, albumin, cholesterol, sodium, and potassium. In addition to general blood work aimed at identifying many secondary causes of chronic diarrhea, specific tests include the measurement of serum concentrations of trypsin-like immunoreactivity (TLI), pancreatic lipase immunoreactivity (PLI), folate, and cobalamin.

2

2.3.3 Division of patients according to the findings on initial evaluation

Patients are divided into two groups according to the case history findings, physical examination, and laboratory results (Figure 2.3). The first group includes patients that show clinical abnormalities in addition to the diarrhea (Group A), while the second group (Group B) does not show any obvious abnormalities except for diarrhea.

2.3.3.1 Patients with obvious abnormalities (A)

Systemic disorders with secondary diarrhea (A1a)

Several systemic diseases lead to secondary chronic diarrhea. Hepatic failure can lead to chronic diarrhea, and abnormally high serum ALT or ALP activities, bilirubin concentrations, or decreased serum albumin, cholesterol, or urea nitrogen concentrations should prompt a further workup. Renal failure can also lead to chronic diarrhea and elevations in serum creatinine and urea nitrogen concentrations may indicate the presence of renal failure. Hypoadrenocorticism in dogs can be associated with hyperkalemia and hyponatremia, but some patients do not have electrolyte abnormalities. The lack of a stress leukogram in a dog with chronic diarrhea should raise a suspicion of possible hypoadrenocorticism and should prompt the clinician to perform an ACTH stimulation test. Other systemic conditions, such as hypothyroidism in dogs and hyperthyroidism in cats can also lead to chronic diarrhea.

Exocrine pancreatic insufficiency (A1b)

Exocrine pancreatic insufficiency (EPI; see 8) is diagnosed by a severely decreased serum trypsin-like immunoreactivity (TLI) concentration (cTLI ≤2.5 µg/L in dogs and fTLI ≤8 µg/L in cats) in association with signs of maldigestion (i.e. polyphagia, weight loss, and/or yellowish loose feces). If the serum TLI concentration is in the questionable range (between 2.5–5.0 µg/L in dogs and between 8–12 µg/L in cats), the measurement should be repeated after approximately 1 month. Repeatedly low serum cTLI concentrations (<5.0 µg/L) have been shown to be highly suggestive of subclinical EPI in German Shepherd dogs and Rough-coated Collies.[1]

Hypoproteinemia (A1c)

Protein-losing enteropathy (PLE) refers to a group of disorders characterized by excessive loss of serum proteins into the gastrointestinal tract. A blood biochemistry profile reveals proportionately equal decreases in albumin and globulin concentrations, often with a total protein concentration <5.5 g/dl. Any number of conditions that lead to alimentary inflammation, infiltration, congestion, or bleeding can result in PLE. Biopsies obtained by endoscopy may reveal a specific etiology in some cases.

Melena and/or anemia (A1d)

Melena describes dark tarry stools, resulting from digested blood and usually originates from bleeding into the stomach or upper small intestine (i.e., ulcers, erosions, or tumors). Black stools can also result from lower small-bowel or upper large-bowel bleeding if the transit time for the blood is sufficiently slow. Microcytic, hypochromic anemia commonly occurs following prolonged gastrointestinal blood loss. Black feces can also rarely be found in normal animals consuming meat-based diets. It is, therefore, essential to take a thorough case history during the initial consultation. Endoscopic examination is necessary for detection of lesions of the upper GI tract that may result in bleeding.

Abnormal abdominal palpation (A1e)

The bowel, when infiltrated with inflammatory or neoplastic cells, may feel thickened upon abdominal palpation. Also, gastrointestinal masses, foreign bodies, and invaginations can sometimes be identified during abdominal palpation.

2.3.3.2 Patients with diarrhea without any other obvious abnormalities (B)

It is essential that the veterinarian explains to the pet owner that since no specific diagnosis has been obtained during the initial examination additional diagnostic tests will need to be performed in order to systematically rule out the different disorders that may cause chronic or intermittent diarrhea. During further workup, the pet owner is asked to evaluate daily the consistency of the feces using a fecal scoring system (Figure 2.4).[2] After every therapeutic trial period, the owner should inform the veterinarian of the patient's health status so that the clinician can plan how to proceed with the workup. Causative factors should be ruled out in the following order:

Endoparasites (B1)

Endoparasites can cause diarrhea and should be ruled out before initiating more complex diagnostic tests. They especially cause diarrhea in young dogs. In some areas, *Giardia* spp. is the most common parasite causing intermittent or chronic diarrhea. Endoparasites can be directly identified using zinc sulfate flotation. Also, *Giardia* antigen, produced by the trophozoites, may be detected in feces using commercially available ELISAs.

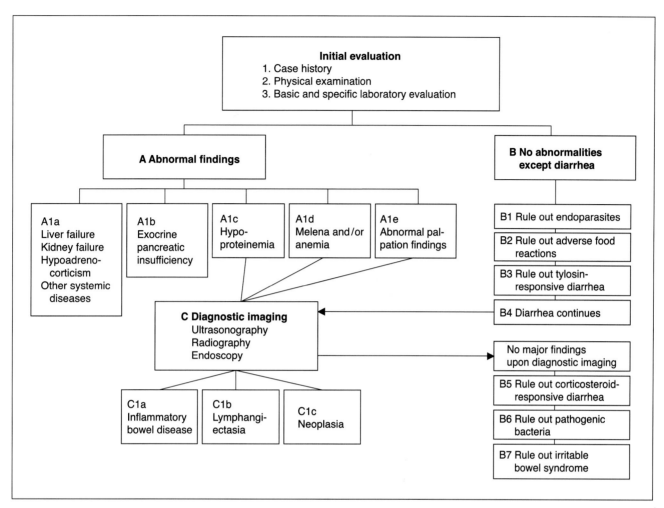

Figure 2.3:
Diagnostic approach for patients with chronic diarrhea. This figure shows the diagnostic approach to dogs and cats with chronic diarrhea as it is used at the Veterinary School in Helsinki, Finland.

Since false-negative results are not uncommon and the collection and examination of fecal samples are to some extent laborious, another option is to treat the patient with fenbendazole at 50 mg/kg q 24 h orally for 5 days, instead of examining fecal samples.

Adverse food reactions (B2)

Diet is probably the most common cause of diarrhea and should be excluded as a cause before empirical treatment trials with drugs are initiated. Potential dietary causes include a sudden change in diet, dietary indiscretion, dietary intolerance, dietary hypersensitivity, or food poisoning. Based on anamnestic data, it is often possible to draw conclusions on the importance of food as a potential cause of the diarrhea.

Opinions vary widely on how the diet should be changed for a dietary treatment trial. Unfortunately, current recommendations are largely based on anecdotal evidence rather than controlled trials. One possible recommendation is to change to a highly digestible, fat-restricted diet. Another possible recommendation is to use a diet with a single novel protein and a single novel carbohydrate source. Sometimes, changing canned food to dry food has a beneficial effect, as does changing a commercial diet to a homemade one. However, homemade diets are often incomplete and should not be fed long-term without consulting with a clinical nutritionist.

Fecal Scoring System

Score 1: Liquid

Liquid stool may not contain any particulate matter. Liquid stools are often deposited in multiple spots instead of a single stool. Liquid stool can also contain mucus or blood. A liquid stool sample is very difficult to collect and a residue is always left on surfaces and gloves.

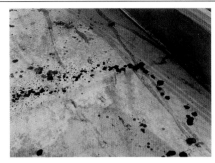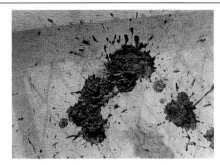

Fecal Score "1". Notice splattered appearance indicative of a liquid consistency. Also, note the large surface area of defecation.

Score 2: Soft, without shape

This stool is soft and does not show any cylindrical shape. Soft stool without shape is also often referred to as cow-patty stool. This stool will lose its original shape when collected and will leave a residue on surfaces and gloves. This stool score is often present with stool of another score, but can comprise the whole stool sample.

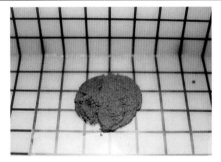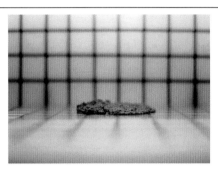

Fecal Score "2". This stool sample clearly appears soft and does not show any cylindrical shape. Notice the increased surface area of the sample, which is commonly referred to as a "cow-patty" appearance.

Score 3: Soft, with shape

This stool is soft, but still has a shape to it. This stool will break apart easily and will leave a residue on surfaces and gloves. The stool often loses the original shape after collection. Soft stool with shape is often present with stool of another score, but can comprise the whole stool sample.

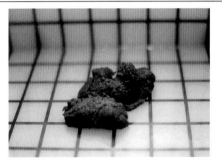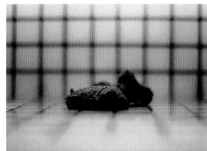

Fecal Score "3". This stool sample exhibits a soft appearance but still has shape to it.

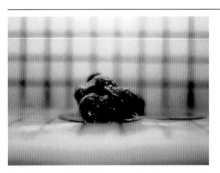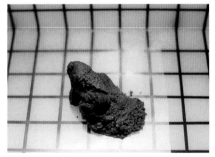

Fecal Score "3/1". Soft, shaped fecal material with a liquid portion.

Fecal Score "3/2". Portions of this stool sample are soft, but shaped, while other portions do not have any shape to it.

Figure 2.4:
Fecal scoring system. This figure shows an example for a scoring system that can be used by dog owners to evaluate fecal consistency (based on a scoring system used by the Iams Company, Dayton, OH, USA).

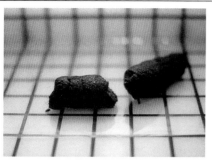 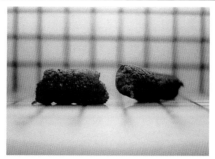

Score 4: Firm (ideal stool)

Firm stool is well shaped and cylindrical. This stool does not break apart easily when picked up, but may leave a residue on surfaces and gloves. Firm stool is often defecated as a single stool and maintains its original shape after collection.

Fecal Score "4". This sample exhibits the standard cylindrical shape. Also, notice the equal of the height of the whole stool sample.

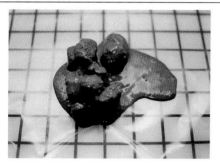 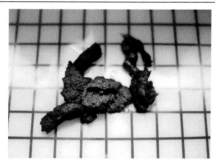 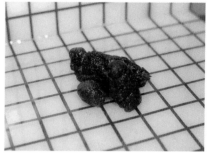

Fecal Score "4/1". This stool sample has portions with a cylindrical shape (score 4), but also contains a liquid portion (score 1).

Fecal Score "4/2". This stool sample shows a clear distinction between some dark cylindrical feces and some lighter and shapeless fecal material.

Fecal Score "4/3". This stool sample contains both cylindrical portions and areas that are softer and less well shaped.

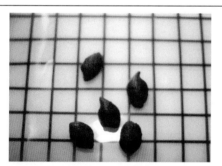 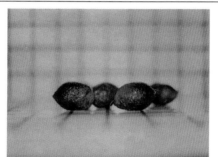

Score 5: Extremely dry

Extremely dry stool is hard and does not stick to surfaces. The stool will roll when pushed. No indentations are made when the stool is picked up and it maintains its original shape after collection. Extremely dry stool is often defecated as multiple fecal balls as opposed to a single stool.

Fecal Score "5". Please note multiple fecal balls as opposed to a single fecal log.

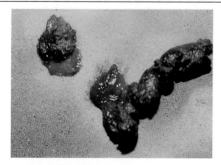

Additional Fecal Observation Codes

11- Blood in stool
15- Foreign object in stool
40- Mucus in stool

Fecal Score "Mucous". Stool of any score can be accompanied by mucus that can be clear or bloody. The mucus may cover the entire stool sample or only a small portion of it.

2

Tylosin-responsive diarrhea (B3)

Different antibiotics such as metronidazole, oxytetracycline, and doxycycline have been used for the treatment of chronic or intermittent diarrhea, and patients responding to such a therapeutic trial are retrospectively diagnosed with antibiotic-responsive diarrhea.

Tylosin is the antibiotic most commonly used for the treatment of chronic diarrhea in Finland. In a recent study, tylosin at 25 mg/kg orally once a day was shown to be effective for the treatment of chronic or intermittent diarrhea in dogs, and patients that responded were diagnosed with tylosin-responsive diarrhea (TRD).[2] Another study indicated that tylosin and a feeding regimen have synergic effects.[3] Dogs that will respond to tylosin treatment will usually do so within 3 days and diarrhea will remain absent as long as the treatment continues. In many dogs, diarrhea will reappear 1–2 weeks after discontinuation of therapy. The effect of tylosin does not appear to diminish even in dogs that have been treated for years and side effects are rarely encountered. The etiology of TRD remains unclear. Little is known about the effect of tylosin in cats with chronic or intermittent diarrhea.

Patients with persistent diarrhea (B4)

Since diagnostic imaging studies are not especially helpful in diagnosing food-related diarrhea or TRD, it is reasonable to perform these studies only after these two entities have been ruled out.

Corticosteroid-responsive diarrhea (B5)

Even if the findings upon diagnostic imaging studies, including histological examination of intestinal biopsies, are only mild or completely absent, it does not rule out the possibility that corticosteroids have a beneficial effect in a patient with chronic diarrhea. Inflammatory changes in the intestine may be localized or may be limited to the deeper layers of the gastrointestinal mucosa.

For empirical corticosteroid treatment, dogs are treated with prednisone at 1–2 mg/kg, twice daily. If side effects (e.g., severe polyuria/polydipsia, panting, or lethargy) are intolerable, other corticosteroids, such as budesonide, a locally active corticosteroid, have been recommended.

Pathogenic bacteria (B6)

Fecal culture, especially for *Salmonella* spp., *Campylobacter* spp., and *Yersinia* spp. is particularly indicated in animals that develop chronic diarrhea after being kenneled with other dogs.

However, it is important to remember that these pathogenic bacteria can sometimes also be found in healthy dogs. Clostridial organisms (*Clostridium perfringens* and *Clostridium difficile*) may also cause chronic diarrhea. However, a cause and effect relationship has not been definitively established. Immunoassays for enterotoxins produced by these organisms are commercially available.

Irritable bowel syndrome (B7)

Stress or psychological disturbances can cause intermittent diarrhea with interspersed periods of remission. The character of the disorder varies widely in different patients. Large breed dogs, especially those used as working dogs (i.e., racing or hunting dogs) and temperamental or easily excitable animals are predisposed. The best therapeutic results are achieved by avoiding stressful situations. If this is not possible, medical therapy using combinations of an anticholinergic and a central nervous system depressant such as clidinium-chlordiazepoxide (Librax) can be effective. If all treatment regimes fail, symptomatic treatment with opioid motility modifiers such as loperamide (Imodium) can be attempted.

2.3.4 Diagnostic imaging (C)

2.3.4.1 Abdominal ultrasonography (see 1.3)

Abdominal ultrasonography is used for evaluating the thickness of the gastrointestinal wall and for guiding the clinician in examining and aspirating abdominal masses and infiltrated organs.

2.3.4.2 Endoscopy (see 1.5)

Gastrointestinal endoscopy allows visualization and sampling of the mucosa from stomach, duodenum, terminal ileum, colon, and rectum. Endoscopy can be used to identify lesions such as ulcers, erosions, inflammation, and lymphangiectasis.

2.3.4.3 Abdominal radiography (see 1.3)

Survey abdominal radiographs and contrast radiography are rarely useful for the diagnosis of an underlying cause in patients with chronic diarrhea. Radiography is, however, helpful in revealing masses and foreign bodies, if present.

Inflammatory bowel disease (C1a; see 9.2)

Intestinal biopsies are required for definitive diagnosis of this disorder. The term inflammatory bowel disease (IBD) refers to a diverse group of chronic enteropathies characterized by idiopathic infiltration of the gastrointestinal mucosa and sometimes the submucosa with inflammatory cells. Infiltrations of either single-cell or mixed-cell populations may be seen. Often, one or two cell types predominate (e.g., in eosinophilic or lymphoplasmacytic enteritis and/or colitis).

Intestinal lymphangiectasia (C1b; see 5.3.9)

Intestinal lymphangiectasia is an obstructive disorder of the intestinal lymphatic system. There are many potential causes of lymphatic obstruction, but in most cases lymphangiectasia is idiopathic. Yorkshire Terriers, Norwegian Lundehunds, and Soft-coated Wheaten Terriers appear to be predisposed. Hypoalbuminemia, hypocholesterolemia, and lymphopenia are common findings. Results obtained upon histological examination of intestinal biopsies often show typical changes. In some circumstances, full-thickness biopsies are needed.

Gastrointestinal neoplasia (C1c)

Lymphosarcoma and adenocarcinoma are the most common intestinal tumors in dogs. Clinical signs usually include weight loss, anorexia, diarrhea, melena, vomiting, and abdominal discomfort. Ultrasound is most useful for evaluating intestinal thickness and aids in revealing non-palpable masses.

⌨ Key Facts

- The etiology of chronic diarrhea in dogs and cats often remains unclear.
- In order to monitor the progress in a patient with chronic diarrhea, it is important that the pet owner daily evaluates the consistency of the feces using a fecal scoring system.
- Diet-related diarrhea should be excluded before treatment trials with drugs are initiated.
- Tylosin can be effective in resolving chronic diarrhea in dogs.

References

1. Westermarck E, Wiberg M. Exocrine pancreatic insufficiency in dogs. *Vet Clin Small Anim* 2003; 33: 1165–1179.
2. Westermarck E, Skrzypczak T, Harmoinen J et al. Tylosin-responsive chronic diarrhea in dogs. *J Vet Intern Med* 2005; 19: 177–186.
3. Westermarck E, Frias R, Skrzypczak T. Effect of diet and tylosin on chronic diarrhea in Beagles. *J Vet Intern Med* 2005; 19: 822–827.

2.4 Clinical Evaluation of Patients with Chronic Weight Loss

Terry L. Medinger

2.4.1 Introduction

A patient presented with the sole complaint of unexplained weight loss can present a significant diagnostic challenge. Obtaining a complete and detailed history in conjunction with performance of a comprehensive physical examination is imperative. Properly performed, these basic clinical tasks will often allow a diagnosis in an expedient and efficient manner. The astute clinician will also realize that clients may unintentionally omit potentially important historical information. The use of probing questions will minimize this occurrence.

Weight loss is considered clinically significant when it equals or exceeds 10% of the patient's normal body weight. Emaciation is defined as a loss of greater than 20% of normal body weight and cachexia, the most advanced state of weight loss, is characterized by severe weakness, anorexia, and an altered mental state.

2.4.2 Pathophysiology

The variety of medical disorders capable of presenting with weight loss as the chief complaint is vast and the ability to obtain a diagnosis can seem daunting. Fundamentally, weight loss occurs when the metabolic demand for energy or the loss of nutrients exceeds energy intake. By keeping this principle in mind, one can systematically and methodically rule out potential causes and achieve the correct diagnosis in most cases.

Inadequate energy intake may occur as a result of feeding an inferior diet containing nutrients of low bioavailability. Alternatively, the patient may not be ingesting a sufficient amount of calories to meet their maintenance energy requirements (MER).[1]

- **Dogs:** MER (metabolizable kcal/day) = $2 [70(wt_{kg}^{0.75})]$.
- **Cats:** MER (metabolizable kcal/day) = $1.4 [70(wt_{kg}^{0.75})]$.

Another cause for weight loss is nutrient malassimilation that can be caused by anorexia, regurgitation, dysphagia, vomiting, maldigestion, or malabsorption. All of these conditions may prevent sufficient caloric intake to meet the patient's energy requirements.

Increased loss of nutrients occurs with disorders such as PLE, PLN, gastrointestinal bleeding, glucosuria (e.g., diabetes mellitus), or in burn victims experiencing extensive loss of protein-rich exudate from skin injuries.

Finally, weight loss may be caused by increased energy utilization due to hypermetabolic states, such as feline hyperthyroidism or due to neoplastic diseases.

2.4.3 Etiology

Determining the underlying cause of weight loss may prove to be challenging and elusive, testing the skills of even the most experienced clinician. Generating a list of differential diagnoses based upon the history and physical examination findings will enable the clinician to proceed in a logical manner.

Firstly, it must be determined whether the weight loss occurred acutely or gradually. Acute weight loss typically occurs secondary to an increased demand for energy or as a result of massive nutrient loss. In both situations, the quantity of energy intake is insufficient to meet the patient's needs.

Secondly, the patient's appetite during the course of the weight loss needs to be established. If the patient is inappetent, it must be established if the inappetence is episodic or ongoing. If episodic, the duration of each episode, the interval between episodes, and the progressiveness of the episodes need to be established. Specifically, it should be determined if the frequency and duration of each inappetence episode is increasing and the time interval between episodes is decreasing.

Causes of weight loss accompanied by inappetence include intestinal disorders (e.g., gastrointestinal ulceration, neoplasia, or IBD), infectious disorders (e.g., pyometra, septicemia, pneumonia, or systemic fungal infections), inflammatory disorders (e.g., immune-mediated disorders or pancreatitis), disorders of the oral cavity (e.g., neoplasia, foreign bodies, uremia-induced oral ulceration, gingivitis, or glossitis), hypoadrenocorticism, cardiac disorders, and various systemic disorders (e.g., renal, hepatic, pancreatic, or neoplastic disorders). Dietary-related issues can also be a factor. Feeding a diet of low palatability or a diet that has spoiled may cause inappetence with accompanying weight loss.

Weight loss occurring in a polyphagic patient may indicate a hypermetabolic state with an increased energy demand. Examples of this include feline hyperthyroidism and neoplasia prior to the onset of anorexia and the cancer cachexia syndrome.[2,3] If the weight-loss patient is febrile, a state of hypercatabolism may exist. Alternatively, the patient may have an increased physiological energy requirement as occurs during gestation, lactation, growth, or strenuous exercise. It should also be remembered that the MER is calculated for a thermoneutral environment. Extreme variations in temperature (i.e., extreme cold or heat) will increase the MER.

Weight loss maybe accompanied by polyphagia and may occur secondary to excessive loss of energy. This situation occurs in disorders such as PLE, PLN, or diabetes mellitus. Protein-losing enteropathies occur when the small intestine is severely diseased resulting in protein leakage into the intestinal lumen. The cause is either one of severe mucosal disease causing increased permeability or defective lymphatic drainage, or a combination of both. When the rate of gastrointestinal protein loss exceeds protein synthesis, hypoproteinemia ensues. Lymphangiectasia is a common cause of PLE. Primary lymphangiectasia is an idiopathic disorder of the lymphatic system in which the normal absorption and flow of lymph is impeded.[4,5] Secondary lymphangiectasia develops in adult animals. The lymph stasis occurs secondary to obstructive lesions. This can be a local phenomenon as is the case in patients with infiltrative intestinal diseases, such as severe IBD or alimentary lymphoma (LSA) or as a result of the development of lipogranulomas within and around the lymphatics.[6,7] Additionally, IBD and alimentary LSA can also cause PLE through small intestinal mucosal injury. Alternatively, systemic venous hypertension resulting from right-sided heart failure can cause lymphatic stasis by interference of normal flow of lymph into the venous circulation.

Protein-losing nephropathy results from disruption of the glomerular filter. The most common glomerular diseases resulting in PLN are glomerulonephritis (GN), glomerulosclerosis, and amyloidosis.

Glucosuria also creates a state of increased energy loss. The most common cause of glucosuria is diabetes mellitus. The weight loss associated with diabetes mellitus is multifactorial in origin but is, in part, caused by loss of glucose in the urine. Glucosuria can also occur during disorders of the proximal renal tubules, such as Fanconi Syndrome or congenital primary renal glucosuria.

Nutrient malassimilation may result from gastrointestinal disorders. Documented causes include IBD, small intestinal bacterial overgrowth (SIBO), EPI, neoplasia, and endoparasitism. Additionally, the feeding of a low quality diet with diminished nutrient bioavailability may prevent proper nutrient assimilation.

It should also be considered that the client may not view the historical occurrence of infrequent or subtle gastrointestinal signs as relevant. These signs may include occasional bouts of vomiting, diarrhea, flatulence, borborygmus, abdominal pain (e.g., assuming the prayer position or walking with a hunched back), belching, or pica. If gastrointestinal signs are present, once again it should be established if the occurrence is episodic or continuous in nature. Also, it should be determined if the patient is clinically normal with the exception of periods when gastrointestinal signs are present or if coexisting clinical signs such as lethargy or weakness are also present.

If diarrhea is present, it should be further classified and worked up (see 2.1.3 and 2.3).

Establishing if pyrexia is present further narrows the list of differential diagnoses. The causes of weight loss accompanied by fever belong to one of the following categories: inflammatory, infectious, immune-mediated, or neoplastic.

Inflammatory and infectious disorders that can cause weight loss include pancreatitis, viral infections such as canine distemper virus (CDV), FIP, FeLV, and FIV accompanied by secondary infectious or neoplastic disorders. Chronic bacterial infections that can cause weight loss include pyelonephritis, endocarditis, and pneumonia. Patients with chronic infections with obligate intracellular parasites such as the various species of rickettsial and ehrlichial organisms also can present with weight loss. Histoplasmosis, coccidioidomycosis, cryptococcosis, and blastomycosis are systemic fungal infections, which may present with fever and weight loss as well as a variety of other clinical signs.

Patients with immune-mediated disorders such as systemic lupus erythematosus (SLE), rheumatoid arthritis, and immune-mediated polyarthropathy may also present with fever and weight loss.

Alimentary LSA, adenocarcinoma, and leiomyosarcoma are the most common primary malignant neoplastic diseases of the intestines.[8–11] Primary intestinal neoplasia and intestinal metastatic disease may both lead to weight loss. The weight loss may result from neoplasia-induced malassimilation of nutrients or may be the result of the cancer cachexia syndrome.

Metabolic disorders resulting in weight loss typically involve one or more major organs, including the kidneys, liver, or pancreas. The biochemical and systemic consequences of uremia include renal secondary hyperparathyroidism, metabolic acidosis, anemia, oral and gastric ulceration, proteinuria, and systemic hypertension, all of which have the potential to contribute to weight loss. Hepatic disorders that can potentially cause weight loss include inflammatory (e.g., cholangiohepatitis and chronic active hepatitis), infectious (e.g., canine adenovirus, leptospirosis), neoplastic (primary or metastatic), and vascular (congenital or acquired) diseases. Pancreatic diseases that can cause weight loss include inflammatory (e.g., acute or chronic pancreatitis), neoplastic, and exocrine and endocrine insufficiency.

Various cardiac abnormalities can induce weight loss. The occurrence of this is referred to as the cardiac cachexia syndrome.[12] Infectious (e.g., endocarditis), inflammatory (e.g., myocarditis or idiopathic pericarditis), neoplastic (primary or metastatic), parasitic (e.g., *Dirofilaria immitis*, *Borrelia burgdorferi*, or *Trypanosoma cruzi*) and various forms of primary myocardial dysfunction can induce the cardiac cachexia syndrome.

2.4.4 Diagnosis

The medical history should include information related to the patient's diet as well as travel history of the patient and other household pets. Any available medical information on the patient's parents or siblings could also prove helpful.

The dietary history should include major dietary components and whether the diet is commercially formulated or home made. Also, the type and quantity of any treats, commercial or table scraps, should be determined. The storage conditions and expiration date of any commercial diet should be noted. If the clinician is unfamiliar with a particular diet, the label indicating the dietary ingredients should be reviewed. It should also be determined if the patient is receiving any dietary supplements or medications. This includes commercially available, holistic, over-the-counter, or prescription medications. This information may help establish if a nutritionally imbalanced diet or a drug interaction is a potential cause for the weight loss. In certain situations, consultation with a veterinary phar-

2

macist, nutritionist, or a veterinarian certified in the practice of complementary medicine may be necessary.

Obtaining an accurate travel history of the patient and housemates is important when infectious diseases are being considered. Diseases indigenous to an area of travel should be identified. This component of the history should also include if the patient has access to the outdoors and, if so, determine if it is in an enclosed area or free roaming. It should also be determined if the patient frequents local parks, has access to bodies of water, and if the potential exists for contact with local wildlife giving consideration to endemic diseases.

Ascertaining previous episodes of ectoparasitism is important especially in areas where tick-borne diseases are endemic. Also, it should be noted whether other pets are kept in the household, especially exotic species and their complete medical history should be recorded. The vaccination and heartworm status of all household pets and preventative measures for ecto- and endoparasitism, including *Dirofilaria immitis*, should also be recorded

If the diagnosis is not apparent after obtaining the signalment and history and performing a thorough physical examination, a minimum data base should be obtained. This includes a CBC, serum biochemistry profile, urinalysis, and feces for floatation and direct smear examination.

Further diagnostics could include fecal assays for the presence of *Giardia* organisms and *Clostridium* enterotoxin, and cytologic examination of a rectal scraping. Finding a suppurative response on cytologic examination of the rectal scraping would support bacterial culture of the feces for specific enteropathogenic organisms. Malignant lymphocytes may be identified suggestive of alimentary LSA. Fungal or algae organisms may be detected indicating systemic infection. A rectal scraping is safe, non-invasive, inexpensive, and easy to perform. Additionally, a presumptive diagnosis can often be made following cytologic examination by the clinician.

Additional tests may include bacterial culture of a urine sample and quantification of the urine albumin concentration. Based on these results more specific tests can be ordered. Depending upon the clinical data of the specific patient, these may include thoracic and abdominal radiographs, a cardiac evaluation (i.e., echocardiogram, ECG), abdominal ultrasound with performance of a fine needle aspiration or a biopsy procedure if indicated, or determining the function of organs such as the liver (see 1.4.3), pancreas (see 1.4.4), adrenal gland (ACTH stimulation test), or kidney (nuclear scintigraphy). Detection of gastrointestinal disease may require determination of serum cobalamin and folate concentrations (1.4.2), fecal alpha-1-protease inhibitor (α_1-PI) concentrations (1.4.2), or endoscopic examination of the gastrointestinal tract with tissue samples obtained for cytological and histopathological examination (see 1.7 and 1.8).

🔑 Key Facts

- Obtaining a complete and detailed history in conjunction with performance of a thorough and comprehensive physical examination is imperative.
- Weight loss occurs when the metabolic demand for energy or the loss of nutrients exceeds energy intake.
- Weight loss is considered clinically significant when it equals or exceeds 10% of the patient's normal body weight.

References

1. *Nutrient Requirements of Dogs.* Washington DC, National Academy of Sciences, 1985; 1–79.
2. Ogilvie GK. Alterations in metabolism and nutritional support for veterinary cancer patients: Recent advances. *Comp Cont Ed Prac Vet* 1993; 15: 925–937.
3. Sigal RK, Daly JM. Enteral nutrition in the cancer patient. In: Rombeau JL, Caldwell MD (eds.), *Clinical Nutrition: Parenteral Nutrition.* Philadelphia, WB Saunders, 1992; 263–275.
4. Sherding RG. Canine intestinal lymphangiectasia. *Proc ACVIM* 1988; 406–408.
5. Mattheeuws D, De Rick A, Thoonen H et al. Intestinal lymphangiectasia in a dog. *Small Anim Pract* 1974; 15: 757–761.
6. Meschter CL, Rakich PM, Tyler DE. Intestinal lymphangiectasia with lipogranulomatous lymphangitis in a dog. *J Am Vet Med Assoc* 1987; 190: 427–430.
7. Van Kruiningen HJ, Lees GE, Hayden DW. Lipogranulomatous lymphangitis in canine intestinal lymphangiectasia. *Vet Pathol* 1984; 21: 377–383.
8. Cotchin E. Some tumors of dogs and cats of comparative veterinary and human interest. *Vet Rec* 1959; 71: 1040–1050.
9. Head KW. Tumors of the lower alimentary tract. *Bull WHO* 1976; 53: 167–186.
10. Birchard SJ, Couto CG, Johnson S. Nonlymphoid intestinal neoplasia in 32 dogs and 14 cats. *J Am Anim Hosp Assoc* 1986; 22: 533–537.
11. Bruecker KA, Withrow SJ. Intestinal leiomyosarcoma in six dogs. *J Am Anim Hosp Assoc* 1988; 24: 281–284.
12. Freeman LM. The role of cytokines in cardiac cachexia. *Proc 14th Ann Vet Med Forum* 1996; 240–242.

Part II

Diseases of the Gastrointestinal Tract

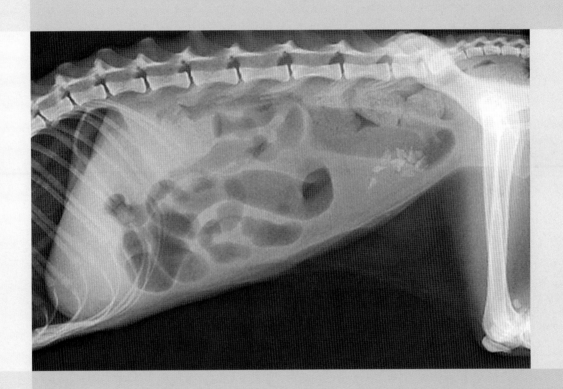

3 Esophagus

3.1 Anatomy[1,2]

LISA E. MOORE

The esophagus is the connection between the oropharynx and the stomach; the major function of which is to carry ingested material from the oral cavity to the stomach. The esophagus is divided into a cervical, thoracic, and abdominal portion. It begins at the upper esophageal sphincter (pharyngoesophageal sphincter), which is comprised of the cricopharyngeus and thyropharyngeus muscles. The cervical portion of the esophagus lies dorsally and to the left of the trachea. The thoracic portion of the esophagus extends from the thoracic inlet to the diaphragmatic hiatus. It lies dorsal to the trachea at the carina, where it then crosses the midline and lies to the right of the aortic arch. From here, it lies very close to the median plane as it passes between the caudal lung lobes. The short terminal portion of the esophagus lies in the abdominal cavity between the diaphragm and stomach.

The esophagus has several layers: adventitia, muscularis, submucosa, and mucosa. In the dog, the muscular layer is comprised of two oblique layers of striated muscle in the form of spiral fibers. These continuous oblique bundles spiral around the esophagus and cross each other at right angles, thus making up the two main muscular layers. About 5–10 cm from the cardia, the muscle fibers of the inner layer become more transverse while those of the outer layer become more longitudinal. The gastroesophageal sphincter is comprised of an outer layer of longitudinal striated muscle and an inner layer of circular smooth muscle. These longitudinal striated fibers continue and partially blend with some of the gastric smooth muscle fibers. In the cat, the muscular layer cranial to the base of the heart is comprised of striated muscle, whereas caudal to the heart it is comprised of smooth muscle. The gastroesophageal sphincter in the cat is comprised solely of smooth muscle.

The submucosal layer loosely attaches the mucosal and muscular layers, and contains mucus glands. In the dog, this loose connection allows the relatively inelastic mucosal layer to be thrown into longitudinal folds. In the cat, the mucosal layer contains longitudinal and transverse folds from the level of the heart base distally. This combination of longitudinal and transverse folds gives the mucosal layer of the esophagus of the cat its characteristic "herringbone" pattern (Figure 3.1). The mucosal layer is comprised of cornified, stratified squamous epithelium, which contains openings of the ducts belonging to the submucosal glands.

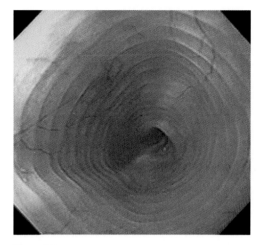

Figure 3.1:
Normal feline esophagus. Endoscopic view of a normal feline distal esophagus showing the "herringbone" pattern of the mucosal folds. (Image courtesy of Dr. David Twedt, Colorado State University, Ft. Collins, CO.)

Branches of the cranial and caudal thyroid arteries serve as blood supply to the cervical portion of the esophagus. The esophageal portion of the bronchoesophageal artery supplies the cranial two-thirds of the thoracic portion of the esophagus, the remaining third being supplied by branches of the dorsal intercostal arteries. The terminal portion of the esophagus is supplied by a branch of the left gastric artery. Venous drainage occurs via satellites of the arteries that supply it. These veins mostly empty into the azygos vein. Lymphatic vessels from the esophagus drain into various lymph nodes including the retropharyngeal, mediastinal, bronchial, and portal nodes. Lymphatics and lymphatic vessels of the esophagus lie in the submucosal layer.

The striated muscle of the upper esophageal sphincter and esophageal body are innervated by branches of the vagus nerve. The vagus nerve also contains autonomic nerves to the smooth muscle and visceral afferents from sensory receptors. Sensory innervation distributes to the spinal segments C1–L2 with the cervical portion reaching segments C2–C6 and T2–T4, the thoracic portion reaching segments T2–T4 and T8–T12, and the lower esophageal sphincter reaching segment T1–L3. Sympathetic nerves also innervate the esophagus.

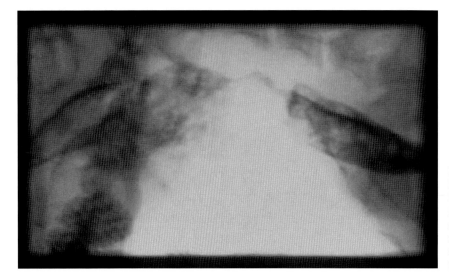

Figure 3.2:
Fluoroscopy of a dog with cricopharyngeal achalasia. Fluoroscopic image of a 6-year-old castrated male mixed-breed dog with adult-onset cricopharyngeal achalasia. The head is to the left. Note the barium remaining in the pharynx after repeated attempts at swallowing. The upper esophageal sphincter fails to relax and allow the barium to pass.

3.2   Physiology[3,4,5]

Swallowing, or deglutition, is a sequence of well-coordinated events to carry ingested material from the mouth to the stomach. Three phases have been described. The first or oropharyngeal phase begins with the prehension of food and the formation of a bolus in the oropharynx, which is then passed to the base of the tongue. This bolus stimulates a series of pharyngeal contractions that move the bolus into the laryngopharynx. At this time, the other pharyngeal openings are closed (the oral cavity, the nasopharynx, and the opening to the trachea) by the actions of various muscle groups and movement of the tongue. These reflex events are initiated by stimulation of various sensory receptors in the laryngopharynx, the nerve fibers of which are located in branches of the trigeminal, glossopharyngeal, and laryngeal nerves. Once the bolus of ingested material is in the oropharynx, the cricopharyngeal and thyropharyngeal muscles relax to allow passage of the bolus into the cranial esophagus. This sphincter closes promptly after passage of the bolus and remains closed at all other times. Once the bolus has passed into the esophagus, the second, or esophageal, phase of swallowing begins. The peristaltic wave that started in the pharynx continues and is propagated throughout the esophagus carrying the bolus aborally to the stomach. This peristaltic wave is termed primary peristalsis. A secondary peristaltic wave can be generated via local esophageal distension to carry out the passage of the bolus into the stomach if the primary wave is inadequate. The third and final phase of swallowing is the relaxation of the gastroesophageal sphincter (GES), which allows passage of the bolus into the stomach. The GES then contracts again to prevent reflux of material back into the esophagus.

Swallowing is mediated by a long and complex neural arc. The reflex response is triggered by sensory receptors in the esophagus via visceral afferent fibers in the trigeminal, vagus, and glossopharyngeal nerves. These impulses are integrated in the nucleus solitarius and the nucleus ambiguus, as well as the swallowing center in the lateral reticular formation. The efferent neurons from the dorsal vagal motor nucleus pass to the pharyngeal and esophageal musculature via the trigeminal, facial, glossopharyngeal, vagus, and the hypoglossal nerves.

3.3   Diseases of the Esophagus

3.3.1   Cricopharyngeal achalasia

Cricopharyngeal achalasia or dysphagia is a disorder characterized by failure of the pharyngoesophageal sphincter (upper esophageal sphincter) to relax during the first phase of swallowing.[6,7] The etiology and pathogenesis of this disease are unknown. The disease has been documented in a number of dog breeds.[8,9] Affected animals have difficulty swallowing, characterized by multiple attempts to swallow and food falling from the mouth. Regurgitation can also be seen as well as nasopharyngeal reflux of ingesta, ptyalism, coughing, gagging, and weight loss. Most dogs show clinical signs from birth, but they may also occur spontaneously in older animals. Older animals often have concurrent acquired disorders such as myasthenia gravis, laryngeal paralysis, or esophageal stricture.[9] Physical examination may reveal a poor body condition, but will likely be unremarkable unless concurrent disease is present. Diagnosis requires the use of contrast videofluoroscopy (Figure 3.2).[6–9] Fluoroscopy shows multiple, unproductive attempts at swallowing. A bolus is formed, but does not pass into the esophagus despite numerous attempts. Eventually, small boluses may be passed into the esophagus.

Most patients diagnosed with this disorder are treated with cricopharyngeal myectomy with relatively good success.[7–9] Patients generally experience immediate relief after surgery. Aspiration pneumonia, if present, should be treated as necessary.

3.3.2 Esophagitis

Esophagitis is an acute or chronic inflammatory disorder of the esophageal mucosa. If severe, esophageal inflammation may extend into the submucosal and muscular layers. Esophagitis can result from ingestion of corrosive or caustic substances, foreign body obstruction, thermal burns, infectious agents, persistent vomiting, and probably most commonly, gastroesophageal reflux (GER).[9–14] The esophageal mucosa has a barrier function to prevent damage by various substances, including gastric acid. This barrier function is provided by the stratified squamous epithelium, tight junctions between the epithelial cells, the mucus layer, prostaglandin production, surface bicarbonate ions, and peristaltic clearance of material from the esophagus.[15]

The clinical signs are often related to the severity and depth of inflammation. Characteristic signs include dysphagia, ptyalism, regurgitation, gagging, varying degrees of inappetence, repeated swallowing motions with extension of the head and neck, odynophagia, lethargy, and weight loss.[11,13,14] The physical examination is often unremarkable, but may show evidence of aspiration pneumonia (i.e., fever and/or increased lung sounds). Diagnostics generally include a minimum database (CBC, serum chemistry profile, urinalysis, and thoracic and/or abdominal radiographs), which is generally unremarkable. The CBC may show a leukocytosis if severe esophagitis or aspiration pneumonia is present. A barium esophagram performed under fluoroscopy may show GER, segmental dilation of the esophagus, an irregular esophageal mucosa, and/or decreased esophageal motility.[13,14] A definitive diagnosis is made via endoscopy and histopathology. At endoscopy, the mucosa may appear hyperemic and irregular, and polypoid masses, nodules, and/or ulcerations with spontaneous bleeding may be seen (Figure 3.3).[11,13,14,16] Loss of distensibility of the esophagus is characteristic for chronic esophagitis.[16] The esophagus can be difficult to biopsy with standard instruments due to its tough stratified squamous epithelium. However, abnormal, eroded, ulcerated, or proliferative esophageal lesions can generally be biopsied easily.[14,16] Histopathology may show an eroded, ulcerated, hyperplastic, or dysplastic epithelium, and/or lymphocytic, plasmacytic, or neutrophilic infiltrates of the submucosa.[13,14]

Mild esophagitis may be treated conservatively by withholding food for 2–3 days. Moderate to severe esophagitis should be treated more aggressively. Withholding food fed by mouth

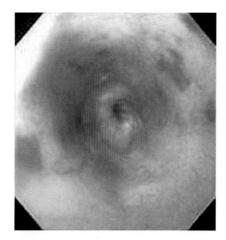

Figure 3.3:
Esophagitis. Endoscopic view of the distal esophagus of a 5-year-old spayed female DSH with protracted vomiting of 5 days' duration. Note the areas of hyperemia and erosion indicating esophagitis.

and providing nutrition via a gastrostomy tube has been recommended for patients with moderate to severe acute esophagitis in the past.[17] However, some authors recommend continuing to feed the animal by mouth throughout treatment.[13,14,18] Whether to place a gastrostomy tube should be decided on an individual basis. Those animals that are completely anorectic, in poor body condition, and those with esophagitis that is in danger of perforating should receive a gastrostomy tube.

Various medical therapies are also recommended. Oral sucralfate suspension has been noted to be one of the most important therapies.[17] Sucralfate has cytoprotective properties when bound to an eroded or ulcerated site.[19,20] However, there are no clinical studies which show that sucralfate is effective in patients with esophagitis. Gastric acid suppression is also recommended. This may be accomplished either using an H_2-receptor antagonist (e.g., cimetidine, ranitidine, or famotidine) or a proton pump inhibitor (e.g., omeprazole). The choice generally depends on the severity of the esophagitis and whether continued GER is present. Proton pump inhibitors may be advantageous in patients with severe erosive esophagitis.[21] Prokinetic agents are also recommended in order to increase lower esophageal sphincter tone and promote gastric emptying, thus decreasing the amount of GER.[12–14] Metoclopramide and cisapride have been used for this purpose. Since cisapride has been removed from the market due to side-effects in humans, it may be difficult to obtain for veterinary patients. However, several compounding pharmacies offer cisapride. Ranitidine and nizatidine have been shown to stimulate gastrointestinal motility by inhibiting acetylcholinesterase activity and may be useful for promotion of gastric emptying in patients with esophagitis.[22]

3

3.3.3 Gastroesophageal reflux

Gastroesophageal reflux disease (GERD) is one of the most commonly diagnosed gastrointestinal disorders in humans. In contrast, GERD has been considered an uncommon disorder in dogs and cats, but is likely more common than previously thought.[13,14,18,23] GER is caused by relaxation of the lower esophageal sphincter leading to reflux of gastric material into the esophagus. Varying degrees of esophagitis may result. Refluxed material may contain acid, pepsin, or even trypsin and bile acids, which may damage the esophageal mucosa. The frequency and content of the reflux determine the severity of the condition.[24] Gastric acid alone may cause mild esophagitis, whereas acid combined with pepsin, trypsin, and/or bile acids may lead to severe esophagitis, and the more frequent the contact, the more likely esophagitis is to develop.[24] The most common cause of GER is general anesthesia, especially in those animals undergoing intra-abdominal procedures.[14,18,23,25] Other disorders such as chronic vomiting, hiatal hernia, and esophageal foreign body may also predispose an animal to GER; but GER may also be idiopathic.[13,18,23]

Clinical signs of GER may mimic those of esophagitis. Animals with mild GER may regurgitate small amounts of material and may be seen to eructate followed by swallowing movements, or may be completely asymptomatic. Regurgitation, odynophagia, multiple attempts at swallowing with extension of the head and neck, and ptyalism may all be seen with moderate to severe disease.[13,14] The owner should be carefully asked whether the animal has recently undergone general anesthesia. The physical examination is often unremarkable and results of the minimum database, including thoracic radiographs, are often within normal limits. A definitive diagnosis is made with a combination of contrast videofluoroscopy and endoscopy. Contrast videofluoroscopy can demonstrate reflux of gastric contents into the distal esophagus, decreased esophageal motility, and potentially may reveal evidence for an underlying condition, such as a hiatal hernia.[13,14] Endoscopy may be normal, but if esophagitis is present, varying degrees of mucosal hyperemia, irregularity, and/or erosion or ulceration may be seen.[13,14] Various agents used to premedicate and induce animals for anesthesia may decrease lower esophageal sphincter tone, which must be taken into consideration when an open lower esophageal sphincter is seen during endoscopy.[26]

Therapy for GER is similar to that for esophagitis. Treatment of esophageal damage is important, as is promoting an increase in lower esophageal sphincter tone and gastric emptying. Therefore, oral sucralfate suspension is used if esophageal erosions or ulcerations are seen, or when the clinician aims to prevent such changes.[20] Additionally, an H_2-receptor antagonist or a proton pump inhibitor along with a prokinetic agent should be administered.[13,14,22,21] In the past, it has been recommended to feed a low fat or fat-restricted diet, as dietary fat may delay gastric emptying and decrease lower esophageal sphincter tone;[17] however, recent evidence in humans has shown that this may not be the case in all patients.[27,28] A fat-restricted diet may be utilized initially, but if the patient does not maintain an adequate body condition, a diet with a moderate amount of fat should be chosen. Any underlying conditions that can be identified should also be corrected. However, the surgical correction of primary GER has not been recommended in veterinary patients to date as has been the case in some human patients.[29]

3.3.4 Esophageal foreign bodies

Esophageal foreign bodies occur relatively frequently in the dog, but less so in the cat. The most commonly encountered esophageal foreign bodies in dogs are bones, fishhooks, and food or compressed chew treats.[30–34] In cats, fishhooks, needles, and trichobezoars are most commonly encountered.[30,35] Foreign bodies generally lodge in those areas of the esophagus that are least distensible, namely the thoracic inlet, the heart base, and the cardia.[16,30–32] The severity of damage produced by the foreign body depends on the duration of the obstruction and the size and angularity of the foreign body.[17] Pressure necrosis of the esophageal wall can occur, and tends to be more severe with larger foreign bodies and those that have been present for a longer duration. Full thickness damage can occur resulting in esophageal perforation, mediastinitis, pleuritis, and on occasion fatal hemorrhage.[33] The clinical signs are those of esophageal obstruction. Most commonly regurgitation, odynophagia, ptyalism, avoidance of food, dysphagia, halitosis, retching, and gagging are seen.[30,32,34] In some cases, the owner may have seen the animal eat the offending object. The physical examination may be normal, but typically will reveal signs of esophageal pain including multiple attempts to swallow with extension of the head and neck, ptyalism, and possibly a hunched appearance.

Diagnosis is often made by historical information and survey thoracic radiographs (Figure 3.4). Occasionally, a contrast study may be needed to detect radiolucent objects. Evidence of esophageal perforation may be present and includes pneumomediastinum, pneumothorax, and mediastinal or pleural fluid, but these findings may be unreliable.[36]

Removal of the foreign body should be immediate or as soon as the patient has been stabilized. Endoscopy is the preferred method of removal if the esophagus has not been perforated (Figure 3.5).[30,32,34,35,37] The foreign object may be removed via the mouth or gently pushed into the stomach and removed via gastrotomy or allowed to be digested (e.g., bones or food). Extreme care must be exercised when attempting to remove an esophageal foreign body via endoscopy. Perforation during endoscopic removal may occur. Once the foreign body has

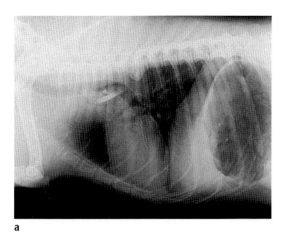

a

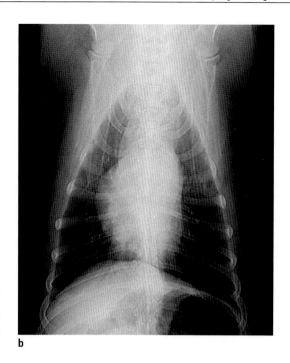

Figure 3.4 a,b:
Esophageal foreign body. Lateral and VD radiographs of a 3-year-old spayed female American Staffordshire Terrier with regurgitation and anorexia for 3 days. The bone esophageal foreign body can be seen on the lateral radiograph at the level of the 3rd and 4th ribs just ventral to the trachea and on the VD radiograph at the level of the 3rd rib to the left of midline.

b

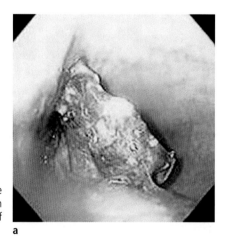

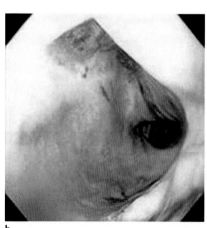

Figure 3.5 a,b:
Esophageal foreign body. Endoscopic views of the bone esophageal foreign body in the same dog shown in Figure 3.4 before and after endoscopic removal of the bone.

a

b

been removed, the esophageal mucosa should be fully evaluated for any potential damage (Figure 3.5b). An erythematous mucosa and mild erosions are common. Thoracic radiography should be repeated after endoscopic removal of a foreign body if a perforation is suspected. Fluoroscope-guided removal has also been used successfully in some patients.[31] Surgical removal may be needed in cases where endoscopic removal is unsuccessful or when a perforation has occurred.[32,34,36,37]

Following removal of the foreign body, animals with no to minimal esophageal damage may not need any medical therapy. Animals with moderate to severe damage should be treated for esophagitis.[17] In addition, broad spectrum antibiotics may also be used preventatively as esophageal mucosal barrier function has been lost. Some clinicians have recommended the use of anti-inflammatory doses of corticosteroids in an attempt to prevent esophageal stricture formation, but this therapy is as of yet unproven. If esophageal damage is severe, the clinician may wish to rest the esophagus and feed the animal through a gastrostomy tube. The prognosis is generally good;

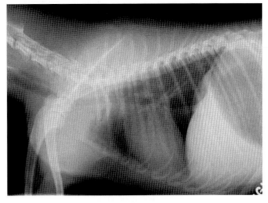

Figure 3.6:
Esophageal stricture. Lateral thoracic radiograph of a 2-year-old castrated male Miniature Pinscher with regurgitation, dysphagia, and anorexia. The dog had been seen to eat a foreign body approximately 2 weeks prior to presentation. A small amount of air can be seen in the mid esophagus.

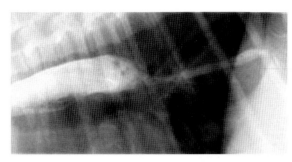

Figure 3.7:
Esophageal stricture. Barium esophagram of the same dog as shown in Figure 3.6. An esophageal stricture can be seen in the mid to distal esophagus.

however, some animals may develop complications, the most common of which is esophageal stricture formation.[18,23,32]

3.3.5 Esophageal strictures

Esophageal strictures occur secondary to damage of the submucosal and muscular layers of the esophagus. Damage to these layers stimulates the production of fibrous connective tissue.[38] Damage to the mucosa alone generally does not result in stricture formation. Benign esophageal strictures have been reported in the dog and cat, and are usually secondary to damage from foreign bodies, ingestion of caustic substances, or most commonly, secondary to GER during an anesthetic procedure.[18,23,32,39,40] Esophageal strictures have also been reported in cats secondary to oral doxycycline administration.[41]

The clinical signs of patients with an esophageal stricture include regurgitation, ptyalism, dysphagia, odynophagia, inappetence, and weight loss.[18,23,38] The physical examination is usually unremarkable, unless aspiration pneumonia has developed, in which case fever and coughing may be seen.

The results of a minimum diagnostic database, including thoracic radiographs, are often normal. Occasionally, a dilated segment of the esophagus may be seen cranial to the stricture on survey thoracic radiographs (Figure 3.6). A definitive diagnosis is made via contrast videofluoroscopy (Figure 3.7) and/or esophagoscopy (Figure 3.8).[23,40] Esophagoscopy allows the clinician to fully evaluate the esophageal mucosa to aid in treatment decisions.

Currently, the treatment of choice for esophageal strictures is balloon dilation (Figure 3.9).[12,18,23,39,40] This is most commonly done under endoscopic guidance, but may also be done under fluoroscopic guidance.[18,23,39,40] Strictures can vary in number, location, and severity.[18,23,39,40] The balloon dilation procedure typically must be repeated an average of 2–4 times per animal.[18,23,39,40] The interval between procedures also varies, but is generally 4–7 days.[18,23] Complications associated with balloon dilation include esophageal perforation and esophageal tears.[18,23,40,42] Placement of a gastrostomy tube has been recommended in cases where the esophageal damage is severe, but this may not be necessary in all cases.[17,18,39] Therapy for esophagitis should be instituted after the balloon dilation procedure. The use of corticosteroids has been advocated to prevent reformation of the stricture.[10] However, the efficacy of such corticosteroid therapy has not been proven in a clinical setting, although it has been reported as an adjunct therapy by some authors.[18,23] Bougienage is also a reported technique for dilation of esophageal strictures, but is not as commonly used as balloon catheters are more readily available and used quite successfully.[12] Surgical removal of strictures and other surgical techniques have been reported, but surgery is generally reserved for refractory cases or those in which perforation has occurred.[43,44] In clinical studies, 70–88% of patients with esophageal strictures had a good to excellent outcome with balloon dilation of the esophageal stricture, returning to eating canned or dry dog food with minimal to no regurgitation.[18,23,39,40]

Figure 3.8 (left):
Esophageal stricture. Endoscopic view of the esophageal stricture of the dog in Figures 3.6 and 3.7. Note the pale to white fibrous tissue. The diameter of the stricture was approximately 3 mm.

Figure 3.9 (right):
Esophageal stricture after balloon dilation. Endoscopic view of the esophageal stricture in the same dog shown in Figures 3.6–3.8 after balloon dilation. The diameter of the strictured area is now approximately 15 mm. Note some hemorrhage and mucosal tearing, which can often be observed after balloon dilation. The dog underwent a total of three balloon dilation procedures and returned to being able to eat canned dog food without regurgitation.

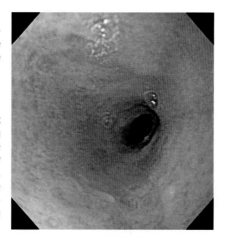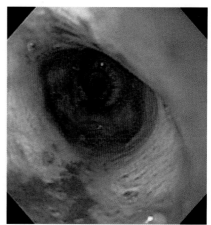

3.3.6 Esophageal diverticula

An esophageal diverticulum is a pouch-like dilation of the esophageal wall. Diverticula may be congenital or acquired and are of two types, pulsion or traction diverticula. Pulsion diverticula represent an outpouching of the esophageal mucosa through a defect in the muscular and adventitial layers of the esophagus.[37,45] It is usually acquired secondary to increased intraluminal pressure and deep esophageal inflammation. Predisposing disorders include esophagitis, esophageal stricture or foreign body, or hiatal hernia.[10] Traction diverticula are generally acquired as a result of inflammation in the thoracic cavity in close proximity to the esophagus. This leads to the formation of fibrous tissue, which then contracts pulling the esophageal wall outwards.[10] This type of diverticulum affects all four layers of the esophageal wall and most commonly occurs secondary to a foreign body perforation.[10] Both types have been reported in the dog while only one case of an esophageal diverticulum has been reported in a cat.[45–47] Clinical signs of small diverticula may not be apparent. Large diverticula allow food trapping, leading to postprandial dyspnea, regurgitation, odynophagia, and anorexia.

The results of a minimum diagnostic database are usually unremarkable. Survey thoracic radiographs usually reveal an air-, fluid-, or food-filled outpouching of the esophagus. Small diverticula must be differentiated from normal esophageal redundancy that occurs in some animals, especially Chinese Shar Peis, young animals, and brachycephalic breeds.[10,17] Contrast radiography can help delineate the diverticulum and differentiate it from other soft tissue structures in the thorax (Figure 3.10). Endoscopy can be used to confirm the diagnosis

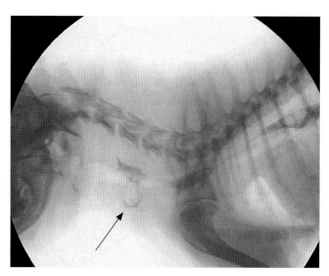

Figure 3.10:
Esophageal diverticulum. Contrast videofluoroscopic image of a 1-year-old castrated male Shih Tzu with a small esophageal diverticulum. The study was performed 1 month after endoscopic removal of a bone foreign body as a follow-up. The dog was asymptomatic for the diverticulum.

and will allow identification of any ulceration or scarring.[16] Small diverticula may be managed with a bland, soft diet fed with the patient in an upright position, and generally carry a favorable prognosis. Large diverticula require surgical excision, justifying a less favorable prognosis, but successful surgical management has been reported.[45,46]

3

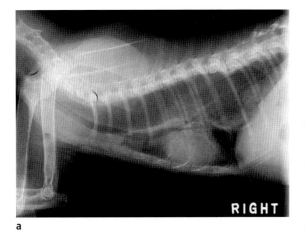

a

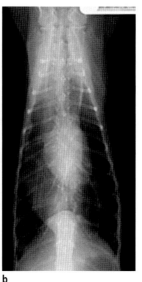

b

Figure 3.11 a,b:
Megaesophagus. Lateral and VD radiographs of a 2-year-old spayed female DSH with chronic regurgitation and weight loss. A complete work-up did not identify a cause for the megaesophagus.

3.3.7 Airway-esophageal fistula

An airway-esophageal fistula is a communication between the esophagus and either the trachea or a main-stem bronchus. They have been reported uncommonly in the dog and cat as either congenital or acquired conditions.[48–51] Acquired airway-esophageal fistulae most commonly develop secondary to foreign body penetration of the esophagus.[50] Congenital airway-esophageal fistulae have been proposed, with Cairn terriers being possibly predisposed.[49,50] The most common clinical sign is coughing or dyspnea after eating or drinking.[49] Other clinical signs include regurgitation and anorexia, fever, or lethargy, with some of these signs being related to aspiration pneumonia.

The results of a minimum diagnostic database typically show leukocytosis with or without a left shift secondary to pneumonia. Survey radiographs may reveal a radiopaque foreign body. However, the foreign body may have already dislodged, and pneumonia may be the only abnormality noted. A definitive diagnosis requires a contrast esophagram, which may show the communication between the esophagus and the airway. It is recommended to use a small amount of barium for the study since iodinated contrast agents are hyperosmolar and may cause pulmonary edema if they reach the airway.[17,49–51] Endoscopy and bronchoscopy may be used as adjunct diagnostic tools.[50]

Treatment requires surgical correction. Lung lobectomy is usually necessary along with repair of the esophageal wall defect.[49,50] The prognosis for a full recovery is good if the animal survives the surgical procedure.

3.3.8 Megaesophagus

Megaesophagus is a dilation of the body of the esophagus associated with poor to no esophageal peristalsis. Megaesophagus has been described as an idiopathic congenital, idiopathic acquired, or secondary acquired disorder.[52–66] Congenital disease has been reported in both the dog and the cat and an inherited basis has been proposed.[52,53,55] The most common underlying disease process that results in a secondary megaesophagus is myasthenia gravis.[63,64,67,68] Other underlying conditions reported include polyneuropathies, lead toxicity, polymyopathies, thymoma (causing a paraneoplastic form of myasthenia gravis), hypoadrenocorticism, dysautonomia, and possibly hypothyroidism, and others.[57–62,65,66] Adult onset, idiopathic megaesophagus was termed esophageal achalasia in the past, as the pathophysiology was thought to be related to failure of a relaxation of the lower esophageal sphincter. This has since been disproven, but as of yet the exact etiology and pathogenesis of primary megaesophagus is still unknown. It has been shown that some dogs have a normal lower and upper esophageal sphincter response to swallowing, but an absent or decreased response of the esophageal sphincters to intraluminal stimuli.[69] This study, along with others, suggest that the underlying defect in dogs with idiopathic megaesophagus may lie in the vagal afferent innervation to the esophagus.[70]

The most common clinical sign, regardless of the cause of the megaesophagus, is regurgitation. Patients with megaesophagus generally maintain their desire to eat, unless they develop aspiration pneumonia. Regurgitation may occur immediately or several hours after eating. Ptyalism and weight loss are common. Physical examination is often unremarkable unless an underlying condition is present (e.g., systemic weakness may be seen with myasthenia gravis). The results of a minimum diagnostic database are often normal. Thoracic radiographs usually show a diffusely dilated esophagus filled with air, food, and/or fluid (Figure 3.11). In questionable cases, contrast videofluoroscopy will help determine the extent of esophageal motility and whether any obstructive lesions are present. A definitive diagnosis involves ruling out other known causes of megaesophagus with appropriate testing, including serum acetylcholine receptor antibody titers, ACTH stimulation testing, lead concentrations, or others.[68] Endoscopy may help rule out an obstructive disease, but is not generally necessary.

If an underlying disease is present, it should be treated appropriately. For example, animals with myasthenia gravis often respond well to immunosuppression and anticholinesterase drugs.[64,71] Other patients, especially those with a focal form, may have spontaneous regression of signs with supportive care.[67] Unfortunately, to date, there is no definitive treatment for congenital or acquired idiopathic forms of megaesophagus, and these patients should be treated with supportive care. Aspiration pneumonia should be treated as it arises. Dietary support should be provided in form of a high quality, high calorie diet either via frequent, small upright feedings or through a gastrostomy tube. Some animals do better with a gruel consistency of the food while others regurgitate less with canned food formed into a meatball shape. Smooth muscle prokinetic agents (i.e., metoclopramide or cisapride) will not stimulate contraction of the canine esophagus as the esophagus is composed entirely of skeletal muscle.[72] These drugs may be helpful in the cat since the distal esophagus consists of smooth muscle, but clinical or experimental efficacy studies are lacking. Surgical treatment of megaesophagus (gastroesophageal myotomy) has been associated with poor results.[10]

The prognosis for congenital or acquired idiopathic megaesophagus is guarded. Some young dogs have been shown to recover esophageal function as they mature.[53] Although adult onset megaesophagus carries a poor prognosis, it has been reported to be transient in rare cases.[73]

3.3.9 Hiatal hernia

A hiatal hernia results from an abnormal or stretched phrenicoesophageal ligament, which allows herniation of the abdominal esophagus, the gastroesophageal junction, parts of the stomach, and/or other abdominal organs into the thoracic cavity via the hiatus. A sliding, axial hiatal hernia occurs when the abdominal esophagus and part of the stomach slide up into the chest as a unit. A paraesophageal hiatal hernia occurs when part of the stomach and/or other abdominal organs enter the chest next to the esophagus.[74] A congenital form of a sliding hiatal hernia has been described in the Chinese Shar Pei and appears to be the most common form.[74,75] Sliding hiatal her-

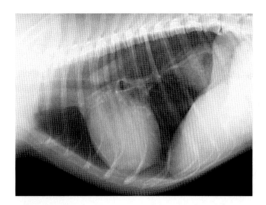

Figure 3.12:
Radiograph of a dog with intermittent vomiting and regurgitation. Lateral thoracic radiograph of a 4-year-old castrated male Beagle with intermittent bouts of vomiting and regurgitation.

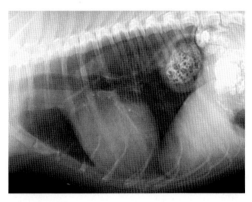

Figure 3.13:
Hiatal hernia. Barium contrast study of the same dog as shown in Figure 3.12 delineating the hiatal hernia.

nias can occur in cats, but are uncommon overall.[76,77] Paraesophageal hiatal hernias are rare. Hiatal hernias can be acquired due to trauma.

The most common clinical signs of hiatal hernias are a result of GER and include occasional or persistent regurgitation, vomiting, dysphagia, dyspnea, and/or ptyalism.[75–77] However, some animals with mild disease may be asymptomatic.[74] The diagnosis may be evident from survey thoracic radiographs. A soft-tissue opacity may be noted in the caudodorsal thorax, in the area of the esophagus (Figure 3.12). Distal esophageal dilation may also be seen. A hiatal hernia is often a dynamic condition so that multiple radiographic exposures may be necessary to yield a diagnosis. In some cases, contrast videofluoroscopy may be needed to confirm the diagnosis (Figure 3.13). The condition is more difficult to diagnose via endoscopy.

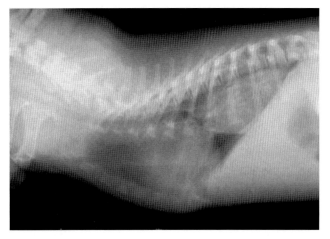

Figure 3.14:
Gastroesophageal intussusception. Lateral thoracic radiograph of a 4-month-old male Labrador Retriever showing a soft tissue mass effect in the area of the distal esophagus. The puppy was diagnosed at endoscopy and surgery with a gastroesophageal intussusception.

The clinical signs are those of esophageal obstruction and include regurgitation, pain, dysphagia, dyspnea, and hematemesis; the signs are usually acute and severe. Death is possible and thought to be mainly due to decreased venous return. Survey radiographs are usually diagnostic showing a soft tissue mass in the distal esophagus and a dilated proximal esophagus (Figure 3.14). Gastric rugal folds may also be seen within the esophagus. Endoscopy may be used as an adjunct diagnostic tool and will reveal rugal folds within the distal esophagus.[16] Surgery is usually required after stabilization of the patient.[79] One report described the successful use of constant air insufflation through an endoscope.[10]

3.3.11 Vascular ring anomalies

Vascular ring anomalies occur when the embryonic aortic arches develop abnormally so that a "vascular ring" is formed that constricts the esophagus. The most common anomaly is a persistent right aortic arch, where the esophagus is entrapped between the heart, the abnormally formed aorta on the right, the pulmonary artery, and the ligamentum arteriosus, which connects the aorta and pulmonary artery.[81,82] Other vascular ring anomalies that have been reported in dogs and cats include a double aortic arch, anomalous right patent ductus arteriosus, and coarctation of the aorta with an aberrant left subclavian artery.[83–86]

The clinical signs are associated with obstruction of the esophagus and aspiration pneumonia, and include onset of regurgitation at the time of weaning, coughing, and lethargy. A dilated esophagus filled with food may be palpated in the cervical region. Diagnosis is made on survey thoracic radiographs, which show a focally distended esophagus with an abrupt narrowing of the esophagus at the heart base. Surgical transection of the constricting bands around the esophagus is the treatment of choice.[82,83,85] This procedure has recently been successfully performed by thoracoscopy.[87] Prognosis for full recovery is good, but some dogs have a persistently dilated esophagus that does not return to normal size or function.[82,83,85,86]

Surgical correction is usually required for animals with congenital disease.[74–77] Those with acquired disease may respond to medical management consisting of small frequent meals, H_2-receptor antagonists, prokinetic agents, and/or sucralfate suspension.[74,77]

3.3.10 Gastroesophageal intussusception

Gastroesophageal intussusception is an invagination of all or parts of the stomach into the thoracic esophagus. In general it occurs uncommonly, but is most frequently seen in puppies, though it has also been reported in adult dogs and cats.[78–80] Predisposing factors may include megaesophagus and incompetency of the gastroesophageal sphincter.

🔑 Key Facts

■ Regardless of the diagnosis, clinical signs of esophageal disease are often similar and include regurgitation, ptyalism, and dysphagia.

■ Videofluoroscopy is the diagnostic test of choice to help diagnose esophageal motility disorders.

■ Esophagoscopy can be an invaluable tool in the diagnosis and therapy of various esophageal diseases.

■ Esophagitis is commonly treated with H_2-receptor antagonists or a proton pump inhibitor, sucralfate suspension, and a prokinetic agent. A gastrostomy tube may be needed for nutritional support in some patients.

References

1. Evans HE. *Miller's anatomy of the dog*. Philadelphia, WB Saunders, 1993; 420–425.
2. Hudson LC, Hamilton WP. *Atlas of feline anatomy for veterinarians*. Philadelphia, WB Saunders, 1993; 149–155.
3. Ganong WF. Regulation of gastrointestinal function. In: *Review of medical physiology, 16th ed*. Norwalk, CT, Appleton and Lange, 1993; 438–467.
4. Doty RW. Neural organization of deglutition. In: Code CF (ed.), *Handbook of Physiology*. Sec. 6; Alimentary canal, Vol 4. Washington, DC, American Physiological Society, 1968; 1861–1902.
5. Miller AJ. Deglutition. *Physiol Rev* 1982; 62: 129–184.
6. Suter PF, Watrous BJ. Oropharyngeal dysphagias in the dog: a cinefluorographic analysis of experimentally induced and spontaneously occurring swallowing disorders. *Vet Radiol* 1980; 21: 24–39.
7. Goring RL, Kagan KG. Cricopharyngeal achalasia in the dog: radiographic evaluation and surgical management. *Compend Contin Educ Pract Vet* 1982; 5: 438–444.
8. Niles JD, Williams JM, Sullivan M et al. Resolution of dysphagia following cricopharyngeal myectomy in six young dogs. *J Small Anim Pract* 2001; 41 (1): 32–35.
9. Warnock JJ, Marks SL, Pollard R et al. Surgical management of cricopharyngeal dysphagia in dogs: 14 cases (1989–2001). *J Am Vet Med Assoc* 2003; 223 (10): 1462–1468.
10. Guilford WG, Strombeck DR. Diseases of swallowing. In: Guilford WG, Center SA, Strombeck DR et al (eds.), *Strombeck's small animal gastroenterology*. Philadelphia, WB Saunders, 1996; 211–238.
11. Mylonakis ME, Rallis TS, Koutinas AF et al. A comparison between ethanol-induced chemical ablation and ivermectin plus prednisolone in the treatment of symptomatic esophageal spirocercosis in the dog: a prospective study on 14 natural cases. *Vet Parasit* 2004; 120: 131–138.
12. Sellon RK, Willard MD. Esophagitis and esophageal strictures. *Vet Clin North Am (Small Anim Pract)* 2003; 33 (5): 945–967.
13. Han E, Broussard J, Baer KE. Feline esophagitis secondary to gastroesophageal reflux disease: Clinical signs, radiographic, endoscopic, and histopathological findings. *J Am Anim Hops Assoc* 2003; 39: 161–167.
14. Han E. Diagnosis and management of reflux esophagitis. *Clin Tech in Small Anim Pract* 18 (4): 231–238.
15. Galmiche JP, Janssens J. The pathophysiology of gastro-oesophageal reflux disease: an overview. *Scand J Gastroenterol* 1983; Suppl 211: 201–208.
16. Gualtieri M. Esophagoscopy. *Vet Clin North Am (Small Anim Pract)* 2001; 31 (4): 605–630.
17. Washabau RJ. Diseases of the Esophagus. In: Ettinger SJ, Feldman EC (eds.), *Textbook of veterinary internal medicine, 4th ed*. Philadelphia, WB Saunders, 2000; 1142–1154.
18. Leib MS, Dinnel H, Ward DL et al. Endoscopic balloon dilation of benign esophageal strictures in dogs and cat. *J Vet Intern Med* 2001; 15: 547–552.
19. Clark S, Katz PO, Wu WC et al. Comparison of potential cytoprotective action of sucralfate and cimetidine: studies with feline esophagitis. *Am J Med* 1987; 83: 56–60.
20. Katz PO, Geisinger KR, Hassan M et al. Acid-induced esophagitis in cats is prevented by sucralfate but not synthetic prostaglandin E. *Dig Dis Sci* 1988; 33: 217–224.
21. Maton PN, Orlando R, Joelsson B. Efficacy of omeprazole versus ranitidine for symptomatic treatment of poorly responsive acid reflux disease – a prospective, controlled trial. *Aliment Pharmacol Ther* 1999; 13: 819–826.
22. Hall JA, Washabau RJ. Diagnosis and treatment of gastric motility disorders. *Vet Clin North Am (Small Anim Pract)* 1999; 29 (2): 377–395.
23. Adamama-Moraitou KK, Rallis TS, Prassinos NN et al. Benign esophageal stricture in the dog and cat: a retrospective study of 20 cases. *Can J Vet Res* 2002; 66: 55–59.
24. Evander A, Little AG, Riddell RH et al. Composition of the refluxed material determines the degree of reflux esophagitis in the dog. *Gastroenterology* 1987; 93 (2): 280–286.
25. Galatos AD, Raptopoulos D. Gastro-oesophageal reflux during anaesthesia in the dog: the effect of age, positioning, and type of surgical procedure. *Vet Rec* 1995; 137 (20): 513–516.
26. Strombeck DR, Harrold D. Effects of atropine, acepromazine, meperidine, and xylazine on gastroesophageal sphincter pressure in the dog. *Am J Vet Res* 1985; 46 (4): 963–965.
27. Penagini R, Mangano M, Bianchi PA. Effect of increasing the fat content but not the energy load of a meal on gastro-oesophageal reflux and lower oesophageal sphincter motor function. *Gut* 1998; 42: 330–333.
28. Pehl C, Waizenhoefer CD, Wendl B et al. Effect of low and high fat meals on lower esophageal sphincter motility and gastroesophageal reflux in healthy subjects. *Am J Gastroenterol* 1999; 94 (5): 1192–1196.
29. Metz DC. Managing gastroesophageal reflux disease for the lifetime of the patient: evaluating the long-term options. *Am J Med* 2004; 117 Suppl 5A: 49S–55S.
30. Michels GM, Jones BD, Huss BT et al. Endoscopic and surgical retrieval of fishhooks from the stomach and esophagus in dogs and cats: 75 cases (1977–1993). *J Am Vet Med Assoc* 1995; 207 (9): 1194–1197.
31. Moore AH. Removal of oesophageal foreign bodies in dogs: use of the fluoroscopic method and outcome. *J Small Anim Pract* 2001; 42 (5): 227–230.
32. Kaiser S, Forterre F, Kohn B et al. Oesophageal foreign bodies in dogs: a retrospective study of 50 cases (1999–2003). *Kleintierpraxis* 2003; 48 (7): 397–400.
33. Cohn LA, Stoll MR, Branson KR et al. Fatal hemothorax following management of an esophageal foreign body. *J Am Anim Hosp Assoc* 2003; 39: 251–256.
34. Spielman BL, Shaker EH, Garvey MS. Esophageal foreign body in dogs: a retrospective study of 23 cases. *J Am Anim Hosp Assoc* 1992; 28: 570–574.
35. Squires RA. Oesophageal obstruction by a hairball in a cat. *J Small Anim Pract* 1989; 30: 311–314.
36. Parker NR, Walter PA, Gay J. Diagnosis and surgical management of esophageal perforation. *J Am Anim Hosp Assoc* 1989; 25: 587–595.
37. Ryan WW, Greene RW. The conservative management of esophageal foreign bodies and their complications: a review of 66 cases in dogs and cats. *J Am Anim Hosp Assoc* 1975; 11 (3): 243–249.
38. Weyrauch EA, Willard MD. Esophagitis and benign esophageal strictures. *Comp Cont Ed Pract Vet* 1998; 20 (2): 203–212.
39. Melendez LD, Twedt DC, Weyrauch EA et al. Conservative therapy using balloon dilation for intramural, inflammatory esophageal strictures in dogs and cats: a retrospective study of 23 cases [1987–1997]. *Eur J Comp Gastroenterol* 1998; 3 (1): 31–36.
40. Harai BH, Johnson SE, Sherding RG. Endoscopically guided balloon dilatation of benign esophageal strictures in 6 cats and 7 dogs. *J Vet Intern Med* 1995; 9 (5): 332–335.
41. Melendez LD, Twedt DC. Esophageal strictures secondary to doxycycline administration in 4 cats. *Feline Pract* 2000; 28 (2): 10–12.
42. Willard MD, Delles EK, Fossum TW. Iatrogenic tears associated with ballooning of esophageal strictures. *J Am Anim Hosp Assoc* 1994; 30 (5): 431–435.
43. Johnson KA, Maddison JE, Allan GS. Correction of cervical esophageal stricture in a dog by creation of a traction diverticulum. *J Am Vet Med Assoc* 1992; 201 (7): 1045–1048.

3

3

44. Gregory CR, Gourley IM, Bruyette DS et al. Free jejunal segment for treatment of cervical esophageal stricture in a dog. *J Am Vet Med Assoc* 1988; 193 (2): 230–232.

45. Lantz GC, Bojrab MJ, Jones BD. Epiphrenic esophageal diverticulectomy. *J Am Anim Hosp Assoc* 1976; 12 (5): 629–635.

46. Faulkner RT, Caywood D, Wallace LJ et al. Epiphrenic esophageal diverticulectomy in a dog: a case report and review. *J Am Anim Hosp Assoc* 1981; 17 (1): 77–81.

47. Fukata T. Esophageal diverticulum-like pouch in a cat with allergic bronchitis. *Vet Med Small Anim Clin* 1984; 79 (2): 175–178.

48. Park RD. Bronchoesophageal fistula in the dog: literature survey, case presentations, and radiographic manifestations. *Comp Cont Ed Pract Vet* 1984; 6 (7): 669–677.

49. Basher AW, Hogan PM, Hanna PE et al. Surgical treatment of a congenital bronchoesophageal fistula in a dog. *J Am Vet Med Assoc* 1991; 199 (4): 479–482.

50. Nawrocki MA, Mackin AJ, McLaughlin R et al. Fluoroscopic and endoscopic localization of an esophagobronchial fistula in a dog. *J Am Anim Hosp Assoc* 2003; 39: 257–261.

51. Freeman LM, Rush JE, Schelling SH et al. Tracheoesophageal fistula in two cats. *J Am Anim Hosp Assoc* 1993; 29 (6): 531–535.

52. Clifford DH, Soifer FK, Wilson CF et al. Congenital achalasia of the esophagus in four cats of common ancestry. *J Am Vet Med Assoc* 1971; 158 (9): 1554–1560.

53. Cox VS, Wallace LJ, Anderson VE et al. Hereditary esophageal dysfunction in the Miniature Schnauzer dog. *Am J Vet Res* 1980; 41 (3): 326–330.

54. Boudrieau RJ, Rogers WA. Megaesophagus in the dog: a review of 50 cases. *J Am Anim Hosp Assoc* 1985; 21 (1): 33–40.

55. Knowles KE, O'Brien DP, Amann JF. Congenital idiopathic megaesophagus in a litter of Chinese Shar Peis: clinical, electrodiagnostic, and pathologic findings. *J Am Anim Hosp Assoc* 1990; 26 (3): 313–318.

56. Rogers WA, Fenner WR, Sherding RG. Electromyographic and esophagomanometric findings in clinically normal dogs and in dogs with idiopathic megaesophagus. *J Am Vet Med Assoc* 1979; 174 (2): 181–183.

57. Shell LG, Jortner BS, Leib MS. Familial motor neuron disease in Rottweiler dogs: neuropathologic studies. *Vet Pathol* 1987; 24 (2): 135–139.

58. Maddison JE, Allan GS. Megaesophagus attributable to lead toxicosis in a cat. *J Am Vet Med Assoc* 1990; 197 (10): 1357–1358.

59. Braund KG, Shores A, Cochrane S et al. Laryngeal paralysis-polyneuropathy complex in young Dalmatians. *Am J Vet Res* 1994; 55 (4): 534–542.

60. Jaggy A, Oliver JE, Ferguson DC et al. Neurological manifestations of hypothyroidism: a retrospective study of 29 dogs. *J Vet Intern Med* 1994; 8 (5): 328–336.

61. Evans J, Levesque D, Shelton GD. Canine inflammatory myopathies: a clinicopathologic review of 200 cases. *J Vet Intern Med* 2004; 18 (5): 679–691.

62. Klebanow ER. Thymoma and acquired myasthenia gravis in the dog: a case report and review of 13 additional cases. *J Am Anim Hosp Assoc* 1992; 28: 63–69.

63. Joseph RJ, Carrillo JM, Lennon VA. Myasthenia gravis in the cat. *J Vet Intern Med* 1988; 2: 75–79.

64. Dewey CW, Bailey CS, Shelton GD et al. Clinical forms of acquired myasthenia gravis in dogs: 25 cases (1988–1995). *J Vet Intern Med* 1997; 11: 50–57.

65. Lifton SJ, King LG, Zerbe CA. Glucocorticoid deficient hypoadrenocorticism in dogs: 18 cases (1986–1995). *J Am Vet Med Assoc* 1996; 209: 2076–2081.

66. Detweiler DA, Biller DS, Hoskinson JJ et al. Radiographic findings of canine dysautonomia in twenty-four dogs. *Vet Radiol Ultrasound* 2001; 42 (2): 108–112.

67. Shelton GD, Willard MD, Cardinet GH et al. Acquired myasthenia gravis: selective involvement of esophageal, pharyngeal, and facial muscles. *J Vet Intern Med* 1990; 4: 281–284.

68. Gaynor AR, Shofer FS, Washabau RJ. Risk factors for acquired megaesophagus in dogs. *J Am Vet Med Assoc* 1997; 211 (11): 1406–1412.

69. Tan BJ, Diamant NE. Assessment of the neural defect in a dog with idiopathic megaesophagus. *Dig Dis Sci* 1987; 32 (1): 76–85.

70. Holland CT, Satchell PM, Farrow BR. Selective vagal afferent dysfunction in dogs with congenital megaesophagus. *Auton Neurosci* 2002; 99 (1): 18–23.

71. Dewey CW, Coates JR, Ducote JM et al. Azathioprine therapy for acquired myasthenia gravis in five dogs. *J Am Anim Hosp Assoc* 1999; 35: 396–402.

72. Washabau RJ, Hall JA. Cisapride. *J Am Vet Med Assoc* 1995; 207 (10): 1285–1288.

73. Hendricks JC, Maggio-Price L, Dougherty JF. Transient esophageal dysfunction mimicking megaesophagus in three dogs. *J Am Vet Med Assoc* 1984; 185 (1): 90–92.

74. Bright RM, Sackman JE, DeNovo C et al. Hiatal hernia in the dog and cat: a retrospective study of 16 cases. *J Small Anim Pract* 1990; 31 (5): 244–250.

75. Callan MB, Washabau RJ, Saunders HM et al. Congenital esophageal hiatal hernia in the Chinese Shar-Pei dog. *J Vet Intern Med* 1993; 7 (4): 210–215.

76. Prymak C, Saunders HM, Washabau RJ. Hiatal hernia repair by restoration and stabilization of normal anatomy. An evaluation in four dogs and one cat. *Vet Surg* 1989; 18 (5): 386–391.

77. Lorinson D, Bright RM. Long-term outcome of medical and surgical treatment of hiatal hernias in dogs and cats: 27 cases (1978–1996). *J Am Vet Med Assoc* 1998; 213 (3): 381–384.

78. Leib MS, Blass CE. Gastroesophageal intussusception in the dog: a review of the literature and a case report. *J Am Anim Hosp Assoc* 1984; 20 (5): 783–790.

79. Greenfield CL, Quinn MK, Coolman BR. Bilateral incisional gastropexies for treatment of intermittent gastroesophageal intussusception in a puppy. *J Am Vet Med Assoc* 1997; 211 (6): 728–730.

80. van Camp S, Love NE, Kumaresan S. Radiographic diagnosis: gastroesophageal intussusception in a cat. *Vet Radiol Ultrasound* 1998; 39 (3): 190–192.

81. Wowk BJ, Olson GA. Megaesophagus produced by persistent right aortic arch in a cat. *Vet Med Small Anim Clin* 1980; 75 (1): 80–83.

82. Muldoon MM, Birchard SJ, Ellison GW. Long-term results of surgical correction of persistent right aortic arch in dogs: 25 cases (1980–1995). *J Am Vet Med Assoc* 1997; 210 (12): 1761–1763.

83. Vianna ML, Krahwinkel DJ. Double aortic arch in a dog. *J Am Vet Med Assoc* 2004; 225 (8): 1196–1197.

84. Yarim M, Gultiken ME, Ozturk S et al. Double aortic arch in a Siamese Cat. *Vet Pathol* 1999; 36: 340–341.

85. Holt D, Heldmann E, Michel K et al. Esophageal obstruction caused by a left aortic arch and an anomalous right patent ductus arteriosus in two German Shepherd littermates. *Vet Surg* 2000; 29 (3): 264–270.

86. White RN, Burton CA, Hale JS. Vascular ring anomaly with coarctation of the aorta in a cat. *J Small Anim Pract* 2003; 44 (7): 330–334.

87. Isakow K, Fowler D, Walsh P. Video-assisted thoracoscopic division of the ligamentum arteriosum in two dogs with persistent right aortic arch. *J Am Vet Med Assoc* 2000; 217 (9): 1333–1336.

3.3.12 Neoplastic conditions of the esophagus

Ann E. Hohenhaus

Introduction

Esophageal tumors represent less than 0.5% of all canine tumors.[1] Both dogs and cats can develop esophageal tumors, which are typically malignant in both species. A strong causal relationship has been reported between infection by the nematode *Spirocerca lupi* and canine esophageal sarcoma in geographical regions where the parasite is enzootic.[2,3] Other than spirocercosis, the etiology of esophageal neoplasms in dogs and cats is unknown.

Histopathology

Many histological types of primary esophageal tumors have been described, including squamous cell carcinoma, adenosquamous carcinoma, adenocarcinoma of the esophageal glands, neuroendocrine carcinoma, plasma cell tumor, and osteosarcoma.[1–11] Benign esophageal tumors such as leiomyoma have been reported in the dog.[12–13] Secondary esophageal tumors originate from locally invasive tumors such as thyroid carcinoma or gastric carcinoma, or via distant metastasis.[1,14] In one study, tumors metastatic to the esophagus were three times more common than primary esophageal tumors (Figure 3.16).[1]

Clinical signs

The clinical signs of esophageal tumors in the dog and cat have been summarized in Table 3.1. Most of the clinical signs associated with esophageal neoplasia can be explained by obstruction of the esophageal lumen by tumor or because of pain during swallowing. An association has been made between chronic upper respiratory signs and papillomatous esophagitis in a cat.[15] This cat was believed to have had chronic reflux into the pharynx and nasal passages resulting in the chronic upper respiratory signs. Esophageal tumors should be suspected in cases of unexplained chronic upper respiratory signs.

Diagnosis

Physical examination findings and routine blood tests are not typically contributory to the diagnosis of esophageal neoplasia unless a cervical mass is present. Diagnostic imaging is required to localize the esophageal tumor and determine the best approach for biopsy and treatment.[14]

Table 3.1: Clinical signs attributed to esophageal neoplasia in the dog

Clinical sign	Dog	Reference	Cat	Reference
Regurgitation / vomiting	√	1, 5, 6, 7, 10, 13	√	4, 6, 8, 9
Anorexia			√	8
Salivation			√	6
Weight loss	√	1, 6	√	6, 8
Bruxism			√	9
Dysphagia			√	9
Hematemesis	√	5		
Blood loss anemia	√	1		
Diarrhea	√	1		

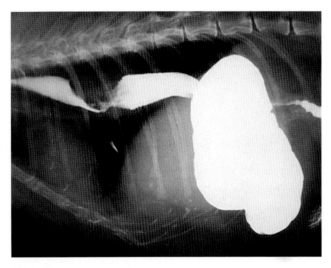

Figure 3.15:
Esophageal tumor in a cat. This contrast esophagram demonstrates a filling defect secondary to an esophageal tumor in a cat.

Plain radiographs are of limited utility in the diagnosis of esophageal neoplasia unless a soft tissue mass associated with the esophagus is seen. Thus, the value of plain radiographs is in eliminating other esophageal disorders, such as foreign bodies and megaesophagus. As a sequela of vomiting and regurgitation, air may be present in the esophagus. Also, pulmonary infiltrates consistent with aspiration pneumonia may be seen. A contrast esophagram will frequently show esophageal dilation proximal to a tumor, a filling defect in the area of the tumor, or leakage of contrast material from an esophageal defect caused by the tumor (Figure 3.15). When interpreting contrast esophagrams, it is important to remember that the

3

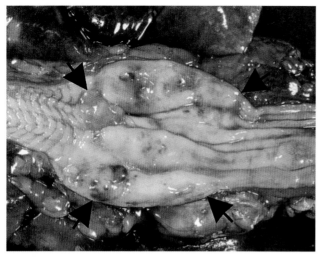

Figure 3.16:
Appearance of striated muscle in a cat esophagus. This Figure shows a metastatic renal sarcoma in the esophagus (arrows) of a cat. Note the normal striated muscle of the distal feline esophagus on the right.

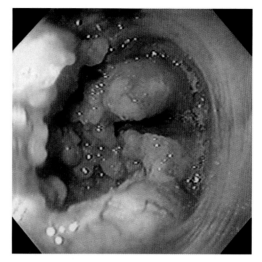

Figure 3.17:
Esophageal squamous cell carcinoma in a dog. This Figure shows an endoscopic view of a squamous cell carcinoma in the esophagus of a dog.

distal portion of the feline esophagus consists of striated muscle and will normally have a regular herringbone appearance (Figure 3.16). Fluoroscopic evaluation of the esophagus is not always necessary for a diagnosis of an esophageal tumor unless an evaluation of esophageal motility is required.

Esophageal tumors are typically intraluminal. Esophagoscopy allows a biopsy to be taken from the luminal surface and is a less invasive procedure than thoracotomy (Figure 3.17). Consequently, esophagoscopy is typically the procedure of choice to obtain a sample for histopathological evaluation of an esophageal tumor. Multiple tissue samples should be obtained with the biopsy forceps to ensure adequate tissue for histological evaluation.

Treatment

Although surgical resection of esophageal tumors has been the treatment modality of choice, rarely is an esophageal tumor amenable to complete resection because the esophagus is incapable of longitudinal stretching and heals poorly under tension. Reconstruction of the esophagus has been attempted by microvascular colon transfer and also by use of a vascular skeletal muscle graft.[16–17] Currently, neither procedure is being widely used.

Only single case reports of other treatment modalities, such as chemotherapy, radiation therapy, and photodynamic therapy for esophageal tumors have been reported. Except for lymphoma, chemotherapy is unlikely to be of benefit in the treatment of esophageal neoplasia. The utility of radiation therapy for the treatment of esophageal tumors is limited by the poor tolerance of normal structures in the thoracic cavity for radiation-induced side effects. Photodynamic therapy, utilizing a photosensitizing dye activated by a laser light source, was administered to a dog with esophageal squamous cell carcinoma.[18] The tumor underwent a partial remission and the dog survived for 9 months before recurrent regurgitation and aspiration pneumonia resulted in euthanasia.

Supportive care

Oral alimentation is compromised by esophageal tumors and a gastrotomy tube should be placed to provide adequate nutrition and decrease the risk of aspiration pneumonia from regurgitation. Naso-esophageal or esophagotomy tubes are not appropriate in patients with esophageal tumors.

Systemic complications of esophageal neoplasia

Paraneoplastic syndromes are sequela of cancer occurring remote from the site of the primary tumor. Hypertrophic osteopathy is a paraneoplastic syndrome of unknown cause associated with esophageal osteosarcoma and also *Spirocerca lupi* infection.[7,19]

Passive congestion of the liver causing ascites and hindlimb edema has been attributed to caudal vena cava compression by an esophageal leiomyoma of the caudal esophagus.[20] Two other complications of esophageal tumors reported include tracheal invasion and aspiration pneumonia.[1,6]

Survival

Typically, esophageal tumors are too advanced at the time of diagnosis to allow successful treatment. Most cases have a reported survival of less than 1 month. An exception is a single reported case of esophageal plasma cell tumor treated with surgery with a survival in excess of 18 months.[5]

🔑 Key Facts

- Esophageal tumors are rare in both dogs and cats.
- Tumors metastatic to the esophagus are more common than primary esophageal tumors.
- Spirocerca lupi is a known cause of esophageal tumors in dogs.
- Clinical signs are most frequently related to esophageal obstruction.
- Resection of the esophageal tumor is rarely possible because the tumor is advanced at the time of diagnosis, leading to short survival times.

References

1. Ridgway RL, Suter PF. Clinical and radiographic signs in primary and metastatic esophageal neoplasms of the dog. *J Am Vet Med Assoc* 1979; 174: 700–704.
2. Colgrove DJ. Transthoracic esophageal surgery for obstructive lesions caused by *Spirocerca lupi* in dogs. *J Am Vet Med Assoc* 1971; 158: 2073–2076.
3. Ivoghli B. Esophageal sarcomas associated with canine spirocercosis. *Vet Med* 1978; 47–48.
4. Patnaik AK, Erlandson RA, Leiberman PH. Esophageal neuroendocrine carcinoma in a cat. *Vet Pathol* 1990; 27: 128–130.
5. Hamilton TA, Carpenter JL. Esophageal plasmacytoma in a dog. *J Am Vet Med Assoc* 1994; 204: 1210–1211.
6. McCaw D, Pratt M, Walshaw R. Squamous cell carcinoma of the esophagus in a dog. *J Am Anim Hosp Assoc* 1980; 16: 561–563.
7. Randolph JF, Center SA, Flanders JA et al. Hypertrophic osteopathy associated with adenocarcinoma of the esophageal glands in a dog. *J Am Vet Med Assoc* 1984; 184: 98–99.
8. Gualtieri M, Monzeglio MG, Di Giancamillo M. Oesophageal squamous cell carcinoma in two cats. *J Small Anim Prac* 1999; 40: 79–83.
9. Shinosuka J, Nakayama H, Suzuki M et al. Esophageal adenosquamous carcinoma in a cat. *J Vet Med Sci* 2001; 63: 91–93.
10. Turnwald GH, Smallwood JE, Helman G. Esophageal osteosarcoma in a dog. *J Am Vet Med Assoc* 1979; 174: 1009–1011.
11. Vernon FF, Roudebusch P. Primary esophageal carcinoma in a cat. *J Am Anim Hosp Assoc* 1980; 16: 547–550.
12. Culbertson R, Branam JE, Rosenblatt LS. Esophageal/gastric leiomyoma in the laboratory Beagle. *J Am Vet Med Assoc* 1983; 183: 1168–1171.
13. Rolfe DS, Twedt DC, Seim HB. Chronic regurgitation or vomiting caused by esophageal leiomyoma in three dogs. *J Am Anim Hosp Assoc* 1994; 30: 425–430.
14. Kleine LJ. Radiologic examination of the esophagus in dogs and cats. *Vet Clin N Am* 1974; 4: 663–686.
15. Wilkinson GT. Chronic papillomatous oesophagitis in a young cat. *Vet Rec* 1970; 87: 355–356.
16. Kuzma AB, Holmberg DL, Miller CW et al. Esophageal replacement in the dog by microvascular colon transfer. *Vet Surg* 1989; 18: 439–445.
17. Straw RC, Tomlinson JL, Constantinescu G et al. Use of a vascular skeletal muscle graft for canine esophageal reconstruction. *Vet Surg* 1987; 16: 155–163.
18. Jacobs TM, Rosen GM. Photodynamic therapy as a treatment for esophageal squamous cell carcinoma in a dog. *J Am Anim Hosp Assoc* 2000; 36: 257–261.
19. Brodey RS. Hypertrophic osteoarthropathy in the dog: a clinicopathologic survey of 60 cases. *J Am Vet Med Assoc* 1971; 159: 1242–1256.
20. Rollois M, Ruel Y, Besso JG. Passive liver congestion associated with caudal vena caval compression due to esophageal leiomyoma. *J Small Anim Pract* 2003; 44: 460–463.

4 Stomach

4.1 Introduction

The stomach is a muscular and glandular organ with its main functions being the storage, mechanical and enzymatic processing, and transportation of partially digested food into the small intestine. The muscular action of the stomach causes mechanical breakdown of food boluses into smaller particles, facilitating duodenal digestion and absorption. The glandular portion of the stomach produces gastric acid, pepsinogen (the precursor of the proteolytic enzyme pepsin), gastric lipase, and several hormones that play an important role in gastric acid secretion. Chemical and enzymatic digestion, particularly of proteins and triglycerides, is initiated in the stomach. The acidic environment in the stomach denatures alimentary protein and provides an optimal pH for activation and proteolytic activity of pepsin. Liquefied food is gradually released into the small intestine for further digestion. Only a few substances (e.g., NSAIDs) are absorbed in the stomach.

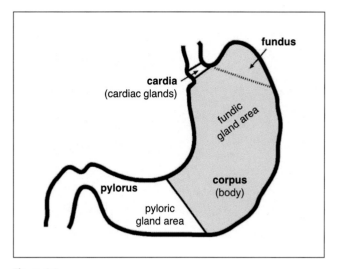

Figure 4.1:
Anatomical division of the stomach. This figure shows the idealized anatomical division of the stomach.

4.2 Anatomy

Jan S. Suchodolski

The stomach can be divided into a proximal and a distal portion. The proximal portion can be further divided into three regions: cardia, fundus, and body (Figure 4.1). The cardia is the thin portion of the stomach that is connected to the intra-abdominal portion of the esophagus. The fundus, which often contains gas that can be seen on abdominal radiographs, follows the cardia, and is located on the left side of the stomach. The corpus is the largest portion of the stomach and connects fundus and pylorus. Gastric fundus and corpus have the ability to dilate in order to accommodate a meal, while maintaining constant intragastric pressure. The proximal portion of the stomach is responsible for the production of most of the gastric juice. The distal portion of the stomach consists of the pyloric antrum, the pyloric canal, and a double sphincter, the pylorus. However, all three areas are often referred to as the pylorus. The major function of the distal portion of the stomach is to grind food particles and to aid in gastric emptying.

The mucosa and the submucosa of the empty stomach are thrown into folds. The mucosal surface is stippled with numerous tiny openings, the gastric pits.

The stomach has three muscular layers: a longitudinal layer (absent in the cranial and caudal portions of the stomach); a circular layer, which is the predominant layer and present in all areas; and an oblique layer. The latter layer is the least developed. The activity of these muscle layers aids in gastric emptying. The pylorus is characterized by a thickening of the circular muscle layer of the distal antrum.

4.3 Gastric physiology

Jan S. Suchodolski

4.3.1 Gastric glands

The gastric mucosa is composed of pits and glands. Located at the base of the pits are the openings of the gastric glands (Figure 4.2). The gastric mucosa contains three different types of glands that are named based on their localization: cardiac glands are located in the gastric cardia, fundic glands (also called oxyntic glands) in the fundus and corpus, and pyloric glands in the pyloric portion of the stomach. Each of these glands contains different secretory cells, which differ in their localization within the gastric glands as well as in the type of products they secrete.

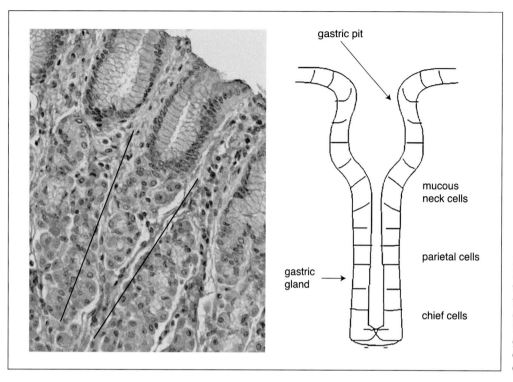

Figure 4.2:
Localization of secretory cells within the gastric gland. This figure shows the idealized localization of the gastric glands on the right and a histopathological view of gastric glands on the left. Please note the orientation of the gastric gland indicated by the two fine lines.

Labels in figure: gastric pit, mucous neck cells, parietal cells, gastric gland, chief cells

Cardiac glands. Cardiac glands consist mainly of mucus-secreting cells.

Fundic glands. Fundic glands are characterized by the presence of mucous neck cells, chief cells, and parietal cells. All these cell types most likely develop from a common progenitor cell.[1] The chief cells are located at the base of the fundic gland and secrete different isoforms of pepsinogen, a precursor of the proteolytic enzyme pepsin. In dogs two distinct groups of pepsinogens have been identified, pepsinogen A and B.[2] The parietal cells are located in the upper third of the fundic gland and secrete hydrochloric acid, R-protein, and in dogs, a glycoprotein called intrinsic factor. R-protein and intrinsic factor are crucial in the absorption of cobalamin (vitamin B12) in the small intestine. In contrast to humans, the stomach appears to be a limited source of intrinsic factor in domestic animals. In the dog, intrinsic factor is almost exclusively produced by the exocrine pancreas and to some extend in the salivary glands, while in the cat intrinsic factor is almost exclusively produced by the exocrine pancreas.[3] Mucous neck cells are scattered between the chief cells and parietal cells. In the dog, the mucous neck cells and mucous pit cells of gastric glands also produce gastric lipase.[4]

Ghrelin is synthesized in the epithelial cells lining the fundus of the stomach, with smaller amounts also produced outside the GI tract. Ghrelin is a peptide hormone that stimulates the release of growth hormone from the anterior pituitary. Ghrelin has a significant effect on appetite and energy balance, and chronic obesity has been reported to be associated with a significant decrease in plasma ghrelin concentration.[5]

Trefoil factors 1 and 2 (TFF 1 and 2) are peptides expressed in the stomach by the mucous neck cells in the gastric fundus and antrum, and by the pyloric glands. Trefoil factors play an important role during epithelial restitution after mucosal damage and/or during inflammation, and decreased expression of TFFs have been implicated in the development of gastric cancer.[6]

Pyloric glands. Pyloric glands contain mainly mucus-secreting cells and gastrin-producing endocrine cells (G cells). Gastrin stimulates gastric acid secretion and has an important trophic influence on the gastric mucosa.

4.3.2 Gastric secretion

Parietal cells have receptors for acetylcholine (ACh), gastrin, and histamine, all of which stimulate hydrochloric acid secretion (Figures 4.3 and 4.4). The secretion of gastric juice occurs in three phases: cephalic, gastric, and intestinal. The cephalic phase, triggered for example by the smell and/or sight of food, is activated through vagal stimuli and neuropeptides, and leads to a direct stimulation of the parietal cells via ACh and gastrin. The histamine-containing enterochromaffin-like cells (ECL cells) in the gastric fundus are also activated through ACh and gastrin. Histamine, released from the ECL cells, subsequently

4

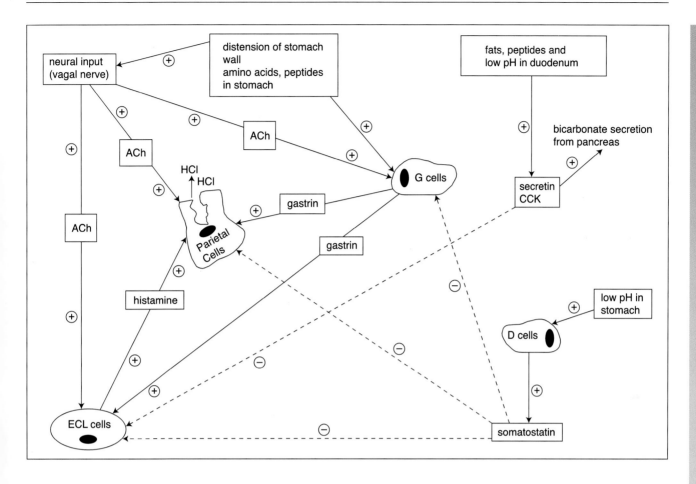

▲
Figure 4.3:
Regulation of gastric acid secretion by the parietal cells. The secretion of gastric acid by the parietal cells is regulated by a complex interaction of stimulatory and inhibitory factors. Stimulatory factors are depicted by "+", while inhibitory factors are depicted by "−". The presence of a particular mixture of stimulatory and inhibitory factors is dependant on the digestive phase of the stomach (interdigestive, cephalic, gastric, or intestinal phase).

Figure 4.4:
Gastric acid secretion by the parietal cell. Carbonic anhydrase catalyzes the reaction that generates H^+ and HCO_3^- from H_2O and CO_2 within the parietal cell. The HCO_3^- ions then diffuse out of the parietal cell and into the vascular space in exchange for the Cl^- ions, which in turn will be secreted into the gastric lumen. This HCO_3^- diffusion into the vascular space leads to an increase in blood pH during gastric acid secretion, producing the alkaline tide after a meal. K^+ moves along its electrochemical gradient into the gastric lumen. The H^+, K^+ ATPase actively secretes H^+ ions into the gastric lumen in exchange for K^+ ions, resulting in HCl accumulation in the gastric lumen. H^+, K^+ ATPase inhibitors (e.g. omeprazole) are the most effective inhibitors of gastric acid secretion.

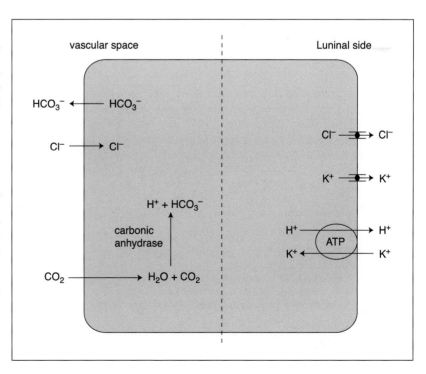

4

binds to parietal cell receptors and potentiates gastric acid secretion.

Distension of the stomach and release of peptides and amino acids from partially digested food marks the beginning of the gastric phase. At this stage, gastrin is released from the antral and duodenal mucosa. The beginning of gastric emptying leads to a decrease in duodenal pH (intestinal phase) and the release of secretin from small intestinal mucosal cells. Secretin stimulates the bicarbonate secretion of the pancreas. A low pH in the gastric antrum also leads to the secretion of somatostatin (from D-cells), which initiates a negative feedback mechanism on gastrin and, therefore, hydrochloric acid secretion. Cholecystokinin (CCK) release is stimulated through fatty acids and the presence of oligopeptides and amino acids in the duodenum. CCK further inhibits gastric acid secretion and stimulates exocrine pancreatic secretion. Pepsinogen release is mainly stimulated by acetylcholine and CCK, and indirectly through gastrin and vagal stimuli.

4.3.3 The gastric mucosal barrier

The gastric mucosa is constantly exposed to damaging insults, such as low pH, mechanical irritation, and digestive enzymes. The gastric mucosa has several defense mechanisms against damage by these insults. The first line of defense consists of the secretion of bicarbonate and mucus by the epithelial cells. For each H^+ that is secreted by a parietal cell into the gastric pit, a hydroxyl group is generated, which combines with CO_2 to form HCO_3^-. This HCO_3^- then reaches the luminal surface through the capillary blood flow from parietal cells, from where it diffuses into the overlaying mucus layer. Mucus secreted by mucous neck cells lines the luminal surface of the epithelial cells and together with the HCO_3^- maintains an alkaline environment, preventing diffusion of gastric acid and pepsin into the tissue.

The structure of the epithelial cells itself constitutes another important defense mechanism against auto-digestion by gastric acid. The apical surface of the epithelial cells contains a high proportion of hydrophobic phospholipids that repel gastric acid. Additionally, the epithelial cells contain a high concentration of intracellular bicarbonate that neutralizes any acid that back-diffuses from the gastric lumen into the epithelial cells. Capillary blood flow in between the epithelial cells provides further support in maintaining the local acid-base balance. Additionally, the gastric mucosa has the ability to self-repair when the above-mentioned defense mechanisms fail and cell injury occurs. The high turnover rate of the epithelial cells leads to a rapid regeneration of injured cells. Also, damaged mucosal cells secrete mucus that forms a protective layer over the gastric mucosa. Epithelial cells from areas adjacent to the injured cells migrate towards the damaged area and cover the lesion by growing over the basement membrane. This proliferation is due to an enhanced expression of epidermal growth factor (EGF), transforming growth factor-alpha (TGF-alpha), trefoil peptides (TFPs), and nitric oxide (NO). Prostaglandins, particularly prostaglandin E_2 and prostacyclin, play a major role in maintaining the integrity of the gastric mucosal barrier. Prostaglandins stimulate mucus and bicarbonate secretion, increase gastric mucosal blood flow, and have an effect on the cell regeneration of epithelial cells.

⌐○ Key Facts

- Mechanical and enzymatic digestion of food is initiated in the stomach.
- The gastric mucosa contains several glands that secrete various secretory products including hydrochloric acid, pepsin, mucus, gastrin, and intrinsic factor in dogs.
- Gastric acid secretion occurs in response to stimulation of histamine, gastrin, and acetylcholine receptors.
- The gastric mucosal barrier protects the stomach from damage by gastric acid and proteolytic enzymes.

References

1. Ge YB, Ohmori J, Tsuyama S et al. Immunocytochemistry and in situ hybridization studies of pepsinogen C-producing cells in developing rat fundic glands. *Cell Tissue Res* 1998; 293: 121–131.
2. Suchodolski JS, Steiner JM, Ruaux CG et al. Purification and partial characterization of canine pepsinogen A and B. *Am J Vet Res* 2002; 63: 1585–1590.
3. Simpson KW, Alpers DH, De Wille J et al. Cellular localization and hormonal regulation of pancreatic intrinsic factor secretion in dogs. *Am J Physiol Gastrointest Liver Physiol* 1993; 265: G178–G188.
4. Steiner JM, Berridge BR, Wojcieszyn J et al. Cellular immunolocalization of gastric and pancreatic lipase in various tissues obtained from dogs. *Am J Vet Res* 2002; 63: 722–727.
5. Jeusette IC, Lhoest ET, Istasse LP et al. Influence of obesity on plasma lipid and lipoprotein concentrations in dogs. *Am J Vet Res* 2005; 66: 81–86.
6. Leung WK, Yu J, Chan FK et al. Expression of trefoil peptides (TFF1, TFF2, and TFF3) in gastric carcinomas, intestinal metaplasia, and non-neoplastic gastric tissues. *J Pathol* 2002; 197: 582–588.

4.4 Diseases of the Stomach

Reto Neiger

4.4.1 Gastritis

Classification

By definition, gastritis is an inflammatory disease of the stomach. Many patients with clinical signs of vomiting or upper GI problems are thought to have some type of mucosal injury; however, as infiltration of the gastric mucosa with inflammatory cells is either not diagnosed or minimal, it might be therefore more accurate to use the term gastropathy for these cases.

The Sydney classification system is the most commonly used scheme for the classification of gastritis in human medicine.[1] Unfortunately, a similar system is, as yet, not available in veterinary medicine. Gastritis is commonly grouped into acute or chronic, based on the duration of the clinical signs and not on histological parameters. If inflammation is deep, a peptic ulcer may ensue.

4.4.1.1 Acute gastritis

Although many conditions have been found to cause acute gastritis, the most common ones are dietary hypersensitivity and dietary indiscretion.[2] Acute gastritis does not have any age predilection and can occur in any dog or cat. It is most often a result of ingestion of inappropriate food (i.e., spoiled or toxic food stuff) or foreign material (e.g., rocks, bones, wood, or weeds). Other possible causes are drugs (e.g., NSAIDs, corticosteroids), chemicals (e.g., fertilizer, herbicide), or heavy metals (e.g., lead, zinc). Several infectious causes also can cause gastritis, such as viral (e.g., parvovirosis, distemper, infectious hepatitis) or parasitic organisms (e.g., *Physaloptera* spp., *Ollulanus* spp.). In human medicine, the discovery of bacterial gastritis due to *Helicobacter pylori* infection has revolutionized the field of gastroenterology.[3] In contrast, in veterinary medicine it is still not clear if *Helicobacter* spp. is indeed pathogenic, or merely a commensal organism, rarely resulting in vomiting in some patients.[4] Most often, only a tentative diagnosis can be reached based on signalment, history, clinical signs, and physical examination findings. During endoscopy, superficial hemorrhage due to erosions and edema can be seen.

Treatment of acute gastritis

Initially, dietary restriction by withholding food for 12–24 hours is all that is needed. Depending on the severity of the clinical signs (i.e., dehydration, continuous vomiting), the animal will also need to be treated with intravenous crystalloids (e.g., lactated Ringer's solution) but no water is given orally. Because most affected animals are hypokalemic, potassium often needs to be supplemented based on the actual serum potassium concentration (see Table 5.3). Water can be introduced 24 hours after vomiting has ceased. If the animal tolerates oral water, a bland commercial or home-cooked diet (e.g., white fish or chicken and rice, cottage cheese), given in small amounts multiple times during the day, is indicated. The animal's regular food can be slowly reintroduced over a 3- to 5-day period after vomiting has ceased.

In some patients, symptomatic treatment with antiemetics is necessary to stop the vomiting. Because antiemetic therapy is based on the neurotransmitter-receptor interactions, it is important to understand these mechanisms (Figure 4.5). Several neurotransmitters and receptors have been identified in the chemoreceptor trigger zone (CRTZ), including receptors that bind dopamine (D_2-dopaminergic), neurokinin$_1$ (NK_1), norepinephrine (α_2-adrenergic), 5-hydroxytryptamine (5-HT_3-serotonergic), acetylcholine (M_1-cholinergic), histamine (H_1- and H_2-histaminergic), or enkephalins (ENK_μ-enkephalinergic). In contrast, the only receptors shown to be present in the vomoting center so far are NK_1, 5-hydroxytryptamine$_3$ and α_2-adrenergic receptors. The α_2-adrenergic receptors in the

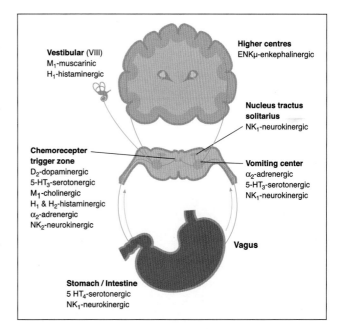

Figure 4.5:
Schematic drawing of the emetic pathways and their receptors. The vomiting center lies in the medulla oblongata and receives input from various stimuli. From the periphery (e.g., the stomach or intestine), the vomiting center is stimulated via sympathetic and parasympathetic nerves. Additional stimulation comes from the chemoreceptor trigger zone, which is located outside the blood-brain barrier. Finally, stimuli might also come from the vestibular apparatus, higher centers, or the nucleus tractus solitarius.

4

emetic center and in the CRTZ may be antagonized by α_2 antagonists (e.g., yohimbine, atipamezole) or by mixed α_1/α_2 antagonists (e.g., prochlorperazine, chlorpromazine). In the vestibular apparatus, muscarinic M_1 receptors and acetylcholine have been demonstrated to be present, and therefore mixed M_1/M_2 antagonists (e.g., atropine, scopolamine) and pure M_1 antagonists, such as pirenzepine, may inhibit motion sickness in dogs and cats. Many receptors are found in the gastrointestinal tract, but the NK_1, 5-HT_3 receptors are likely to play the most important role in the initiation of vomiting. Cytotoxic agents cause the release of 5-HT from enterochromaffin cells in the gastrointestinal tract, which then activate the 5-HT_3 receptors on afferent vagal fibers. Thus, vomiting induced by the activation of 5-HT_3 receptors can be completely abolished by treating the patient with a 5-HT_3 antagonist, such as dolasetron, ondansetron, granisetron, or tropisetron. Another antagonist of 5-HT_3 receptors is metoclopramide, but only at high concentrations. Recently, the administration of substance P has been found to result in emesis by binding to the NK_1 receptor. NK_1-receptor antagonists block central and peripheral vomiting both in dogs and ferrets.[5]

Several antiemetic drugs are directed at the neurotransmitter-receptor system just described (Table 4.1). These antagonists are classified as α_2-adrenergic, D_2-dopaminergic, NK_1, H_1-histaminergic, H_2-histaminergic, M_1-muscarinic-cholinergic, 5-HT_3-serotonergic, and 5-HT_4-serotonergic. Some of these drugs have several mechanisms of action as an antiemetic agent. For example, the phenothiazines (e.g., prochlorperazine, chlorpromazine) are antagonists of α_1- and α_2-adrenergic, D_2-dopaminergic, H_1- and H_2-histaminergic, and muscarinic-cholinergic receptors. Phenothiazines are very potent but should be avoided in dehydrated or hypotensive animals without first resuscitating the patient with intravenous fluid administration. Also, these drugs are contraindicated in animals with a known seizure history. Metoclopramide blocks receptors in the CRTZ, increases the threshold in the emetic center, and also has an effect on the viscera. Metoclopramide increases the lower esophageal sphincter tone, decreases the pyloric sphincter tone, and increases the frequency and amplitude of gastric and duodenal contractions. All these functions combined make metoclopramide useful for controlling vomition that is due to nonspecific gastritis or gastric motility disorders. The prokinetic activity of metoclopramide seems to be limited to the liquid phase of gastric emptying as a study showed no effect on the gastric emptying rate of digestible solids.[6] Metoclopramide can be given orally, intravenously, or as a constant rate infusion.

Table 4.1: Antiemetic medications. This table shows a comprehensive summary of antiemetic medications with their commonly recommended dosages.

Classification	Example	Site of action	Dosage	Side effects
α_2-adrenergic antagonists	■ atipamezole ■ chlorpromazine ■ prochlorperazine ■ yohimbine	■ CRTZ, emetic center ■ CRTZ, emetic center ■ CRTZ, emetic center ■ CRTZ, emetic center	■ Unknown ■ 0.2–0.4 mg/kg SC, IM q 8 h ■ 0.1–0.5 mg/kg SC, IM q 6–8 h ■ 0.25–0.5 mg/kg SC, IM q 12h	■ hypotension, sedation ■ hypotension, sedation ■ hypotension, sedation ■ hypotension, sedation
D_2-dopaminergic antagonists	■ chlorpromazine ■ domperidone ■ metoclopramide ■ prochlorperazine ■ trimethobenzamide	■ CRTZ ■ GI smooth muscle ■ CRTZ, GI muscles ■ CRTZ ■ CRTZ	■ 0.2–0.4 mg/kg SC, IM q 8 h ■ 0.1–0.3 mg/kg IM, IV q 12 h ■ 0.2–0.4 mg/kg PO, SC, IM q 6 h ■ 0.1–0.5 mg/kg SC, IM q 6–8 h ■ 3 mg/kg IM q 8–12 h	■ tremors, shivering ■ none reported ■ extrapyramidal signs ■ sedation, hypotension ■ allergic reaction
NK_1-receptor antagonist	■ maropitant	■ CRTZ, emetic center	■ 2 mg/kg PO q 24 h ■ 1 mg/kg SC q 24 h	■ none reported
H_1-histaminergic antagonists	■ chlorpromazine ■ dimenhydrinate ■ diphenhydramine ■ prochlorperazine	■ CRTZ ■ CRTZ ■ CRTZ ■ CRTZ	■ 0.2–0.4 mg/kg SC, IM q 8 h ■ 4–8 mg/kg PO q 8 h ■ 2–4 mg/kg PO, IM q 8 h ■ 0.1–0.5 mg/kg SC, IM q 6–8 h	■ tremors, shivering ■ sedation ■ sedation ■ sedation, hypotension
M_1-cholinergic antagonists	■ chlorpromazine ■ pirenzepine ■ prochlorperazine ■ scopolamine	■ CRTZ ■ vestibular, CRTZ ■ CRTZ ■ vestibular, CRTZ	■ 0.2–0.4 mg/kg SC, IM q 8 h ■ unknown ■ 0.1–0.5 mg/kg SC, IM q 6–8 h ■ 0.03 mg/kg SC, IM q 6 h	■ hypotension, sedation ■ unknown ■ hypotension, sedation ■ sedation, xerostomia
5-HT_3-serotonergic antagonists	■ dolasetron ■ granisetron ■ metoclopramide ■ ondansetron	■ CRTZ ■ CRTZ, vagal afferents ■ CRTZ, GI muscles ■ CRTZ, vagal afferents	■ 0.3–0.6 mg/kg IV, SC, PO q 8–12 h ■ unknown ■ 0.2–0.4 mg/kg PO, SC, IM q 6 h ■ 0.5–1 mg/kg PO q 12–24 h	■ unknown ■ sedation, head shaking ■ extrapyramidal signs ■ sedation, head shaking
5-HT_4-serotonergic antagonists	■ cisapride	■ myenteric neurons	■ 0.1–0.5 PO q 8 h	■ none reported

IM = muscular administration; IV = intravenous administration; PO = oral administration; SC = subcutaneous administration

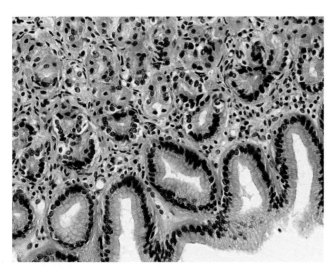

Figure 4.6:
Lymphoplasmacytic gastritis. This figure shows a histopathological image of the gastric mucosa of a 5-year-old female mixed-breed dog with lymphoplasmacytic gastritis. There are large aggregates of lymphocytes and a smaller number of plasma cells infiltrating the gastric mucosa in this patient. (HE staining, 120x; image courtesy of Dr. Thomas Bilzer, University of Düsseldorf, Germany.)

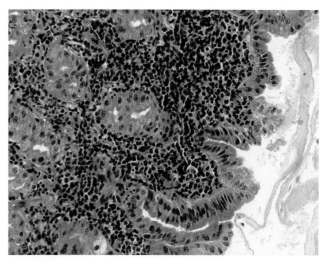

Figure 4.7:
Eosinophilic gastritis. This figure shows a histopathological image of the gastric mucosa of a 13-year-old male cat with inappetence and weight loss. Note the abundant presence of eosinophils throughout this section of gastric mucosa. Histological diagnosis: eosinophilic gastritis. (HE staining, 120x; image courtesy of Dr. Thomas Bilzer, University of Düsseldorf, Germany.)

A new NK$_1$-receptor antagonist, maropitant, will soon become available and licensed for dogs. In various licensing studies, maropitant has been highly effective in abolishing vomiting induced through peripheral emetogenic stimuli, such as cisplatin administration or central emetogenic stimuli, such as apomorphine.[7] Even travel-sickness-induced vomiting was successfully suppressed by the administration of maropitant.

4.4.1.2 Chronic gastritis

The pathogenesis of chronic gastritis in dogs and cats is not fully understood. In some cases, a cause, such as parasitism or a metabolic disorder (e.g., uremia, hepatopathy), can be identified. Several dog breeds are at risk for chronic gastritis, including the Basenji, the Drentse Patrijshond, and the Norwegian Lundehund.[8] In most cases, however, chronic gastritis is idiopathic and an immune-mediated condition is hypothesized to be responsible for the inflammatory infiltrate in the gastric mucosa. Experimentally, chronic gastritis in dogs can be induced by mucosal irritants, systemic administration of gastric juice, or prenatal thymectomy;[9] however, each of these experimental models disturbs oral tolerance. Chronic idiopathic gastritis is probably part of the inflammatory bowel disease (IBD) syndrome and may arise as an adverse reaction to food or bacterial antigens. The presence of *Helicobacter* spp. in the stomach of dogs almost certainly does not cause chronic gastritis.[4] In cats the clinical role of gastric *Helicobacter* spp. is less clear.[10]

Clinical signs in dogs and cats with chronic gastritis are characterized by chronic persistent or intermittent vomiting of variable frequency and character. Because inflammation impairs gastric motility and delays gastric emptying, animals with chronic gastritis may retain food in the stomach for long periods of time. A definitive diagnosis of chronic gastritis requires a mucosal biopsy. The gastritis can then be classified based on the histopathological findings as lymphoplasmacytic gastritis, eosinophilic gastritis, hypertrophic gastritis, or atrophic gastritis.

4.4.1.2.1 Lymphoplasmacytic gastritis

Most patients with chronic gastritis have some infiltration of the gastric mucosa with lymphocytes and/or plasma cells (Figure 4.6). This form of gastritis is often part of the more diffuse IBD complex and has likely a similar etiopathogenesis. Abnormal or increased food antigens, intestinal bacterial antigens, or both together and/or an abnormal or overwhelmed tolerance of the host might play an integral part. There are no typical clinical, laboratory, or diagnostic imaging findings in dogs and cats with gastritis. Since no uniform criteria to evaluate gastric biopsies exist so far, there must be good communication between the clinician and pathologist to ensure that neither over- nor under-interpretation of the biopsy specimen occurs. Severe lymphoplasmacytic infiltration is often difficult to distinguish from gastric lymphoma, especially when the biopsy specimens are small.

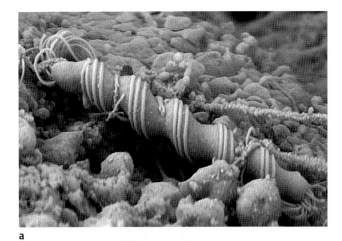

a

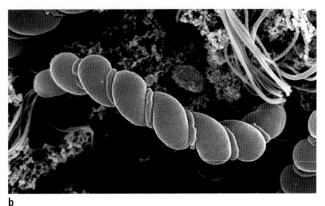

b

Figure 4.8:
Electron microscopic views of *Helicobacter* spp. **a:** This picture shows a scanning electron microscopic view of *Helicobacter felis* from an experimentally infected mouse. Please note the typical three periplasmic filaments and the spiral shape. *H. felis* measures 4–6 µm in length and approximately 0.5 µm in thickness. (Image courtesy of Dr. M. Stoffel, Bern, Switzerland). **b:** Scanning electron microscopic image of *H. bizzozeronii* from an experimentally infected mouse. While the most common type of *H. bizzozeronii* lack the periplasmic fibers, some show a filament running along the groove of the spirals. (Image courtesy of Dr. M. Stoffel, Bern, Switzerland.)

4.4.1.2.2 Eosinophilic gastritis

Eosinophilic gastritis is an uncommon disorder of unknown etiology that is characterized by diffuse eosinophilic infiltration of the distal portion of the stomach (Figure 4.7) and is also often associated with eosinophilic infiltration of the small bowel or colon. Gastric infiltration is usually restricted to the mucosa but in some patients may extend into the muscularis and even the serosa. Mucosal involvement causes enlargement of the rugal folds. The diseased mucosa may become ulcerated, which leads to bleeding or leakage of plasma proteins into the gastric lumen. Peripheral eosinophilia is a common finding, but its severity can vary markedly. Some pets also have a history of either urticaria or vomiting that may be associated with the ingestion of a specific diet.

4.4.1.2.3 Hypertrophic gastritis

Chronic hypertrophic gastritis is a rare disorder that appears either as diffuse, generalized mucosal hypertrophy or, more frequently, as a localized hypertrophy of the antral mucosa that may cause intermittent or chronic pyloric obstruction. Causative factors that may lead to gastric mucosal hypertrophy include chronic inflammation, foreign bodies, or long-term use of proton pump inhibitors. Hypergastrinemia can also have a trophic effect on the mucosa, as seen in chronic renal disease, chronic gastric distension, gastrin-secreting tumors (gastrinoma), and idiopathic hypertrophy of antral G cells. Boxers and Basenjis have a predilection for the diffuse form of hypertrophic gastritis. In contrast, the localized form has a predilection for miniature and toy dog breeds (e.g., Lhasa Apso, Maltese, Pekingese, and Shih Tzu). The hypertrophic mucosa is inflamed and causes delayed emptying, chronic vomiting, anorexia, and lethargy.

4.4.1.2.4 Atrophic gastritis

Atrophic gastritis is a rare disorder in which the gastric mucosa atrophies and loses its secretory functions. Atrophic gastritis has been reported in the Norwegian Lundehund. The cause is unknown, but the condition occurs mainly in older dogs and may be mediated through the immune system. Atrophic gastritis may also be a sequel to chronic reflux gastritis in dogs. The predominant complaint is chronic intermittent vomiting. Mucosal degeneration is thought to result in achlorhydria, which may predispose to bacterial overgrowth in the proximal small intestine. This can lead to malabsorption, chronic diarrhea, and/or loss of body weight and condition.

4.4.1.2.5 Helicobacter infection

Helicobacter spp. are gram-negative, microaerophilic, curved to spiral-shaped, motile bacteria. Their main location is the stomach, however, they can also be found in the intestine and the liver.[11–13] To date, over 30 organisms with typical characteristics of *Helicobacter* spp. have been described, with new species being published constantly. Most gastric *Helicobacter*-like organisms (GHLO) found in dogs and cats are large spiral organisms (0.5 × 5–10 µm) that cannot be distinguished by light microscopy. To date *H. felis, H. bizzozeronii, H. salomonis, Flexispira rappini, H. bilis,* and "*H. heilmannii*" have all been reported to have been present in the stomach of dogs,[14–16] while *H. felis, H. pametensis, H. pylori, H. bizzozeronii, H. salomonis,* and "*H. heilmannii*" have been reported to be present in the stomach of cats (Figures 4.8 a and b).[13,15,17,18] Mixed infections with two or more *Helicobacter* spp. appear to be common in dogs and cats.[15,16]

Several studies showed a high prevalence of GHLO in cats and dogs (Table 4.2) with up to 100% infection rate amongst laboratory animals, 50–100% amongst healthy pets, and 41–100% among vomiting pets. Housing conditions and age appear to play an important role with pets living in shelters or colonies having a higher prevalence, while young animals may be less often colonized than adults, but this is controversial.[14,17]

The mode of transmission of *Helicobacter* spp. is still unclear. Fecal-oral transmission is hypothesized by some, since *H. pylori* can be cultured from cat feces. Oral-oral transmission is hypothesized by others, because *H. pylori* can be found in the saliva of infected humans. Also, the spouses of infected individuals also were shown to have a higher prevalence.

In human patients, there is extensive evidence implicating *H. pylori* in the pathogenesis of chronic superficial gastritis. Eradication of *H. pylori* by use of antimicrobial therapy may cure gastritis and the titer of anti-*H. pylori* antibodies decreases with time. A plethora of reports have shown many putative mechanisms by which *H. pylori* alters gastric physiology;[19] e.g., through the induction of gastric inflammation (by secretion of IL-8, platelet activating factor, urease, etc.), through the disruption of the gastric mucosal barrier (by disrupting phospholipases, secreting vacuolating cytotoxins, inducing apoptosis, etc.), or through altering the gastric-secretory axis (by decreasing somatostatin release, inducing hypergastrinemia, diminishing the responsiveness of parietal cells, etc.). Infection with *Helicobacter* spp. also predisposes humans to the development of gastric cancer.

In pets with naturally acquired *Helicobacter* colonization, however, the pathogenic role of this organism is still highly debated. Obvious clinical signs of infection are absent in the majority of infected cats and dogs, and few studies have investigated the cellular and immunological consequences of infection. In dogs, a mild gastritis with infiltration of the gastric mucosa involving lymphocytes and plasma cells was most commonly found,[4,14] but no correlation between the histopathological changes and the occurrence of GHLOs as well as a clear pathologic role due to enlarged canaliculi and pyknotic parietal cells has been reported. In some cats, normal gastric mucosa was found in several GHLO-colonized animals, while others reported mild chronic gastritis irrespective of GHLO colonization.[17,20,21] In dogs with naturally acquired *Helicobacter* spp. infection, a variety of secretory function tests, such as unstimulated gastric pH, fasting, post-prandial and bombesin-stimulated plasma gastrin concentrations as well as

Table 4.2: Prevalence of gastric *Helicobacter*-like organisms in cats and dogs

Status	% infected	# of pets	Species	Reference
Healthy	100	12	cat	Weber et al. *Am J Vet Res* 1958; 19: 677–680
	100	30	dog	Henry et al. *Am J Vet Res* 1987; 48: 831–836
	41	29	cat	Geyer et al. *Vet Rec* 1993; 133: 18–19
	86	55	cat	Otto et al. *J Clin Microbiol* 1994; 32: 1043–1049
	91	54	dog	Eaton et al. *J Clin Microbiol* 1996; 34: 3165–3170
	100	25	cat	El-Zataari et al. *J Med Microbiol* 1997; 46: 372–376
	100	15	cat	Papasouliotis et al. *Vet Rec* 1997; 140: 369–370
	90	10	cat	Yamasaki et al. *J Am Vet Med Assoc* 1998; 212: 529–533
	86	21	dog	Yamasaki et al. *J Am Vet Med Assoc* 1998; 212: 529–533
	94	32	cat	De Majo et al. *Europ J Comp Gastroenterol* 1998; 3: 13–18
	91	58	cat	Neiger et al. *J Clin Microbiol* 1998; 36: 634–637
	100	25	dog	Happonen et al. *J Vet Med Assoc* 1998; 43: 305–315
	100	15	cat	Norris et al. *J Clin Microbiol* 1999; 37: 189–194
	93	68	dog	Neiger et al. *Microbiol Ecol Health Dis* 1999; 11; 234–240
Diseased	57	60	cat	Geyer et al. *Vet Rec* 1993; 133: 18–19
	74	42	dog	Geyer et al. *Vet Rec* 1993; 133: 18–19
	76	127	cat	Hermanns et al. *J Com Pathol* 1995; 112: 307–318
	82	122	dog	Hermanns et al. *J Com Pathol* 1995; 112: 307–318
	100	24	cat	Papasouliotis et al. *Vet Rec* 1997; 140: 396–370
	64	33	cat	Yamasaki et al. *J Am Vet Med Assoc* 1998; 212: 529–533
	61	56	dog	Yamasaki et al. *J Am Vet Med Assoc* 1998; 212: 529–533
	95	21	dog	Happonen et al. *J Vet Med A* 1998; 43: 305–315

4

pentagastrin-stimulated maximal acid output and titratable acidity, were similar when compared to a SPF, *Helicobacter*-free control group.[22]

There are only a few studies on experimental infection of dogs and cats with *Helicobacter* spp. While experimentally infected gnotobiotic dogs showed chronic gastritis and an increase in fasting gastric pH in some, there was no relationship between *H. felis* infection and gastric inflammation in SPF dogs after six months in others.[23] The gastric secretory axis, assessed by fasting and meal-stimulated plasma gastrin concentration, mucosal gastrin and somatostatin immunoreactivity, fasting gastric pH and pentagastrin-stimulated gastric acid secretion functioned similarly in both the infected and uninfected SPF dogs.[23] Conventional puppies infected with *H. pylori* showed some clinical signs shortly after inoculation and the gastric mucosa initially demonstrated acute gastritis changing to chronic gastritis with time. In another investigation, SPF, *Helicobacter*-free cats were studied before and for one year after inoculation with *H. felis*.[24] Uninfected cats were used as controls. Lymphoid follicular hyperplasia, atrophy, and fibrosis were observed primarily in the pylorus of the infected cats.

Seroconversion of experimentally infected dogs and cats was observed in all of these studies. *H. felis*- and *H. pylori*-infected gnotobiotic dogs showed a fairly rapid and uniform seroconversion 3 weeks after infection, while *H. felis*-infected SPF dogs showed a more gradual and variable seroconversion over a six-month period after infection.[23]

Diagnostic tests for GHLO are either invasive (i.e., rapid urease tests, histopathology, touch cytology, culture, polymerase chain reaction of biopsies, or electron microscopy) requiring a biopsy sample or they can also be non-invasive (i.e., urea breath and blood tests, serology, and fecal PCR testing).

Invasive tests for Helicobacter spp.

The rapid urease test (also called CLO test for *Campylobacter*-like organism test) is based on the production of urease by all gastric *Helicobacter* spp. A tissue sample is incubated in a broth containing urea and phenol red as a pH indicator. As the urease breaks down urea into ammonia, the pH rises and a color change occurs (Figure 4.9). The results can often be obtained within one to three hours, but may take up to 24 hours.

Histopathology relies on the visualization of *Helicobacter* organisms in gastric biopsy samples. Special staining such as Warthin-Starry silver, Giemsa, or toluidine blue stain will enhance the visibility of GHLOs (Figure 4.10). Due to the patchy distribution of the *Helicobacter* organisms, several biopsies from the antrum and corpus should be evaluated. Touch cytology stained with Gram's or Diff Quick stain is a simple, rapid, and sensitive diagnostic test; however, the extent of a

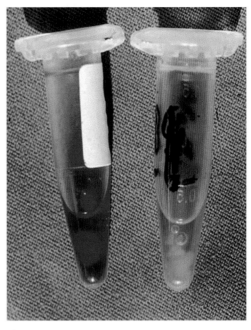

Figure 4.9:
Rapid urease test. This figure shows examples of a positive (red) and negative (yellow) rapid urease test that is used for the diagnosis of *Helicobacter* spp. Rapid urease tests are based on a color change, which is caused by a change in pH that is due to the production of ammonium by urease-producing organisms in a biopsy sample.

concurrent gastritis cannot be evaluated based on cytological evaluation alone (Figure 4.11).

Culture for GHLOs is cumbersome and the least sensitive method for diagnosing these organisms; however, a positive culture is highly specific. Gastric *Helicobacter* spp. are difficult to isolate *in vitro*. Polymerase chain reaction (PCR) of DNA extracted from a biopsy specimen permits definitive identification of the *Helicobacter* strain present. Electron microscopy can be used to differentiate *Helicobacter* spp. on the basis of typical morphological criteria. Five cultured canine *Helicobacter* spp. could be differentiated based on transmission and scanning electron microscopy (Figures 4.8a and 4.8b).[25] Overall, the rapid urease test, histopathology with special stains, and touch cytology are associated with a high accuracy for diagnosing a *Helicobacter* spp. colonization in dogs and cats (Table 4.3).

Non-invasive tests

The urea breath and blood tests use labeled urea (mostly labeled with non-radioactive ^{13}C). Ingested urea is metabolized in the stomach by bacterial urease to ammonia and the released carbon atoms are absorbed into the systemic circulation

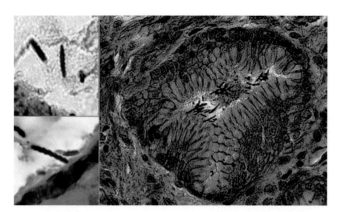

Figure 4.10:
Helicobacter spp. in a Warthin-Starry silver stain of a gastric biopsy. This picture shows a gastric biopsy stained with Warthin-Starry silver stain. This biopsy was taken from a naturally infected cat. Multiple large spiral-shaped organisms can be seen in a gastric pit. The spiral morphology is clearly visible under higher magnification.

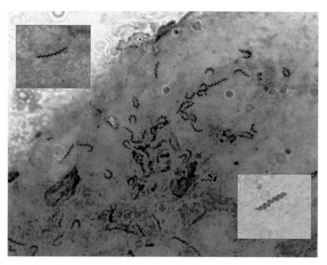

Figure 4.11:
This figure shows multiple *Helicobacter* spp. organisms in a Gram-stained gastric touch cytology. The proteinaceous background is due to gastric mucous. The enlargements clearly delineate the spiral structure of these bacteria.

and finally exhaled. The exhaled air is collected and the ratio of $^{12}CO_2$ to $^{13}CO_2$ is measured.[17,26] Since the urea breath test demonstrates the actual colonization with *Helicobacter* spp. organisms, it is the preferred non-invasive method to document a successful eradication in both humans and animals.

Serology by ELISA or Western blotting is used extensively in human epidemiological studies and IgG or IgA can be quantified in both serum and gastric fluid. Dogs and cats harbor several *Helicobacter* spp. but not *H. pylori*, and thus serum samples of pets cannot be analyzed by commercially available serological tests. Amplification of *Helicobacter* DNA from canine fecal samples has recently been described.[12] With this technique, gastric as well as intestinal *Helicobacter* DNA could be identified in dogs. Also, the treatment success could be monitored non-invasively by this method.

4.4.1.2.6 Parasitic gastritis

Physaloptera spp. are nematodes with an indirect live cycle requiring an intermediate host to develop into the infective stage. Suitable intermediate hosts (e.g., cockroaches, field crickets, canal crickets, or flour beetles) ingest the eggs, which have been shed by the definite hosts (e.g., cats, dogs). The first-stage larvae hatch in the intestine of intermediate hosts, migrate to the outer layer of the intestine, encyst and molt to second-, and finally, infective third-stage larvae. After the intermediate hosts are ingested by either paratenic (e.g. frogs, snakes, or mice) or definite hosts, the adults develop and attach to the gastric or duodenal mucosa.[27]

Table 4.3: Accuracy of various tests for the diagnosis of gastric *Helicobacter* spp. in dogs and cats

Test	Sensitivity	Specificity
Based on morphology		
Gram's stain	95%	92%
Warthin-Starry stain	90%	100%
Based on urease activity		
Rapid urease tests	93%	92%
Urea breath test	90%	73%
Based on molecular genetics		
PCR of gastric biopsy	94%	92%

4

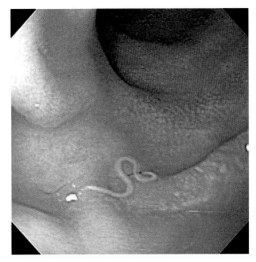

Figure 4.12:
Physaloptera. This figure shows an endoscopic picture of the stomach of a dog with a single *Physaloptera* specimen. (Image courtesy of Dr. Mike Willard, Texas, USA.)

It is unclear if *Physaloptera* are always pathogenic and how many stomach worms are required for clinical signs to ensue. Besides histological evidence of gastritis, these parasites can also result in delayed gastric emptying, possibly due to altered electromechanical activity.[28] Other clinical signs are chronic or intermittent vomiting, diarrhea, regurgitation, weight loss, melena, and lethargy.[27] Diagnosis can be difficult as fecal flotation is frequently falsely negative. Speculated reasons for this include that the adults only produce low numbers of eggs, the fact that a single-sex infection produces no eggs at all, or the fact that the specific gravity of the fecal flotation medium is too close to that of the eggs and thus the eggs do not float well.[28] Identification of worms in the vomit or endoscopic visualization of stomach worms (1–6 cm in length, stout, cream-colored to white, straight or coiled; Figure 4.12) appears to be most successful in the diagnosis of this parasite.

Ollulanus tricuspis is a common gastric nematode of cats with a prevalence of up to 20% that also occurs rarely in dogs.[29] After oral ingestion of third-stage larvae, the complete life cycle occurs within the stomach of the host, where the parasite attaches to the gastric mucosa. Infective larvae are vomited up and survive in the environment for up to 15 days, where they can infect another animal. Common clinical signs are inappetence, intermittent vomiting, and weight loss. Gastric erosions, increased mucous production, mucosal hyperplasia, and infiltration with inflammatory cells can be seen histopathologically. Diagnosis is best achieved by examining vomited material (possibly induced by the administration of xylazine or metedomidine) or gastric lavage solution. Rarely, parasites can be found in gastric biopsy samples by histopathology. Fecal flotation is rarely diagnostic.

If possible, the underlying cause of the gastric inflammation should be managed first (e.g., removal of foreign body, cessation of drug administration). Diagnosis of infestation with a stomach worm (i.e., *Physaloptera* spp. in dogs and *Ollulanus tricuspis* in cats) maybe challenging and routine therapy with a broad-spectrum anthelminthic agent that is effective in eradicating stomach worms (i.e., in dogs: pyrantel pamoate at 15 mg/kg PO repeated in 2–3 weeks; in cats: fenbendazole at 50 mg/kg PO q 24 h for 3 days) is prudent before recommending more expensive diagnostic tests.[27] However, most cases of chronic gastritis are idiopathic and treatment of the underlying cause is thus rarely possible. In cases of idiopathic chronic gastritis, rational treatment options include dietary management, immunosuppressive therapy, inhibition or neutralization of gastric acid secretion (see 4.4.1.3; Table 4.1; 4.4.1.1).

Dietary management is based on the concept that antigens in the food may be responsible for an exaggerated immune response of the body. Feeding single novel protein and carbohydrate sources, to which the animal has not yet been exposed to, is the cornerstone of this treatment concept. Although commercial "hypoallergenic" diets are very useful, on rare occasions it is necessary to feed a home-cooked novel protein source (e.g., kangaroo or horse). In most cases, some response should be seen after a 2-week strict dietary trial.

Immunosuppressive drug therapy is indicated in those dogs and cats that do not respond to dietary management alone (e.g., those with lymphoplasmacytic or eosinophilic gastritis). Corticosteroids, in addition to their immunosuppressive and anti-inflammatory properties, have regenerative effects on the gastric parietal cells. The ulcerogenic property of corticosteroids is of concern only in dogs that are exposed to a marked synergistic ulcerogenic effect (e.g., NSAID administration or hypotension). Initially, prednisone is given at a dose of 1–2 mg/kg PO q 12 h for 5 to 7 days. This dose is then gradually tapered in decremental doses of 50% over a period of several months. Other immunosuppressive drugs, such as azathioprine and cyclophosphamide, have only been used sporadically in dogs with chronic gastritis and should not be used for this purpose in cats.

4.4.1.3 Gastric ulceration

By definition, an ulcer is an area of damaged gastric mucosa to the level of the lamina muscularis mucosae or deeper; more superficial damage is called erosion. Erosions or ulcers occur when the »aggressive forces« (i.e., acid, pepsin, and/or trauma) are more potent than the »protective forces« (i.e., mucosal microcirculation, epithelial turnover, gastric mucus, and prostaglandins). Epithelial cells have a rapid turnover and need an abundant blood circulation to ensure the transport of nutrients and oxygen and the removal of back-diffused hydrogen ions. The entire gastric surface is replaced every 2 to 3 days. Epithelial cells are produced in the crypts and then migrate towards the gastric lumen, where they are shed. Gastric mucus neck cells produce a viscous gel of glycoprotein (5%) and water (95%), which adheres to the surface of the mucosa. This mucus protects against mechanical abrasion and acts as a barrier against digestive enzymes. In addition, bicarbonate is secreted actively into this layer. A pH gradient forms from the lumen to the epithelium, which neutralizes gastric acid. Finally, prostaglandins, which are derived from arachidonic acid via the enzyme cyclooxygenase (COX), have a protective role for the gut mucosa. They increase gastric mucus and bicarbonate secretion, maintain mucosal blood flow by causing vasodilation, and inhibit acid secretion. They may possibly stimulate mucosal cell turnover and migration by acting as an intercellular messenger. Prostaglandin-inhibiting drugs, such as NSAIDs, can counteract all these protective mechanisms and lead to the formation of gastric ulcers.

Peptic ulcers of the gastric and duodenal mucosa are not commonly seen in dogs or cats, but several underlying mechanisms can lead to the formation of this type of ulcer (Table 4.4). NSAIDs (e.g., aspirin, flunixin, ibuprofen, indomethacin, ketoprofen, meloxicam, naproxen, phenylbutazone, or piroxicam) inhibit the COX-1 enzyme, thereby limiting prostaglandin production. Even though these drugs have been implicated as a common cause of peptic ulcers in dogs, only a few reports of NSAID-induced peptic ulcers in pets exist.[30,31] Eicosanoids produced by COX-2 are mainly responsible for the inflammatory and pain properties of the gastric mucosa, while those produced by COX-1 are mainly responsible for its protective mechanisms. Unspecific COX inhibition increases the ulcerogenic risk dramatically. However, newer NSAIDs are COX-2 specific (e.g., carprofen) and have a lower, although not abolished, ulcerogenic effect.[32]

Corticosteroids also decrease the production of protective eicosanoids. Nevertheless, they are only responsible for peptic ulcers in dogs with concurrent problems, such as severe hypotension or if they are also given NSAIDs.[33] Mast cell tumors have long been thought to be responsible for peptic ulcers because of their histamine-containing granules, which can cause hyperacidity in the stomach.[34] However, no series of dogs or cats with mast cell tumor and peptic ulceration or even gastritis has been published as of yet. Most dogs with acute intervertebral disk diseases have endoscopic signs of gastric erosions, and surgical interventions with or without corticosteroid administration greatly increases the risk for peptic ulcers.[35] The gastrointestinal tract is the shock organ of dogs and therefore, hypovolemia, shock, and sepsis are common, but frequently overlooked, causes of gastric ulceration. Thus all critically ill patients should be considered at risk for developing gastric ulcers.[36] Gastrinoma (see 9.4.3) arising from the

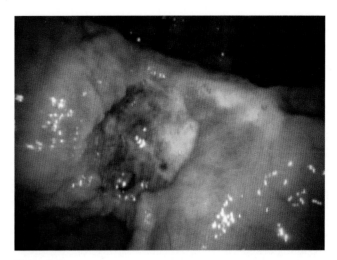

Figure 4.13:
Large ulcer at the incisura angularis. An 8-year-old male Basset hound presented with a 7-week history of hematemesis. During gastroscopy a peptic ulcer with a hard rim could be seen. Histopathology of the biopsies revealed the cause of this ulcer to be a gastric adenocarcinoma.

Table 4.4: Causes of peptic ulcers in dogs and cats

Drugs
- NSAIDs
- Corticosteroids (only when concurrent risk factors are present; e.g., NSAID administration)

Infiltrative Disease
- Gastric neoplasia
- Pythiosis in endemic areas
- Inflammatory bowel disease

Metabolic Disease
- Hepatopathy
- Renal failure (common in older cats)

Gastric hyperacidity
- Gastrinoma
- Mast cell tumor (rarely causes gastric ulcers)
- APUDoma

Other Causes
- Chemical toxins
- Disseminated intravascular coagulation
- Foreign objects (might worsen pre-existing gastritis or ulceration)
- Hypovolemia
- Pancreatitis
- Septic shock
- Stress?

APUDoma = amine precursor uptake and decarboxylation tumors

4

pancreas can secrete excessive amounts of gastrin and the resultant hyperacidity may also cause peptic ulceration.

Large ulcers in the pyloric antral region, often near the incisura, are commonly seen in dogs with gastric tumors (Figure 4.13). In a study on cats, 14 of 33 peptic ulcers were due to gastric neoplasia, mostly gastrointestinal lymphoma or gastric adenocarcinoma.[31]

Clinical signs

Clinical signs of peptic ulceration are poorly defined. Chronic vomiting is probably the most frequent sign, with or without hematemesis. Unlike humans, dogs do not secrete acid continuously and blood in the vomitus does, therefore, not always appear digested. Melena and pale mucous membranes may also be observed if bleeding is severe. Inappetence and anorexia are also common. Because of the important pathogenic role of medications, a careful history should include specific questions about any medications the owner may be administering to the animal.

Any changes in routine blood work are nonspecific. However, routine blood work is used to rule out other causes of vomiting. Chronic blood loss may result in anemia that can sometimes be non-regenerative and appear typical for iron deficiency (i.e., hypochromic, microcytic). Blood biochemistry results may show some electrolyte abnormalities as a consequence of profound vomiting.

Minor blood loss from gastric ulceration may not lead to gross melena and a fecal occult blood test may be required to identify such cases. However, some fecal occult blood tests can be affected by red meat in the diet. Fecal occult blood test kits are based on one of two different test principles. Guaiac-based tests contain guaiaconic acid, which when oxidized by hemoglobin leads to the development of a blue quinone. O-toluidine-based tests contain tetramethylbenzidine, which when oxidized by hemoglobin also leads to the generation of a blue compound. Both kit types can give positive test results when exposed to red meat or peroxidase-rich foods, such as turnip and cauliflower, present in the diet. However, in one study an o-toluidine-based test was associated with far fewer false positive results due to diet than a guaiac-based test. In another study, the same o-toluidine-based test was also slightly more sensitive than a guaiac-based test at 12 hours after oral administration of hemoglobin. But ideally patients should be fed a meat-free diet for at least 3 days prior to testing.[37]

Although gastroscopy is by far the best tool to diagnose gastric ulcers, this is often not necessary if the history (i.e., administration of NSAIDs, hematemesis) and clinical findings are indicative of gastric ulcers. Diagnosis can also be made based on contrast radiographic studies or exploratory laparotomy. The latter has the disadvantage that the gastric mucosa is not easily evaluated from the exterior of the stomach.

Treatment

The goals of therapy of gastric ulceration are to eliminate clinical signs, complications, and relapses (Table 4.5). To that end, it is vital to avoid ulcerogenic drugs. If the peptic ulcer might be due to decreased mucosal blood flow, the animal should be given sufficient amounts of intravenous fluids. Antacids act by neutralizing gastric acid. Calcium carbonate ($CaCO_3$), sodium bicarbonate ($NaHCO_3$), magnesium hydroxide ($Mg[OH]_2$), or aluminum hydroxide ($Al[OH]_3$) all contain an H^+-binding group. The neutralizing reaction with gastric acid produces water and a neutral salt. Antacids are also of benefit in that they bind to bile acids, decrease pepsin activity in the stomach, and stimulate the secretion of endogenous prostaglandins. However, the requirement of frequent dosing and poor palatability make antacids an inconvenient choice for animals.

The cornerstone of peptic ulcer therapy is the reduction of gastric acid secretion as Schwartz' dictum from 1910 "no acid, no ulcer" remains valid today. There are a variety of drugs available and the two most commonly prescribed drug classes in veterinary medicine are histamine$_2$-receptor antagonists and proton pump inhibitors. H$_2$-receptor antagonists (H$_2$-RA) block the secretion of gastric acid by blocking histamine H$_2$ receptors located on the surface of acid-producing parietal cells within the gastric glands (Figure 4.14). Cimetidine and ranitidine are used equally frequently in veterinary medicine. While ranitidine is 5 to 12 times more potent than cimetidine and has a longer half-life allowing for a decreased frequency of administration, a recent study indicated that ranitidine at the

Table 4.5: Therapeutic agents used for gastric diseases

Generic name	Class of drug	Dosages
aluminum hydroxide	antacid	dogs: 100–200 mg PO q 4–6 h cats: 50–100 mg PO q 4–6 h
bismuth subsalicylate	mucosal protectant	0.25–2.0 ml/kg PO q 4–6 h
cimetidine	H$_2$-receptor antagonist	5–10 mg/kg PO, IV q 8 h
famotidine	H$_2$-receptor antagonist	0.5–1 mg/kg PO, IV q 12–24 h
misoprostol	prostaglandin analogue	2–5 µg/kg PO q 8–12 h
nizatidine	H$_2$-receptor antagonist prokinetic agent	5 mg/kg PO q 24 h
omeprazole	proton-pump inhibitor	0.7 mg/kg PO q 24 h
ranitidine	H$_2$-receptor antagonist prokinetic agent	1–2 mg/kg PO, IV q 12 h
sucralfate	mucosal protectant	0.5–1 g PO q 8 h

PO = oral administration; IV = intravenous administration

regular dose (2 mg/kg IV q 12 h) was not different from saline administration in increasing the intragastric pH. In comparison, famotidine (0.5 mg/kg IV q 2 h) was significantly more effective than saline.[38] Another H$_2$-RA is nizatidine which, together with ranitidine, also possesses prokinetic activity in the stomach. In addition to their blockade of the histamine H$_2$ receptors of parietal cells, the H$_2$-RA increase the luminal secretion of bicarbonate and mucus as well as raising mucosal blood flow. These effects may be related to a stimulation of prostaglandin synthesis. In addition, it has been suggested that cimetidine increases *in vitro* cell-mediated immunity by blocking the H$_2$ receptors on T lymphocytes. Cimetidine decreases hepatic perfusion and is recognized as an inhibitor of hepatic P-450 and P-488 enzymes.[39] Drugs metabolized by these enzyme systems may be cleared more slowly and may reach a higher plasma concentration (e.g., cyclosporin) when administered together with cimetidine. Other histamine H$_2$-receptor antagonists do not show this interaction and may be preferred in animals receiving multiple drugs.

Omeprazole, a substituted benzimidazole, belongs to the class of proton pump inhibitor drugs (PPIs). By blocking the H$^+$/K$^+$-APTase enzyme at the luminal membrane of the parietal cell (Figure 4.14), acid secretion is inhibited regardless of the secretagogue (i.e., histamine, gastrin, or acetylcholine). Compared with cimetidine, omeprazole is about 20 times more potent and has a longer duration of action because it accumulates in a pH-dependent manner. Newer PPIs include lansoprazole or pantoprazole, but experience with these newer PPIs in veterinary patients is limited.[38]

Sucralfate is a gastromucosal protectant. It is a basic salt of a sulfate disaccharide with many aluminum hydroxide groups. Sucralfate dissociates after oral ingestion to sucrose octasulfate and aluminum hydroxide, which buffers H$^+$. Sucrose octasulfate reacts in the stomach with hydrochloric acid to form a paste-like complex that has greater affinity for damaged tissue than the normal mucosa. This adhering complex prevents further damage of the gastric mucosa by pepsin, acid, or bile. Sucralfate may also have some cytoprotective effects, possibly by stimulation of prostaglandin synthesis. Systemic absorption of sucralfate is minimal, and it is extremely well tolerated. Since sucralfate is effective at an acidic to almost a neutral pH, antisecretory drugs can be used concurrently. Other, orally administered drugs, however, should be given 2 hours apart as sucralfate can affect their absorption.[39]

Finally, misoprostol is a synthetic analog of prostaglandin E$_1$ (PGE$_1$). Although orally administered, it has to be absorbed into the circulation to be effective. Its effect is the same as those of endogenous prostaglandins. Although the prophylactic effect of misoprostol in dogs receiving corticosteroids or undergoing spinal surgery is debatable, this drug appears to be of little use in dogs that already have a peptic ulcer. Misoprostol can cause abortion and should be avoided in pregnant

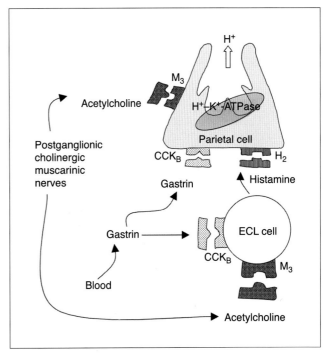

Figure 4.14:
Physiological mechanism of gastric acid secretion. The parietal cell contains receptors for gastrin (CCK$_B$), acetylcholine (M$_3$), and histamine (H$_2$). In addition, gastrin and acetylcholine can also interact with their receptors on enterochromaffin-like cells (ECL-cells) and release histamine.

animals. Also, women in child-bearing age should use gloves when administering misoprostol to their pet.[40]

Other means of decreasing gastric acid concentration have been developed, but are not yet available for routine use (e.g., gastrin-receptor antagonists, gastrin-releasing peptide receptor antagonists). A class of drugs which might be of future interest is the class of potassium-competitive acid blockers (P-CABs). These drugs block the action of the H$^+$-K$^+$-ATPase by competing with K$^+$.[41] Soraprazan and raveprazan are currently under investigation, but no information in dogs or cats is yet available.

4.4.2 Gastric dilation-volvulus

Acute gastric dilation/volvulus (GDV) is a sudden and often fatal GI disorder that particularly affects large, deep-chested breeds (e.g., Great Danes, German Shepherd dogs, Standard Poodles, large mixed-breed dogs).[42] It has been estimated that there are as many as 60,000 cases of GDV in the United States each year, with an overall mortality of about 15% to 20% depending on the time from the onset of clinical signs to treat-

4

ment. Although GDV may occur at any age, there is a greater risk of occurrence in older dogs.[43] Gastric dilation from rapid distension of the stomach with food, fluid, and especially gas (from swallowed air and/or fermentation) may progress to volvulus. This occurs because the forces exerted on the distended canine stomach cause it to rotate either to the right or the left (most often to the left in a clockwise direction) on an axis that is at a right angle to a line between the esophageal and pyloric sphincters. However, it is not entirely clear if the stomach first becomes distended or if the stomach rotates first.[44]

A single causative agent for the pathogenesis of acute GDV has not yet been identified. Several intrinsic physical risk factors (i.e., body size and thoracoabdominal dimension) and environmental risk factors (i.e., diet, accumulation of gastric gas, anesthesia, stress, being asleep) have been identified, and many more intrinsic anatomic (i.e., gastric ligament laxity, gastric volume and position, gastric hormones such as gastrin) and pathological (i.e., gastric rhythm, motility, and emptying) risk factors are suspected.[43–45] However, in one study feeding and exercise patterns did not alter the incidence of GDV in a large population of military dogs.

Clinical signs

The onset of clinical signs is usually acute or peracute. Abdominal distension is associated with progressive restlessness, unproductive retching, salivation, dyspnea, and gastric tympany, leading to severe pain and shock. Prolonged gastric distension markedly decreases the prognosis because mucosal ischemic changes may be irreversible. Death from hypovolemic and cardiogenic shock may occur within a few hours of the onset of clinical signs.

Rapid gastric distension adversely affects the function of the lower esophageal sphincter and appears to impair gastric motility and emptying. It has been postulated that distension occludes the gastroesophageal junction, precluding emptying by either eructation or emesis. Distension decreases gastric motility by impairing normal contraction and by reflex nervous inhibition. Following dilation, the gastric mucosa and later the gastric smooth muscle undergoes potentially irreversible ischemic necrosis. There is also an accumulation and sequestration of gastric secretions. The distended stomach occludes venous return from the rear limbs and caudal abdomen, thereby precipitating hypovolemic and cardiogenic shock. Lactic acid and other metabolic by-products accumulate in the poorly perfused hind limbs and viscera to cause severe metabolic acidosis, especially after relief of the gastric dilation. During ischemia the pancreas produces a "myocardial depressant factor", which, together with the acid-base and electrolyte disturbances may lead to a reduced cardiac contractility.[46] Signs of reperfusion injury, endotoxemia, DIC, and fatal cardiac arrhythmias often occur. Splenic torsion with infarc-

tion and necrosis is also a common sequel.[44] Due to the reduced perfusion, animals often go into prerenal oliguria and renal failure, which, together with the lactic acidosis and endotoxemia will result in multiple organ failure and finally death of the patient.

Diagnosis

Diagnosis is made from history, signalment, and physical examination findings. In dogs that are presented with unproductive vomiting, retching and hypersalivation, a distended abdomen is often clearly seen. In more severe cases, animals are laterally recumbent and show clinical signs of tachypnea and shock. With progression of the disease, animals will eventually decompensate, and bradycardia, hypothermia, white mucous membranes and cold extremities are coupled with a poor prognosis. While emergency blood work is rarely needed, baseline values should be obtained to direct acid-base and electrolyte replacements. Marked hemoconcentration, hypokalemia, azotemia, and increased liver enzymes are commonly seen. Plasma lactate concentrations are often elevated and have been used as predictor of perfusion and possibly even survival.[47] A coagulation profile may show evidence of hypercoagulability (reduction in prothrombin and activated thrombin times) or evidence of DIC (prolongation of coagulation times, thrombocytopenia).[48]

Treatment

Management of hypovolemia (to prevent or treat shock) is the primary goal of emergency treatment of patients with GDV. Fluid therapy should be started at a rate of 90 ml/kg/hour intravenously through large-bore catheters with crystalloid fluid solutions (e.g., lactated Ringer's solution) until the animal is stabilized. This fluid bolus is followed by high-volume administration of crystalloid fluids (e.g., 20 ml/kg/hour) for the following time period. A combination of colloids (e.g., hetastarch) combined with crystalloids can also be used; the former may prolong the effects of crystalloid fluids by increasing the oncotic pressure. Gastric decompression is attempted only after the correction of hypovolemia is well under way.

Gastric decompression can usually be achieved by orogastric intubation in unsedated patients using an equine nasogastric tube with large end and side holes. If orogastric intubation is unsuccessful, aseptic right- or left-sided gastrocentesis with a large-bore catheter or needle should be performed. Radiography is not necessary to diagnose gastric dilation but is invaluable in diagnosing gastric volvulus (Figure 4.15). Radiographs should only be taken after the patient has been stabilized. Radiographs in right-lateral recumbency are required to show the typical double-bubble image (i.e., air in both the pylorus and fundus), since the pylorus is displaced to the left-hand side of the abdominal cavity in a dorsocranial position with respect to the fundus. Free gas in the abdomen indicates a ruptured viscus.

When its vital signs are stable, the patient should be taken to surgery as quickly as possible for decompression and reversal of the volvulus. Small amounts of induction agents (e.g., thiopental, propofol) are given to effect, and anesthesia should be maintained with isoflurane or sevoflurane in oxygen. Nitrous oxide, if part of the anesthetic protocol, is not given until complete gastric decompression has been achieved. After the stomach has been decompressed, the torsion is reversed, the viability of the stomach and spleen are evaluated, a partial gastrectomy or splenectomy is performed as needed, and the stomach is pexied to prevent reoccurrence. Both, an incisional or belt-loop gastropexy have been described – if a gastropexy is not performed, recurrence rates of up to 80% have been reported.[49,50]

Cardiac arrhythmias, such as premature ventricular contractions or ventricular tachycardia, occur frequently in GDV patients. They can be seen up to 3 days after surgical correction, and require treatment if there is evidence of poor cardiac performance. Electrolyte and acid-base disturbances must be identified and corrected if present. Follow-up management includes feeding of a meat-based, canned, highly digestible diet at least three times daily. It is important to note that pyloroplasty does not influence the rate of recurrence.[44] Prophylactic gastropexy might be indicated in some dogs that are considered to be at increased risk for GDV and can be achieved by minimally-invasive laparoscopy.[51]

4.4.3 Motility disorders

Gastric emptying is a highly coordinated physiological response to the presence of food in the stomach and can be impaired during a range of different disease processes. In general, there are three separate gastric motility disorders: accelerated gastric emptying, retrograde transit, and delayed gastric emptying. Delayed gastric emptying can be due to mechanical or functional obstruction of the pylorus. Causes of mechanical obstruction are pyloric stenosis, chronic hypertrophic pyloric gastropathy, foreign bodies, pyloric or duodenal neoplasia, chronic hypertrophic gastritis, or intra-abdominal masses causing external compression of the pylorus. Functional disorders of gastric emptying result from one or more abnormalities of gastric motility. These motility disorders are often not associated with any morphological changes. Many different diseases, such as inflammatory and infiltrative lesions, gastric ulceration, IBD, altered electrolyte concentrations, acid-base disturbances, recent abdominal surgery, diabetes mellitus, and several drugs all can affect gastric motility.[52]

In normal monogastric animals, the pylorus serves as a sieve during the postprandial period. Liquids easily pass through the

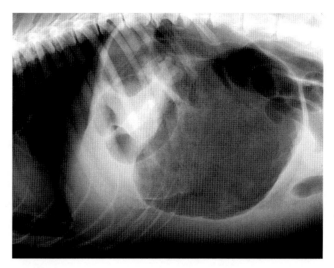

Figure 4.15:
Radiographic view of a gastric dilation-volvulus. This figure shows a radiographic view of a 10-year-old male German Shepherd dog. The radiographic image shows a large amount of air in the gastric fundus (dorsal "bubble") and the pyloric antrum (ventral "bubble"; "double-bubble is trouble") with gas-filled and dilated intestinal loops.

pylorus and empty relatively rapidly from the stomach by first-order kinetics. The rate of liquid expulsion from the stomach is proportional to its volume and the greater the gastric fluid volume, the more rapidly it is expelled. Solids are handled differently, requiring reduction to a small particle size (<2 mm in diameter) before they can pass through the pyloric canal.[53] In dogs, large food particles are normally retained in the stomach after feeding and pass into the duodenum only during the interdigestive period. During this period, called the migrating motor complex or housekeeper contraction, a special mechanism exists to expel these larger particles together with swallowed saliva, a small amount of mucous secretion, and cellular debris. One migrating motility complex, which lasts about 2 hours, is divided into four phases, the third causing intense bursts of action potentials resulting in powerful distal gastric peristaltic contractions that lead to the emptying of larger particles. Abnormal gastric emptying is assumed to affect solid-phase gastric contents rather than liquids.

Diagnosis

Diagnosis of a mechanical obstruction of the stomach is generally straightforward, whereas a functional obstruction, causing delayed gastric motility, may be more difficult to confirm. Several methods are available for evaluating gastric emptying (Table 4.6). Contrast radiographic techniques are the most commonly available means for diagnosing gastric motility disorders in small animals. Gastric emptying times for liquids, including barium suspension, are relatively short (about 1 hour

4

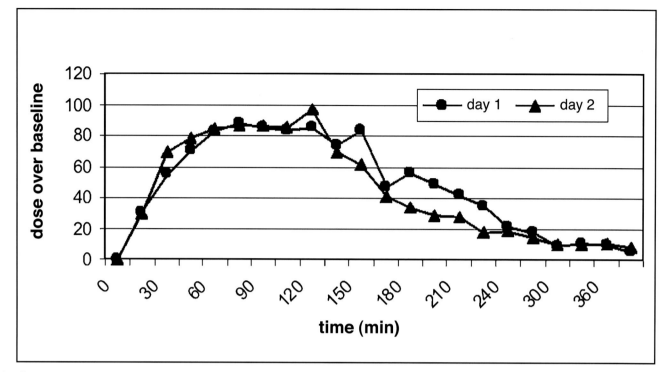

Figure 4.16:
Graph of a ^{13}C-sodium acetate breath test in a healthy dog. The test was performed on two consecutive days in the same dog. Note the repeatability of the curve for both experiments. There is an initial plateau phase at about 90 minutes and a more-or-less linear emptying thereafter. Gastric emptying is complete after 5 hours.

in cats, up to 3 hours in dogs). Studies using barium mixed with food have shown gastric emptying times varying from 4 to 16 hours in the dog and 4 to 17 hours in the cat, depending on the composition of the food, thus making it difficult to diagnose an emptying disorder unless gastric emptying times are markedly prolonged.[54] Furthermore, when solid meals are

Table 4.6: Methods for assessing gastric emptying

Technique	Information gained	Availability in pets
Plain radiographs	+	+++
Contrast radiographs (barium)	+++	+++
Contrast radiographs (BIPS)	++	+++
Ultrasonography	+	++
Endoscopy	++	++
^{13}C-based tests	++	+ – ++
Scintigraphy	+++	+ (referral institutions only)
Computed tomography (CT)	+	+ (referral institutions only)
Manometry	++	+ (referral institutions only)

BIPS = barium-impregnated polyethylene spheres

mixed with barium granules or suspension, the barium can dissociate from the food and redistribute into the liquid phase of the gastric contents. A few years ago, barium-impregnated polyethylene spheres (BIPS) were introduced and their use for the assessment of gastric emptying in dogs and cats has been described.[55] BIPS are produced in two diameters: 1.5 mm and 5 mm. The small BIPS are designed to empty with small particles, thereby mimicking solid-phase gastric emptying. Large BIPS tend to be retained in the stomach longer than small BIPS, often remaining after the test meal has passed into the duodenum and then leaving the stomach once the migrating motor complex begins. The BIPS should accumulate immediately orad to an obstructing lesion. Interpretation of gastric emptying of BIPS has some of the same limitations as that of barium studies and the use of BIPS may be more helpful in documenting a mechanical rather than a functional obstruction.[54]

Recently, ultrasonography has been used as an alternative method for assessing gastric emptying times.[56] Finding more than just a small amount of fluid in the stomach 18 hours after feeding provides evidence for delayed gastric emptying in the dog. Gastric emptying can also be evaluated by means of ^{13}C-breath or blood testing.[52] The main advantages of ^{13}C-based

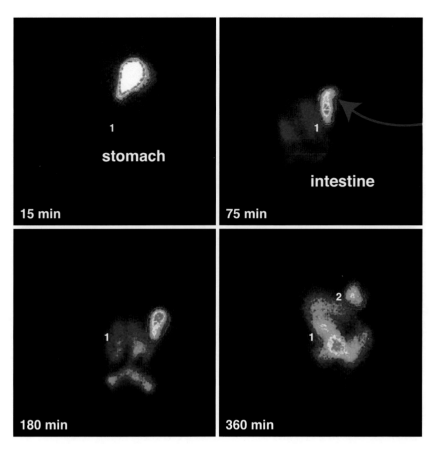

— ROI

4

Figure 4.17:
Scintigraphic assessment of gastric emptying in a healthy dog. Fifteen minutes after feeding of a radioactively-labeled meal, radioactivity can only be observed in the stomach. As time passes, the radioactively-labeled food moves into the small intestine and after 6 hours, there is only a small amount of radioactivity detectable in the stomach. The region of interest (ROI; see arrow) is drawn manually around the stomach to calculate gastric emptying.

tests are that no radiation is required, the tests are non-invasive and non-operator dependent, and they can be performed several times in the same subject without any biological hazard. ^{13}C-based breath or blood tests involve the detection of an increased fraction of $^{13}CO_2$ in comparison to $^{12}CO_2$ after the ingestion of a labeled meal or administration of a labeled substrate. The substrate or meal is rapidly digested and absorbed at the site of interest by enzymatic or microbial digestion and the rate and appearance of the isotope in the breath or blood is a direct reflection of the GI transit of the substrate. The ^{13}C-octanoic acid breath (^{13}C-OBT) or blood tests and the ^{13}C-sodium acetate breath test are all based on the administration of a substrate with a functional group containing ^{13}C. On leaving the stomach, the ^{13}C-octanoic acid or ^{13}C-sodium acetate is rapidly absorbed in the duodenum and metabolized in the liver. Following oxidation, the resulting $^{13}CO_2$ diffuses into the blood and is excreted in the breath, either of which can be collected and measured by isotope mass spectrometry. Because gastric emptying is the rate-limiting step in the process of absorption and metabolism of the labeled substrate, the appearance of the ^{13}C in the exhaled breath or blood is a direct reflection of the rate and pattern of gastric emptying (Figure 4.16). Finally, scintigraphy is considered the gold standard technique for assessing gastric emptying (Figure 4.17).[52]

Patients with abnormalities of gastric motility appear normal except for intermittent postprandial vomiting. The vomitus is characteristically undigested or only partly digested, and occasionally contains mucus. It may also have an acidic pH, but bile is absent. The precise interrelationship between pyloric stenosis and pylorospasm is unclear. Signs of gastric outlet obstruction vary with the degree of obstruction. Vomiting is the predominant clinical sign and may occur at any time after a meal. The time for complete emptying of a normal meal from the stomach is 7 to 8 hours in dogs fed once daily. Vomiting of all or part of a meal at periods more than 10 hours after ingestion suggests delayed gastric emptying and the probability of a gastric, pancreatic, or proximal duodenal lesion.

Treatment

In addition to a dietary trial, prokinetic therapy is often needed. A low-fat, highly digestible blended or liquid diet fed over multiple feedings may be beneficial. Dopaminergic agonists (e.g., metoclopramide) have GI prokinetic and antiemetic properties because they inhibit peripheral and/or central dopamine receptors. The mechanism of the prokinetic activity of metoclopramide is not entirely clear but may also be due to

4

other pharmacological properties (e.g., 5-HT_3-receptor or 5-HT_4-receptor antagonism).[57] Metoclopramide increases the amplitude and frequency of antral contractions, inhibits fundic receptive relaxation, and coordinates gastric, pyloric, and duodenal motility, all of which result in accelerated gastric emptying. Erythromycin, an antibiotic, has motilin-like action and at low doses increases the pressure of the gastroesophageal sphincter and accelerates gastric emptying by inducing antral contractions similar to phase III of the migrating motility complex.[57] The prokinetic dose (1 mg/kg PO q 12 h) is much lower than the antimicrobial dose. Some histamine H_2-receptor antagonists (e.g., ranitidine and nizatidine) also have acetylcholinesterase-inhibiting properties, thereby stimulating gastric emptying and small intestinal and colonic motility.

Cisapride was used to treat several GI motility disorders in dogs and cats throughout the 1990s. Because of unexplained deaths in humans, cisapride has been taken off the market and is currently only available through compounding pharmacies. There has been little clinical experience with the newer prokinetic agents, such as tegaserod (Zelnorm [USA], Zelmac [Europe], Novartis) and prucalopride (R093877, Janssen). Tegaserod is a potent partial nonbenzamide agonist of 5-HT_4 receptors and a weak agonist of 5-HT_{1D} receptors with known prokinetic effects in the canine colon. *In vitro* studies suggest that tegaserod does not delay cardiac repolarization or prolong the QT interval of the electrocardiogram as had been occasionally reported with cisapride. Its clinical efficacy has been demonstrated in human motility disorders. Gastric and intestinal effects of tegaserod have not been reported in the dog and this drug may not prove as useful as cisapride in stimulating proximal GI motility in small animal patients. Prucalopride is also a potent partial benzamide agonist of 5-HT_4 receptors but has no effect on other 5-HT receptors and lacks cholinesterase enzyme activity. Unlike tegaserod, prucalopride appears to stimulate gastric emptying in the dog. Prucalopride is not commercially available at this time.

The only effective treatment for pyloric hypertrophy is pyloroplasty. In some patients, the outlet obstruction may be sufficiently severe that nutritional homeostasis cannot be sustained on any kind of diet, and enteral or parenteral nutrition will become necessary.

🔑 Key Facts

- Dolasetron and maropitant are highly efficacious as antiemetic agents.
- A diagnosis of gastritis can only be achieved after a gastric biopsy has been analyzed histopathologically.
- Gastric ulceration is an uncommon albeit serious complication of NSAID treatment and should be aggressively treated with sucralfate and either a histamine$_2$-receptor antagonist or a proton pump inhibitor.
- In dogs with gastric dilation-volvulus (GDV), aggressive intravenous fluid therapy should be initiated before the stomach is decompressed.
- Gastric motility disorders are best diagnosed by scintigraphy or ^{13}C-based breath or blood tests.

References

1. Price AB. Classification of gastritis. *Verh Dtsch Ges Pathol* 1999; 83: 52–55.
2. DeNovo RC. Diseases of the stomach. In: Tams TR (ed.), *Handbook of Small Animal Gastroenterology, 2nd ed*. Philadelphia, WB Saunders, 2003; 159–194.
3. Marshall BJ, Warren JR. Unidentified curved bacilli in the stomach of patients with gastritis and peptic ulceration. *Lancet* 1984; 1(8390): 1311–1315.
4. Neiger R, Simpson KW. *Helicobacter* infection in dogs and cats: Facts and fiction. *J Vet Intern Med* 2000; 14: 124–133.
5. Watson JW, Gonsalves SF, Fossa AA et al. The anti-emetic effect of CP-99,994 in the ferret and the dog: role of the NK_1 receptor. *Brit J Pharmacol* 1995; 115: 84–94.
6. Gue M, Fioramonti J, Bueno L. A simple double radiolabeled technique to evaluate gastric emptying of a canned food meal in dogs. Application to pharmacological tests. *Gastroenterol Clin Biol* 1988; 12: 425–430.
7. de la Puente-Redondo V, Clemence RG, Ramsey DS. Maropitant (Cerenia) provides robust preventative and therapeutic anti-emetic efficacy in dogs from 30 minutes to 24 hours after a single dose. *J Vet Intern Med* 2006; 20: (abstract)
8. Kolbjornsen O, Press CM, Landsverk T. Gastropathies in the Lundehund. 1. Gastritis and gastric neoplasia associated with intestinal lymphangiectasia. *APMIS* 1994; 102: 647–661.
9. Whittingham S, Mackay IR. Autoimmune gastritis: historical antecedents, outstanding discoveries, and unresolved problems. *Int Rev Immunol* 2005; 24: 1–29.
10. Simpson KW, Neiger R, DeNovo R et al. ACVIM-Consensus statement: The relationship of *Helicobacter* spp. infection to gastric disease in dogs and cats. *J Vet Intern Med* 2000; 14: 223–227.
11. Fox JG, Lee A. The role of *Helicobacter* species in newly recognized gastrointestinal tract diseases of animals. *Lab Anim Sci* 1997; 47: 222–255.
12. Shinozaki JK, Sellon RK, Cantor GH et al. Fecal polymerase chain reaction with 16S ribosomal RNA primers can detect the presence of gastrointestinal *Helicobacter* in dogs. *J Vet Intern Med* 2002; 16: 426–432.
13. Greiter-Wilke A, Scanziani E, McDonough PL et al. Are *Helicobacter* spp. associated with inflammatory liver disease in cats? *J Vet Intern Med* 2002; 16: 328 (abstract).
14. Eaton KA, Dewhirst FE, Paster BJ et al. Prevalence and varieties of *Helicobacter* species in dogs from random sources and pet dogs: animal and public health implications. *J Clin Micro* 1996; 34: 3165–3170.

15. Jalava K, On SLW, Vandamme P et al. Isolation and identification of *Helicobacter* spp. from canine and feline gastric mucosa. *Applied Environ Micro* 1998; 64: 3998–4006.

16. Neiger R, Tschudi ME, Burnens AP et al. Diagnosis and identification of gastric *Helicobacter* species by polymerase chain reaction in dogs. *Microbial Ecol Health Dis* 1999; 11: 234–240.

17. Neiger R, Dieterich C, Burnens AP et al. Detection and prevalence of *Helicobacter* infection in pet cats. *J Clin Micro* 1998; 36: 634–637.

18. Handt LK, Fox JG, Dewhirst FE et al. *Helicobacter pylori* isolated from the domestic cat: Public health implications. *Infect Immun* 1994; 62: 2367–2374.

19. Kusters JG, van Vliet AHM, Kuipers EJ. Pathogenesis of *Helicobacter pylori* infection. *Clin Micro Reviews* 2006; 19: 449–560.

20. Norris CR, Marks SL, Eaton KA et al. Healthy cats are commonly colonized with »*Helicobacter heilmannii*« that is associated with minimal gastritis. *J Clin Micro* 1999; 37: 189–194.

21. Yamasaki K, Suematsu H, Takahashi T. Comparison of gastric lesions in dogs and cats with and without gastric spiral organisms. *J Am Vet Med Assoc* 1998; 212: 529–533.

22. Simpson KW, Strauss-Ayali D, McDonough PL et al. Gastric function in dogs with naturally acquired gastric *Helicobacter* spp. infection. *J Vet Intern Med* 1999; 13: 507–515.

23. Simpson KW, McDonough PL, Strauss-Ayali D et al. *Helicobacter felis* infection in dogs. Effect on gastric structure and function. *Vet Pathol* 1999; 36: 237–248.

24. Simpson KW, Strauss-Ayali S, Scanziani E et al. *Helicobacter felis* infection is associated with lymphoid follicular hyperplasia and mild gastritis but normal gastric secretory function in cats. *Infect Immun* 2000; 68: 779–790.

25. Stoffel MH, Friess AE, Burnens A et al. Distinction of gastric *Helicobacter* spp. in humans and domestic pets by scanning electron microscopy. *Helicobacter* 2000; 5: 232–239.

26. Cornetta A, Simpson KW, Strauss-Ayali D et al. Evaluation of a ^{13}C-urea breath test for detection of gastric infection with *Helicobacter* spp. in dogs. *Am J Vet Res* 1998; 59: 1364–1369.

27. Campell KL, Graham JC. *Physaloptera* infection in dogs and cats. *Comp Cont Edu* 1999; 21: 299–314.

28. Theisen SK, LeGrange SN, Johnson SE et al. *Physaloptera* infection in 18 dogs with intermittent vomiting. *J Am Anim Hosp Assoc* 1998; 34: 74–78.

29. Eckert J, Friedhoff KT, Zahner H et al. *Lehrbuch der Parasitologie für die Tiermedizin*. Stuttgart, Enke, 2005; 259–260.

30. Stanton ME, Bright RM. Gastroduodenal ulceration in dogs. Retrospective study of 43 cases and literature review. *J Vet Intern Med* 1989; 3: 238–244.

31. Liptak JM, Hunt GB, Barrs VDR et al. Gastroduodenal ulceration in cats: eight cases and a review of the literature. *J Feline Med Surg* 2002; 4: 27–42.

32. Lascelles BDX, Blikslager AT, Fox SM et al. Gastrointestinal tract perforation in dogs treated with a selective cyclooygenase-2 inhibitor: 29 cases (2002–2003). *J Am Vet Med Assoc* 2005; 227: 1112–1117.

33. Neiger R. Gastric ulceration. In: Bonagura JD (ed.), *Kirk's Current Veterinary Therapy XIV*. Philadelphia, WB Saunders, (in press).

34. Misdrop W. Mast cells and canine mast cell tumours. A review. *Vet Quarterly* 2004; 26: 156–169.

35. Neiger R, Gaschen F, Jaggy A. Endoscopically detectable gastric mucosal lesions in dogs with acute intervertebral disc disease: prevalence and effects of omeprazole and misoprostol. *J Vet Intern Med* 2000; 14: 33–36.

36. Hinton LE, McLoughlin MA, Johnson SE et al. Spontaneous gastroduodenal perforation in 16 dogs and seven cats (1982–1999). *J Am Anim Hosp Assoc* 2002; 38: 176–187.

37. Tuffli SP, Gaschen F, Neiger R. Effect of dietary factors on the detection of fecal occult blood in cats. *J Vet Diagnost Invest* 2001; 13: 177–179.

38. Bersenas AM, Mathews KA, Allen DG et al. Effects of ranitidine, famotidine, pantoprazole, and omeprazole on intragastric pH in dogs. *Am J Vet Res* 2005; 66: 425–431.

39. Plumb DC (ed.), *Plumb's Veterinary Drug Handbook*. Iowa, Blackwell Publishing, 2005.

40. Zikopoulos KA, Papanikolaou EG, Kalantaridou SN et al. Early pregnancy termination with vaginal misoprostol before and after 42 days gestation. *Hum Repro* 2002; 17: 3079–3083.

41. Mössner J, Caca K. Developments of the inhibition of gastric acid secretion. *Europ J Clin Invest* 2005; 35: 469–475.

42. Brockman DJ, Washabau RJ, Drobatz KJ. Canine gastric dilation/volvulus syndrome in a veterinary critical care unit: 295 cases, 1986–1992. *J Am Vet Med Assoc* 1995; 207: 460–464.

43. Brockman DJ, Holt DE, Washabau RJ. Pathogenesis of acute canine gastric dilation-volvulus syndrome: is there a unifying hypothesis. *Compend Contin Educ Pract Vet* 2000; 22: 1108–1114.

44. Monnet E. Gastric dilation-volvulus syndrome in dogs. *Vet Clin North Am* 2003; 33: 987–1005.

45. Glickman LT, Glickman NW, Perez CM et al. Analysis of risk factors for gastric dilation and dilation volvulus in dogs. *J Am Vet Med Assoc* 1994; 204: 1465–1471.

46. Orton EC, Muir WW. Isovolumetric indices and humoral cardioactive substance bioassay during clinical and experimentally induced gastric dilation-volvulus in the dog. *Am J Vet Res* 1983; 44: 1516–1520.

47. De Papp E, Drobatz KJ, Hughes D. Plasma lactate concentration as a predictor of gastric necrosis and survival among dogs with gastric dilation-volvulus: 102 cases (1995–1998). *J Am Med Vet Assoc* 1999; 215: 49–52.

48. Millis DL, Hauptman JG, Fulton RBJ. Abnormal hemostatic profiles and gastric necrosis in canine gastric dilation-volvulus. *Vet Surg* 1993; 22: 93–97.

49. Eggertsdottir AV, Stigen YO, Lonaas L et al. Comparison of the recurrence rate of gastric dilation with and without volvulus in dogs after circumcostal gastropexy versus gastrocolopexy. *Vet Surg* 2001; 30: 546–551.

50. Wingfield WE, Betts CW, Greene RW. Operative techniques and recurrence rates associated with gastric volvulus in the dog. *J Small Anim Pract* 1975; 16: 427–432.

51. Rawlings CA, Mahaffey MB, Bement S et al. Prospective evaluation of laparoscopic-assisted gastropexy in dogs susceptible to gastric dilation. *J Am Vet Med Assoc* 2002; 221: 1576–1581.

52. Wyse CA, McLellan J, Dickie AM et al. A review of methods for assessment of the rate of gastric emptying in the dog and cat: 1898–2002. *J Vet Intern Med* 2003; 17: 609–621.

53. Ganong WF (ed.), *Review of Medical Physiology, 22nd ed.* New York, Lange Medical Books, 2005.

54. Lamb CR. Recent developments in diagnostic imaging of the gastrointestinal tract of the dog and cat. *Vet Clin N Am* 1999; 29: 307–342.

55. Sparkes AH, Papasouliotis K, Barr FJ et al. Reference ranges for gastrointestinal transit of barium-impregnated polyethylene spheres in healthy cats. *J Small Anim Pract* 1997; 38: 340–343.

56. Chalmers AF, Kirton R, Wye CA et al. Ultrasonographic assessment of the rate of solid-phase gastric emptying in dogs. *Vet Rec* 2005; 157: 649–652.

57. Washabau RJ. Gastrointestinal motility disorders and gastrointestinal prokinetic therapy. *Vet Clin N Am* 2003; 33: 1007–1028.

4.4.4 Neoplastic conditions of the stomach

Ann E. Hohenhaus

Introduction

Gastric tumors are rare in dogs. Typically, dogs with gastric tumors are older, with a median age of 10 years, but dogs less than 5 years old have also been reported. A sex predilection has not been consistently reported. Some case series report an equal male to female ratio, but most report a male predominance.[1–8] Breed predispositions for gastric tumors include the Chow Chow, Staffordshire Bull terrier, and Rough Collie for gastric carcinoma, and the Belgian Shepherd for mucinous adenocarcinoma of the lesser curvature.[1,4,6]

Tumors can occur in any region of the canine stomach and there does not appear to be an anatomical predisposition for any particular region. One early case series found neoplastic tissue extending into both the body and pylorus of the stomach of most dogs with gastric tumors.[7] More recently, the lesser curvature of the stomach has been a frequently described location for gastric tumors.[4,8,9] Carcinoma, leiomyoma, and leiomyosarcoma have been found to occur in the pyloric antrum.[2]

Gastric tumors are exceedingly rare in cats. Lymphoma, which is a rare gastric tumor in the dog, is the most common gastric tumor in the cat. Three published case series including 96 cats with gastrointestinal tumors report a total of 3 cases of gastric carcinoma.[8,10,11] However, age, breed, and sex predilections cannot be determined from such a small number of cases.

Histology

Three major histological types of gastric tumors have been described: carcinomas, sarcomas, and round cell tumors, which are most commonly lymphoma. Although most gastric tumors in dogs are malignant, benign gastric tumors have also been reported.[2,9,12,13] Morphologically, carcinomas can be classified as intestinal (also called tubular) or diffuse (Table 4.7).[5] The intestinal type of gastric carcinoma can be further differentiated into papillary, acinar, and solid. Also, the diffuse type of gastric carcinoma can be further differentiated into adenocarcinoma (glandular carcinoma) and the undifferentiated carcinoma. Signet ring cells containing mucin are characteristic of undifferentiated carcinomas. The scirrhous nature of gastric carcinomas is the result of desmoplasia induced by the malignant epithelium. Both types of diffuse carcinomas show desmoplasia, while intestinal type gastric carcinomas tend to be less scirrhous. A gastric carcinoid tumor has been reported in both a dog and a cat.[14,15]

Table 4.7: Histological types of gastric carcinoma

Subtype	Form
Intestinal (tubular) type	■ Acinar ■ Papillary ■ Solid
Diffuse type	■ Adenocarcinoma ■ Undifferentiated carcinoma (signet ring)

Clinical signs

The clinical signs of gastric neoplasia are similar to those seen with other gastric disorders. Vomiting is common and in many cases is due to gastric outflow obstruction. Malignant ulceration occurs in more than 50% of dogs with a gastric carcinoma (Figure 4.18). Hematemesis, melena, and pallor due to anemia are also commonly seen.[5,7] Tumor-associated nausea can be responsible for anorexia, weight loss, cachexia, and ptyalism.

Clinical pathology

The results of clinical pathology testing are not specific for gastric tumors in general or for a specific histological type of gastric neoplasia. Clinicopathological abnormalities are, in general, due to gastric inflammation, gastric outflow obstruction, malabsorption, or blood loss. Hypoproteinemia and elevated liver enzymes are common.[1,3] In dogs with tumor-induced gastric outflow obstruction and vomiting, a hypochloremic metabolic alkalosis with paradoxical aciduria may develop.[3] Frequently, a CBC demonstrates an inflammatory leukogram and anemia.[1,3] If the gastric bleeding is acute, the ensuing anemia will be regenerative, but if the hemorrhage is chronic, the anemia will become non-regenerative.

Diagnostic imaging

Diagnostic imaging is extremely important in determining the presence of a gastric mass and the extent of involvement of the surrounding organs. Unfortunately, the features of both benign and malignant gastric masses as well as the various histological types of gastric neoplasia overlap and neither abdominal radiography nor abdominal ultrasonography are useful in differentiating the specific tumor types.

Radiography

In some patients with gastric tumors, the survey radiographs may be normal. Abnormal findings include excessive fluid or gas in the stomach despite fasting.[3] A mass or caudal displacement of the gastric axis on the lateral radiograph has been described in dogs with gastric tumors.[2]

The use of contrast agents facilitates the radiographic visualization of gastric wall thickening, distortion of the gastric lumen, presence of a filling defect, and derangement of the rugal folds caused by tumor infiltration. While the normal gastric emptying time is not well defined, delayed emptying is common with gastric tumors.[2,3] The stomach may also appear rigid and non-distensible, which is termed "linitis plastica" or "leather bottle stomach". Ulcers can also be highlighted by contrast material.[7]

Ultrasonography

Both benign and malignant gastric tumors can be associated with mural thickening, loss of normal wall layering, and decreased or absent motility in the area of the tumor.[1,3,12,16] The echogenicity of gastric tumors may be hypoechoic, hyperechoic, or mixed regardless of the histologic type.[12,16] Carcinomas and lymphomas may appear as sessile masses or diffuse in distribution, while leiomyomas and leiomyosarcomas are typically focal in distribution.[12] An ultrasound finding termed pseudolayering appears to correlate with an uneven intramural distribution of tumor cells seen histologically in dogs with gastric carcinoma.[1] Extension of the tumor through the serosal surface of the stomach has been identified in dogs with carcinoma.[12]

The accuracy of ultrasonography increases with the expertise of the ultrasonographer. The utility of ultrasound in identifying gastric masses is decreased when the patient is uncooperative or gas and ingesta obscure the stomach wall. In addition, non-neoplastic gastric disorders such as gastritis can appear identical to gastric neoplasia in some cases.[9] Ultrasonography is also useful to identify regional lymphadenopathy; although finding enlarged lymph nodes is not specific for metastatic gastric neoplasia.

Biopsy techniques

Although clinical signs, laboratory data, and diagnostic imaging may be suggestive of a gastric tumor, a biopsy is essential for a definitive diagnosis. Exploratory laparotomy can be used to obtain tissue samples for biopsy. Multiple samples can easily be obtained and are typically adequate in size for arriving at an accurate diagnosis, but the procedure is invasive. Gastroscopy, using a fiberoptic or video endoscope, allows collection of a tissue sample and visualization of the gastric lesion prior

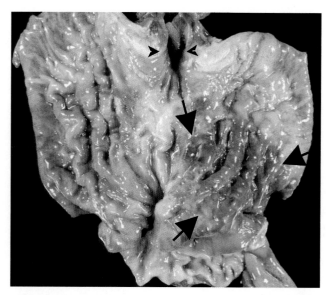

Figure 4.18:
Gastric adenocarcinoma in a dog. The arrows mark the outline of a gastric adenocarcinoma. The entrance of the esophagus into the stomach is shown by the arrowheads.

to any therapeutic surgical procedure. Samples tend to be small and 10–20% of samples may be inadequate for obtaining an accurate diagnosis. Ultrasound-guided percutaneous fine needle aspiration of gastric masses to obtain cytologic samples has been reported; and this procedure appears to be useful for the diagnosis of gastric tumors in some patients.[1,3,17]

Treatment

Because gastric tumors are rare and, in many cases, advanced at the time of diagnosis, reports of treatment are limited to single case reports. Surgery has been the primary treatment modality used in most cases. A relief of gastric outflow obstruction by side-to-side gastrojejunostomy has been achieved.[2] Total gastrectomy or gastroduodenostomy have been attempted to achieve complete tumor resection.[2,18] One dog undergoing gastroduodenostomy was provided nutrition through a jejunostomy tube and was also treated with chemotherapy using a combination of cisplatin, 5-fluorouracil, doxorubicin, and cyclophosphamide.[2] Photodynamic therapy has also been reported for the treatment of a gastric carcinoma in a single case.[4]

Systemic complications of gastric neoplasia

Hypochloremic metabolic alkalosis resulting in paradoxical aciduria occurs in dogs with gastric carcinoma and severe vomiting.[3] Vomiting leads to the loss of hydrogen and chloride

4

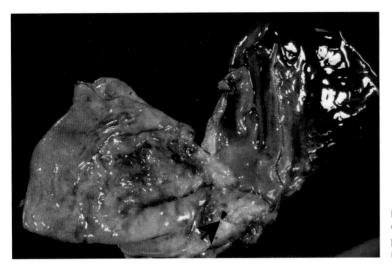

Figure 4.19:
Gastric perforation in a dog with gastric adenocarcinoma. The arrow points to a gastric perforation as a result of a gastric adenocarcinoma in a dog.

ions, alkalosis, and volume depletion. Normally, the renal tubules will resorb sodium ions in exchange for chloride ions in response to alkalosis and hypovolemia. However, when chloride is depleted, the kidneys resorb sodium and excrete hydrogen ions instead of chloride in order to maintain electrical neutrality, leading to a paradoxical aciduria.

Iron deficiency anemia results when gastric tumors cause ulceration and chronic GI blood loss. Loss of iron into the feces and inadequate intake of replacement iron due to vomiting and anorexia result in a microcytic, hypochromic, non-regenerative anemia.

Paraneoplastic hypoglycemia with a low serum insulin concentration has been described in a dog with a gastric leiomyosarcoma.[19] The diagnostic investigation of this patient suggested the synthesis of an unidentified hypoglycemic factor by the tumor. Non-islet cell tumors associated with hypoglycemia such as this one are typically large and palpable on physical examination.[19] Pneumoperitoneum results when the tumor erodes through the entire gastric wall (Figure 4.19).[20]

Tumor invasion and metastasis

All histological types of gastric tumors are highly metastatic. Gastric carcinomas most commonly metastasize to the regional lymph nodes, but they can also widely disseminate to other abdominal organs, the central nervous system, the myocardium, mediastinum, long bones, and testicular connective tissue.[2,4,16,21,22] The single case of a gastric carcinoid tumor in a cat was found to have metastasized to the kidney, brain, liver, spleen, lung, and lymph node.[11] Gastric leiomyosarcomas have been shown to metastasize to the liver and duodenum [2].

Survival

In general, the survival of dogs with gastric cancer is poor. One case series reported a median survival time of 3 days with a range of 0 days to 10 months.[2] Occasionally, longer survival times have been reported in single cases. Survivals of 240 days and 9 months were reported in two dogs undergoing gastrectomy.[18,23]

🔑 Key Facts

- Most gastric tumors are malignant and are highly metastatic.
- Diagnostic imaging, plain radiography, contrast radiography, and ultrasonography contribute to the diagnosis of gastric tumors; however, a biopsy is required to make a definitive diagnosis and to determine if the tumor is benign or malignant.
- Tissue samples can be obtained via exploratory laparotomy or endoscopy.
- Between 10–20% of the time, a sample obtained via endoscopy will be inadequate to diagnose gastric cancer.
- In general, survival in dogs and cats with gastric neoplasia is poor due to the advanced stage of disease at the time of diagnosis.

References

1. Penninck DG, Moore AS, Gliatto J. Ultrasonography of canine gastric epithelial neoplasia. *Vet Radiol Ultrasound* 1998; 39: 342–348.
2. Swann HM, Holt DE. Canine gastric adenocarcinoma and leiomyosarcoma: a retrospective study of 21 cases (1986–1999) and literature review. *J Am Anim Hosp Assoc* 2002; 38: 157–164.
3. Rivers BJ, Walter PA, Johnston GR et al. Canine gastric neoplasia: utility of ultrasonography in diagnosis. *J Am Anim Hosp Assoc* 1997; 33: 144–155.
4. Fonda D, Gualtieri M, Scanziani E. Gastric carcinoma in the dog: a clinicopathological study of 11 cases. *J Am Small Anim Prac* 1989; 30: 353–360.
5. Patnaik AK, Hurvitz AI, Johnson GF. Canine gastric adenocarcinoma. *Vet Pathol* 1978; 15: 600–607.
6. Sullivan M, Lee R, Fisher EW et al. A study of 31 cases of gastric carcinoma in dogs. *Vet Rec* 1987; 120: 79–83.
7. Sautter JH, Hanlon GF. Gastric neoplasms in the dog: a report of 20 cases. *J Am Vet Med Assoc* 1975; 166: 691–696.
8. Gualtieri M, Monzeglio MG, Scanziani E. Gastric neoplasia. *Vet Clin North Am* 1999; 29: 415–440.
9. Easton S. A retrospective study into the effects of operator experience on the accuracy of ultrasound in the diagnosis of gastric neoplasia in dogs. *Vet Radiol Ultrasound* 2001; 42: 47–50.
10. Brodey RS. Alimentary tract neoplasms in the cat: a clinicopathologic survey of 46 cases. *Am J Vet Res* 1966; 27: 74–80.
11. Turk MAM, Gallina AM, Russell TS. Nonhematopoietic gastrointestinal neoplasia in cats: a retrospective study of 44 cases. *Vet Pathol* 1981; 18: 614–620.
12. Lamb CR, Grierson J. Ultrasonographic appearance of primary gastric neoplasia in 21 dogs. *J Small Anim Prac* 1999; 40: 211–215.
13. Kapatkin AS, Mullen HS, Matthiesen DT et al. Leiomyosarcoma in dogs: 44 cases (1983–1988). *J Am Vet Med Assoc* 1992; 201: 1077–1079.
14. Albers TM, Alroy J, McDonnell JJ. A poorly differentiated gastric carcinoid in a dog. *J Vet Diagn Invest* 1998; 10: 116–118.
15. Rossmeisl JH, Forrester SD, Tobertson JL et al. Chronic vomiting associated with a gastric carcinoid in a cat. *J Am Anim Hosp Assoc* 2002; 38: 61–66.
16. Kaser-Hotz B, Hauser B, Arnold P. Ultrasonographic findings in canine gastric neoplasia in 13 patients. *Vet Radiol Ultrasound* 1996; 37: 51–56.
17. Crystal MA, Penninck DG, Matz ME et al. Use of ultrasound-guided fine-needle aspiration biopsy and automated core biopsy for the diagnosis of gastrointestinal diseases in small animals. *Vet Radiol Ultrasound* 1993; 34: 438–444.
18. Sellon RK, Bissonnette K, Bunch SE. Long-term survival after total gastrectomy for gastric adenocarcinoma in a dog. *J Vet Intern Med* 1996; 10: 333–335.
19. Bellah JR, Ginn PE. Gastric leiomyosarcoma associated with hypoglycemia in a dog. *J Am Anim Hosp Assoc* 1996; 32: 283–286.
20. Mellanby RJ, Baines EA, Herrtage ME. Spontaneous pneumoperitoneum in two cats. *J Small Anim Pract* 2002; 43: 543–546.
21. Esplin DG, Wilson SR. Gastrointestinal adenocarcinomas metastatic to the testes and associated structures in three dogs. *J Am Anim Hosp Assoc* 1998; 34: 287–290.
22. Wang FI, Lee JJ, Liu CH et al. Scirrhous gastric carcinoma with mediastinal invasion in a dog. *J Vet Diagn Invest* 2002; 14: 65–68.
23. Beck C, Slocombe RF, O'Neill T et al. The use of ultrasound in the investigation of gastric carcinoma in a dog. *Aust Vet J* 2001; 79: 332–334.

4

5   Small Intestine

5.1   Anatomy

Craig G. Ruaux

5.1.1   Introduction

The intestinal tract is the point of entry of all metabolic energy into the animal. The processes of digestion and absorption undertaken in the intestinal tract need to be carried out over a large surface area. Many of the anatomical features of the intestine act to increase the surface area exposed and available for carrying out the major intestinal functions.

The intestinal tract has numerous functions, all of which are necessary for normal digestion. The five main digestive functions of the intestinal tract are:

- Motility – The movement of ingesta through the intestinal tract from the stomach to the colon/rectum and eventual expulsion as feces.
- Secretion – Secretion of fluid, enzymes, and electrolytes into the GI lumen.
- Digestion – Degradation of ingesta occurs in the cranial small intestine, mediated largely by pancreatic digestive enzymes. The small intestinal mucosa also has a role in the further digestion of food material at the brush border (see below).
- Absorption – Following degradation of ingested foodstuffs, the resulting nutrients need to be assimilated and introduced into the animal's circulation. Fluid and electrolytes secreted during the processes of digestion are reabsorbed during the formation of feces.
- Barrier Function – Prevention of the translocation of intestinal bacteria and digestive enzymes into the circulation as well as the prevention of loss of plasma proteins.

In addition to the digestive functions listed above, the intestinal tract has an important role in normal immune function, antigen processing and presentation, and a role in the endocrine regulation of digestive enzyme synthesis and release by other digestive organs, such as the pancreas. In this section, the anatomical structure of the intestinal tract is described, particularly with reference to the anatomical features contributing to the large surface area of the small intestine. The endocrine and immunological features of intestinal function are described in 5.2.

5.1.2   Gross anatomy of the intestinal tract

The intestinal tract is essentially a muscular tube, with a varying diameter and mucosal structure in the different sections of the tract. The variations in diameter, mucosal structure and function relate to the differing physiological role of each area; for instance, the stomach is readily distensible, while the small intestine is much less distensible.

The intestinal wall is divided into four discrete layers. The four layers are visible on cut sections of the intestine and can be readily distinguished by differences in echogenicity during ultrasound examination of the intestinal tract.

Proceeding from the lumen outwards to the serosa, the four layers of the intestinal tract visible during ultrasound examination are:

- Mucosa (slightly hypoechoic)
- Submucosa (hyperechoic)
- Muscularis (hypoechoic)
- Serosa (brightly hyperechoic)

In addition to the four physical layers described above, a very narrow hyperechoic layer is usually visible at the interface between the mucosa itself and the intestinal lumen.

5.1.2.1   Anatomical features of the small intestine

5.1.2.1.1   Increasing available surface area

There are several anatomical features that increase the available surface area of the intestinal epithelium (Figure 5.1).

The inward folding of the mucosa into grossly visible folds or rugae increases the available surface area by a factor of approximately 3 over a plain tube of equivalent diameter. The mucosa is arranged into finger-like structures called villi, which increase the surface area by an additional factor of approximately 10.

Enterocytes have a microscopic brush-border modification of their luminal cell membrane called microvilli. These microvilli increase the available surface area for digestion and absorption of nutrients by a factor of nearly 20 over the surface area of the villous projections.

5

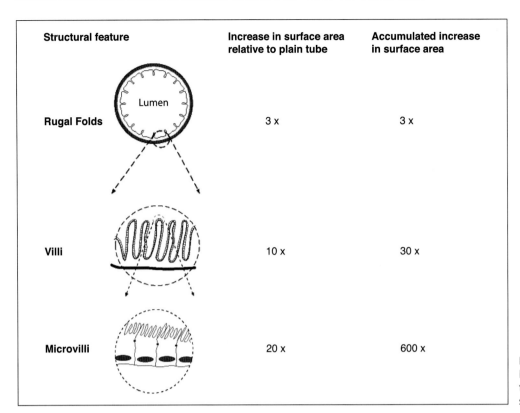

Structural feature	Increase in surface area relative to plain tube	Accumulated increase in surface area
Rugal Folds	3 x	3 x
Villi	10 x	30 x
Microvilli	20 x	600 x

Figure 5.1:
Macroscopic and microscopic anatomical structures increasing the surface area of the intestine.

In combination the three structural elements of rugae, villi, and microvilli increase the effective surface area of the intestinal mucosa by a factor of approximately 600 compared to a plain tube of the same diameter. The loss of one element, for instance villous blunting, as occurs with some viral enteropathies or IBD, will dramatically alter the function of the small intestine.

5.1.2.1.2 Microscopic anatomy of the intestinal tract

The villus is the functional unit of the small intestinal mucosa. Enterocytes arise from the division of stem cells in crypts at the base of the villus. They then migrate and mature along the length of the villus and are finally shed from the villous tip into the lumen. As enterocytes migrate along the villus their function alters, starting from a mainly secretory function in the crypt and lower villus, maturing to a mostly absorptive function in the upper part of the villus (see 5.2.2).

5.1.2.1.3 Spatial variation in intestinal structure

The small intestine has three major anatomical divisions. Proceeding from oral to aboral, these are the duodenum, the jejunum, and the ileum. The specific function of these three regions varies, with digestion of nutrients primarily occurring in the duodenum. The jejunum has both transport and absorptive functions, and the ileum is almost exclusively absorptive. The size and structure of the villi vary down the length of the small intestine, with duodenal villi being short and blunt, while the villi of the jejunum are long and narrow. In the duodenum, the ratio of the villus length to crypt depth is nearly equal, while the jejunal and ileal villi are much longer than the crypt depth. This anatomical difference reflects the greater need for increased surface area for the absorptive processes in the jejunum and ileum.

🔑 Key Facts

- The small intestine in dogs and cats is relatively short and simple, reflecting a predominantly carnivorous diet.
- The small intestine has several anatomical features that increase its effective surface area.
- Small intestinal anatomy varies along its length, reflecting the differing functions of different sections of the small intestine.

5.2 Intestinal Physiology

CRAIG G. RUAUX

5.2.1 Introduction

The normal regulation of the small intestine is carried out by a highly complex, interconnecting group of physiological mechanisms. Normal functioning of the intestine requires the production and secretion of digestive enzymes, pancreatic juice, bile acids, normal motility of the intestines and associated organs, mixing and compartmentalization of the gut contents, feedback regulation of the stomach and pancreas, and the regulation of food intake. To achieve these various functions, the GI tract produces and responds to a large number of hormonal substances.

The GI tract also possesses a complex enteric nervous system, receiving efferent inputs from the central nervous system (CNS) and providing afferent signals to the CNS.

The GI tract provides an enormous surface area that is in constant contact with dietary and environmental antigens. A complex system of gut-associated lymphoid tissue (GALT) regulates the GI mucosal immune responses to potential pathogens and dietary allergens, as well as regulating the expression of immune mechanisms and antibodies on other mucosal surfaces in the body.

The small intestine contains a complex population of microorganisms that play a role in maintaining the normal structure and function of the intestine. The small intestine is also in direct, if circuitous, contact with the external environment of the animal, and thus represents a major potential point of entry for bacteria, viruses, and allergens.

5.2.2 Secretion, digestion, and absorption: function of the villus

The villus is the functional unit of the small intestinal mucosa. Enterocytes arise from stem cell division in crypts at the base of the villus, then migrate and mature along the length of the villus, and are finally shed from the villus tip into the lumen. As enterocytes migrate along the villus their function alters, from a mainly secretory function in the crypt and lower villus, maturing to a mostly absorptive function in the upper part of the villus. The normal physiology of GI epithelial cell generation and maturation is discussed in detail elsewhere.[1] Figure 5.2 shows an idealized illustration of a typical villus.

Enterocytes have a microscopic brush-border modification of the luminal cell membrane, the microvilli. These microvilli increase the available surface area for digestion and absorption of nutrients by a factor of nearly twenty over the surface area of the villous projections.

As the function of the enterocytes varies with their location, the pathological effect of diseases affecting the small intestinal mucosa varies depending upon which part of the villus is predominantly affected. Rotaviral and coronaviral diarrheas are typically mild and self-limiting, affecting the older enterocytes and thus reducing the absorptive capacity of the small intestine, but sparing the younger enterocytes. This contrasts with the effects of the *Parvovirus*, which damages much younger enterocytes than in the rotaviral and coronaviral enteritides. This loss of younger enterocytes compromises mucosal permeability, promotes bacterial translocation and GI bleeding, and also leads to a loss of absorptive function, as the enterocytes are no longer present to mature. Consequently, feline and canine parvoviral enteritides are severe diseases that are associated with high morbidity and mortality.

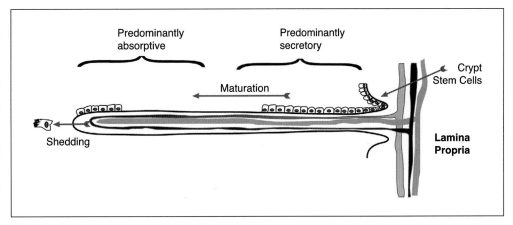

Figure 5.2:
Diagrammatic representation of the structure and function of the small intestinal villus. Gastrointestinal epithelial cells (enterocytes) arise from stem cells in the mucosal crypts. As they mature, they migrate along the length of the villus. During maturation the function of the cell changes, from predominantly secretory at the base of the villus to predominantly absorptive at the tip of the villus. Enterocytes are shed into the gastrointestinal lumen from the tip of the villus.

The brush border of the enterocytes of the apical villus provides an enormous increase in the surface area of the villus. This large surface area provided by the brush border promotes contact of the partially digested intestinal contents with the brush border enzymes that carry out many of the last steps of digestion. The large surface area also promotes the absorption of nutrients, both by increasing the number of receptors and carrier molecules available and by promoting the passive diffusion of simple compounds, water, and some electrolytes.

Loss of the brush border will reduce the uptake of fluids secreted by the villus crypts and younger enterocytes, thus leading to an increased fluid content in the intestinal tract. Visualization of the brush border is difficult with routine histopathological examination, thus subtle alterations in brush border morphology and function may not be detected by routine histopathology.

5.2.3 Regulation of secretion, absorption, and motility: gastrointestinal hormones

The GI tract is the largest endocrine organ in the body, both in terms of the total mass of hormone-producing cells and the total number of hormonal substances produced.[2,3] The vast majority of GI hormones are small peptides, rather than the steroidal compounds produced by the gonads and adrenal cortex. Regardless of this difference in structure from the gonadal/adrenal hormones, GI hormones are "true" hormonal compounds. These compounds are liberated from hormone-producing cells into the circulation, manifesting a physiological effect on tissues distant from the cells that produce the hormone. Representative examples of the best-known and most thoroughly charac-

terized hormones are listed in Table 5.1. The GI tract regulates its own motility and secretory processes in response to food input and changes in the luminal environment.

Secretin, a 23-amino-acid peptide hormone produced in the mucosa of the duodenum, was the first hormone to be isolated and its function described. This hormone, produced by the "S" cells in the duodenal mucosa in response to acidification of the duodenal lumen, stimulates the pancreas into producing pancreatic juice with a high concentration of bicarbonate, neutralizing the acid in the duodenal lumen. Bicarbonate production and neutralization of the gastric acid is necessary for the optimum function of exocrine pancreatic and duodenal mucosal digestive enzymes, most of which have pH optima near neutrality (pH 7.0).

After the observation of secretin activity in duodenal extracts, other workers demonstrated an endocrine activity of gastric antral mucosal extracts on gastric acid secretion. The responsible substance was originally called "gastric secretin", but was subsequently abbreviated to gastrin.[3] Gastrin is a 17-amino-acid peptide, produced by "G" cells in the antral mucosa in response to the presence of protein and fat in the distal gastric antrum. Gastrin acts upon enterochromaffin-like cells to increase the production of histamine by these cells. Histamine released by the enterochromaffin-like cells then stimulates gastric acid production by the chief cells. Entry of food into the small intestine stimulates the production of cholecystokinin (CCK). CCK is released from duodenal "I" cells, stimulating the emptying of the gall bladder and the production of digestive enzymes by the pancreatic acinar cells.

These three "classical" GI hormones were isolated and their predominant functions identified in the early decades of the twentieth century. As all three are stimulatory, elucidation of their effects on the GI tract and associated organs was rela-

Table 5.1: Examples of endocrine compounds with major effects on the gastrointestinal tract

Hormone	Source	Function(s)
"Classical" GI Hormones		
Cholecystokinin	Duodenal mucosa, "I" cells	Stimulates gall-bladder contraction and pancreatic enzyme secretion
Gastrin	Gastric antrum, "G" cells	Stimulates gastric acid secretion
Secretin	Duodenal mucosa, "S" cells	Stimulates pancreatic bicarbonate secretion
"Modern" GI Hormones		
Enteroglucagon	Distal small intestine, "L" Cells	Enhances release of insulin in response to glucose
Gastric Inhibitory Peptide	Proximal small intestine	Inhibits gastric motility and acid secretion
Ghrelin	Gastric epithelium	Stimulation of growth hormone release, regulation of appetite
Motilin	Proximal small intestine	Stimulates migrating motor complexes
Pancreatic Polypeptide	Pancreatic acinar cells	Affects pancreatic secretion, complex effects on GI motility
Somatostatin	Pancreas, enteric nervous system, GI epithelium	Inhibits secretion of many other GI hormones

tively simple. Inhibitory hormones, whose effects are manifest as decreases in GI secretion or motility, are more difficult to demonstrate in whole-animal studies, and the major hormone with inhibitory effects on the GI tract, somatostatin, was not isolated and identified until nearly forty years later.

The small intestinal mucosa is the source of motilin, a peptide hormone that stimulates GI motility. Motilin is released into the circulation during the interdigestive phase. This pulsatile release of motilin stimulates cyclical muscle contractions that sweep the length of the intestine. These cyclical "housekeeping" contractions are called the migrating motor complex.

Sensations of hunger and satiety are important in the regulation of food intake. Ghrelin, another peptide hormone produced in the gastric mucosa, is released into the circulation when the stomach is empty. Ghrelin acts on the CNS to regulate hunger and satiety, with circulating concentrations increasing during the interdigestive period, which then rapidly decrease after feeding. Ghrelin's name is derived from another important systemic function of this hormone, acting as a growth-hormone-releasing hormone (GhRH) in the pituitary. Ghrelin acts in concert with somatostatin and GhRH to regulate the release of growth hormone. Ghrelin is a potent stimulator of growth hormone release, while somatostatin is a suppressor of growth hormone release. The actions and release patterns of ghrelin and somatostatin, in concert with GhRH from the hypothalamus, lead to a highly pulsatile release of growth hormone. Thus, the stomach mucosa, and the state of GI filling, play an important role in the integrated regulation of body-wide physiology by its production and release of ghrelin, and hence its influence on growth hormone production.

Ghrelin concentrations are lower in obese humans than in lean controls. Conversely, in patients with Prader-Willi syndrome, extremely high circulating concentrations of ghrelin are observed in association with a severely increased, uncontrollable, voracious appetite and extreme obesity.[4] Studies of ghrelin in companion animals are currently lacking, thus it is not known if similar changes occur in dogs or cats with obesity.

5.2.4 Gut-associated lymphoid tissue and the immune system

As the largest area of mucosal tissue exposed to the external environment, it is understandable that the GI tract plays an important role in the regulation of the immune system. The GI tract is a major component of the "common mucosal immune system". Exposure to antigens in the GI tract is associated with increased production of secretory IgA at other mucosal sites, and IgG systemically. Conversely, exposure to potential GI pathogens at other mucosal surfaces will lead to increased production of secretory IgA in the GI mucosa.[5]

Immune system cells occur throughout the GI tract. Intraepithelial lymphocytes are widely distributed in the GI mucosa, where they may mediate antibody-dependant cellular cytotoxicity, or act as natural killer cells. Mast cells are also scattered diffusely throughout the mucosa, submucosa, and lamina propria of the intestine. Particularly in the ileum, immune cells of the GI tract may be organized in lymphoid follicles, forming Peyer's patches. Specialized mucosal cells in the epithelium over the Peyer's patches endocytose antigens. The antigens are passed to dendritic cells and macrophages, which act as antigen-presenting cells within the lymphoid follicle. Immunocompetent T cells produced within the Peyer's patch can subsequently migrate to other mucosal surfaces, where they produce IgA. Some T cells, after exposure to antigen within the Peyer's patch, will migrate into the GI mucosa where they become cytotoxic T cells, directed against potential pathogens.

The GI tract is constantly exposed to a vast number of antigens. These may be derived from food proteins, the intestinal microflora, or the host organism itself. It has been said that the GI tract exists normally in a constant state of inflammation, but excessive inflammatory cell activation will lead to disease, such as IBD or colitis. The normal regulation of the immune system's reactivity to antigenic challenge is carried out by a complex system of cytokines and regulatory cells, which have been reviewed elsewhere.[5]

Increased GI immune system responsiveness to either endogenous antigens or bacterial proteins has been postulated to be an underlying cause of IBD in many veterinary patients. It is unclear whether the underlying problem is one of inappropriate reactivity, IgE-mediated allergic disease, suppressed downregulation of immune cells, or some combination of multiple predisposing causes that lead to the pathological process referred to as IBD.

The predominant immunoglobulin subtype produced by the GI tract is IgA. Dimeric and polymeric IgA molecules are produced by plasma cells within the lamina propria, then taken up by enterocytes, complexed with a secretory component and released into the intestinal lumen. Within the lumen, IgA binds with surface proteins of many potential pathogens, helping to prevent their adhesion to the mucosa and subsequent bacterial invasion of the epithelium.

Secretory IgA deficiency is the most common immune deficiency of human beings, and has also been described in some dog breeds, such as the German Shepherd.[6,7] While secretory IgA deficiency in dogs has been associated with an increased incidence of intestinal disease by some authors,[6] the actual prevalence of IgA deficiency in both healthy and diseased dogs, and the role of IgA deficiency in veterinary gastroenterology is an area of active research.

5.2.5 Intestinal bacteria

The GI tract is home to a vast population of microbes, particularly in the more distal parts of the intestine. Gastrointestinal microbes are an important source of some vitamins. For example, it has been estimated that approximately 1/4 of the total body folate in humans is derived from the bacterial flora of the gut. Also, the presence of a normal GI microflora is necessary for the development of normal intestinal mucosal structure. Finally, many species of bacteria assist in the fermentation and digestion of dietary fiber. *Lactobacillus* and *Bifidobacter* spp., for instance, are able to ferment complex polysaccharides such as inulin and fructo-oligosaccharides, generating short-chain fatty acids that are used as an energy source by the enterocytes.

The GI tract microflora is made up of a mixture of aerobes, microaerobes, as well as facultative and obligate anaerobic bacteria. Much of the anaerobic flora is found in close association with the GI mucosa, making reproducible sampling of this flora difficult.

The normal canine intestinal microflora is highly complex, varying markedly from individual to individual and at differing points within the GI tract.[8] Each individual appears to have a unique bacterial flora present within its GI tract, and based on longitudinal studies in several species, this flora is apparently quite stable in healthy individuals.

The normal bacterial content in the feline small intestine has not been thoroughly explored, but it appears that, in comparison to dogs, the total number of bacteria in the small intestine and the proportion of obligate anaerobic bacteria are greater in the cat.[9,10] While the actual organisms present were not defined, experimental work investigating the effects of diet and antibiotic therapy on serum markers of intestinal bacterial biomass in cats, such as serum cobalamin and folate concentrations, suggest that the normal flora in the cat is stable and resilient, with serum markers returning to pre-treatment concentrations rapidly after withdrawal of antibiotic therapy.[11]

While the GI microflora is an integral part of the normal intestinal physiology, it also contains many organisms that are potential pathogens. Bacterial translocation across the GI mucosa is a major cause of sepsis in critically ill patients. The GI tract itself is susceptible to infection by specific, identified pathogens from contaminated food or the environment, such as *Salmonella* spp., which can lead to GI disease.

The presence of an increased biomass of bacteria in the GI tract may also be associated with intestinal disease (see 5.3.8). This increase in biomass may occur due to the loss of normal regulatory mechanisms that control the size of the intestinal bacterial population. Loss of gastric acid (for instance, from the long-term use of antacid medications), loss of antibacterial pancreatic secretions in exocrine pancreatic insufficiency, secretory IgA deficiency, and suppression of mucosal cellular immunity may all be associated with an increase in the total bacterial biomass present within the small intestine. This increased bacterial biomass may then exert adverse effects on the host animal through increased competition for limiting nutrients, increased production of toxic metabolites from bile acids and nutrients, or direct invasion of the mucosa and production of bacterial exotoxins.[12]

🔑 Key Facts

- Physiological regulation of the intestine involves complex interactions between the endocrine, neural, and immune systems that are specific to the intestine.
- The villus is the functional unit of the small intestine. Diseases affecting the villus are associated with diarrhea and malabsorption.
- The gastrointestinal microflora plays an integral part in normal intestinal physiology.

References

1. Pageot LP, Perreault N, Basora N et al. Human cell models to study small intestinal functions: recapitulation of the crypt-villus axis. *Microsc Res Tech* 2000; 49: 394–406.
2. Holst JJ, Fahrenkrug J, Stadil F et al. Gastrointestinal endocrinology. *Scand J Gastroenterol* 1996; 216: 27–38.
3. Rehfeld JF. The new biology of gastrointestinal hormones. *Physiol Rev* 1998; 78: 1087–1108.
4. Korbonits M, Grossman AB. Ghrelin: update on a novel hormonal system. *Eur J Endocrinol* 2004; 151 Suppl 1: S67–S70.
5. Castro GA. Gut immunophysiology: regulatory pathways within a common mucosal immune system. *News Physiol Sci* 1989; 4: 59–64.
6. Batt RM, Barnes A, Rutgers HC et al. Relative IgA deficiency and small intestinal bacterial overgrowth in German Shepard dogs. *Res Vet Sci* 1991; 50: 106–111.
7. German AJ, Hall EJ, Day MJ. Relative deficiency in IgA production by duodenal explants from German Shepherd dogs with small intestinal disease. *Vet Immunol Immunop* 2000; 76: 25–43.

8. Suchodolski JS, Ruaux CG, Steiner JM et al. Application of molecular fingerprinting for qualitative assessment of small-intestinal bacterial diversity in dogs. *J Clin Microbiol* 2004; 42: 4702–4708.

9. Johnston KL, Lamport A, Batt RM. An unexpected bacterial flora in the proximal small intestine of normal cats. *Vet Rec* 1993; 132: 362–363.

10. Johnston KL, Swift NC, Forster-van Hijfte M et al. Comparison of the bacterial flora of the duodenum in healthy cats and cats with signs of gastrointestinal tract disease. *J Am Vet Med Assoc* 2001; 218: 48–51.

11. Johnston KL, Lamport A, Proud J et al. The effect of diet and metronidazole on the bacterial flora and permeability of the feline small intestine. *J Vet Intern Med* 1994; 8: 149.

12. Mathias J, Clench M. Review: Pathophysiology of diarrhea caused by bacterial overgrowth of the small intestine. *Am J Med Sci* 1985; 289: 243–248.

5.3 Small Intestinal Disease

Karin Allenspach, Frédéric P. Gaschen

5.3.1 Introduction

The small intestine plays an essential role in the digestion and absorption of nutrients. Absorption is made possible by the very high mucosal surface area. Most pathological processes affecting the small intestine cause some degree of structural mucosal damage, resulting in a reduction of the mucosal surface area. This may lead to decreased absorption and cause further intestinal dysfunction, accompanied by clinical signs such as diarrhea, vomiting, dehydration, weight loss, and lethargy. Small bowel diarrhea is characterized by a normal or slightly increased defecation frequency and a large volume of feces passed at each defecation. If there is blood in the stool, the feces will usually be of dark color (melena).

Intestinal parasites are the most common cause of small intestinal disease in dogs and cats, followed in dogs by dietary indiscretion. However, a wide array of disease processes can affect the small intestine of small animals including other infectious agents, such as viruses, bacteria, or fungal organisms, adverse reactions to food (i.e., food allergy or intolerance), IBD, or neoplasia. This chapter provides an overview of some of these small intestinal diseases.

5.3.2 Infectious causes of small intestinal disease

5.3.2.1 Viral infections

5.3.2.1.1 Canine parvovirus enteritis

Canine parvovirus (CPV) is a small, non-enveloped DNA virus that is highly resistant in the environment. Disinfection of contaminated areas must be performed with sodium hypochlorite (i.e., household bleach). There are two known strains of CPV: CPV-1 and CPV-2.[1,2] For the most part, clinically important disease is caused by CPV-2 infection in dogs below 6 months of age. In the 1980s, CPV-2 evolved into two different strains, CPV-2a and CPV-2b.[2] During this evolution, the virus became more pathogenic and developed a higher capacity to replicate in susceptible tissues. CPV-2 is a highly contagious virus that is transmitted predominantly by contaminated feces. The incubation period in the field is 7–14 days. Rottweilers, Doberman Pinschers, Labrador Retrievers, American Staffordshire Terriers, German Shepherd dogs, and Alaskan Sled dogs have been reported to be at an increased risk for infection.[3]

The virus enters through oronasal lymphoid tissue and spreads by way of the lymphoid system to other organs with rapidly dividing cell lines, mainly intestinal crypt epithelium and the bone marrow. The virus destroys intestinal crypt cells, which leaves the epithelium more susceptible to secondary bacterial infections, especially with gram-negative bacterial organisms.[4,5] After contact with CPV-2, most older puppies and adult dogs undergo a subclinical infection. Puppies with severe infections are usually under 12 weeks of age at the time of infection. Vomiting, foul-smelling and often bloody diarrhea, anorexia, and dehydration develop 2–5 days after infection. Fever associated with secondary bacterial infection due to leukopenia and the breakdown of the intestinal barrier is also frequently seen.[6] Myocarditis can be observed in puppies that have been infected in utero or up to 8 weeks after birth.[7] A preliminary clinical diagnosis of CPV-2 infection is likely when the typical signs of acute vomiting, bloody diarrhea, and dehydration are seen in a young dog with an uncertain vaccination history.

An in-house fecal ELISA test is available to diagnose CPV infection. The ELISA test is only positive during the time of viral shedding, which is up to 10–12 days post infection. However, the test can be falsely positive if the dog has been vaccinated with an attenuated live vaccine.[8] The only possibility to differentiate between an infection and a vaccine strain in these cases is by PCR-based detection of viral DNA in feces.[9]

5

Table 5.2: Fluid therapy. This table shows guidelines for designing fluid therapy in patients with acute gastrointestinal disease.[78] Please note that for every patient all three components need to be estimated. The total volume of fluids given per hour is the sum of volumes given for each of the three components on an hourly basis.

Replacement of deficit
Dehydration (%) x body weight (kg) x 10 = ml of fluid to be administered over 4–6 hours

Maintenance fluid requirement
40–60 ml/kg body weight/24 hours

Ongoing losses
Estimate ongoing losses through vomiting and/or diarrhea and replace with maintenance fluids

5

Table 5.3: Potassium supplementation. Guidelines for potassium supplementation in patients with acute gastrointestinal disease.[78]

plasma K (mmol/L)	mmol KCl/250 ml	mmol KCl/500 ml	mmol KCl/1000 ml	maximum fluid rate ml/kg/h
<2.0	20	40	80	6
2.0–2.5	15	30	60	8
2.6–3.0	10	20	40	12
3.1–3.5	7.5	15	30	16

Treatment is directed towards restoration of fluid and electrolyte balance (Tables 5.2 and 5.3). Earlier recommendations included GI rest (i.e., nothing per os, NPO) until the vomiting has stopped, but newer studies show that early enteral nutrition is beneficial for earlier weight gain and decreased mortality.[10] Other supportive measures include broad-spectrum antimicrobial agents against gram-positive as well as gram-negative bacteria; for example, amoxicillin-clavulanic acid at 12.5 mg/kg IV twice a day. If the patient is sufficiently rehydrated, some clinicians choose to add gentamycin at 5 mg/kg IV once a day. However, a urinalysis must be evaluated on a daily basis to monitor the patient for occurrence of granular casts, an early sign of renal toxicity. Ticarcillin-clavulanic acid maybe a safer, broad-spectrum choice and can be given at a dosage of 40–50 mg/kg q 8 h. Antiemetic drugs are indicated if vomiting persists (e.g., maropitant 1 mg/kg/day SC for up to 5 days, metoclopramide at 0.1–0.4 mg/kg/h as a constant rate infusion, or dolasetron at 0.3–0.6 mg/kg IV or SC once or twice per day). Plasma or whole blood transfusions are indicated if the patient develops severe hypoalbuminemia and/or anemia. Further treatment options include the use of feline interferon omega (only available in Europe and Japan at the moment), hyperimmune serum, recombinant human granulocyte-colony stimulating factor (G-CSF), or anti-endotoxin serum. However, except for feline interferon omega, none of these therapies have been shown to improve survival or shorten hospitalization time.[4,11,12,13]

Puppies surviving an infection with CPV-2 are protected from re-infection for at least 20 months, if not lifelong. Inactivated CPV-2 vaccines protect vaccinated dogs only for a short period of time (i.e., several weeks) and must therefore be given repeatedly to increase protection to up to 15 months. In contrast, a single attenuated live vaccine is safe and protects vaccinated dogs for several years. Vaccination failure is mainly seen when the vaccine interferes with maternal antibodies present in vaccinated puppies.[4] Maternal antibody titers may persist up to 16 weeks after birth if the antibody titer of the bitch is very high. To prevent interference with maternal antibodies, it has been recommended to apply a low-titer attenuated live vaccine at 8, 12, 16, and 20 weeks of age and annually thereafter. For high-titer attenuated live vaccines, which are highly immunogenic, the recommended regimen includes vaccinations at 6–8 weeks of age, then every 3–4 weeks until 16 weeks of age, followed by a booster at one year of age. Revaccination every 3 or more years is considered protective.

5.3.2.1.2 Canine distemper virus infection

Canine distemper virus (CDV) is an enveloped, single-stranded RNA virus. Most infections occur at the age of 3–6 months. The severity of the infection depends on the virus strain with which the dog is infected, with certain virulent strains being more pathogenic than others.[15] After infection, the virus usually spreads from macrophages in the upper respiratory tract to the lymphatic tissue of the stomach, intestines, and liver. At this stage, most infected dogs show leukopenia and fever. At about 14 days post infection, the virus is either entirely cleared from the body or spreads to the epithelial tissues of the skin, exocrine and endocrine glands, GI tract, as well as the respiratory and genitourinary tract. At this time, most dogs show severe clinical signs consistent with persistence of the virus in affected tissues. Spread to the CNS is dependent on the degree of systemic immune response of the dog.

CDV infection should be suspected in unvaccinated 3- to 6-month-old puppies with clinical signs of the respiratory and gastrointestinal tracts, which are followed by neurological signs. Maternal antibodies can persist in puppies up to 14 weeks after birth.[15] Vaccination schedules for CVD therefore should include booster vaccinations every 3–4 weeks until the puppies are 16 weeks of age.

5.3.2.1.3 Feline coronavirus infection

Feline coronavirus (FeCoV) infection can manifest itself as two different syndromes: a transient, most often mild diarrhea or as a disseminated granulomatous disease, feline infectious peritonitis (FIP). The disseminated disease is believed to be caused by a mutation of the FeCoV resulting in increased tropism for macrophages.[16] It has also been speculated that repetitive infection with large doses of the virus associated with stress and a crowded environment may lead to FIP in young cats.[17] The virus is transmitted by ingestion or inhalation. It primarily infects intestinal epithelial cells, but can spread to macrophages if it carries a gene that encodes a specific spike protein. This may then lead to FIP by initiating an immune-complex disease.[16] The intestinal infection is mainly seen as a mild, transient disease. It is sometimes associated with vomiting, and is usually self-limiting with supportive care alone.

5.3.2.1.4 Feline panleukopenia

Feline panleukopenia is caused by the feline parvovirus (FPV), a very stable virus without an envelope that survives in the environment for up to 1 year. However, disinfection can be achieved with sodium hypochlorite (i.e., household bleach, undiluted), 4% formaldehyde, and 1% glutaraldehyde. The virus is shed in the feces for up to 6 weeks after infection. Most infections with FPV are subclinical. The virus usually spreads from the tonsils to other lymphoid tissues, the bone marrow, and intestinal crypt cells. The most severe clinical signs are seen in 3- to 5-month-old unvaccinated kittens. Fever, depression, anorexia, vomiting, severe dehydration, bloody diarrhea, and oral ulcerations are most commonly seen. In pregnant queens, the clinical signs can include infertility, mummified fetuses, and abortions. If the infection occurs during late pregnancy, the developing kittens can suffer cerebellar damage causing a typical hypermetric gait and intention tremors in neonates.[18]

A presumptive diagnosis of FPV infection is made based on the clinical signs along with a severe leukopenia (50–3000 leucocytes/ml). An ELISA test similar to the one available for CPV is useful to confirm infection.[19]

Treatment is mostly supportive, with parenteral fluid therapy as a mainstay. Broad-spectrum antibiotic treatment in febrile neutropenic kittens is important and amoxicillin, cephalosporins, and/or gentamycin have been recommended. However, gentamycin should be used cautiously and should be avoided in patients that are dehydrated. In addition, antiemetic therapy with metoclopramide, dolasetron, or thiethylperazine is often necessary. Colostral antibodies against FPV persist in kittens for 12 to 14 weeks, and vaccination regimens with vaccinations as early as 6 weeks of age, then every 3–4 weeks until 16 weeks of age, followed by a booster at one year of age are recommended. Thereafter, revaccinations every 3 or more years are protective.

5.3.2.1.5 Feline leukemia virus (FeLV) and feline immunodeficiency virus (FIV)

Cats infected with FeLV or FIV predominantly show signs of immune-suppression, lymphoma, leukemia, and non-regenerative anemia. Diarrhea is often a sign of general immuno-suppression associated with secondary infections with enteral viruses, bacteria, or fungal organisms.[20] Aggressive symptomatic therapy may control the clinical signs, but the long-term prognosis in these patients is poor.

5.3.2.2 Bacterial Infections

The small intestinal lumen naturally harbors a limited number of a variety of bacteria. This resident bacterial flora has important functions in preserving anatomical structures and enhancing the physiological processes necessary for the proper digestion and absorption of dietary components. The small intestinal flora also plays a role in preventing colonization by pathogenic bacteria, and positively influences the development of the enteric immune system. The composition of the resident bacterial flora can be modulated by diet and/or pre- and probiotic agents.

Although not the most common etiology of small intestinal disease, bacterial infections with pathogenic bacterial species have been documented in small animals. Responsible enteropathogens include *Campylobacter* spp., *Clostridium perfringens* and *difficile*, *Salmonella* spp., *Yersinia* spp., and some strains of *E. coli*. However, some of these bacterial species have not only been isolated in feces of dogs and cats with diarrhea, but also in healthy animals.[21] To further complicate matters, pathogenic bacteria may just be opportunistic in patients with intestinal diseases due to an unrelated cause. If enteropathogenic bacteria are not the actual source of the animal's clinical signs and it is assumed that they represent an incidental finding, indiscriminate use of antibiotics is not recommended as it may lead to the development of resistant strains with possible public health relevance. Even though the pathogenicity of many of these bacteria is subject to controversy, a risk for the development of zoonotic infections in humans after contact with an infected pet does exist. More importantly, such a risk also exists when the infected pet is healthy, but is shedding enteropathogens. These facts often make diagnostic and therapeutic decisions difficult. Additional research is needed to more clearly establish the role of the small intestinal microflora in general, and enteric pathogens in particular, in both canine and feline intestinal disease.

5

5

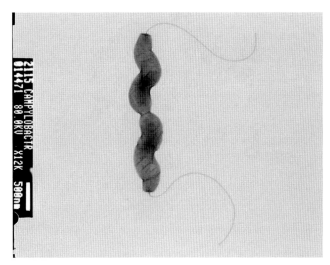

Figure 5.3:
Campylobacter spp. This figure shows an electron-microscopic image of a *Campylobacter* spp. organism. Note the spiral shape of the flagellated organism (12,000x; image courtesy of Dr. Mary Parker, Institute of Food Research, Norwich, UK).

5.3.2.2.1 Campylobacter spp.

Campylobacter spp. are slender and curved gram-negative rods with polar flagella that typically appear in spiral shapes (Figure 5.3). These microorganisms are motile, and grow under microaerophilic conditions. *Campylobacter spp.*, such as *C. jejuni* may attach to and invade host enterocytes and produce soluble components with enterotoxin-like activity.[22]

Numerous reports have shown that *C. jejuni, C. upsaliensis,* and other enteric *Campylobacter* spp. may be present in the feces of healthy as well as diarrheic dogs and cats.[21,23] *Campylobacter* infections appear to be less frequent in cats than in dogs.[24,25] Interestingly, studies performed in Europe yielded a higher incidence of *Campylobacter* spp.-positive pets in the investigated populations than those reported in studies from North America.[26] Based on a recent epidemiological study from Switzerland, *Campylobacter spp.* could be detected in the feces of approximately 42% of healthy dogs and cats presented for vaccination.[27] A longitudinal study of healthy 3-month-old pet dogs in Denmark revealed that 60% of the dogs evaluated carried *Campylobacter* spp. in their fecal matter. At one year of age, nearly 100% of the dogs were shown to be positive. At 2 years of age, the microorganisms could be isolated in 67% of the population.[28] Moreover, 21% of healthy dogs < 12 months of age were reported to shed *Campylobacter* spp., and shedding was more than twice as common in young dogs with diarrhea as in healthy dogs.[28]

Clinical signs in dogs and cats, if present, may vary widely. Diarrhea can be mild with occasional loose stools, moderate, or severe with watery or bloody feces with or without mucus. Clinical disease may be precipitated by stressful situations (i.e., boarding, concurrent diseases, etc.). Cytological evaluation of a rectal swab may reveal *Campylobacter*-like organisms with their typical slender curved rod or seagull-shaped appearance (Figure 5.3). Moreover, the presence of leukocytes indicates intestinal inflammation. Diagnosis is made by cultural identification of *Campylobacter* spp. in fresh fecal samples or rectal swabs. Shipping of fecal samples is usually not a problem as *Campylobacter* spp. remain stable for at least 3 days at room temperature, and 1 week if refrigerated. Alternatively, PCR-based assays for the detection of pathogenic *Campylobacter* strains in fecal samples are available (www.cvm.tamu.edu/gilab).

The therapeutic approach to dogs with proven fecal shedding of *Campylobacter* spp. depends on the health status of the patient (i.e., healthy vs. showing signs of GI disease). Healthy patients that are found to be positive and are sharing a home with immune-compromised people or with infants should probably be treated. For all other situations, the necessity of antibiotic treatment in healthy dogs is controversial. In animals showing diarrhea, vomiting, and/or other signs compatible with small intestinal disease, appropriate antibiotic therapy is recommended, even though the causal relationship of *Campylobacter* spp. infection and the clinical signs may be difficult to establish. The antibiotics of choice for treating campylobacteriosis in dogs and cats are erythromycin or fluoroquinolones (Table 5.4). The prognosis for full recovery is generally good. If an infection occurs secondary to another underlying intestinal disease, recovery may also depend on the identification and treatment of that condition.

Campylobacter spp. can also infect humans, and cause abdominal discomfort, fever, and diarrhea, which may be bloody. Recovery frequently occurs spontaneously but antibiotic treatment may be required. In several countries, *Campylobacter* infections have now become the most common intestinal infection observed.[27] Based on recent studies, risk factors for human infection include eating poultry cooked at home, drinking water from a well, lake or river, and daily contact with a dog.[29] Therefore, fecal shedding of *Campylobacter* spp. by healthy infected pets may represent a source of infection in people. Dogs and cats seem to function as reservoir hosts for *C. upsaliensis* and *C. helveticus* (with 30% and 35% prevalence, respectively) with an increased risk of fecal shedding in animals < 3 years of age. However, the role of these organisms in the epidemiology of *C. jejuni* infections is deemed to be negligible as the prevalence of isolates is low.[27]

5.3.2.2.2 Clostridium spp.

Clostridia are large gram-positive bacteria that produce endospores. Most pathogenic *Clostridia* are strict anaerobes. Some *Clostridia* are part of the normal intestinal microflora; however,

Table 5.4: Antimicrobials. Recommended antimicrobials for the treatment of small intestinal bacterial infections.

	Campylobacter spp.	*Clostridium perfringens*	*Clostridium difficile*	*E. coli*	*Salmonella* spp.[5]
Amoxicillin 10–20 mg/kg PO q 12 h	no	yes	no	yes	no
Aminoglycosides (i.e., gentamicin: 4–6 mg/kg IV, SC q 24 h)	no	no	no	yes	yes
Erythromycin[1] 20 mg/kg PO q 12 h (dog) 10 mg/kg PO q 8 h (cat)	yes[2]	yes	no	no	no
Fluoroquinolones (e.g., enrofloxacin: 5 mg/kg PO q 12 h)	yes	no	no	yes	yes
Metronidazole 8–15 mg/kg PO q 8–12 h	no	yes	yes[4]	no	no
Tetracyclines 10–20 mg/kg PO q 8 h	yes[3]	no	no	yes	yes
Trimethoprim-sulfonamides 12–15 mg/kg PO q 12 h	no	no	no	yes	yes
Tylosin 10–20 mg/kg PO q 12–24 h	no	yes	no	no	no

[1] Vomiting is a relatively frequent side effect after administration of erythromycin to dogs and cats. [2] First choice for therapy of *Campylobacter* spp. infections. [3] Tetracyclines are also frequently effective for the treatment of *Campylobacter* spp. infections if erythromycin or fluoroquinolones cannot be used. [4] *C. difficile*-associated diarrhea is best treated with metronidazole. [5] Antimicrobial treatment should be based on the results of *in vitro* sensitivity testing.

5

C. perfringens type A as well as *C. difficile* may be responsible for GI disease and enterotoxemia in dogs or cats.[30,31]

Clostridium perfringens. *C. perfringens* is widespread in the environment and can be present in feces of healthy animals. The two main toxins produced by *C. perfringens* type A are major toxin α and enterotoxin (also called *C. perfringens* enterotoxin or CPE). Enterotoxigenic *C. perfringens* are commonly associated with food poisoning in humans. CPE can be detected in fecal samples using immunoassays. Although *C. perfringens* could be cultivated from canine fecal samples in 76–86% of healthy and 71–75% of diarrheic dogs, only 5–14% of isolates from healthy dogs and 15–34% of those from dogs with diarrhea were enterotoxigenic.[30] Enterotoxigenic strains have been associated with nosocomial diarrhea, hemorrhagic enteritis, and acute or chronic large and/or small bowel diarrhea.[32] Since CPE may also be present in the feces of healthy, non-diarrheic dogs, it is possible that enteritis only develops if large enough concentrations of CPE are present in the intestinal lumen. However, currently available immunoassays do not allow for a quantitative assessment of fecal CPE.

Isolation of *C. perfringens* in feces is not sufficient for the diagnosis of *C. perfringens*-associated disease. Endospore counts performed on fecal smears are also unreliable. The clinical value of CPE assays as an accurate marker of pathogenicity of *C. perfringens* remains to be determined, but, as mentioned above, fecal CPE has been detected in a larger proportion of diarrheic than healthy dogs. Options for antimicrobial treatment are summarized in Table 5.4.

Clostridium difficile. *Clostridium difficile* produces two major toxins (toxins A and B). Infections with toxin-producing species are a common cause of nosocomial and antimicrobial-associated enteric infections in human beings and may lead to a potentially fatal pseudomembranous colitis, even though asymptomatic carriage has also been reported in humans. In various studies, *C. difficile* was cultured from the feces of healthy puppies and their dams, healthy adult dogs and cats, and diarrheic dogs and cats presented to veterinary clinics. *C. difficile* has also been isolated from the feces of dogs with nosocomial diarrhea, and was recovered during environmental surveys of veterinary hospitals where nosocomial clostridial infections had occurred.[32,33] Also, toxins A and/or B were detected significantly more frequently in diarrheic pets than in healthy pets. Therefore, a causal relationship between enterocolitis and *C. difficile* should only be suspected if toxins A and/or B can be detected in a fecal sample. Recommendations for antimicrobial therapy are summarized in Table 5.4.

5

5.3.2.2.3 Enterobacteriaceae

This family of enteric gram-negative rods contains numerous genera and species. The major gastrointestinal pathogens in small animals that belong to this family are *Escherichia coli* and *Salmonella* serovars.

5.3.2.2.4 Pathogenic E. coli

Shortly after birth, *E. coli* from environmental sources colonize the mammalian intestinal tract where they persist as an important member of the normal flora. Most strains have a low virulence and may occasionally cause infections in extra-intestinal locations such as the urogenital tract. Pathogenic *E. coli* have a variety of virulence factors such as adhesins, which allow their adhesion to mucous membranes; capsular polysaccharides that interfere with phagocytosis by host cells; and endotoxin, a lipopolysaccharide cell wall component.[34]

Shiga-toxin-producing *E. coli* (STEC) could be isolated with a similar frequency from healthy and diarrheic dogs, which suggests that they are not pathogenic in dogs. Canine enteropathogenic *E. coli* (EPEC) have been described in young dogs with diarrhea, but their actual clinical significance remains unknown.[35] In a study of 122 dogs with diarrhea at the time of death, 44 dogs had EPEC. Of those dogs, 29 were affected by concurrent enteric pathogens such as parvovirus.[35] In contrast, enterotoxin-producing *E. coli* (ETEC) could only be isolated from young dogs with diarrhea, and not from healthy animals. Based on the paucity of published reports, intestinal infections with *E. coli* do not seem to play an important role in canine and feline patients. Theoretically, asymptomatic canine carriers of STEC could be a source for human infections. However, the general risk of zoonotic transmission appears to be low.

5.3.2.2.5 Salmonellae

Salmonella serovars occur worldwide and may infect mammals, birds, and reptiles. The majority of *Salmonellae* of veterinary importance are serotypes of *S. enterica* subspecies *enterica*. In humans, the most common route of infection is by ingestion of contaminated food, especially chicken eggs and other egg products, but also meat products from pigs and chickens. Recently, serotype *infantis* cultured from dried pig ears marketed as dog treats was determined to be the cause of an outbreak of human disease in Canada and the USA.[36] In humans, the disease is characterized by diarrhea, fever, and abdominal cramps, often with a mild to moderate and self-limiting course.

Generally, healthy adult carnivores are considered resistant to salmonellosis. In recent prevalence studies, *Salmonella* serotypes could only very rarely be cultured from the feces of healthy or diarrheic dogs and cats. Only up to 2.3% of dogs and 1% of cats shed *Salmonella* spp. in their feces. However, in a study from Belgium, the frequency of *Salmonella* spp. isolation was much higher.[37] This study evaluated group-housed kittens (isolation frequency: 51.4%) and cats that had died or were euthanized due to incurable disease (isolation frequency: 8.6%).[37]

Although pets are rarely confirmed as the source of human salmonellosis, occasional outbreaks of *Salmonella* infections may be associated with visits to a veterinary clinic.[38] Thus, the practice of good hygiene is strongly recommended, especially when dealing with highly susceptible individuals such as infants, the elderly, and immune-compromised people.[39]

Clinical signs in dogs and cats with salmonellosis include fever, vomiting, diarrhea, anorexia, weight loss, and lethargy. Sepsis was reported as a complication of clinical salmonellosis in two cats fed a raw meat diet.[40] In another report, several kittens died of systemic salmonellosis, shortly after vaccination with a modified live panleukopenia vaccine.[41]

Diagnosis is made on the basis of fecal isolation of *Salmonella* serotypes in a patient with compatible clinical signs. The CBC may reveal changes suggestive of sepsis.

Treatment consists of fluid therapy and other supportive measures. Administration of antimicrobials is only recommended in pets with systemic infection, and is based on the sensitivity results of the isolated *Salmonella* strain (Table 5.4). In pets recovering from clinical salmonellosis, chronic carriage of *Salmonella* over several weeks post recovery may occur as a result of organisms remaining in the local lymph nodes. This may require long-term parenteral administration of an appropriate antibiotic. Because they are resistant to many environmental factors, *Salmonella* organisms may survive for long periods of time in the environment.[42]

5.3.2.2.6 Other bacteria

Ileocolitis associated with *Anaerobiospirillum* infection was reported in six cats from California.[43] This organism belongs to a genus of small, spiral, gram-negative motile bacteria that had been previously isolated from the throat and feces of normal dogs and cats. Three infected cats had gastrointestinal signs, two of which had diarrhea, one cat was anorectic and lethargic, and two cats had clinical signs unrelated to the GI tract. All six cats were euthanized or died, and ileitis and/or colitis were confirmed histologically. Using light and electron microscopy as well as PCR amplification, *Anaerobiospirillum* spp. was demonstrated in the intestinal lumen of all six cats.[43] The exact role of these bacteria in the pathogenesis of intestinal disease remains to be elucidated.

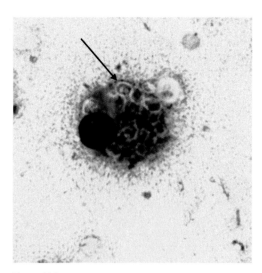

Figure 5.4:
Histoplasma capsulatum. The image shows a single macrophage with several phagocytized *Histoplasma* organisms from a rectal scrape in a dog. Please note that only one of the phagocytized organisms (see arrow) shows the typical eccentric location of the nucleus (Wright's stain, 165x; image courtesy of Dr. Steve Gaunt, Louisiana State University, Baton Rouge, LA).

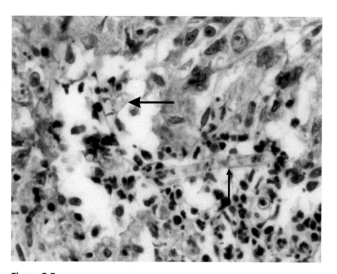

Figure 5.5:
Pythiosis. This figure shows a histological image of the intestinal wall from an 18-month-old Boxer presented with a 1-month history of vomiting and weight loss. A jejunal mass was palpated on abdominal palpation and was surgically resected with a 15- to 20-cm piece of small intestine. The image shows three hyphal structures (two hyphal structures are marked by arrows), one of them septate (large arrow). A severe mixed inflammatory response with macrophages, granulocytes, and necrotic material in the background can be appreciated. The granulocytes were identified as eosinophils with H&E staining. An infection with *Pythium insidiosum* was diagnosed. (Immunohistochemistry with polyclonal anti-*P. insidiosum* antibody, 600x; image courtesy of Dr. Andrew David, Louisiana State University, Baton Rouge, LA.)

5

5.3.2.3 Fungal and algae infections

5.3.2.3.1 Histoplasmosis

Histoplasma capsulatum is a dimorphic soil-borne fungus that can be found throughout the world in temperate and subtropical climates. Infection occurs mostly in young dogs and cats through the inhalation or ingestion of microconidia. Localized *H. capsulatum* infection in dogs can affect the respiratory tract, but if the disease is disseminated, it typically involves the GI tract.[44] Common signs include large-bowel diarrhea and tenesmus, hematochezia, and mucus in the feces. The small bowel may be infiltrated as well, with signs such as weight loss, intractable diarrhea, and sometimes protein-losing enteropathy (PLE). Histoplasmosis is most reliably diagnosed by identifying the organism on cytologic smears (Figure 5.4) from lymph node aspirates, rectal scrapings, or histological samples. Treatment consists of itraconazole (10 mg/kg PO q 24 h), which should be continued for 4–6 months and at least 2 months beyond the resolution of clinical signs.[44]

5.3.2.3.2 Pythiosis

Pythiosis is caused by the aquatic pathogen *Pythium insidiosum* that belongs to the class Oomycetes. Large breed male dogs are affected most commonly, probably because of their increased risk of exposure. In some areas of the USA, the GI form of the disease predominates in the dog, while in other areas the skin form is more prevalent.[45,46] The history can be suggestive of upper GI obstruction with a palpable abdominal mass or chronic diarrhea and weight loss, or sometimes also be suggestive of lower bowel disease. Histologically, eosinophilic granulomatous to pyogranulomatous enteritis can be found in the deep layers of the intestinal wall (Figure 5.5). The diagnosis is confirmed by isolation of the organism. Serology using ELISA or immunoblot has been shown to be very sensitive and specific. Antibody titers can be monitored during therapy and should significantly decrease in dogs that respond to treatment.[45] However, the prognosis is poor, unless complete resection of the affected GI area is possible during surgery.[45,47] If resection is incomplete, medical therapy can be attempted with itraconazole (10 mg/kg PO q 24 h) and terbinafine (5–10 mg/kg PO q 24 h), but treatment is not often successful.[45]

5

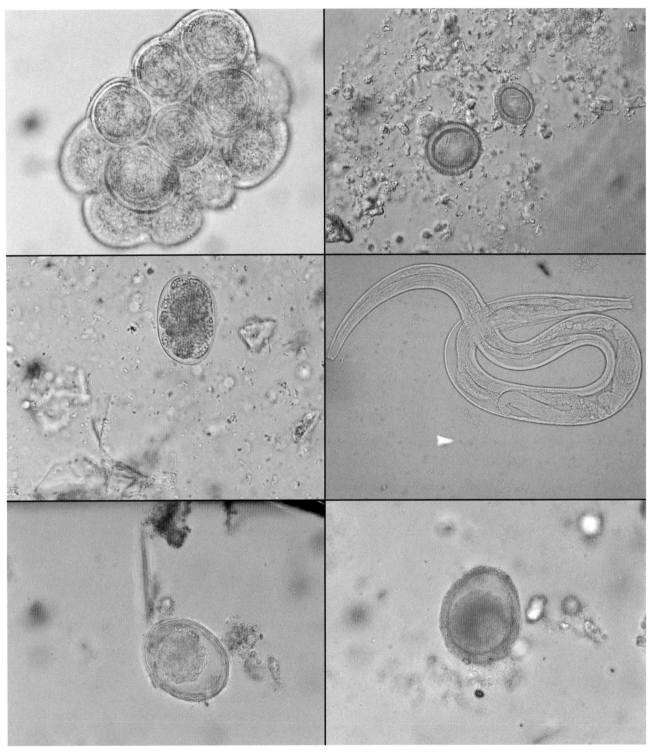

Figure 5.6:
Helminths. This figure shows ova and adult helminths commonly found in fecal samples from dogs and cats. Upper left: *Dipylidium canis* egg; upper right: *Echinococcus* sp. egg; middle left: *Ancylostoma* egg; middle right: *Ollulanus tricuspis* adult; lower left: *Toxascaris leonina* egg; lower right: *Toxocara* egg.

5.3.2.4 Parasitic diseases

5.3.2.4.1 Helminths

Parasitism is common in both dogs and cats. All dogs with acute vomiting and/or diarrhea should be evaluated for parasites. The diagnosis of a helminthic infection is based on the demonstration of ova during fecal flotation (Figure 5.6). Several anthelminthics may be considered, with some being more effective than others for specific helminths (Table 5.5). Cestodes, *Taenia* spp., and *Echinococcus* spp. are not very pathogenic in small animals, but can pose a significant zoonotic threat (especially *Echinococcus* infection in humans). Nematodes are more likely to cause clinical disease in dogs and cats.

Ollulanus tricuspis

The feline stomach worm is transmitted by infectious vomitus. These worms are usually located in the fundic area of the stomach in cats and may cause inappetence, vomiting, weight loss, and diarrhea.[48]

Ancylostoma caninum

The hookworm, *Ancylostoma caninum*, causes significant disease in puppies in temperate climates. In subtropical areas, *A. braziliense* and *A. ceylanicum* may also infect the small intestine. Other hookworms such as *Uncinaria* spp. are mainly found in the colon, but can also sometimes cause small intestinal disease. After oral infection with *Ancylostoma* larvae, the parasite develops into the adult stage in the stomach and duodenum. The larvae can also penetrate into blood vessels and travel to the lungs, where they are coughed up and swallowed back into the GI tract. Percutaneous infections occur mainly in puppies. The larvae can travel to different organs, where they can persist in a hypobiotic state. These dormant stages can be reactivated during pregnancy and can then be secreted in the milk.[49] Typical clinical signs in young puppies are blood loss, diarrhea, dehydration, PLE, and anemia. Effective anthelminthics are listed in Table 5.5. Milbemycin-oxime at 0.5–1 mg/kg PO every 30 days may be used for chemoprophylaxis in areas with a high infectious pressure.

Ascarids

***Toxocara canis* and *Toxocara mystax*.** Both of these parasites may cause significant disease in puppies and kittens, respectively. As is the case with hookworm infections, the parasite can travel from the wall of the GI tract into blood vessels and to the lungs or other organs and can also be transmitted through the colostrum. In fact, the lactogenic route is epidemiologically most important. Possible clinical signs include

Table 5.5: Treatment for helminth infections. This table shows commonly used anthelminthic agents used for the treatment of helminth infections in dogs and cats

Anthelminthic agent	Commonly used dosage
Ascarids and hookworms	
■ Fenbendazole	50 mg/kg PO once daily for three consecutive days
■ Pyrantel pamoate	5–10 mg/kg PO once; consider repeating after 2–4 weeks
■ Febantel	10–20 mg/kg PO once daily for 3 days
■ Moxidectin (1) for prevention of infection with hookworms (2) for prevention of reactivation of dormant *Ancylostoma* and *Toxocara canis* larvae and their transmission to puppies	(1) 0.5 mg/kg SC (sustained release formulation; currently not available) (2) 1 mg/kg PO administered on day 55 (hookworms) or days 40 and 55 (ascarids) of pregnancy
■ Milbemycin oxime	0.5–1 mg/kg PO once
Taenia, echinococcus, and dipylidium	
■ Praziquantel	5–10 mg/kg PO, SC; repeat in 3 weeks

vomiting; diarrhea, sometimes with hematochezia and the presence of mucus in the feces; a distended and painful abdomen; dehydration; anemia and fever. In puppies, *T. canis* infection may also cause clinical signs due to larval migration to different organs, and clinical signs due to pneumonia and/or hepatic disease may also be seen.

***Toxascaris leonina*.** *Toxocara leonina* causes small intestinal disease in dogs and cats. The development of the parasite occurs entirely in the intestinal tract. Clinically, enteritis can be seen, but the symptoms are rarely as severe as with *Toxocara* infections. Treatment options for ascarid infections are summarized in Table 5.5.

Strongyloides spp.

Strongyloides stercoralis and *S. planiceps* infect dogs, while *S. felis* and *S. tumefaciens* are seen in cats. Most infections are subclinical, but the presence of a high worm burden in puppies or kittens may be associated with hemorrhagic enteritis.

5.3.2.4.2 Protozoal infections

The two main protozoal parasites affecting the intestinal tract in dogs and cats are *Giardia* spp. and *Cryptosporidium* spp. Recently, another protozoal organism, *Tritrichomonas foetus* (see

5

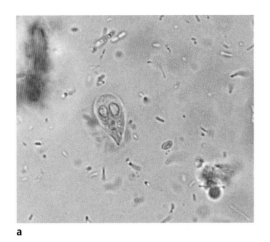

a

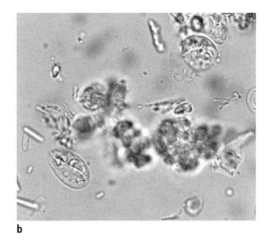

b

Figure 5.7:
Giardia. **a.** *Giardia* trophozoite in a smear from canine feces. **b.** *Giardia* cysts in a fecal flotation specimen from a dog. (Images courtesy of Dr. Heinz Sager, Institute for Parasitology, University of Bern, Switzerland.)

6.4.2.3), has been described as a pathogenic organism in the GI tract in cats, but this organism mainly affects the large intestines.

Giardia spp.

Giardia duodenalis exists in two forms, a motile trophozoite of piriform to ellipsoidal shape with two nuclei, four pairs of flagella, and one pair of median bodies (Figure 5.7a), and a cyst form that is highly resistant in the environment (Figure 5.7b). The cysts are absorbed with contaminated food or water, and release trophozoites into the small intestinal lumen where they attach to the mucosal epithelium and cause disease by affecting epithelial permeability. Trophozoites multiply by cell division and become encysted in the large bowel. *Giardia* cysts have four nuclei, a thin envelope, and are surrounded by a convolute of flagella. Under favorable conditions, they can persist for 3 weeks or even longer in the environment.[50]

Giardia spp. are globally distributed and are responsible for approximately 280 million cases of human giardiasis per year worldwide.[51] Symptoms of giardiasis in humans include acute or chronic diarrhea, dehydration, abdominal pain, and weight loss. Giardiasis is one of the most common parasitic diseases diagnosed in people living in North America. This protozoan is also encountered in dogs and cats, where the infection may remain subclinical, or may cause GI signs similar to those observed in humans. Consumption of water contaminated with *Giardia* cysts is the main origin of infection in people; however, the zoonotic potential of giardiasis in pets remains a subject of controversy. *Giardia* isolates are further divided into several different genotypes or assemblages with specific host ranges. Al-though assemblages infecting humans and pets are different, several anecdotal reports describe infections with similar genotypes in pets and people sharing a common environment.[50]

Several diagnostic tests are available for the diagnosis of *Giardia* infections in dogs and cats. These diagnostic tests include the direct examination of fecal smears for motile trophozoites (low sensitivity); concentration techniques including centrifugation with zinc sulfate (ZSFC), sodium acetate / acetic acid / formaldehyde (SAF), or merthiolate / iodine / formaldehyde (MIF) for detecting cysts (moderate to high sensitivity); fecal immunoassays such as ELISA or IFA for group specific antigens (moderate to high sensitivity); and fecal polymerase chain reaction (PCR; highly sensitive, but not recommended for routine diagnosis). Successful detection of *Giardia* using fecal flotation is operator-dependent. The retrieval of cysts significantly increases from 70% to more than 90% if two or more fecal samples collected at 2–3 days intervals are examined.[52] The SNAP *Giardia* Test Kit (Idexx Laboratories) has a comparable accuracy to fecal immunoassays, and can be helpful for in-clinic screening of dogs with compatible clinical signs.[53]

Studies concerning the prevalence of giardiasis in the canine and feline population report different rates in healthy pets, pets presented for veterinary care, and cats and dogs kept in shelters. Using ZSFC, *Giardia* cysts were detected in 7.2% of dogs presented to a veterinary clinic in Canada.[54] In another study, *Giardia* cysts were found in 12% of feline and 16% of canine fecal samples submitted to a laboratory in Germany.[55] The frequency of fecal ELISA-positive cases in dogs from shelters in Rome, Italy, was reported to be between 21% and 74%.[56] The prevalence is greatest in patients that live in high density group housing, especially when recommended disinfecting protocols are not carried out optimally. In such cases, *Giardia* cysts can easily survive in the environment and continuously infect new animals or re-infect animals after they have been treated.

Several pharmaceutical agents have been successfully used for the treatment of giardiasis in dogs and cats. In dogs, metronidazole at 25–30 mg/kg PO q 12 h for 5–8 days and fenbendazole at 50 mg/kg PO q 24 h for 3 days are most commonly used.[57] Albendazole (25 mg/kg PO q 12 h for 4 doses) can also be used successfully, but may lead to bone marrow toxicity in both dogs and cats.[58,59] In cats, metronidazole benzoate given at a dosage of 25 mg/kg PO q 12 h for 7 days was well tolerated and eliminated cyst shedding within 7–10 days of treatment.[60] Results of another study in cats about the use of fenbendazole were less convincing.[61] An increased rate of resistance of *Giardia* spp. to metronidazole and other antigiardial agents has been reported in human patients. However, no published data concerning drug resistance in canine or feline giardiasis are currently available. Dogs kept in group housing should be removed from their runs, shampooed, and rinsed with quaternary-ammonium-based disinfectants. The runs should be cleaned and disinfected before reuse. Quaternary-ammonium-containing disinfectants have shown an excellent efficacy for inactivating *Giardia* cysts in a short period of time.

Vaccines against *Giardia* spp. are commercially available for dogs and cats in North America. The prophylactic efficacy of vaccination was shown in kittens and puppies, but routine vaccination is not recommended at this time.[62] The vaccine may be useful in kennels and catteries with recurring infections. In some studies, investigators have attempted to use the vaccine therapeutically in infected dogs and cats. However, the results were not convincing, particularly in cats.[63]

Cryptosporidium spp.

Cryptosporidium spp. are obligate intracellular parasites that infect enterocytes. The cycle of the parasite is complex and consists of asexual and sexual stages. Oocysts are produced during the sexual stage and enclose four sporozoites protected by a wall that is resistant to many environmental factors, but sensitive to desiccation and heat above 60 °C. Sporulated oocysts are passed with the feces and are infectious to appropriate hosts.[64] In humans, immunocompetent people develop a self-limiting infection that typically lasts for 4–7 days, characterized by voluminous and watery diarrhea, possibly accompanied by other GI signs. The parasites are usually restricted to the lower small bowel. However, in immunocompromised patients, infections may spread throughout the whole bowel and become chronic and/or life-threatening.

In a seroprevalence study conducted in cats from different regions of the USA, 8.3% cats were positive for *Cryptosporidium*. The lowest prevalence was in the mid-Atlantic states (1.3%)

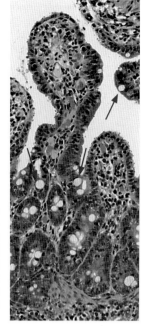

Figure 5.8:
Cryptosporidium parvum. This image shows small intestinal villi infected with *Cryptosporidium parvum.* The organisms can be seen on the immediate surface of the villi (see arrows). *Cryptosporidium* oocysts are difficult to see on direct fecal smears as they are translucent and very small. (H&E; image courtesy of Dr. Jody Gookin, North Carolina State University, Raleigh, NC.)

and the highest in the south-eastern region (14.7%).[65] Prevalence rates between 0% and 38.5% (median 5.4%) have been reported in different feline populations, while prevalence rates reported in dogs were 0–44.8% (median 7.1%).[66]

As is the case in humans, cryptosporidial infections may be associated with diarrhea in dogs and cats. In some instances, chronic or intermittent diarrhea, anorexia, and weight loss may occur. However, in many cases, clinical signs go unnoticed. Several diagnostic tests for *Cryptosporidium* spp. are available and have recently evaluated in kittens.[67,68]

The oocysts are small (approximately 4–6 mm in diameter; Figure 5.8) and difficult to see in fecal preparations. When only one fecal sample was examined, two of the three investigated commercial enzyme immunoassays were the most sensitive (ProSpecT *Cryptosporidium* microplate assay, Remel Inc, Lenexa, KS and Premier *Cryptosporidium* enzyme immunoassay, Meridian Diagnostics Inc, Cincinnati, OH). However, when two consecutive fecal samples were examined, a modified Ziehl-Neelsen acid-fast stain was as sensitive as the immunoassays.[67] In addition, a PCR-based test developed for the detection of *Cryptosporidium* spp. in cat feces has been shown to be more sensitive than the available immunoassays.[68]

In humans, most infections are water-borne, and many drinking-water-related outbreaks have been reported. However, most of the *Cryptosporidium* spp. are not strictly species-specific and zoonotic transmission involving pet dogs and cats may represent a serious risk to immunocompromised human patients.

5

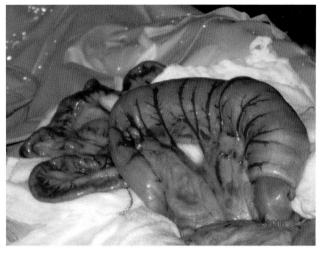

Figure 5.9:
Intestinal intussusception. Surgical image of a dog with a small intestinal intussusception following severe parvoviral infection. (Image courtesy of Dr. Bennito DeLaPuerta, Royal Veterinary College, London, UK.)

In humans, nitazoxanide (NTZ), a nitrothiazole benzamide, appears to be the treatment of choice. NTZ was used in laboratory cats naturally infected with *Cryptosporidium* at a dosage of 25 mg/kg PO q 12 h. The drug caused vomiting and foul-smelling dark diarrhea. However, *Cryptosporidium* shedding resolved immediately after the NTZ treatment was initiated.[69] Paromomycin (150 mg/kg PO q 12 to 24 h for 5 days in dogs and cats) has also been used in small animals. However, it has been reported to not consistently stop oocyst shedding, and was also associated with severe renal failure in cats.[70]

Coccidia

Coccidial infections are more likely to occur in puppies and kittens than in adult dogs and cats. The general prevalence of coccidiosis in dogs is reported to be between 3% and 38%, and is highest in stray dogs.[71] However, it is unclear if coccidia actually cause diarrhea under natural conditions in dogs, as most case reports describe concurrent viral or bacterial infections. *Coccidia* spp. found in dogs include *Isospora canis* and the *I. ohioensis* complex. In cats, between 3% to 36% of individuals are reported to excrete *I. rivolta* or *I. felis* oocysts, with the highest prevalence among stray cats. Coccidiosis is not thought to be a common clinical problem in cats. Also, cats develop immunity after infection with coccidia.

The diagnostic test of choice for coccidia in dogs and cats is fecal flotation with Sheather's sugar solution. In coprophagic dogs, special attention must be paid to the possible presence of coccidia oocysts from other animals.

Treatment consists of the administration of sulfonamides such as sulfadimethoxine (50 mg/kg PO q 24 h for 10–14 days) or a combination therapy of ormetoprim (11 mg/kg PO q 24 h) and sulfadimethoxine (55 mg/kg PO q 24 h), or trimethoprim-sulfamethoxazole (30–60 mg/kg PO q 24 h for 6 days).[72] The anticoccidial drugs toltrazuril (15 mg/kg PO q 12 h for 3 days) and diclazuril (25 mg/kg PO, single dose) are also effective in the treatment of *Isospora* spp. in kittens and puppies, although some animals may need to be re-treated 10 days after the initial therapy.[73]

5.3.2.4.3 Other protozoal parasites

Cats are the definitive host for several other enteric protozoa such as *Toxoplasma gondii*, *Hammondia* spp., *Besnoitia* spp., or *Sarcocystis* spp. These protozoa are of low significance in feline medicine, but may be clinically relevant in intermediate hosts.

5.3.3   Dietary indiscretion (garbage can intoxication)

Acute vomiting and diarrhea after ingestion of garbage occurs commonly in dogs. It has been speculated that bacterial toxins are responsible for the clinical signs. Treatment is mainly supportive. A more in-depth discussion of adverse reactions to food can be found in chapter 9.1.

5.3.4   Intestinal obstruction – intestinal foreign bodies, intussusception, and intestinal torsion

Small intestinal obstruction most often results from foreign bodies such as peach pits, corn cobs, toys, and fish hooks in dogs and linear foreign bodies in cats. Other differential diagnoses for intestinal obstruction include intussusception, intestinal torsion, and neoplasia. The clinical findings of intestinal obstruction are related to the site, severity, and cause of the obstruction. Complete upper intestinal obstruction results in severe acute vomiting, which is associated with fluid loss and dehydration and, if left untreated, can lead to circulatory shock. Partial obstructions can be more challenging to diagnose, as they often present with an insidious onset of vomiting and intermittent chronic diarrhea. The history is sometimes helpful in raising the suspicion of a foreign body. Intussusceptions are commonly seen in young animals, particularly in conjunction with severe acute enteritis, such as parvovirus infection (Figure 5.9) or ascarid infestation, but can also be seen in cases of chronic diarrhea, such as IBD.[74] Intestinal neoplasia (see 5.3.10 and 9.3) is more commonly seen in middle-aged to older animals, but single lymphoma lesions can also be seen in young patients, particularly in cats. Intestinal torsion (volvulus) is a rare disorder in dogs, which involves intestinal rotation at the root of the mesentery, with complete occlusion of the cranial mesenteric artery. This results in bowel necrosis, release of toxins and life-threatening shock. Most cases have been reported in adult, medium to large breed male dogs.[75]

A thorough physical examination is important in all cases, which includes a meticulous examination of the base of the tongue for linear foreign bodies, especially in cats. Abdominal palpation sometimes reveals the site of intestinal obstruction. Immediate radiographic and/or ultrasonographic examination is also indicated (see 1.3). Complete intestinal obstruction and intestinal volvulus are readily visible on abdominal radiographs by the presence of diffusely distended bowel loops. It is important to identify signs of a possible bowel perforation, such as decreased serosal detail and free abdominal gas. A minimum blood chemistry database to characterize the fluid and electrolyte losses should be performed and fluid therapy should be initiated before exploratory laparotomy.

Treatment of intestinal obstruction involves removal or resection of the cause of the obstruction. Antibiotics should be given to patients with signs of intestinal perforation or those at risk of intestinal bacterial translocation. Antibiotic protocols vary, but one example is the combination of ampicillin and metronidazole. The prognosis depends on the cause of obstruction and the severity of complications associated with it. For intestinal volvulus, the prognosis is usually grave unless immediate exploratory laparotomy is performed.[75]

5.3.5 Hemorrhagic gastroenteritis (HGE)

Hemorrhagic gastroenteritis is an acute GI disease of unknown etiology in dogs. Anaphylactic reactions to enteric toxins have been suspected as being involved in the pathogenesis. The clinical signs are mostly seen in small breed dogs and can occur peracutely. Early signs are vomiting, depression, hematemesis, bloody diarrhea, and extreme hemoconcentration (i.e., PCV of up to 70–80%). Treatment consists of aggressive fluid therapy to prevent further dehydration and additional supportive care as indicated by the clinical status of the patient. Complications, including leukopenia, sepsis, and coagulation abnormalities can also be seen, but the prognosis is generally good if patients are supported aggressively.

5.3.6 Short bowel syndrome

Short bowel syndrome occurs when more than two thirds of the entire length of the small intestine have been surgically removed. The clinical hallmark is intractable small intestinal diarrhea resulting from severe malabsorption due to the massively reduced mucosal surface area. If the ileum had to be resected as well, malabsorption of bile salts and cobalamin can occur.[76] If the ileocolic valve has been resected, antibiotic treatment is necessary because of bacterial overgrowth of the small intestine. Tylosin (25 mg/kg PO q 12 h) or metronidazole (10 mg/kg PO q 12 h) can be used in these cases. Fluid and electrolyte replacement is important in the immediate post-operative period, but oral feeding should be continued as well to prevent starvation of the remaining mucosal epithelial cells. A fat-restricted oligomeric liquid diet should be fed at first, with gradual transition to more solid food. If the ileum has been removed, the patient should also receive cobalamin supplementation as cobalamin is exclusively absorbed in this region of the bowel. The prognosis depends on the patient's response to therapy. Some animals will have life-long intractable diarrhea.

5.3.7 Motility disorders

Intestinal motility disorders are not very well characterized as a primary cause of small intestinal disease in dogs and cats. However, secondary alterations in the motility of the small intestine occur in many diseases. Most often, hypomotility of the intestines and ileus are seen after abdominal surgery, or during ischemic or inflammatory conditions, such as peritonitis, pancreatitis, or parvovirus infection. In malabsorptive disorders, undigested and osmotically active particles in the intestinal lumen can decrease the transit time. Dietary management should be attempted at first. Small amounts of a low-fat, low-protein diet given at frequent intervals can help reduce the symptoms of delayed gastric emptying. Medical therapy can be attempted if dietary management alone is unsuccessful (Table 5.6). Metoclopramide or domperidone act peripherally at

Table 5.6: Prokinetic agents. This table shows a list of commonly used gastric and small intestinal prokinetic agents.[79]

Compound	Commonly used dose
Cisapride	0.1–0.5 mg/kg PO q 8–12 h
Erythromycin	0.5–1 mg/kg PO q 8 h
Metoclopramide	0.2–0.5 mg/kg PO or SC q 8 h 0.01–0.02 mg/kg/h as a CRI
Nizatidine	2.5–5 mg/kg PO q 24 h
Ranitidine	1–2 mg/kg PO or IV q 12 h

5

dopaminergic receptors and promote antral contractions. These compounds are contraindicated if an intestinal obstruction is suspected. Cisapride has also been successfully used for the treatment of delayed gastric emptying. While this drug has been withdrawn from the market, it can still be acquired through compounding pharmacies and can be used at dosages of 0.1–0.5 mg/kg PO q 8 h. Erythromycin at lower dosages than those recommended for antibacterial treatment regimens (1 mg/kg PO q 12 h) can also stimulate gastric emptying by inducing an interdigestive motor pattern. This causes larger particles to pass into the duodenum faster than with normal antral contractions and may lead to a worsening of the symptoms if the motility disorder is primarily located in the small intestine as erythromycin also stimulates small intestinal motility. Newer prokinetic agents are ranitidine and nizatidine, which act as acetylcholinesterase inhibitors in the stomach and the small intestine. Hypothyroidism in dogs and hyperthyroidism in cats may also alter intestinal transit time and cause diarrhea.

Feline dysautonomia is caused by a degeneration of autonomic ganglia and can cause constipation and decreased anal tone among other signs of sympathetic and parasympathetic dysfunction, such as dysuria, mydriasis, vomiting, regurgitation, and diarrhea.[77] Treatment is largely supportive and the overall prognosis is poor.

⌦ Key Facts

■ Important viral infections that can cause primary intestinal disease are canine parvovirosis and canine distemper in unvaccinated puppies. Supportive care, including antibiotic therapy for the prevention of septicemia, is the treatment of choice.

■ Helminthic parasite infections are common in both dogs and cats. Ancylostoma and ascarids can cause significant disease in small animals.

■ Many enteropathogenic bacteria can be isolated from the feces of healthy dogs and cats and when such pathogens are found in the feces in animals with diarrhea, it is often difficult to distinguish primary infections from opportunistic secondary infections.

■ Many bacterial infections in the gut are self-limiting and the indiscriminate use of antibiotics is not advised.

■ Although dogs and cats do not appear to play a central role in the epidemiology of gastrointestinal infections in humans, caution is warranted when pets, shedding potential bacterial or protozoal pathogens, have close contact with immune-compromised individuals.

■ The diagnosis of gastrointestinal protozoal infections may be challenging and requires the examination of several fecal samples and/or using immunoassays or PCR-based assays on fecal material.

References

1. Parrish CR, Have P, Foreyt WJ et al. The global spread and replacement of canine parvovirus strains. *J Gen Virol* 1988; 69: 1111–1116.
2. Parrish CR, O'Connell PH, Evermann JF et al. Natural variation of canine parvovirus. *Science* 1985; 230: 1046–1048.
3. Glickman LT, Domanski LM, Patronek GJ et al. Breed-related risk factors for canine parvovirus enteritis. *J Am Vet Med Assoc* 1985; 187: 589–594.
4. Otto CM, Drobatz KJ, Soter C. Endotoxemia and tumor necrosis factor activity in dogs with naturally occurring parvoviral enteritis. *J Vet Intern Med* 1997; 11: 65–70.
5. Turk J, Miller M, Brown T et al. Coliform septicemia and pulmonary disease associated with canine parvoviral enteritis: 88 cases (1987–1988). *J Am Vet Med Assoc* 1990; 196: 771–773.
6. Pollock RV, Coyne MJ. Canine parvovirus. *Vet Clin North Am Small Anim Pract.* 1993; 23: 555–568.
7. Waldvogel AS, Hassam S, Weilenmann R et al. Retrospective study of myocardial canine parvovirus infection by in situ hybridization. *Zentralbl Veterinarmed B.* 1991; 38: 353–357.
8. Hoskins JD Gourley KR, Taylor HW. Evaluation of a fecal antigen ELISA test for the diagnosis of canine parvovirus. *J Vet Int Med* 1996; 10: 159–164.
9. Senda M, Parrish CR, Harasawa R et al. Detection by PCR of wild-type canine parvovirus, which contaminates dog vaccines. *J Clin Microbiol,* 1995; 33: 110–113.
10. Möhr AJ, Leisewitz AL, Jacobson LS et al. Effect of early enteral nutrition on intestinal permeability, intestinal protein loss, and outcome in dogs with severe parvoviral enteritis. *J Vet Intern Med* 2003; 17: 791–798.
11. Otto CM, Jackson CB, Rogell EJ et al. Recombinant bactericidal/permeability-increasing protein (rBPI21) for treatment of parvovirus enteritis: a randomized, double-blinded, placebo-controlled trial. *J Vet Intern Med* 2001; 15: 355–360.
12. Rewerts JM, McCaw DL, Cohn LA et al. Recombinant human granulocyte colony-stimulating factor for treatment of puppies with neutropenia secondary to canine parvovirus infection. *J Am Vet Med Assoc* 1998; 213: 991–992.
13. De Mari K, Maynard L, Eun HM et al. Treatment of canine parvoviral enteritis with interferon-omega in a placebo-controlled field trial. *Vet Rec* 2003; 152: 105–108.
14. O'Brien SE, Roth JA, Hill BA. Response of pups to modified live canine parvovirus component in a combination vaccine. *J Am Vet Med Assoc* 1986; 188: 699–701.
15. Greene CE, Appel MJ. Canine Distemper. In: Greene CE (ed.), *Infectious diseases of the dog and cat, 3rd ed.* St. Louis, MO, Saunders Elsevier, 2006; 25–31.
16. Rottier PJ, Nakamura K, Schellen P et al. Acquisition of macrophage tropism during the pathogenesis of feline infectious peritonitis is determined by mutations in the feline coronavirus spike protein. *J Virol* 2005; 79: 14122–14130.

17. Addie DD, Jarrett O. A study of naturally occurring feline coronavirus infections in kittens. *Vet Rec* 1992; 130: 133–137.
18. Inada S, Mochizuki M, Izumo S et al. Study of hereditary cerebellar degeneration in cats. *Am J Vet Res* 1996; 57 (3): 296–301.
19. Esfandiari J, Klingeborn B. A comparative study of a new rapid and one-step test for the detection of parvovirus in faeces from dogs, cats and mink. *J Vet Med B Infect Dis Vet Public Health* 2000; 47: 145–153.
20. Reinacher M. Diseases associated with spontaneous feline leukemia virus (FeLV) infection in cats. *Vet Immunol Immunopathol* 1989; 21: 85–95.
21. Burnens AP, Angeloz-Wick B, Nicolet J. Comparison of *Campylobacter* carriage rates in diarrheic and healthy pet animals. *Zentralbl Veterinarmed B* 1992; 39: 175–180.
22. Murinda SE, Nguyen NT, Nam HM et al. Detection of sorbitol-negative and sorbitol-positive Shiga toxin-producing *Escherichia coli*, *Listeria monocytogenes*, *Campylobacter jejuni*, and *Salmonella* spp. in dairy farm environmental samples. *Foodborne Pathog Dis* 2004; 1:97–104.
23. Hald B, Madsen M. Healthy puppies and kittens as carriers of *Campylobacter* spp., with special reference to *Campylobacter upsaliensis*. *J Clin Microbiol*, 1997; 35: 3351–3352.
24. Spain CV, Scarlett JM, Wade SE et al. Prevalence of enteric zoonotic agents in cats less than 1 year old in central New York State. *J Vet Intern Med* 2001; 15: 33–38.
25. Sandberg M, Bergsjo B, Hofshagen M et al. Risk factors for *Campylobacter* infection in Norwegian cats and dogs. *Prev Vet Med* 2002; 55: 241–253.
26. Hackett T, Lappin MR. Prevalence of enteric pathogens in dogs of north-central Colorado. *J Am Anim Hosp Assoc* 2003; 39: 52–56.
27. Wieland B, Regula G, Danuser J et al. *Campylobacter* spp. in dogs and cats in Switzerland: risk factor analysis and molecular characterization with AFLP. *J Vet Med B* 2005; 52: 183–189.
28. Hald B, Pedersen K, Waino M et al. Longitudinal study of the excretion patterns of thermophilic *Campylobacter* spp. in young pet dogs in Denmark. *J Clin Microbiol* 2004; 42: 2003–2012.
29. Kapperud G, Skjerve B, Bean NH et al. Risk factors for sporadic *Campylobacter* infections: results of a case-control study in southeastern Norway. *J Clin Microbiol* 1992; 30: 3117–3121.
30. Weese JS, Staempfli HR, Prescott JF et al. The roles of *Clostridium difficile* and enterotoxigenic *Clostridium perfringens* in diarrhea in dogs. *J Vet Intern Med* 2001; 15: 374–378.
31. Marks SL, Kather EJ, Kass PH et al. Genotypic and phenotypic characterization of *Clostridium perfringens* and *Clostridium difficile* in diarrheic and healthy dogs. *J Vet Intern Med* 2002; 16: 533–540.
32. Weese JS, Armstrong J. Outbreak of *Clostridium difficile*-associated disease in a small animal veterinary teaching hospital. *J Vet Intern Med* 2003; 17: 813–816.
33. Weese JS, Staempfli HR, Prescott JF. Isolation of environmental *Clostridium difficile* from a veterinary teaching hospital. *J Vet Diagn Invest* 2000; 12: 449–452.
34. Turk J, Maddox C, Fales W et al. Examination for heat-labile, heat-stable, and *Shiga*-like toxins and for the eaeA gene in *Escherichia coli* isolates obtained from dogs dying with diarrhea: 122 cases (1992–1996). *J Am Vet Med Assoc* 1998; 212: 1735–1736.
35. Beutin L. *Escherichia coli* as a pathogen in dogs and cats. *Vet Res* 1999; 30: 285–298.
36. Clark C, Cunningham J, Ahmed R et al. Characterization of *Salmonella* associated with pig ear dog treats in Canada. *J Clin Microbiol* 2001; 39: 3962–3968.
37. Van Immerseel F, Pasmans F, De Buck J et al. Cats as a risk for transmission of antimicrobial drug-resistant *Salmonella*. *Emerg Infect Dis* 2004; 10: 2169–2174.
38. Cherry B, Burns A, Johnson GS et al. *Salmonella typhimurium* outbreak associated with veterinary clinic. *Emerg Infect Dis* 2004; 10: 2249–2251.
39. Tauni MA, Osterlund A. Outbreak of *Salmonella typhimurium* in cats and humans associated with infection in wild birds. *J Small Anim Pract* 2000; 41: 339–341.
40. Stiver SL, Frazier KS, Mauel MJ et al. Septicemic salmonellosis in two cats fed a raw-meat diet. *J Am Anim Hosp Asso*, 2003; 39: 538–542.
41. Foley JE, Orgad U, Hirsh DC et al. Outbreak of fatal salmonellosis in cats following use of a high-titer modified-live panleukopenia virus vaccine. *J Am Vet Med Assoc* 1999; 214: 67–4.
42. Wall PG, Davis S, Threlfall EJ et al. Chronic carriage of multidrug resistant *Salmonella typhimurium* in a cat. *J Small Anim Pract* 1995; 36: 279–281.
43. De Cock HE, Marks SL, Stacy BA et al. Ileocolitis associated with *Anaerobiospirillum* in cats. *J Clin Microbiol* 2004; 42: 2752–2758.
44. Greene CE. Histoplasmosis. In: Greene CE (ed.), *Infectious diseases of the dog and cat, 3rd ed.* St. Louis, MO, Saunders Elsevier, 2006; 577–583.
45. Grooters AM, Foil CS. Miscellaneous fungal infections. In: Greene CE (ed.), *Infectious diseases of the dog and cat, 3rd ed.* St. Louis, MO, Saunders Elsevier, 2006; 637–649.
46. Grooters AM. Pythiosis, lagenidiosis, and zygomycosis in small animals. *Vet Clin North Am Small Anim Pract* 2003; 33: 695–720.
47. Grooters AM, Taboada J. Update on antifungal therapy. *Vet Clin North Am Small Anim Pract* 2003; 33: 749–758.
48. Hasslinger MA. [Research on the cat stomach worm, *Ollulanus tricuspis*]. *Tierarztl Prax* 1985; 13: 205–215.
49. Stoye M. [Biology, pathogenicity, diagnosis and control of *Ancylostoma caninum*]. *Dtsch Tierarztl Wochenschr* 1992; 99: 315–321.
50. Thompson RC. The zoonotic significance and molecular epidemiology of *Giardia* and giardiasis. *Vet Parasitol* 2004; 126: 15–35.
51. Marshall MM, Naumovitz D, Ortega Y et al. Waterborne protozoan pathogens. *Clin Microbiol Rev* 1997; 10: 67–85.
52. Zimmer JF, Burrington DB. Comparison of four techniques of fecal examination for detecting canine giardiasis. *J Am Anim Hosp Assoc* 1986; 22:161–167.
53. Dryden MW, Pane PA, Smith V. Accurate diagnosis of *Giardia* spp. and proper fecal examination procedures. *Vet Ther* 2006; 7: 4–14.
54. Jacobs SR, Forrester CP, Yang J. A survey of the prevalence of *Giardia* in dogs presented to Canadian veterinary practices. *Can Vet J* 2001; 42: 45–46.
55. Barutzki D, Schaper R. Endoparasites in dogs and cats in Germany 1999–2002. *Parasitol Res* 2003; 90 Suppl 3: S148–S150.
56. Papini R, Gorini G, Spaziani A et al. Survey on giardiasis in shelter dog populations. *Vet Parasitol* 2005; 128: 333–339.
57. Barr SC, Bowman DD, Heller RL. Efficacy of fenbendazole against giardiasis in dogs. *Am J Vet Res* 1994; 55: 988–990.
58. Barr SC, Bowman DD, Heller RL et al. Efficacy of albendazole against giardiasis in dogs. *Am J Vet Res* 1993; 54: 926–928.
59. Stokol T, Randolph JF, Nachbar S et al. Development of bone marrow toxicosis after albendazole administration in a dog and cat. *J Am Vet Med Assoc* 1997; 210: 1753–1756.
60. Scorza AV, Lappin MR. Metronidazole for the treatment of feline giardiasis. *J Feline Med Surg* 2004; 6: 157–160.
61. Keith CL, Radecki SV, Lappin MR. Evaluation of fenbendazole for treatment of Giardia infection in cats concurrently infected with *Cryptosporidium parvum*. *Am J Vet Res* 2003; 64: 1027–1029.
62. Olson ME, Morck DW, Ceri H. Preliminary data on the efficacy of a *Giardia* vaccine in puppies. *Can Vet J* 1997; 38: 777–779.
63. Olson ME, Morck DW, Ceri H. The efficacy of a *Giardia lamblia* vaccine in kittens. *Can J Vet Res* 1996; 60: 249–256.

5

64. Chappell CL, Okhuysen PC. Cryptosporidiosis. *Curr Opin Infect Dis* 2002; 15: 523–527.

65. McReynolds CA, Lappin MR, Ungar B et al. Regional seroprevalence of *Cryptosporidium parvum*-specific IgG of cats in the United States. *Vet Parasitol* 1999; 80: 187–195.

66. Lindsay DJ, Zajac AM. Cryptosporidium infections in cats and dogs. *Compend Cont Educ Pract Vet* 2004; 864–874.

67. Marks SL, Hanson TE, Melli AC. Comparison of direct immunofluorescence, modified acid-fast staining, and enzyme immunoassay techniques for detection of *Cryptosporidium* spp. in naturally exposed kittens. *J Am Vet Med Assoc* 2004; 225: 1549–1553.

68. Scorza AV, Brewer MM, Lappin MR. Polymerase chain reaction for the detection of *Cryptosporidium spp.* in cat feces. *J Parasitol* 2003; 89: 423–426.

69. Gookin JL, Levy MG, Law JM et al. Experimental infection of cats with *Tritrichomonas foetus*. *Am J Vet Res* 2001; 62: 1690–1697.

70. Gookin JL, Riviere JE, Gilger BC et al. Acute renal failure in four cats treated with paromomycin. *J Am Vet Med Assoc* 1999; 215: 1821–1823.

71. Lindsay DS, Dubey JP, Blagburn BL. Biology of *Isospora* spp. from humans, nonhuman primates, and domestic animals. *Clin Microbiol Rev* 1997; 10: 19–34.

72. Kirkpatrick CE, Dubey JP. Enteric coccidial infections. *Isospora, Sarcocystis, Cryptosporidium, Besnoitia,* and *Hammondia*. *Vet Clin North Am Small Anim Pract* 1987; 17: 1405–1420.

73. Lloyd S, Smith J. Activity of toltrazuril and diclazuril against *Isospora* species in kittens and puppies. *Vet Rec* 2001; 148: 509–511.

74. Patsikas MN, Jakovljevic S, Moustardas N et al. Ultrasonographic signs of intestinal intussusception associated with acute enteritis or gastroenteritis in 19 young dogs. *J Am Anim Hosp Assoc* 2003; 39: 57–66.

75. Junius G, Appledoorn AM, Schrauwen M. Mesenteric volvulus in the dog: a retrospective study of 12 cases. *J Small Anim Pract* 2004; 45: 104–107.

76. Yanoff SR, Willard MD. Short bowel syndrome in dogs and cats. *Semin Vet Med Surg Small Anim* 1989; 4: 226–231.

77. Cave TA, Knottenbelt C, Mellor DJ et al. Outbreak of dysautonomia (Key-Gaskell syndrome) in a closed colony of pet cats. *Vet Rec* 2003; 153: 387–392.

78. DiBartola S. *Fluid Therapy in Small Animal Practice*. St. Louis, MO, Saunders Elsevier, 2000; 271–277.

79. Washabau RJ. Gastrointestinal motility disorders and gastrointestinal prokinetic therapy. *Vet Clin North Am Small Anim Pract* 2003; 33: 1007–1028.

5.3.8 Alterations in the small intestinal microflora (Small intestinal bacterial overgrowth)

JAN S. SUCHODOLSKI

Introduction

In humans, small intestinal bacterial overgrowth (SIBO) is defined as a clinical syndrome caused by an increased number of microorganisms in the small intestine.[1] In dogs, the existence of SIBO, as defined in humans, is currently under debate. In an early study by Batt et al.,[2] bacterial counts in dogs with diarrhea were significantly higher compared to healthy dogs and the authors of this study defined SIBO as $>10^4$ anaerobic or $>10^5$ total bacterial colony-forming units (cfu)/mL of fasting duodenal juice. However, these criteria for dogs are now controversial, because substantially higher bacterial counts have been found in duodenal juice of healthy dogs since the report by Batt et al.[2] Recent studies performed in dogs with chronic enteropathies found no correlation between the number of bacterial colonies in the duodenum and clinical signs. Some dogs with suspected SIBO had counts that were substantially lower than 10^5 cfu/ml.[3] Since this condition usually responds to antibiotic treatment, some authors propose the term "antibiotic-responsive diarrhea" (ARD) rather than SIBO.[4] Recently, the term "tylosin-responsive diarrhea" (TRD) was proposed for a subgroup of dogs with antibiotic-responsive diarrhea that is specifically responsive to tylosin.[5] However, at this time, it is unclear if these terms (SIBO, ARD, and TRD) can be used synonymously as some dogs diagnosed with SIBO based on findings traditionally associated with SIBO do not respond to antibiotic therapy and some dogs that respond to antibiotic therapy do not have findings that have traditionally been associated with SIBO. Currently, there is no consensus on the definition and diagnostic criteria for SIBO. While it is generally accepted that a subgroup of dogs with small intestinal disease shows alterations of the small intestinal microflora, it is controversial if this is truly caused by an abnormal increase in bacterial numbers. In humans, there are several known risk factors for SIBO (Table 5.7). One of these risk factors is a decreased intestinal motility, which may result in an increase in bacterial numbers.[1] The same mechanisms implicated in humans could potentially also lead to bacterial overgrowth in dogs. It is important to distinguish SIBO/ARD/TRD from GI disorders caused by potentially pathogenic bacteria such as *Salmonella* spp., *Campylobacter* spp., and enterotoxigenic *Clostridium perfringens* and *difficile*. SIBO has not been reported in cats as healthy cats appear to have much higher duodenal bacterial counts compared to healthy dogs, and these numbers do not differ from cats with enteropathies.[6]

The small intestinal microflora

Based on bacterial culture results, bacterial counts in the small intestine range from 0 to $>10^9$ cfu/mL for aerobic bacteria and from 0 to $>10^8$ cfu/mL for anaerobic bacteria in clinically healthy dogs, with a progressive increase in total bacterial numbers and microbial diversity from the duodenum to the ileum.[7] Today, it is recognized that the majority of bacterial species are not amenable to routine bacterial culture techniques.[8] Using molecular biology methods that are based on identification of 16S ribosomal DNA, many previously uncharacterized bacterial species from canine small intestinal samples have now been identified.[8] Additionally, the use of molecular profiling of the GI flora of dogs has recently demonstrated that the small intestinal microflora in dogs is highly variable and unique to each individual dog.[9]

The resident intestinal microflora offers nutritional benefits to the host by the production of short-chain fatty acids (e.g., butyrate, propionate, and acetate), which stimulate mucosal growth and epithelial cell proliferation. Lactate, produced by microbial fermentation, also serves as an energy source for the host. In addition, the normal intestinal microflora plays a major role in the protection of the host from invasion by harmful bacteria through the exclusion of potentially pathogenic organisms. The implicated defense mechanisms against these harmful bacterial species include competition for oxygen and nutrient substrates, competition for mucosal adhesion sites, creation of a physiologically restrictive environment for non-resident bacterial species (e.g., production of substances that are toxic to other bacteria, changes in pH and redox potential, or hydrogen sulfide production), and secretion of antimicrobial substances (e.g., bacteriocins).[10]

Pathophysiology

There are several physiological mechanisms that regulate bacterial colonization in the small intestine, including secretion of gastric acid and antibacterial factors (i.e., pancreatic and biliary secretions), and most importantly, intestinal motility. Failure of one or more of these control mechanisms may lead to alterations in the small intestinal microflora resulting in clinical signs associated with SIBO.

Based on the underlying mechanism, SIBO can be divided into primary or idiopathic SIBO and secondary SIBO. Secondary SIBO occurs more frequently than primary SIBO. Table 5.7 summarizes the causes for secondary SIBO.

Most, but not all, bacteria ingested orally are destroyed by gastric acid. Human patients with atrophic gastritis or those who undergo acid suppressant therapy (e.g., therapy with a proton pump inhibitor) show an increase in small intestinal bacterial counts.[11] The pancreatic juice also contains antimicrobial substances that suppress excessive bacterial growth in the proximal small intestine. Dogs with experimentally induced exocrine pancreatic insufficiency (EPI) show significantly increased bacterial counts in the small intestine.[12] The ileocolic valve serves as a natural barrier between the small and large intestine in dogs.[13] This barrier, together with intestinal motility, is believed to prevent retrograde migration of bacteria from the highly populated large intestine into the less populated small intestine. Also, the formation of blind and stagnant small

Table 5.7: Conditions associated with secondary SIBO

Small intestinal stasis
- Anatomic abnormalities
  - Congenital blind loops
  - Small bowel diverticula, strictures, or adhesions
  - Surgical resection of the ileo-colic valve
  - Surgical blind loops (end-to-side anastomosis)
- Partial obstructions of the small intestine
  - Neoplasia
  - Foreign bodies
  - Chronic intussusception
- Motility disorders
  - Hypothyroidism
  - Diabetic autonomic neuropathy
  - Scleroderma
  - Abnormal migrating motor complexes

Decreased gastric acid output
- Atrophic gastritis
- Administration of acid-suppressing drugs (H_2-blockers, omeprazole)

Exocrine pancreatic insufficiency
- Decreased output of pancreatic antimicrobial factors

Miscellaneous
- Decreased mucosal immunity

intestinal loops are a common site of bacterial overgrowth in humans.[14]

There are several mechanisms that may lead to GI disease due to an alteration of the small intestinal microflora. Many bacterial species are able to deconjugate bile acids, which in severe cases may lead to fat malabsorption. Also, some bacterial species (i.e., *Clostridium hiranonis* and *C. scindens*) have $7\alpha/\beta$-dehydroxylating activity, changing primary into secondary bile acids, which can be associated with increased toxic effects to epithelial cells.[15] Bacterial toxins and metabolites can damage enterocytes. Bacterial metabolites may also cause destruction of the intestinal brush border and damage carrier proteins, resulting in malabsorption. Competition between bacteria and host cells for nutrients (e.g., cobalamin) may lead to malnutrition. Increased fat metabolism within the GI tract may lead to the production of toxic short-chain fatty acids, which can act as potent pro-inflammatory agents. Hydroxylation of fatty acids may further contribute to diarrhea. SIBO can lead to sufficient mucosal damage to cause PLE.

While some breeds (i.e., German Shepherd dogs and Chinese Shar Peis) have anecdotally been reported to be at an increased risk for developing SIBO, no genetic basis has yet been identified. Also, IgA deficiency, which was commonly suspected to be associated with SIBO in German Shepherd dogs, has not been conclusively confirmed. A genetic susceptibility for a dysregulation in the cell-mediated immune response to a normal luminal microflora is suspected to occur in human beings with idiopathic SIBO and a similar mechanism may lead to chronic enteropathies in dogs.

Clinical signs

The clinical signs of an abnormal intestinal microflora may include chronic intermittent small and/or large bowel diarrhea. Affected dogs are usually active, but show a variable appetite ranging from poor to excessive (i.e., polyphagia). Weight loss or poor growth is frequently observed. Owners often report borborygmus and/or flatulence. Mild to moderate steatorrhea may be observed in some cases due to chronic fat malabsorption. Occasionally, dogs may show clinical signs related to the underlying cause of SIBO, such as vomiting secondary to chronic partial obstruction due to an intestinal tumor.

Diagnosis

A definitive diagnosis of SIBO is difficult to arrive at. A tentative diagnosis can be established based on clinical signs and altered serum cobalamin and/or folate concentrations, and by response to an antibiotic therapeutic trial. It must be noted that other conditions, such as undetected intestinal pathogens, may respond to antibiotic therapy, and a positive response to therapy does not necessarily confirm the presence of SIBO.

Other differential diagnoses, such as maldigestion due to EPI and causes for malabsorption such as IBD, intestinal lymphoma, lymphangiectasia, or food intolerance should be ruled out. It is also important to evaluate the patient for intestinal parasites such as *Giardia* spp. and known bacterial pathogens (i.e., enterotoxigenic *Clostridium* spp., *Campylobacter* spp., *Salmonella* spp., or enterotoxigenic *E. coli*).

The histopathology of the small intestinal mucosa is typically unremarkable as SIBO is usually not associated with morphological changes of the small intestinal mucosa.[16] Occasionally, villous blunting or shortening may be observed.[17] Diagnostic imaging may reveal causes of secondary SIBO such as anatomical abnormalities. Findings on routine CBC, blood chemistry, and urinalysis are unrewarding in most patients. The measurement of serum cobalamin and folate can be useful for the diagnosis of SIBO.

Serum cobalamin and folate concentrations

The assessment of serum cobalamin and folate concentrations is currently the most useful aid for the diagnosis of SIBO. Serum cobalamin may be decreased and serum folate may be increased in dogs with this condition. If both serum vitamin

concentrations are altered, this is considered highly suggestive of SIBO; however, both have a rather poor sensitivity and specificity for the diagnosis of SIBO.[4] The reported sensitivity of serum cobalamin concentration for a diagnosis of SIBO ranges from 25% to 55% and from 50% to 66% for serum folate concentration.[4]

Aberrations in the small intestinal microflora may lead to an increased competition for cobalamin, resulting in decreased absorption of this vitamin. *Bacteroides* spp. are the principle organisms involved in the competition for cobalamin since they can utilize cobalamin-intrinsic factor complexes, while other bacteria can only bind free cobalamin, which is present in lower concentrations in the intestinal lumen.[16]

Bacteria present in the distal small intestine and large intestine produce large quantities of folic acid. However, as folate carriers responsible for folate uptake are located exclusively in the proximal small intestine, folate produced in distal sections of the intestine will not be absorbed but will instead be excreted in the feces. If folate-producing bacteria migrate upwards into the proximal small intestine, folate of bacterial origin can be absorbed by the host resulting in increased serum folate concentrations.

However, cobalamin and folate uptake from the small intestine is highly complex and can be affected by several mechanisms (see 1.4.2.2). For example, a diet high in folate may lead to falsely increased serum folate concentrations, while inflammation of the ileum may damage cobalamin receptors and thus may lead to cobalamin malabsorption. Dogs with EPI have a decreased secretion of antibacterial substances with subsequent small intestinal bacterial overgrowth.[17,18] As a consequence, dogs with EPI often have increased serum folate concentrations. Thus, in dogs with an abnormal serum concentration of cobalamin and/or folate, serum trypsin-like immunoreactivity (TLI) should be evaluated to rule out EPI as a secondary cause of SIBO.

Recently, it has been demonstrated that administration of tylosin does not lead, as would be expected, to a decrease in serum folate and an increase in serum cobalamin concentrations.[19] Therefore, serum folate concentrations may not reflect therapeutic success and serum folate concentrations should always be evaluated together with the clinical picture.

Quantitative bacterial culture

Quantitative aerobic and anaerobic bacterial cultures have traditionally been considered the gold standard for the diagnosis of SIBO, but it is now recognized that there is no correlation of bacterial counts and disease status.[4] Also, each dog harbors a very unique small intestinal microflora, making the determination of a normal or abnormal microflora difficult.

Miscellaneous tests

Many other tests have been proposed for the evaluation of patients suspected of having SIBO. However, many of these tests, such as the measurement of serum unconjugated cholic acid concentration (SUCA), ^{13}C-xylose absorption test, ^{13}C-bile acid absorption test, urinary indican test, or the hydrogen breath test, are associated with a high degree of variation between healthy animals, making them unrewarding for the diagnosis of SIBO.[4]

Treatment

General guidelines

It should be noted that while the altered bacterial population in the GI tract of the patient is not optimal, the resident bacterial populations are stable and able to resist acute changes or insults, such as a short course of antibiotics or temporary changes in diet. While such interventions may be associated with a transient alteration in the intestinal flora and some degree of clinical improvement, the aberrant microflora is likely to repopulate after the withdrawal of short-term therapy.[10] Therefore, in most cases long-term therapy is required.[5]

The treatment of choice for SIBO is the administration of a broad-spectrum antibiotic that is effective against both aerobic and anaerobic bacteria. Tylosin, metronidazole, and oxytetracycline are the most commonly used antibiotics for the treatment of SIBO (Table 5.8). Some patients may require several days to weeks of therapy before responding. However, if no clinical response is observed within two weeks, a therapeutic regimen with another antibiotic should be considered. The initial treatment period should last for 6 weeks. Thereafter, antibiotic treatment should be reinstated when clinical signs recur.

Underlying factors predisposing dogs to secondary SIBO (Table 5.7) should be corrected if they can be identified. For example, in most dogs with EPI and clinical signs of SIBO, the microflora returns to normal within a few weeks after initiation of enzyme replacement therapy. However, some patients may require antibiotic therapy.

Tylosin

Tylosin is often proposed as the antibiotic of choice in patients with suspected derangements of the intestinal microflora.[5] Tylosin is a macrolide antibiotic, which inhibits bacterial protein synthesis by binding to the 50S ribosomal subunit. Tylosin has antibiotic activity predominantly against gram-positive bacteria (e.g., *Staphylococcus* spp., *Streptococcus* spp., and *Clostridium* spp.) and also against some *Mycoplasma* and *Chlamydia* spp.

Table 5.8: Antibiotic agents used for the treatment of ARD/SIBO

■ Tylosin	25 mg/kg PO q 12 h for 6 weeks
■ Oxytetracycline	20 mg/kg PO q 8–12 h for 6 weeks
■ Metronidazole	10–20 mg/kg PO q 8–12 h for 6 weeks

While tylosin also has an effect against some gram-negative bacteria (e.g., *Campylobacter* spp., *Helicobacter pylori, Hemophilus* spp., *Pasteurella* spp., and *Legionella* spp.), it has no effect against members of the *Enterobacteriaceae* group (e.g., *Escherichia coli* and *Salmonella* spp.). It is speculated that tylosin also may exhibit immunomodulatory effects, however, no mode of action has yet been identified.[5]

Tylosin is very well tolerated and considered safe for long-term use. Several dosages of tylosin have been reported in the literature, underlining its broad therapeutic safety. Tylosin can be purchased as a powder for use in poultry and can be mixed into the food. Due to its broad dynamic and safety range, the dosage can be roughly estimated. For small patients, however, compounding of the powder may be necessary. Most commonly used dosages range between 15–25 mg/kg PO q 12 h. However, recent data would suggest that tylosin is only bactericidal at higher dosages and the author recommends a dosage of 25 mg/kg PO q 12 h for routine use. The initial treatment period should last at least for 6 weeks, unless adding tylosin into the treatment protocol does not lead to any improvement, in which case tylosin can be discontinued after 2 weeks. Some patients may have a recurrence after treatment is discontinued. Such patients should be further evaluated for any underlying cause of SIBO, but if one cannot be identified, long-term therapy can be initiated. After improvement of clinical signs, a reduction in the frequency of administration or a reduction in dosage, to the lowest frequency and/or dosage necessary to control clinical signs, may be attempted.

Oxytetracycline

Oxytetracycline is an excellent antibiotic choice for the treatment of SIBO due to its unusual metabolism. Oxytetracycline (administered at a dosage of 20 mg/kg PO q 8–12 h) is secreted in the bile and undergoes enterohepatic circulation, reaching high penetration in the small intestine and bile. Oxytetracycline can have some side-effects, and should thus not be administered in very young or pregnant animals. Also, calcium in the diet chelates oxytetracycline, rendering it ineffective. Oxytetracycline should, therefore, not be administered with food. As for tylosin, oxytetracycline should initially be given for a period of 6 weeks if the antibiotic therapy leads to an improvement in the clinical signs. It should also be noted that the oral formulation of oxytetracycline has limited availability, currently only being available in some European countries.

5

5

Metronidazole

Because of its activity against anaerobic bacteria, metronidazole at a dosage of 10–20 mg/kg PO q 8–12 h, is a commonly used antibiotic for the treatment of SIBO. In addition to its antibiotic properties, it also has been proposed that metronidazole exhibits immunomodulatory functions with beneficial effects in the treatment of intestinal inflammation. Metronidazole has, however, potential side effects and long-term therapy, as often required in patients with SIBO, may not be optimal. *In vitro* studies have shown the mutagenic properties of metronidazole.[20] While no conclusive data about the mutagenic potential of metronidazole *in vivo* are available, given the fact that tylosin is a safe and effective alternative for long-term administration, it appears prudent that prolonged administration of metronidazole should only be attempted if tylosin has proven to be ineffective for controlling clinical signs.

Cobalamin supplementation

Dogs with SIBO may be cobalamin (Vitamin B12) deficient and parenteral supplementation of cobalamin (cyanocobalamin) is indicated. The typical dose in small dogs (5–15 kg) is 500 μg cobalamin SC per injection; in dogs > 15 kg, the typical dose is 500 to 1,200 μg cobalamin SC per injection depending on body size. Supplementation should be given for several weeks using the following dose regimen: one dose weekly for six weeks, one dose every other week for six weeks, and one more dose a month later. Serum cobalamin concentration should be re-evaluated a month after the last dose and if the serum cobalamin concentration is in the lower part of the reference range, supplementation should be continued.

Dietary management

Dietary management may be useful in some patients with SIBO. A highly digestible, fat restricted diet, containing a prebiotic can be offered to these patients. A recent study showed that feeding a diet containing fructo-oligosaccharides, as a prebiotic agent, had similar effects as did antibiotic therapy.[21] The use of a diet containing a prebiotic is aimed at promoting the growth of beneficial bacteria in the gut and limiting the growth of more harmful species. While the study compared two treatment groups that received either antibiotic therapy or dietary management, it seems prudent to combine antibiotic and dietary management in clinical patients. If combined antibiotic and dietary management leads to amelioration of the clinical signs, the antibiotic can be discontinued after 6 weeks. However, dietary management should be continued long-term.

Probiotics

Empirical administration of a probiotic compound (e.g., *Lactobacillus* spp. or *Bifidobacterium* spp.) may be considered as an ancillary treatment. However, it should be noted that no studies evaluating the clinical utility of probiotics in canine patients with SIBO have been published.

Prognosis

The prognosis for patients with secondary SIBO is excellent if the underlying cause can be effectively treated. However, it should be noted that an underlying cause can rarely be identified in dogs with SIBO. In dogs with primary SIBO that respond to treatment but show recurrent clinical signs after withdrawal of antibiotics, clinical signs can often be controlled with long-term administration of antibiotics.

🔑 Key Facts

- SIBO is a clinical syndrome that is difficult to definitively diagnose.
- Patients diagnosed with SIBO need to be evaluated for an underlying cause.
- Serum cobalamin may be decreased and serum folate may be increased in patients with SIBO. If both serum vitamin concentrations are altered, this is highly suggestive of SIBO.
- Empirical administration of a broad-spectrum antibiotic effective against both aerobic and anaerobic bacteria in combination with dietary management is the treatment of choice for SIBO.
- The treatment should be re-evaluated after approximately six weeks; many dogs will require repeated or long-term treatment to control clinical signs.

References

1. King CE, Toskes PP. Small intestine bacterial overgrowth. *Gastroenterol* 1979; 76: 1035–1055.
2. Batt RM, Needham JR, Carter MW. Bacterial overgrowth associated with a naturally occurring enteropathy in the German Shepherd dog. *Res Vet Sci* 1983; 35: 42–46.
3. Johnston KL. Small intestinal bacterial overgrowth. *Vet Clin North Am Small Anim Pract* 1999; 29: 523–550.
4. German AJ, Day MJ, Ruaux CG et al. Comparison of direct and indirect tests for small intestinal bacterial overgrowth and antibiotic-responsive diarrhea in dogs. *J Vet Intern Med* 2003; 17: 33–43.

5. Westermarck E, Skrzypczak T, Harmoinen J et al. Tylosin-responsive chronic diarrhea in dogs. *J Vet Intern Med* 2005; 19: 177–186.

6. Johnston KL, Swift NC, Forster-van Hijfte M et al. Comparison of the bacterial flora of the duodenum in healthy cats and cats with signs of gastrointestinal tract disease. *J Am Vet Med Assoc* 2001; 218: 48–51.

7. Benno Y, Nakao H, Uchida K et al. Impact of the advances in age on the gastrointestinal microflora of Beagle dogs. *J Vet Med Sci* 1992; 54: 703–706.

8. Suchodolski JS, Ruaux CG, Steiner JM et al. Molecular identification of intestinal bacteria in healthy dogs. *J Vet Intern Med* 2005; 19: 473 (abstract).

9. Suchodolski JS, Ruaux CG, Steiner JM et al. Assessment of the qualitative variation in bacterial microflora among compartments of the intestinal tract of dogs by use of a molecular fingerprinting technique. *Am J Vet Res* 2005; 66: 1556–1562.

10. Kanauchi O, Matsumoto Y, Matsumura M et al. The beneficial effects of microflora, especially obligate anaerobes, and their products on the colonic environment in inflammatory bowel disease. *Curr Pharm Des* 2005; 11: 1047–1053.

11. Camilo E, Zimmerman J, Mason JB et al. Folate synthesized by bacteria in the human upper small intestine is assimilated by the host. *Gastroenterology* 1996; 110: 991–998.

12. Simpson KW, Batt RM, Jones D et al. Effects of exocrine pancreatic insufficiency and replacement therapy on the bacterial flora of the duodenum in dogs. *Am J Vet Res* 1990; 51(2): 203–206.

13. Griffen WO, Jr., Richardson JD, Medley ES. Prevention of small bowel contamination by ileocecal valve. *South Med J* 1971; 64: 1056–1058.

14. Greenlee HB, Gelbart SM, DeOrio AJ et al. The influence of gastric surgery on the intestinal flora. *Am J Clin Nutr* 1977; 30: 1826–1833.

15. Kitahara M, Takamine F, Imamura T et al. *Clostridium hiranonis* sp. nov., a human intestinal bacterium with bile acid 7alpha-dehydroxylating activity. *Int J Syst Evol Microbiol* 2001; 51: 39–44.

16. Abrams GD. Microbial effects on mucosal structure and function. *Am J Clin Nutr* 1977; 30: 1880–1886.

17. Williams DA, Batt RM, McLean L. Bacterial overgrowth in the duodenum of dogs with exocrine pancreatic insufficiency. *J Am Vet Med Assoc* 1987; 191: 201–206.

18. Simpson KW, Morton DB, Sorensen SH et al. Biochemical changes in the jejunal mucosa of dogs with exocrine pancreatic insufficiency following pancreatic duct ligation. *Res Vet Sci* 1989; 47: 338–345.

19. Ruaux CG, Suchodolski JS, Berghoff N et al. Alterations in markers assessing the canine small intestinal microflora in response to altered housing and tylosin administration. *J Vet Intern Med* 2005; 19: 441 (abstract).

20. Mudry MD, Carballo M, Labal de V et al. Mutagenic bioassay of certain pharmacological drugs: III. metronidazole (MTZ). *Mutat Res* 1994; 305: 127–132.

21. Ruaux CG, Tetrick MA, Steiner JM et al. Fecal consistency and volume in dogs with suspected small intestinal bacterial overgrowth receiving broad spectrum antibiotic therapy or dietary fructo-oligosaccharide supplementation. *J Vet Intern Med* 2004; 18: 425 (abstract).

5.3.9   Protein-losing enteropathies

SHELLY L. VADEN

Introduction

Protein-losing enteropathy (PLE) refers to a syndrome characterized by the non-selective and excessive loss of proteins into the intestinal lumen. This loss may be due to increased mucosal permeability secondary to cell damage or cell loss, mucosal erosion or ulceration, or altered lymphatic drainage. Hypoproteinemia occurs when protein loss exceeds protein synthesis. Panhypoproteinemia in an animal with clinical evidence of intestinal disease typifies this syndrome. However, animals with PLE may have normal stool frequency and consistency. Prompt diagnosis and treatment of PLE is important because affected animals with severe hypoalbuminemia can deteriorate rapidly and develop life-threatening complications, such as thromboembolism, pleural effusion, or both.

Causes of protein-losing enteropathy

PLE is more commonly diagnosed in dogs than in cats. Whether this is because of a lower prevalence of PLE in cats than in dogs or because diagnostic modalities for the diagnosis of PLE in cats are insensitive remains to be determined. Currently, PLE in cats is most often associated with gastrointestinal lymphoma. Conversely, in dogs, PLE is associated with a variety of GI diseases and some systemic disorders (Table 5.9). Basenjis, Chinese Shar Peis, German Shepherd dogs, Norwegian Lundehunds, Rottweilers, Soft-coated Wheaten Terriers, and Yorkshire Terriers have all been reported to be at increased risk for PLE.[1]

Intestinal lymphangiectasia (IL) is believed to be one of the most common disorders associated with PLE in dogs.[2] Dilated lymphatics, found in the deeper portion of the mucosa or between the mucosa and submucosa, result in ruptured lacteals, leading to loss of proteins, lymphocytes, and chylomicrons into the intestinal lumen.[3] IL can be primary or secondary. In people, primary or congenital IL, due to lymphatic malformation, may be associated with diffuse lymphatic disease.[4] Similarly, in dogs, intestinal lymphangiectasia has been reported in association with chylothorax.[4] Inflammatory cell infiltrates can be found in a patchy distribution along the intestines in dogs with primary IL. Lipogranulomatous lymphangitis is associated with dilated lymphatics in the submucosa, serosal surface, and mesentery.[5] These inflammatory lesions may develop in dogs with primary IL in response to stagnated chyle and fat leakage into adjacent tissues. Inflammatory bowel disease (IBD) also is considered to be a common cause of PLE in dogs (see 9.2). Secondary IL develops when inflammatory infiltrates or granulomas obstruct lymphatic flow in patients with IBD.

5

Table 5.9: Diseases associated with PLE in dogs

Inflammatory bowel disease
- Lymphoplasmacytic
- Eosinophilic
- Granulomatous

Adverse food reactions
- Food allergy
- Food intolerance
- Gluten enteropathy

Systemic immune-mediated disease
- Systemic lupus erythematosus

Viral gastroenteritis
- Parvovirus

Bacterial gastroenteritis
- Small intestinal bacterial overgrowth
- Salmonellosis

Intestinal fungal infections
- Histoplasmosis
- Pythiosis

Intestinal neoplasia
- Lymphosarcoma
- Adenocarcinoma

Mechanical enteropathy
- Chronic foreign body
- Chronic intussusception

Gastrointestinal ulceration
- Non-steroidal anti-inflammatory drugs

Altered Lymphatic Drainage
- Lymphangiectasia
  - Primary or congenital

Venous hypertension
- Constrictive pericarditis
- Right-sided heart failure
- Portal vein thrombosis
- Budd-Chiari syndrome

Pathophysiology of serum protein abnormalities

All serum proteins are lost at the same rate in patients with PLE, regardless of their molecular size. When proteins are lost into the GI tract, they are digested into their constituent amino acids, reabsorbed, and reused for protein synthesis. When losses exceed the intestinal reabsorptive capacity as well as the body's synthetic capacity, hypoproteinemia occurs. However, the reduction in serum concentrations of the various proteins may differ markedly. Proteins that normally have a long half-life (e.g., IgG, IgM, and IgA) are more substantially impacted than those with shorter half-lives (e.g., insulin and IgE).[6] Other factors that may impact plasma protein concentrations include the ability of the liver to produce proteins, the rate of endogenous protein degradation, and the degree of stimulation of globulin production.

Because the liver is only able to increase albumin synthesis to about twice the normal production, hypoalbuminemia is common in patients with PLE. Decreased plasma colloidal osmotic pressure becomes clinically relevant when serum albumin concentration decreases to between 1–2 g/dl; with peripheral edema, ascites, or pleural effusion often developing once serum albumin concentrations are below 1.5 g/dL. While hypoglobulinemia is most often found in patients with PLE, serum globulin concentrations are more variable than are serum albumin concentrations. Hypoglobulinemia can sometimes be evident before hypoalbuminemia, as has been seen in Soft-coated Wheaten Terriers (Vaden, unpublished data), because globulin regeneration occurs more slowly than the hepatic synthesis of albumin. Alternatively, normal serum globulin concentrations or hyperglobulinemia may be present in patients with PLE that have an increased globulin production as a result of their primary disease process (i.e., histoplasmosis or immunoproliferative disease in the Basenji).

Diagnosis

PLE should be suspected in dogs and cats that have hypoproteinemia and clinical signs of GI disease (Table 5.10). Chronic, intermittent, small bowel diarrhea is common in animals with PLE. Most affected animals also have a reduced appetite, weight loss, and vomiting. However, it should be noted that some affected patients do not have these clinical signs.[1] Animals with PLE may present for evaluation of dyspnea, which can be due to thromboembolism or pleural effusion. Other animals will have ascites or peripheral edema. Signs of neuromuscular disease may occur secondary to thromboembolic disease or hypocalcemia. Neurological signs secondary to vitamin E deficiency also have been reported in humans with intestinal lymphangiectasia, but have not yet been described in animals.[2] Abdominal palpation may reveal thickened loops of bowel, lymphadenopathy, or findings compatible with a chronic foreign body or an intussusception. Animals with PLE resulting from venous hypertension due to cardiac disease may have distended jugular veins and an abnormal thoracic auscultation.

In addition to the serum protein abnormalities described above, animals with PLE may have lymphopenia and hypocholesterolemia due to excessive intestinal loss of lymphocytes and chylomicrons, respectively. Hypomagnesemia and decreased ionized serum calcium concentrations may also be present, particularly in Yorkshire Terriers.[7] Intestinal loss and malabsorption of these minerals and/or abnormalities of vitamin D and parathyroid hormone metabolism are speculative causes.

The diagnostic evaluation of animals with PLE must be designed to allow for the exclusion of other causes of hypoalbuminemia. These include decreased synthesis (hepatic failure), increased loss (i.e., glomerular disease, blood loss, and severe exudative skin disease), and rarely inadequate intake (i.e., starvation). Therefore, fasting and post-prandial serum bile acid concentrations, a complete urinalysis, a urine protein/creatinine ratio, and a CBC should be performed. Combined PLE and protein-losing nephropathy has been reported in Soft-coated Wheaten Terriers and also may occur in Yorkshire Terriers at a higher frequency than expected in the general canine population (Vaden, unpublished data).[8]

^{51}Cr-albumin clearance, determined by intravenous administration of ^{51}Cr, can be used to document excessive GI protein loss. However, the use of a radionuclide and the need to collect the animal's feces for 3–5 days makes this test impractical for confirming canine PLE.

Alpha$_1$-proteinase inhibitor (α_1-PI) is a serum proteinase inhibitor that is of approximately the same size as albumin and is, therefore, lost at about the same rate as is albumin in patients with PLE. As a proteinase inhibitor, α_1-PI is not digested or degraded by digestive or bacterial proteases and is therefore excreted intact.[9] Fecal α_1-PI concentrations have been used as a marker for PLE in humans and dogs, and may prove to be of most value in the early detection of this syndrome. There is a high degree of intra-individual variability in fecal α_1-PI concentrations.[10] Therefore, three separate naturally voided fecal specimens should be collected into specific specimen tubes provided by the laboratory (Gastrointestinal Laboratory, Texas A&M University, College Station, TX). Samples should be immediately frozen after collection and shipped overnight on ice because substantial degradation occurs within 72 hours at room temperature. Both the mean and the maximum concentrations should be considered, with a mean above 8–9 µg/g feces or a maximum above 15 µg/g feces being considered abnormal. Care should be taken not to digitally remove the feces from the rectum as this may falsely increase fecal α_1-PI concentrations. An assay for the measurement of feline α_1-PI in cat feces has recently been developed and validated, but the clinical usefulness of this test for the diagnosis of feline PLE has not yet been determined.

Gastrointestinal biopsies can be collected via endoscopy, laparoscopy, or laparotomy. Laparotomy allows for full-thickness biopsies to be obtained from sites that may not be reached via endoscopy. Biopsy specimens of other organs (e.g., liver, kidney) can be obtained if needed by either laparotomy or laparoscopy. However, animals with PLE may be at greater risk for developing complications post-operatively, including dehiscence, delayed wound healing, and thromboembolism. Serosal patch grafting of the biopsy site may reduce the likelihood of dehiscence or peritonitis. Care should be taken to minimize the loss of abdominal fluid during laparotomy or laparoscopy. Rapid fluid shifts that can occur post-operatively when ascites rapidly reforms can lead to central volume depletion, further complicating patient recovery. Endoscopy is associated with fewer complications than is laparotomy or laparoscopy, making it a good first choice in most patients. However, endoscopy may not be indicated if abdominal ultrasound leads to the identification of lesions that are believed to be beyond the reach of the endoscope (e.g., jejunum). At least eight quality biopsy samples should be obtained from each accessible site: stomach, duodenum, ileum, and colon.[11] Endoscopically-obtained biopsies may not be diagnostic if the mucosal pathology is not reflective of the deeper intestinal layers. Although finding expanded white villi via endoscopy is suggestive of lymphangiectasia, endoscopically obtained biopsies may not be diagnostic in some animals with lymphangiectasia. Feeding a high fat meal (e.g., corn oil or cream) the night before endoscopy can make lymphangiectasia more evident during endoscopy and also during histopathologic evaluation of the biopsy specimens.

Treatment

The first step in the management of PLE is the implementation of appropriate treatment for the primary disease process. Dietary management is a cornerstone to the management of both IL and IBD.[12] Diets should be highly digestible and low

Table 5.10: Clinical abnormalities associated with protein-losing enteropathy in dogs and cats

Historical Findings
- Diarrhea (96%*)
- Vomiting (56%*)
- Weight loss (>52%*)
- Anorexia
- Polyuria/polydipsia (5%*)

Physical Examination Findings
- Ascites (41%*)
- Pleural effusion (5%*)
- Peripheral edema (7%*)
- Signs of thromboembolism (10%*)
- Neuromuscular signs (4%*)
- Thickened bowel loops
- Distended jugular veins**

Clinicopathological Findings
- Hypoalbuminemia
- Hypoglobulinemia
- Hypocalcemia
- Hypomagnesemia
- Hypocholesterolemia
- Lymphopenia
- Increased fecal alpha$_1$-proteinase inhibitor concentration

*Reported percentage in 134 dogs with PLE.[1]

**In animals with venous hypertension from cardiac disease.

5

in fat. When serum albumin is <1.5 g/dL, intestinal mucosal edema may contribute to further malassimilation. In these animals feeding a hydrolyzed protein or elemental diet may be required until the animal's condition stabilizes. Administration of medium chain triglyceride (MCT) oil is sometimes suggested, although seldom used because it can be difficult to administer, can cause diarrhea, and is rarely needed to maintain body condition if the primary disease process is appropriately controlled. Glucocorticoids or other immunosuppressive agents are generally indicated in dogs with PLE due to IBD and may be indicated in some dogs with IL if there is secondary inflammation. Sodium cromoglycate has been shown in children to reduce gut permeability following oral administration.[13] Sodium cromoglycate acts by inhibiting the degranulation of mast cells, thereby blocking the release of biochemical mediators.[14] Clinical improvement has also been seen in a few Soft-coated Wheaten Terriers with PLE that had failed traditional management following sodium cromoglycate administration (100 mg, administered PO 3–4 times daily; Vaden, unpublished data). The drug is believed to be minimally absorbed from the normal GI tract and has a low incidence of toxicity but more studies are needed to validate the efficacy and safety of this drug in dogs with PLE.

Plasma transfusions or the administration of hetastarch or dextran may be needed in order to increase plasma oncotic pressure prior to anesthesia, but will not provide long-term benefits. Spironolactone may be more effective and safer than furosemide in the long-term management of edema or effusions.

🔑 Key Facts

■ PLE can result from any disease that causes increased mucosal permeability, mucosal ulceration, or altered lymphatic drainage.

■ Most dogs and cats with PLE have diarrhea, anorexia, and weight loss, although some dogs with PLE do not exhibit these clinical signs.

■ Most affected animals have panhypoproteinemia, but some patients may only have hypoalbuminemia.

■ Care should be taken to exclude other causes of hypoalbuminemia: hepatic failure, glomerular disease, blood loss, and severe exudative skin disease.

■ Prompt diagnosis and treatment of PLE is important because affected animals with severe hypoalbuminemia can deteriorate rapidly and develop life-threatening complications.

References

1. Peterson PB, Willard MD. Protein-losing enteropathies. *Vet Clin Small Anim* 2003; 33: 1061–1082.
2. Fossum TW. Protein-losing enteropathy. *Sem Vet Med Surg* 1989; 4: 219–225.
3. Suter MM, Palmer DG, Schenk H. Primary intestinal lymphangiectasia in three dogs: a morphological and immunopatholgical investigation. *Vet Pathol* 1985; 22: 123–130.
4. Fossum TW, Sherding RG, Zach PM et al. Intestinal lymphagiectasia associated with chylothorax in two dogs. *J Am Vet Med Assoc* 1987; 190: 61–64.
5. Van Kruiningen HJ, Lees GE, Hayden DW et al. Lipogranulomatous lymphangitis in canine intestinal lymphangiectasia. *Vet Pathol* 1984; 21: 377–383.
6. Kim KE. Protein-losing gastroenteropathy. In: Feldman M, Scharschmidt BF, Sleisenger MH (eds.), *Sleisenger & Fordtran's Gastrointestinal and Liver Disease Pathophysiology / Diagnosis / Management*, 7th ed. Philadelphia, WB Saunders, 2002; 446–375.
7. Kimmel SE, Waddell LS, Michel KE. Hypomagnesemia and hypocalcemia associated with protein-losing enteropathy in Yorkshire Terriers: Five cases (1992–1998). *J Am Vet Med Assoc* 2000; 217: 703–706.
8. Littman MP, Dambach DM, Vaden SL et al. Familial protein-losing enteropathy and/or protein-losing nephropathy in Soft-Coated Wheaten Terriers: 222 cases (1983–1997). *J Vet Intern Med* 2000; 14: 68–80.
9. Murphy KF, German AJ, Ruaux CG et al. Fecal α_1-proteinase inhibitor concentration in dogs with chronic gastrointestinal disease. *Vet Clin Path* 2003; 32: 67–72.
10. Steiner JM, Ruaux CG, Miller MD et al. Intra-individual variability of fecal α_1-proteinase inhibitor concentration in clinically healthy dogs. *J Vet Intern Med* 2003; 17: 445 (Abstract).
11. Willard MD, Lovering SL, Cohen ND et al. Quality of tissue specimens obtained endoscopically from the duodenum of dogs and cats. *J Am Vet Med Assoc* 2001; 219: 474–479.
12. Zoran DL. Nutritional management of gastrointestinal conditions. In: Ettinger SJ, Feldman EC (eds.), *Textbook of Veterinary Internal Medicine, 6th ed.* St. Louis, Elsevier Saunders 2005; 570–573.
13. Falth-Magnusson K, Kjellman NI et al. Intestinal permeability in healthy and allergic children before and after sodium cromoglycate treatment assessed with different sized polyethylene glycols. *Clin Allergy* 1984; 14: 277–286.
14. Sogn D. Medications and their use in the treatment of adverse reactions to foods. *J Allergy Clin Immunol* 1986; 78: 238–243.

5.3.10 Neoplastic diseases of the small intestines

Carolyn J. Henry

Introduction

Small intestinal (SI) neoplasia is uncommon, noted in 0.3% and 0.7% of all canine and feline necropsy submissions, respectively, each year.[1] Of the non-lymphoid SI tumors (see 9.3 for lymphoid tumors), carcinomas predominate in both species.[2] Leiomyosarcomas comprise the second most commonly reported non-lymphoid gastrointestinal malignancy in dogs.[2–4] Other reported canine SI tumors include leiomyomas, fibrosarcomas, undifferentiated sarcomas, mast cell tumors (MCT), carcinoids (see 9.4.6), neurilemomas, and extramedullary plasmacytomas.[1,2,5–7] Although uncommon, leiomyosarcomas have been reported in cats, as have MCTs, hemangiosarcomas, adenomatous polyps, and extraskeletal osteosarcomas.[8–16]

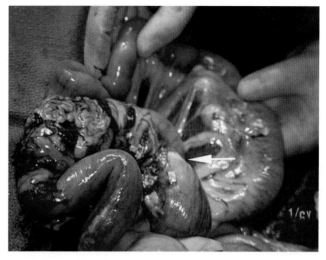

Figure 5.10:
Intestinal adenocarcinoma. This figure shows an adenocarcinoma located in the ileum of a dog. The mesentery is adhered to the affected portions of intestine. The lesion is tubular in nature and causes annular narrowing of the bowel noted by a white band of constriction (arrow).

Incidence

Although the small intestine comprises 90% of the length of the intestinal tract, most canine non-lymphoid intestinal tumors, other than MCTs, are located in the colon or rectum, not in the more proximal segments.[1,5,17] This is true in human beings as well, where small bowel tumors account for only 3% of all GI malignancies.[18] In contrast, previous reports have indicated that 90% of feline intestinal tumors occur in the small intestines.[1] However, more recent data suggest that this reported site predilection in cats may no longer hold true (personal unpublished data). Multiple hypotheses have been proposed to explain the low incidence of SI tumors in dogs and humans. Proposed factors include the rapid transit time of potential carcinogens in the proximal segments compared to the colon, an inability of the SI flora to transform procarcinogens into their active metabolites, the presence of microsomal enzymes in the small intestine that detoxify carcinogens, and local immunosurveillance by IgA-secreting lymphocytes and B cells in the distal ileum.[19] However, the reason for the previously reported SI site predilection in cats remains unexplained. A role for retroviral diseases in the etiology of feline non-lymphoid intestinal cancer has not been identified.[1,2,20] Any segment of the canine SI may be affected, although sarcomas occur more often in the jejunum than in other segments. The jejunum and ileum are affected more often in cats than is the duodenum.[1,11,20,21]

Small intestinal neoplasia is generally a disease of older animals, occurring at a mean age of approximately 9 years in dogs and a mean and median age of 8.7 and 11 years, respectively, in cats.[2,3,11,20] Some tumor types, especially leiomyosarcomas, have been reported in very young animals.[22] Accordingly, age should not be used to exclude a diagnosis of SI neoplasia. No clear breed predispositions have been identified for canine SI cancer except with MCT, for which miniature breeds, especially the Maltese, are at increased risk.[5] Siamese cats appear to be predisposed to intestinal cancer.[2,11,20,21] Conflicting views exist regarding gender predispositions for intestinal cancer in both species, with some reports indicating a male predisposition and others noting a female predisposition.[1–3,21,22] In humans, there is a slight male predominance for malignant small bowel tumors.[19]

The most common primary SI tumor in both species, with the exception of lymphoma, are those of epithelial origin, the majority of which are malignant.[1] Of the four types of malignant epithelial tumors (adenocarcinoma, mucinous adenocarcinoma, signet ring cell carcinoma, and undifferentiated or solid carcinoma) adenocarcinomas predominate. The tumors often cause annular constriction (Figure 5.10) and may become quite large before they are clinically detectable. Feline intestinal adenocarcinomas (ACA) have been histologically subtyped as tubular, undifferentiated, or mucinous.[11,20,23] Of these, mucinous ACA are the least common.[23] Approximately one third of feline intestinal ACAs have areas of osseous or cartilaginous metaplasia.[1] Tumor grading based on degree of cellular differentiation may not be clinically relevant. In a series of cats with intestinal ACAs, papillary ACAs were described as the most differentiated tumors, yet they were associated with the highest rate of metastasis.[21]

5

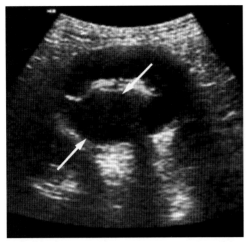

Figure 5.11:
Ultrasonographic appearance of a small intestinal mass. Transverse sonogram of a hypoechoic circumferential mural lesion in the small intestine. The hyperechoic central portion represents the bowel lumen and arrows indicate the extent of wall thickening due to neoplasia.

Leiomyomas and leiomyosarcomas originate from smooth muscle and are the most common mesenchymal tumors affecting the canine GI tract.[2,4,24] Over 50% of dogs with intestinal leiomyosarcoma have intra-abdominal metastasis at the time of diagnosis, thus emphasizing the need for presurgical tumor staging.[25] Metastatic disease may occur through hematogenous or lymphatic routes, as well as by transcoelomic spread and tumor seeding.[1] Metastatic lesions are occasionally found in the testes, although the route by which this occurs is unclear.[7,26]

Clinical signs

Weight loss, vomiting, and anorexia are the most common presenting complaints associated with SI cancer in dogs and cats.[2,3,20,23] In dogs, weight loss and vomiting are more common with duodenal or jejunal lesions whereas in cats, there is equal site distribution for masses associated with these presenting complaints.[2] Diarrhea and tenesmus are more typical for ileal or colonic masses than for proximal SI lesions.[2] Other signs reported with SI cancer include melena, abdominal distension, and lethargy.[2,3,20,25,27] Paraneoplastic syndromes have been reported with smooth muscle tumors and include hypoglycemia (leiomyoma and leiomyosarcoma) and nephrogenic diabetes insipidus (leiomyosarcoma).[25,27,28] Dogs with paraneoplastic hypoglycemia may present with CNS signs including seizures and ataxia.[25,29,31] Hypoglycemia may also occur secondary to tumor-related peritonitis, especially with smooth muscle tumors, which are prone to grow quite large

and can subsequently rupture.[25] Polyuria and polydipsia (PU/PD) were noted in over one third of the dogs with GI leiomyosarcoma in one report and have been described in other reports of smooth muscle tumors.[25,28,31] In one case, the cause of PU/PD was apparently tumor-related nephrogenic diabetes insipidus; however, the cause has remained undetermined in others.[25,28,31]

Diagnostics

Physical examination findings may aid in the diagnosis, as a palpable mass is found in approximately half of all cases.[2,3,20] Plain radiographs are generally less sensitive than palpation or abdominal ultrasound for detection of intestinal masses, especially in cats.[2,20] However, plain radiographs were sufficient to warrant surgical exploration in 65% of cats in one report.[23] Contrast radiography may enhance tumor visualization and was diagnostic for tumor-related obstruction in 13 of 15 cats in one study.[20] Abdominal ultrasound is becoming the gold standard for imaging intestinal neoplasia as it permits more accurate assessment of intestinal wall layering and facilitates the differentiation of neoplasia from nonspecific enteritis.[32] Abdominal ultrasound did permit identification of intestinal neoplasia in 87% to 90% of cases in two reported case series.[3,32] Dogs in which intestinal wall layers are no longer visible (Figure 5.11) are reportedly over 50 times more likely to have intestinal neoplasia than nonspecific enteritis.[32] Segmental intestinal wall thickening of mixed echogenicity in cats supports a diagnosis of ACA over that of lymphoma.[33] However, definitive diagnosis is generally made by fine needle aspiration of a palpable or ultrasound-imaged mass or by histopathological examination of a tissue biopsy collected during laparoscopy or exploratory laparotomy.

Preoperative lab work should include a CBC, serum chemistry profile, and urinalysis. Anemia and leukocytosis are the predominant CBC abnormalities noted in both species.[2,20] The leukocytosis is generally characterized by neutrophilia.[2] Lymphopenia was noted in 7 of 11 affected cats in one report.[23] Decreased neutrophil numbers, a degenerative left shift, or toxic changes in neutrophils should alert the clinician to the likelihood of tumor rupture and peritonitis, and is commonly reported with leiomyosarcomas.[25] Biochemical abnormalities in dogs may include hypoproteinemia due to protein loss or decreased production, and hypoglycemia occurring either as a paraneoplastic syndrome or secondary to sepsis or hepatic failure.[3,25] In cats, hypoproteinemia, hyperglycemia, azotemia, hypercholesterolemia, and increased activities of alanine transaminase and alkaline phosphatase have been reported.[2,20,23]

36. Takahashi T, Kadosawa T, Nagase M et al. Visceral mast cell tumors in dogs: 10 cases (1982–1997) *J Am Vet Med Assoc* 2000; 216: 222–226.

37. Thomson M. Alimentary tract and pancreas. In: Slatter D (ed.), *Textbook of Small Animal Surgery, 3rd ed.* Philadelphia, WB Saunders, 2003; 2368–2378.

38. Bezuidenhout AJ. The lymphatic system. In: Miller ME, Evans HE (eds.), *Anatomy of the Dog.* Philadelphia, WB Saunders, 1993; 717–757.

39. LaRock RG, Ginn PE. Immunohistochemical staining characteristics of canine gastrointestinal stromal tumors. *Vet Pathol* 1997; 34: 303–311.

40. Sandusky GE, Wightman KA, Carlton WW. Immunocytochemical study of tissues from clinically normal dogs and of neoplasms, using keratin monoclonal antibodies. *Am J Vet Res* 1991; 52 (4): 613–618.

41. Paolini M, Penninck DG, Moore AS. Ultrasonographic and clinicopathologic findings in 21 dogs with intestinal adenocarcinoma. *Vet Radiol & Ultrasound* 2002; 43: 562–567.

42. Gibbs C, Pearson H. Localized tumours of the canine small intestine: a report of twenty cases. *J Small Anim Pract* 1986; 27: 507–519.

5

6   Large Intestine

6.1   Introduction

Michael S. Leib

Diseases of the large intestine are common in both dogs and cats. The clinical signs are obvious and unpleasant to owners and usually result in a prompt visit to the veterinarian. The most common clinical sign of large intestinal disease is diarrhea, usually characterized by increased frequency of defecation, decreased quantity of stool per defecation, tenesmus, hematochezia, and excess mucus. Concurrent involvement of the small intestine may additionally result in melena and weight loss. Vomiting and reduced appetite may also accompany some large bowel diseases. Constipation, the second major clinical sign of large intestinal disease, may be associated with a variety of dietary and environmental factors, neurological or musculoskeletal disorders, and may progress to megacolon. This chapter will discuss the normal anatomy and physiology of the large intestine and many of the common colonic diseases of dogs and cats.

6.2   Anatomy

The large bowel ranges in length from 28–90 cm in dogs and 20–45 cm in cats.[1,2] It begins at the ileocolic junction and terminates at the anus. Anatomically, the large bowel is divided into the cecum, colon, and rectum. The cecum is a sigmoid-shaped diverticulum of the proximal colon and joins the colon through the cecocolic orifice. This junction is in close proximity to the ileocolic orifice, also referred to as the ileocolic valve (Figure 6.1). The cecum is variable in length and measures 8–30 cm in dogs and 2–4 cm in cats (Figure 6.2).

6

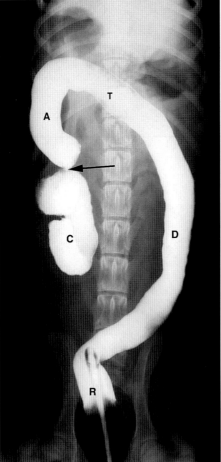

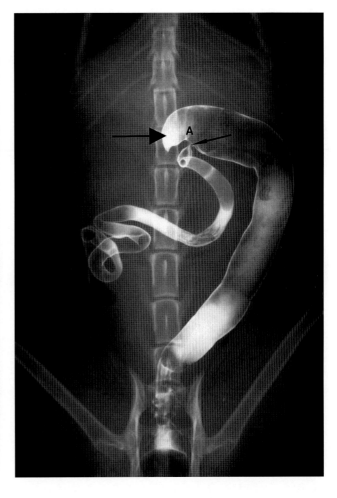

Figure 6.1 (left): Barium enema in a dog. This figure shows a ventro-dorsal abdominal radiograph after a barium enema in a dog showing the cecum (C), ascending colon (A), transverse colon (T), descending colon (D), rectum (R), and cecocolic junction (arrow).

Figure 6.2 (right): Barium enema in a cat. Ventrodorsal abdominal radiograph after a barium enema in a cat showing the ileocolic junction (thin arrowhead), the short cecum (thick arrowhead), and the short ascending colon (A).

6

The colon is divided into ascending, transverse, and descending portions and their connecting flexures. These subdivisions are identified on the basis of their relative position within the body. The ascending colon is a short segment that begins at the ileocolic sphincter and courses cranially to the right (hepatic) colic flexure. Spatially, the cecum and ascending colon lie to the right of the median plane and are in close association with the descending duodenum, right limb of the pancreas, and stomach. From the right colic flexure, the transverse colon runs, cranial to the root of the mesentery, to the left (splenic) colic flexure, where it joins the descending colon. The transverse colon is in close proximity to the left limb of the pancreas, stomach, and loops of small intestine. The descending colon, the longest segment, passes caudally, following the left lateral abdominal wall into the pelvic inlet, where the rectum begins. It is usually covered by the greater omentum and lies adjacent to the ascending portion of the duodenum. The uterus or prostate and the urinary bladder lie ventral to its terminal portion.

Blood is supplied to the large bowel by the cranial and caudal mesenteric arteries. Venous drainage occurs through the cranial and caudal mesenteric veins, which empty into the portal vein. Lymphatic drainage occurs through the right, middle, and left colic lymph nodes.

Histologically, the large bowel is similar to the small bowel, and contains mucosal, submucosal, muscular, and serosal layers. The anatomical modifications of the colonic mucosa, which increase its absorptive surface area, are not as distinctive as those in the small bowel. The colonic mucosa is devoid of villi, and the microvilli of colonic epithelial cells are less abundant than their counterparts in the small bowel. Despite the absence of villi, there are numerous crypts that extend from the absorptive surface through the entire thickness of the mucosa. These crypts of Lieberkühn, contain epithelial, mucus, and endocrine cells. Compared to the small bowel, mucus cells are more prominent and endocrine cells are fewer in number. The deeper portion of the crypts consist mainly of undifferentiated cells, which migrate along the crypts as they proliferate and mature, ultimately giving rise to the aforementioned epithelial, mucus, and endocrine cells. At the mucosal surface, the cells undergo apoptosis, degenerate, and are sloughed into the lumen. Cell turnover in the colon is slower than in the small intestine, requiring 4–7 days. Within the lamina propria moderate numbers of diffusely distributed lymphocytes and plasma cells can be found.[3,4]

Both the intrinsic and extrinsic nervous systems regulate large bowel function. Intrinsic innervation occurs through the intramural network of neurons contained in the myenteric plexus, which lies between the longitudinal and circular muscle layers, and the submucosal plexus. Intrinsic control allows the large bowel to autonomously regulate functions based on intraluminal conditions, such as the degree of distension and the type and quantity of fluid and other intraluminal contents. Extrinsic neural control occurs through the autonomic nervous system. Parasympathetic innervation to the proximal portion of the large bowel is through the vagus nerve with the remainder of the large bowel supplied by the pelvic nerves. Sympathetic innervation arises from the paravertebral ganglia and follows the splanchnic nerves to the wall of the large intestine. Parasympathetic preganglionic fibers and sympathetic postganglionic fibers synapse on cell bodies and neurons of the intrinsic nervous system, respectively.

6.3 Physiology

The major functions of the large intestine are extraction of water and electrolytes from the ileal effluent, storage of feces, and defecation. In addition, microbial fermentation of organic matter that escapes digestion and absorption in the small intestine also occurs in the large intestine. Absorptive processes and microbial metabolism occur in the proximal colon whereas fecal storage and elimination occur in the distal colon. These functional differences may be attributed to regional differences in patterns of colonic motility.

6.3.1 Motility

The majority of muscular contractions arising in the proximal colon are retrograde peristaltic contractions, which are initiated in the transverse colon and are propagated towards the cecum.[2] Termed antiperistalsis, this type of motility slows the transit of colonic contents and enhances mucosal absorption of fluid and electrolytes. The transverse colon plays the most important role in the proximal colon for mixing, storage, and dehydration of fecal contents.

Throughout the colon, rhythmic segmentation, originating in the circular muscle layer, moves the contents short distances in both antegrade and retrograde directions, preventing rapid transit. This promotes absorption of the remaining water and electrolytes. Coordinated peristalsis can be observed in any part of the colon, but is the predominant pattern of motility in the mid-portion of the colon. Peristaltic waves are tonic rings of constriction, transmitted by the longitudinal muscle layer, which serve to move colonic contents aborally.

Spontaneous giant migrating contractions, or mass movements, are the predominant form of motility in the distal large intestine. These powerful smooth muscle contractions originate in the proximal colon and migrate in an aborad direction over a segment or the entire length of the colon, moving colonic contents towards the rectum in preparation for defecation.[5]

Intrinsic smooth muscle properties, intrinsic neurons, extrinsic nerves, and neuroendocrine polypeptides influence colonic contractile activity. Control of peristalsis and rhythmic segmentation in the colon is determined by slow wave activity, which is an inherent myoelectric property of smooth muscle. Slow waves are generated by ion fluxes across the smooth muscle cells. The frequency of slow wave activity determines the rate of contraction, while the number of spike potentials superimposed upon slow waves and generated during the depolarization phase determines the strength of contractions. Slow waves are less frequent in the proximal colon than in the distal colon, which helps to impede transit and promotes the extraction of water and electrolytes. In contrast to the small bowel, slow waves in the large bowel are generated in the circular muscle layer. There are multiple pacemakers in the colon that propagate slow waves over a short distance. However, a single pacemaker exists in the transverse colon, from which slow waves are spread most often in an orad direction and are associated with antiperistalsis. Giant migrating contractions result from prolonged bursts of electrical activity, which span several slow wave cycles and appear to be independent of slow wave activity. Differences in the intrinsic mechanical properties of colonic longitudinal and circular smooth muscle have been demonstrated in cats and contribute to regional specialization of motility. This is most notable in the proximal colon where antiperistaltic activity of the longitudinal smooth muscle layer predominates over the segmental activity of the circular muscle layer.

The intrinsic nervous system is essential for normal colonic motility and can function independently of the extrinsic nervous system. Reflexes mediated through efferent cholinergic neurons stimulate segmental contractions and peristalsis. Stimulation of mechanoreceptors in the muscular layers that respond to distension, or of chemoreceptors within the mucosa that respond to luminal contents result in muscular contractions.

In addition to acetylcholine and norepinephrine, a variety of other neurotransmitters have been identified that are released from the neurons of the intrinsic nervous system. Many of these are peptides and include neurotensin, cholecystokinin, substance P, somatostatin, and 5-hydroxytryptamine.[6,7] The response of colonic smooth muscle to neurotransmitters varies throughout the colon. Regional differences have been observed in smooth muscle responses to neurotensin and cholecystokinin, both of which are more potent stimuli of proximal than distal colonic smooth muscle activity.[8] These differences may, in part, explain the different motility patterns and functions in the proximal and distal colon.

Extrinsic neural and hormonal regulation of colonic motility is poorly understood. In general, extrinsic parasympathetic activity stimulates and sympathetic activity inhibits segmental contractions. The major function of the extrinsic nervous system is in the distal colon, where it participates in the defecation reflex.

The defecation reflex may be initiated in response to ingestion of a meal (gastrocolic reflex) as well as luminal distension in the distal colon and rectum. Increased tension in the rectal wall stimulates intramural receptors that transmit impulses along afferent parasympathetic pathways within the pelvic nerve to the sacral spinal cord. Efferent nerve fibers contained within the pudendal, hypogastric, and pelvic nerves complete the reflex arc. Stimulation of these fibers initiates a motor response that causes contraction of colonic and rectal smooth muscle, and relaxation of the internal and external anal sphincters, allowing evacuation of the rectum and distal colon. Defecation is usually preceded by giant migrating contractions of the distal colon.[5] The defecation reflex can be inhibited by voluntary contraction of the external anal sphincter. Receptive relaxation of the distal colon and rectum accommodates fecal storage until the next defecation reflex is initiated.

6.3.2 Water and electrolyte transport

The large intestine normally absorbs a smaller quantity of water than the small intestine, but does so much more efficiently. Approximately 90% of the water entering the large bowel is absorbed.[2,9] Water absorption in the large bowel occurs passively across an osmotic gradient principally created by the absorption of sodium. The large bowel has a maximum absorptive capacity for water. When fluid flow from the small intestine exceeds this absorptive capacity, when there is excessive colonic fluid secretion, or when colonic absorption is decreased, diarrhea ensues. Therefore, the capacity of the large bowel to absorb water principally determines whether or not diarrhea is present with either small or large bowel diseases.

Sodium absorption in the proximal colon appears to occur principally via chloride-coupled sodium transport. This process results from two separate ion transport mechanisms working in concert to facilitate the movement of sodium and chloride across the apical membrane of the epithelial cells. An even exchange of sodium with potassium and chloride with bicarbonate maintains electrical neutrality.

The large bowel secretes potassium by way of an active conductance mechanism at the apical membrane of the colonocytes. In contrast, active potassium absorption occurs in the distal colon through a K^+/H^+ exchange.

Mineralocorticoids and glucocorticoids stimulate sodium absorption and potassium secretion in the distal colon. These substances affect colonic transport by increasing the permeability of the apical membrane to sodium and potassium, and by enhancing the activity of the Na^+/K^+ ATPase pump. Colonic epithelial cells also secrete bicarbonate. Bicarbonate neutralizes the acid produced by colonic bacteria, which can be irritating to the mucosa. The secretion of bicarbonate is cou-

6

pled to the absorption of equal numbers of chloride ions and may occur independently of sodium absorption.

6.3.3 Mucus secretion

Mucus is the principal secretory product of the large bowel. Mucus acts as a lubricant and facilitates the passage of large bowel contents and protects the mucosa from mechanical or chemical injury. Various agents (microorganisms, enterotoxins) can be bound by mucus, thus preventing their attachment, entry into, or their adverse effects upon the colonic mucosa.[9,10] Direct tactile stimulation of the mucus cells by luminal contents and intramural reflexes primarily regulate the production of mucus. The large bowel is capable of secreting large volumes of mucus, water, and electrolytes when inflamed. This response serves to dilute the irritating factor and promote colonic distension and evacuation of colonic contents. Marked increases in mucus secretion can also be caused by stimulation of parasympathetic activity.

6.3.4 Colonic microflora

The large bowel contains the highest concentration of bacteria within the GI tract, with a single gram of feces containing up to 10^{11} organisms.[2] Nearly 50% of the dry weight of feces consists of bacteria. Anaerobic (spore- and non-spore-forming) bacteria predominate, accounting for up to 90% of the large intestinal microflora. *Bifidobacterium* spp. and *Bacteroides* spp. are found in the highest numbers, with lesser numbers of *Clostridia* spp. The predominant aerobic bacteria found in the large bowel are *Lactobacillus* spp., *Enterobacteriacea* spp., and *Streptococcus* spp.

The physiological mechanisms that are important to maintain a normal colonic microflora and to prevent disease induced by bacterial overgrowth or colonization with pathogenic organisms include normal colonic motility, maintenance of the mucosal barrier, and local immune factors. Interactions of resident microflora, diet, and orally administered or enterohepatically circulated antibacterial agents also influence the colonic microflora.

The normal large intestinal microflora resist colonization by other, potentially pathogenic, organisms by producing metabolic products that inhibit growth of other bacteria and by competing for mucosal attachment sites and nutrients. The use of antibiotics with an anaerobic or broad spectrum may upset this sensitive balance and may result in an overpopulation of potential pathogens.

Colonic bacteria metabolize carbohydrates, proteins, and lipids. Carbohydrates are fermented into acidic short-chain fatty acids (acetate, propionate, and butyrate) and gases (hydrogen, methane, and carbon dioxide). Luminal bicarbonate neutralizes most of the acids, resulting in the production of carbon dioxide and water. Luminal fatty acids may inhibit replication of pathogenic bacteria. Absorbed fatty acids are either metabolized by the colonic epithelium (butyrate) or are transported to other tissues and used as an energy source (acetate, propionate, or butyrate).

6.3.5 Immune function

The immune functions of the intestinal tract are extremely complex and our knowledge of them is constantly expanding.[2,11] The major functions of intestinal immunity include: tolerance to orally administered antigens, locally protective responses, and systemic and mucosal dissemination of stimulated B- and T-lymphocytes.[12] Natural intestinal defense mechanisms include both mechanical and immunological factors, which act in concert to protect the host.[1] These mechanisms are particularly important because of ingestion and digestion of nutrients, ingestion of potentially pathogenic organisms and foreign substances, and the extensive resident bacterial flora contained within the intestines. Important mechanical factors include the mucosal epithelial barrier, intestinal motility, mucus production, and the normal resident bacterial flora.

The gut-associated lymphoid tissue (GALT) is compartmentalized into afferent and efferent sites.[12] The afferent arm of the GALT consists of mucosal lymphoid follicles, Peyer's patches, and the mesenteric lymph nodes. Effector functions are performed in the lamina propria and intestinal epithelium.[10,12] The function of the lymphoid follicles is to capture and process antigens in order to initiate an appropriate immunological response. The GALT contains both B- and T-lymphocytes and antigen-processing cells, such as macrophages and dendritic cells. The germinal centers of the lymphoid follicles contain IgA-producing B-lymphocytes. Specialized epithelial cells, termed membranous or M-cells overlie the lymphoid follicles. These cells trap soluble or particulate antigens and whole microorganisms and channel them towards the antigen-processing cells.[11]

Intraepithelial lymphocytes (IEL) are principally suppressor T-cells, many of which are CD8+.[12] Mast cell progenitors are also found in this compartment. In the mucosal lamina propria, IgA-producing B-cells predominate the B-cell subtype, while the majority of the T-cells are of the helper subset, many of which being CD4+.[12] Plasma cells, mast cells, macrophages, and eosinophils are also present in the lamina propria. Besides mediating immediate hypersensitivity, mast cells also may play a role in delayed hypersensitivity, inflammation, cytotoxicity, and immunoregulation.

Plasma cells within the mucosa produce IgA, which is bound to a secretory component on the epithelial cell membrane and released into the gut lumen. Secretory IgA prevents the attachment and uptake of antigens by the intestinal mucosa by binding them. IgA in combination with protective mechanical factors serve to exclude antigenic material from the mucosa.

Antigens captured by M-cells or those penetrating the mucosal epithelium initiate an immune response. Following antigen processing, the immune system undergoes regulated expansion to produce clones responsible for cell-mediated immunity, humoral immunity, immune memory, and immunoregulation. The immune response results in sensitivity (elimination) of or tolerance to the antigen.

Cell-mediated immunity involves cellular cytotoxicity and synthesis of cytokines. When stimulated, T-helper-1 lymphocytes secrete IL-2, IFN-γ, and TNF-α, which support the cell-mediated immune response.[12] Lymphocytes in the epithelial and mucosal compartments possess cytotoxic potential. Macrophages also may become cytotoxic. T-helper-2 lymphocytes secrete IL-4, IL-5, and IL-10, which support antibody production.[12]

Following antigen penetration of the mucosal barrier, non-IgA immunoglobulins become involved in the humoral immune response. IgM, IgG, and IgE participate in host defense by the processes of opsonization, complement fixation, and promotion of an inflammatory response, all properties that IgA lacks. IgE is also important in the mediation of immediate hypersensitivity. When antigen binds to IgE molecules fixed to mast cells, degranulation of the mast cells occurs, releasing inflammatory mediators (e.g., histamine, serotonin, leukotrienes, and others). This release of inflammatory mediators by mast cells may be important in the expulsion of parasites.

Immunological tolerance is an important feature of the GI immune system. Tolerance results from the induction of IgA, T-cell deletion, anergy, and immunosuppression.[11] Most intraluminal antigens processed via M-cells induce tolerance. Both IL-10 and TGF-β are down-regulatory cytokines that help to promote tolerance.[12] However, potentially harmful antigens that penetrate the mucosal barrier stimulate lymphocytes producing IgM, IgE, IgG, and proinflammatory cytokines, such as IFN-γ, IL-12, and IL-6.[11] Tolerance is necessary to prevent mucosal and systemic injury as a result of a continuous inflammatory response to benign, persistent intraluminal antigens. A breakdown of this tolerance response may be involved in the pathogenesis of inflammatory bowel disease (IBD).

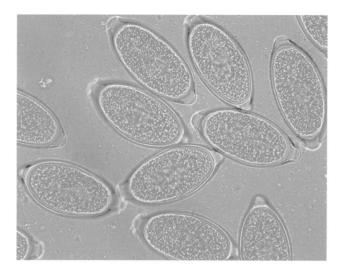

Figure 6.3:
Whipworm eggs. Close up of a group of whipworm eggs in a fecal flotation.

6.4 Diseases of the Large Intestine

6.4.1 Whipworms

Trichuris vulpis infestation is one of the most common causes of acute or chronic large bowel diarrhea in dogs.[2,13] Puppies and dogs that live in contaminated environments are commonly affected and often reinfected. Cats rarely have whipworms.

Clinical signs

Diarrhea with hematochezia and excess mucus occurs frequently. Abdominal pain, vomiting, inappetence, and weight loss can also be observed.[14] The diarrhea may be intermittent in chronic cases. Anemia can result in pale mucous membranes and lethargy.

Pathophysiology

The parasite's life cycle is direct. Adult worms shed eggs intermittently, which can result in false-negative fecal examinations. The eggs have thick, yellow-brown shells, are barrel-shaped, with polar plugs, and are approximately 80 × 35 μm (Figure 6.3). Whipworm eggs can persist for years in the environment, but prolonged sunlight will kill them. Areas that cannot be easily cleaned, such as lawns and dirt kennels, can become contaminated, providing a source for reinfection. Under optimal environmental conditions, the eggs embryonate in as few as 10 days. After a dog ingests the infective eggs, the larvae

6

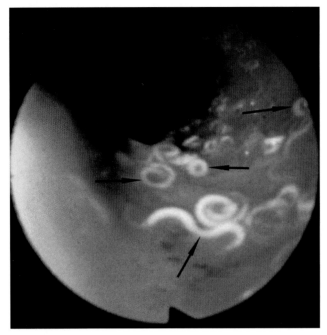

Figure 6.4:
Whipworms. Endoscopic appearance of adult whipworms (arrows) in the ascending colon of a dog.

hatch in the small intestine and burrow into the mucosa for 2–10 days, emerge again, and attach to the mucosa in the cecum and ascending colon, where they complete their maturation.[14] Female worms begin producing eggs 70–107 days after the infection has been acquired. Estimates of daily egg production range from 1,000–4,000. Adult worms may live up to 18 months.

Pathogenicity is related to the tunneling of the thin anterior portion of the adult worm into the epithelium of the cecum or ascending colon, producing localized inflammation, mucosal hyperplasia, and in some cases focal granulomatous reactions.[14,15] Adult worms measure 45–75 mm in length (Figure 6.4). The worms feed on tissue fluid, blood, and cellular debris. The parasites may be found throughout the large intestine in dogs harboring large numbers of worms.

Many infected dogs will not show any clinical signs. The factors contributing to the development of clinical signs include the number of worms present, the location of worms, degree of inflammation produced, level of anemia or hypoproteinemia, nutritional status of the host, and the presence of other GI parasites.[14]

Although infrequent, infections of human beings with *Trichuris vulpis* may occur.[14,15] Clients should be warned of the possible public health significance and appropriate sanitary measures should be taken when disposing of fecal material.

Diagnosis

Whipworm eggs can be identified using routine fecal flotation procedures. Zinc sulfate flotation (with centrifugation) has been demonstrated to be more sensitive than other flotation techniques for identifying whipworm eggs.[16] However, if multiple fecal examinations fail to identify eggs, treatment for whipworms should be instituted prior to performing additional diagnostic tests. A presumptive diagnosis of whipworm infection can be made if clinical signs improve within 2–3 days of appropriate anthelminthic therapy. Adult worms may be seen in the cecum and ascending colon during colonoscopy if a dog with an occult infection has not been treated prior to performing colonoscopy (Figure 6.4).[17] Eosinophilia may be present. Anemia and hypoproteinemia may develop in cases with severe infestation.

Treatment

There are numerous therapeutic agents that are effective against whipworms in dogs.[15] Commonly used treatments include fenbendazole (Panacur® at 50 mg/kg PO q 24 h for three days) and a combination of febantel, pyrantel pamoate, and praziquantel (Drontal® Plus at 25 mg/kg febantel PO once).[18]

Fenbendazole is a safe and efficacious drug with broad-spectrum activity against common GI nematodes, *Giardia*, and some tapeworms. Febantel is converted to fenbendazole in the liver. The combination of febantel and pyrantel is synergistic and allows treatment with a single dose. When both are combined with praziquantel, they offer broad-spectrum activity against common GI nematodes and tapeworms.

Treatment should be repeated after three weeks and again after three months. The effects of most anthelminthics on the larval stages of whipworms remain unknown.[14] After anthelminthic administration has removed the adult worms, larvae still develop into adult parasites and may reestablish infestation. Frequent disposal of feces will help reduce the risk of reinfection. In severe, recurrent cases, heartworm prophylaxis with milbemycin oxime (Interceptor® at 0.5 mg/kg PO q 1 month) will help control the whipworm infection.[19]

Prognosis

Clinical signs rapidly resolve following appropriate therapy. Reinfestation is common in dogs that live in contaminated environments.

6.4.2 Colitis

Acute and chronic colonic inflammation (colitis) commonly results in large bowel diarrhea in dogs and cats. Signs of colitis include excess fecal mucus, hematochezia, tenesmus, increased frequency of defecation, and reduced volume of feces per defecation. Vomiting, anorexia, dehydration, and abdominal pain may also be observed. With concurrent small bowel involvement, melena and weight loss (chronic cases only) may also occur.

Acute colitis is most commonly caused by dietary indiscretion or intolerance (see 9.1), toxin or foreign body ingestion, drug administration (antibiotics or NSAIDs), whipworm infestation (dogs only), *Clostridium perfringens* enterotoxicosis, or may be idiopathic. Infections with *Salmonella* spp. or *Campylobacter* spp. are uncommon causes of acute colitis, and may cause both small and large bowel diarrhea. Diagnosis is based on history, fecal examination, and response to dietary management with a highly digestible, low fat, and low fiber diet, or exclusion of a source of dietary indiscretion. Colonoscopy and mucosal biopsy are rarely performed, so histological documentation of colonic inflammation is not often acquired, and the speculative diagnosis of acute colitis is based on the rapid resolution of diarrhea.

Chronic colitis is usually associated with IBD (see 9.2), or *Clostridium perfringens* enterotoxicosis (see below). Uncommon causes of colitis include histiocytic ulcerative colitis (see below), pythiosis (phycomycosis), and colitis associated with histoplasmosis, the colorless unicellular alga *Prototheca* spp., or *Heterobilharzia americana* (schistosomiasis).

6.4.2.1 Histiocytic ulcerative colitis of Boxers

Histiocytic ulcerative colitis (HUC) is an uncommon, chronic, idiopathic disease characterized by progressive colitis and ulceration (Figure 6.5), which is histologically associated with an inflammatory mucosal infiltrate of plasma cells, lymphocytes, and distended PAS-positive macrophages.[20,21] The immunohistochemical characteristics of the inflammatory response have recently been characterized.[4] The disease occurs most commonly in young Boxer dogs, less than 2 years of age, but has also been reported in a French Bulldog, a Mastiff, an Alaskan Malamute, and a Doberman Pinscher.[22]

Weight loss and debilitation occur as a result of chronic intestinal blood and protein loss. A corrugated, thickened mucosa, hemorrhage, or pain may be evident on digital rectal examination.

Traditionally, treatment similar to that for IBD described in 9.2.2.4 has been suggested, with sulfasalazine being the drug of choice. Recently, preliminary evidence is accumulating that

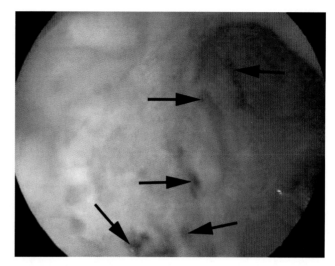

Figure 6.5:
Histiocytic ulcerative colitis. Endoscopic appearance of the descending colon in a 2-year-old Boxer with histiocytic ulcerative colitis. Erosions (arrows) and ulcers were present throughout the entire colon.

treatment with enrofloxacin at 2.5–5.0 mg/kg PO q 12 h for 4–8 weeks, may be more effective.[23] However, more cases with a longer follow-up period need to be studied. Traditionally, if signs of HUC are severe at the time of diagnosis, a poor prognosis is warranted. Dogs with mild signs may respond well to traditional therapy.[24]

6.4.2.2 Clostridium perfringens enterotoxicosis

A preliminary review has associated large bowel diarrhea with *Clostridium perfringens* type A enterotoxin.[34] The disorder occurs most commonly in dogs, but can occasionally be seen in cats. Both naturally occurring and hospital acquired cases have been described.[35] Recently, several epidemiological studies have characterized the prevalence of *Clostridium perfringens* fecal enterotoxin in dogs with diarrhea, hospitalized dogs without diarrhea, and healthy outpatients.[36–39] A concise description of this syndrome that is universally accepted has not yet emerged, and some of the syndrome's characteristics remain controversial. The author believes that *Clostridium perfringens* enterotoxicosis is a common cause of chronic large bowel diarrhea in dogs and may also be an important cause of acute diarrhea. Many questions will hopefully be answered after the completion of case-based studies in which a definitive diagnosis is reached, the animals treated with appropriate antibiotics, and the clinical outcome is assessed.

6

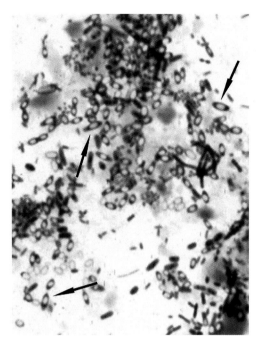

Figure 6.6:
Clostridium perfringens endospores. Huge numbers of clostridial endospores (arrows) in a rectal cytology specimen stained with a rapid Wright stain.

Pathophysiology

Clostridium perfringens is an anaerobic, spore-forming, gram-positive bacillus.[39] Five toxigenic types have been differentiated based on the production of one to four major toxins. In addition, each type can also produce other toxins. The majority of enterotoxin is produced by type A strains. A vegetative form of *C. perfringens* is a normal inhabitant of the colon.[39] The enterotoxin is produced during sporulation and causes intestinal fluid accumulation, mucosal inflammation, alterations in mucosal tight junctions, increased mucosal paracellular permeability, and diarrhea.[40] In some experimental models, the enterotoxin has its greatest effects within the small intestine. The stimuli for sporulation and enterotoxin production are unknown.

Clinical signs

Acute and chronic large bowel diarrhea commonly occur with *Clostridium perfringens* enterotoxicosis. Vomiting, weight loss, flatulence, and abdominal pain are seen less frequently. Small bowel diarrhea may also occur, but a causal relationship with *C. perfringens* is somewhat controversial. A syndrome of acute hemorrhagic diarrhea in dogs has been strongly associated with the presence of both *C. perfringens*

and *C. difficile* enterotoxins in their feces.[36] The syndrome described in that study was characterized by acute hemorrhagic diarrhea, hematemesis, severe dehydration, and necrotizing hemorrhagic enteritis and mesenteric lymphadenopathy on necropsy.

Diagnosis

The diagnosis is confirmed by identifying the enterotoxin in the feces from a dog or cat with typical clinical signs, which lack evidence of another large bowel disease. The clinical signs should rapidly improve following antibiotic administration. The only test currently available is a qualitative ELISA (Tech-Lab, Blacksburg, VA). The test is available through some commercial diagnostic laboratories. In animals with intermittent signs, fecal samples should be collected when diarrhea is present, as the enterotoxin may not be found during asymptomatic periods. There is some suspicion that refrigeration may lead to unreliable results.[41]

In the past, it has been suggested that diagnosis of this enterotoxicosis should be suspected when more than 3–5 spores per oil immersion field are seen in a rectal cytology specimen. The spores are larger than most bacteria and assume a "safety pin" appearance (Figure 6.6). However, recent epidemiological studies have not demonstrated a consistent relationship between the number of fecal spores and the presence of enterotoxin.[37,38] However, dogs with signs of large bowel diarrhea have been associated with large numbers of spores on rectal cytology.[36] In the author's experience, large numbers of spores on rectal cytology samples from dogs with typical clinical signs and diagnostic findings are usually associated with a positive test for fecal enterotoxin and rapid clinical response to antibiotic treatment. However, the presence of fecal enterotoxin, typical clinical signs, and response to antibiotic treatment may also occur in dogs without an increase in spores on a rectal cytology sample. Although endoscopic examination of affected animals has been infrequently performed, the colon may be grossly and histologically normal or may show a hyperemic, hemorrhagic, or ulcerated mucosa with histopathological findings of catarrhal or suppurative colitis.[34]

Treatment

Clinical signs in acute cases may resolve spontaneously. Affected animals usually respond to antibiotic therapy rapidly, within 3–5 days. Metronidazole at 6 mg/kg PO q 8–12 h, ampicillin at 22 mg/kg PO q 8 h, or amoxicillin at 11–22 mg/kg PO q 8–12 h, for 7–10 days are all effective.[34] Animals that develop recurrent clinical signs after treatment may require repeat therapy (1 or 2 additional times) or long-term therapy with tylosin (Tylan® powder) for 3–6 months, at 10–20 mg/kg PO q 12 h. Tylosin powder has a bitter taste and may need to

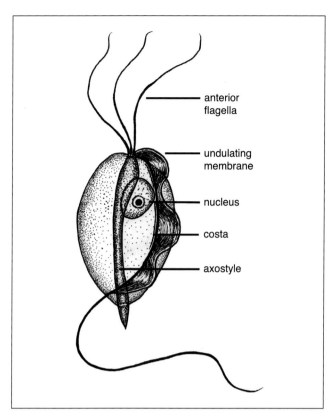

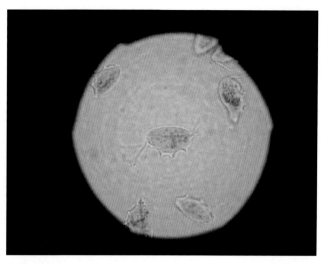

Figure 6.8:
Tritrichomonas foetus. Appearance of an individual *T. foetus* organism stained with Lugol's iodine solution. Three anterior flagellae and an undulating membrane that runs the length of the body can be seen. (Image reproduced with permission from www.fabcats.org; photograph by Andy Sparkes.)

Figure 6.7:
Tritrichomonas foetus. This line drawing shows a detailed outline of a *Tritrichomonas foetus* organism. As seen in Figure 6.8, the three flagellae and the undulating membrane are defining characteristics that can be used to differentiate *T. foetus* from other protozoal organisms on fecal examination. (Image reproduced with permission from supplemental visual material posted on the www for Biology 625 at Kansas State University; original line drawing by Jarrod Wood.)

be mixed with a small quantity of canned food or placed into a gelatin capsule. Some chronic recurrent cases benefit from feeding a high fiber diet. The proposed mechanisms of action for dietary fiber include bacterial fermentation of fiber, leading to acidification of the colon, which may inhibit sporulation, or an alteration of bacterial flora that inhibits *C. perfringens* proliferation.

Prognosis

The prognosis for patients with *Clostridium perfringens* enterotoxicosis is excellent. Most affected animals respond to therapy within several days. At the present time, clinical findings have not been identified that can predict which patients will require long-term therapy.

6.4.2.3 Tritrichomonas foetus infection

JAN S. SUCHODOLSKI

Recently, *Tritrichomonas foetus* (Figures 6.7 and 6.8), a flagellated protozoal parasite that is usually associated with venereal trichomoniasis in cattle has been identified as an intestinal pathogen in cats.[42,43] Diarrhea has been reported in cats after both experimental and natural infection. Although the true prevalence of *T. foetus* infection in cats is unknown, it is suspected to be relatively high. In one study, 31% of 117 cats examined at an international cat show were found to be infected with *T. foetus*.[44]

While cats of any age, breed, or sex can be infected, young cats that are densely housed (e.g., cats in catteries, animal shelters, or multi-cat households) seem to be at an increased risk.[43]

6

Infection is most commonly seen in young cats (i.e., those that are less than 12 months of age) but older cats may also be infected. *Tritrichomonas foetus* primarily colonizes the surface of the colonic mucosa, leading to chronic large bowel diarrhea. Without appropriate treatment cats usually remain persistently infected. While the diarrhea may spontaneously resolve, infected cats will often experience recurrent bouts of diarrhea after being exposed to stress. Indeed, cats infected with *T. foetus* generally appear healthy but show an increased frequency of defecation with loose to liquid stools, which may contain blood and/or mucus. Fecal incontinence is frequently observed. The anal region often appears edematous and may become painful with severe diarrhea. A rectal prolapse may occur in some cases.

Diagnosis

Diagnosis of a *T. foetus* infection can be made by the identification of trophozoites on a direct fecal smear examination (Figure 6.8), fecal culture, PCR analysis of fecal material, or by colonic mucosal biopsy. The disadvantages of direct fecal smear examination include a low sensitivity (14%), low specificity (*T. foetus* can be misdiagnosed as *Giardia* spp. or the non-pathogenic *Pentatrichomonas hominis*), and the fact that only fresh fecal samples can be used.

Tritrichomonas foetus can also be cultured in-house using the commercially available culture system In Pouch™ TF (Biomed Diagnostics, San Jose, CA). The pouches should be inoculated with less than 0.1 g of freshly voided feces and then incubated at 25°C. The pouches need to be evaluated under a microscope every couple of days. Results are usually obtained between 1 and 11 days after setting up a pouch. Although fecal culture is more sensitive than direct fecal smear examination, difficulties in the interpretation of results, the necessity of using freshly voided feces, and the fact that the results might not be available for up to 11 days, are important disadvantages of this method.

Tritrichomonas foetus DNA can be amplified from fecal samples by PCR.[45] PCR has been shown to be the most sensitive method for detecting *T. foetus* in fecal samples, and is ideally suited for the direct diagnosis of *T. foetus* infection.[45] The advantages of PCR testing compared to culture include a higher sensitivity, faster turnaround time, and easier handling and storing of samples since DNA is relatively stable at various temperatures.

Therapy

Until recently, a successful treatment strategy for *T. foetus* infections in cats was not available. However, a recent study has shown that administration of ronidazole (30–50 mg/kg PO q

12 h for two weeks) is effective in both resolving diarrhea and eradicating *T. foetus*.[46] There has been some anecdotal evidence that ronidazole may cause neurological side effects. However, these side effects appear to be reversible once therapy is discontinued. It should also be noted that ronidazole is not approved for use in domestic animals and it is recommended to obtain signed consent from the owner before initiating therapy. Recently, several compounding pharmacies have started offering ronidazole.

6.4.3 Irritable bowel syndrome

Irritable bowel syndrome (IBS) is a commonly diagnosed, but poorly understood functional disorder in dogs.[2] Other terms used to describe this syndrome include spastic colon, nervous colitis, and mucus colitis.[25] It has been estimated that 10–15% of dogs with chronic large bowel diarrhea have IBS.[26] Approximately 15% of human adults in the United States report symptoms consistent with a diagnosis of IBS.[27] IBS is defined by colonic dysfunction in the absence of identifiable structural, biochemical, or microbiological abnormalities. There are no data-based clinical reports of this syndrome in the veterinary literature.

In dogs, IBS is a diagnosis of exclusion and known causes of large bowel diarrhea must be eliminated before a diagnosis of IBS can be made. It is possible that dogs diagnosed with IBS: 1) may truly have a syndrome similar to IBS in human beings, 2) may have another colonic disorder that has not been correctly diagnosed, or 3) may have one of several newly described conditions, such as fiber-responsive large bowel diarrhea or *Clostridium perfringens* enterotoxicosis.

Pathophysiology

There have been no pathophysiological studies concerning IBS in dogs. Studies in human beings have investigated the role of low fiber diets, food allergy or intolerance, abnormal GI motility, altered pain and visceral perception, psychosocial factors, and an imbalance of GI neurotransmitters.[27] Abnormal myoelectrical activity leads to abnormal intestinal motility, which is likely the ultimate cause of the clinical signs.[25]

Clinical signs

In dogs, the most common clinical sign of IBS is intermittent large bowel diarrhea with excess fecal mucus, tenesmus, urgency to defecate, and increased frequency of defecation.[25] Intermittent bloating, nausea, vomiting, and abdominal pain may also occur, but hematochezia is uncommon. Often, stressors can be identified in the history and they may be associated with the development of cyclic clinical signs. Affected dogs may be hyperexcitable, unmanageable, or possess abnormal personality traits. However, dogs without these abnormalities can also develop IBS.[26]

Diagnosis

It cannot be overemphasized that IBS in dogs is a diagnosis of exclusion. A thorough diagnostic plan must be followed before a diagnosis of IBS can be made. Fecal examinations must be negative for parasite infestations and laboratory evaluation should eliminate the possibility of any systemic disorder. Also a dietary trial with a highly digestible low-fat diet and deworming against whipworms should be instituted before making a diagnosis of IBS. Finally, colonoscopic examination and mucosal biopsy must be normal (Figure 6.9). In some cases of IBS, spasm of the colonic wall may occur after contact with the endoscope. In the author's experience, response to a high fiber diet does not eliminate the presence of IBS, but it may support a diagnosis of fiber-responsive large bowel diarrhea instead. The potential relationship between IBS and fiber-responsive large bowel diarrhea will be discussed in the next section.

Treatment

The intermittent nature of clinical signs often makes assessment of IBS therapy difficult. Multiple treatments often need to be tried before a control of the clinical signs is achieved. If a stress factor or abnormal personality trait can be identified, behavioral modification can be beneficial. Unfortunately, many stressors cannot be eliminated, and many clients are unable or unwilling to alter their own behavior or attempt to alter their pet's behavior. Thus, dietary and pharmacological therapy is commonly utilized. The author has recommended supplementing highly digestible diets with a source of soluble fiber. In many cases, feeding high fiber diets can lead to a reduction in dosages and frequency of administration of pharmacological agents required or may totally eliminate the need for drug therapy. An in-depth discussion of dietary fiber can be found in the next section on fiber-responsive large bowel diarrhea.

The severity and frequency of diarrhea can also be reduced by motility modifying agents, such as loperamide or diphenoxylate. These drugs reduce diarrhea by increasing colonic segmentation. They can often be given for several days and discontinued after the diarrhea resolves.[25] Pain can often be relieved by antispasmodic agents and the effects of stressors can be reduced by sedatives. Librax® contains the sedative chlordiazepoxide (5 mg) and clidinium bromide (2.5 mg), an anticholinergic agent. A suggested dosage is 0.1–0.25 mg/kg of clidinium or 1–2 capsules of Librax® PO q 8–12 h.[25,28] The

drug can be given when the owner first notices abdominal pain or diarrhea, or when stressful conditions are anticipated or encountered, and can usually be discontinued after a few days. Other anticholinergics such as propantheline (Pro-Banthine®) at 0.25 mg/kg PO q 8–12 h, hyoscyamine (Levsin®) at 0.003–0.006 mg/kg PO q 8–12 h, or dicyclomine (Bentyl®) at 0.15 mg/kg PO q 8–12 h have also been suggested.[2,25] Anticholinergics can decrease or inhibit GI motility, which may worsen the diarrhea. Other side-effects are uncommon. In human patients with IBS, the side effects include xerostomia, urinary retention, blurred vision, headache, psychosis, nervousness, and drowsiness. On occasion, nausea and vomiting prevent the administration of oral medications. Parenteral antiemetics can be given to relieve nausea and vomiting and allow administration of oral medications 1–2 days later.[25]

Prognosis

The prognosis for a cure of IBS in dogs is guarded. Affected dogs may have intermittent clinical signs for years. Environmental, dietary, and pharmacological therapy often results in control or a reduction of clinical signs. Those dogs that respond to fiber supplementation have a good prognosis for reduction or elimination of their clinical signs (see next section).

6.4.4 Fiber-responsive large bowel diarrhea

Some dogs with chronic idiopathic large bowel diarrhea can be successfully managed by feeding a highly digestible diet supplemented with soluble fiber. Such patients are diagnosed as having fiber-responsive large bowel diarrhea (FRLBD). Most of these dogs are middle-aged.[29]

Pathophysiology

Some of the dogs with FRLBD (especially those with abnormal personality traits or environmental stressors identified in the history) can be diagnosed with IBS. Presently, the relationship between IBS and FRLBD is unclear and an overlap of cases may exist. However, many of the dogs with FRLBD have hematochezia, a clinical sign considered uncommon in dogs with IBS.[25,26] In addition, dogs with IBS only rarely have been described as responding to dietary fiber supplementation alone.[25] Thus, it is possible that dogs with FRLBD may represent a separate syndrome or a subset of IBS patients that respond to dietary fiber supplementation. Some of the dogs with FRLBD also may have *Clostridium perfringens* enterotoxicosis (see below). The pathophysiology of FRLBD is unknown.

6

6

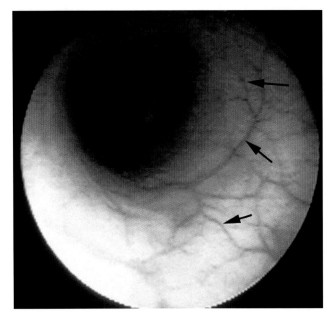

Figure 6.9:
Normal colonic mucosa. Endoscopic appearance of normal colonic mucosa in a dog with idiopathic large bowel diarrhea. The mucosa is smooth and glistening, and submucosal blood vessels are clearly visible (arrows).

Clinical signs

The predominant clinical sign of dogs with FRLBD is chronic intermittent large bowel diarrhea, with hematochezia, excess fecal mucus, and tenesmus. Some dogs may have continuous diarrhea. Occasionally, vomiting and decreased appetite can occur. Abnormal personality traits and environmental stress factors are found in approximately 38% of affected dogs. Only rarely do owners describe their dogs as nervous or highly strung. Separation anxiety, submissive urination, noise sensitivity, fear of thunderstorms, or aggression occur rarely. In most cases, it is not possible to relate stressors or personality traits to the development or intensification of the diarrhea. Some stressful factors that have been identified include: household visitors, travel, moving, construction, installation of an invisible fence, death of another household pet, or visits to the groomer, veterinarian, or a dog show.

Diagnosis

The diagnosis of FRLBD is based on exclusion of known causes of large bowel diarrhea after a thorough diagnostic evaluation, including colonoscopy (Figure 6.9) and mucosal biopsy. If no cause of diarrhea is identified, the diagnosis of idiopathic large bowel diarrhea is made. If the diarrhea re-

sponds to fiber supplementation, the diagnosis is amended to FRLBD.

Treatment

Dietary fiber is a collective term for a wide variety of plant polysaccharides and lignins that are resistant to mammalian digestive enzymes.[30] There are many types of dietary fiber, each with diverse chemical, physical, and physiological properties.[30] Water-soluble fibers include pectin, gums, mucilages, and some hemicelluloses.[30] They are found in the parenchymatous portions of fruits and vegetables, and in the seeds of leguminous plants. Water-insoluble fibers include cellulose, lignin, and some hemicelluloses, and are found in cereal grains and seed coats.

Dietary fiber supplementation has been shown to normalize colonic myoelectrical activity and colonic motility in humans. There are several potential mechanisms by which dietary fiber supplementation results in clinical improvement in dogs with FRLBD. Soluble fibers adsorb a large quantity of water, improving fecal consistency. Colonic bacteria, which make up approximately 40–55% of the dry stool mass, ferment soluble fiber, which results in a vast increase in the numbers (but not types) of colonic bacteria and quantity of bacterial byproducts.[31,32] Bacterial fermentation of fiber leads to the production of short-chain fatty acids, of which butyrate serves as an energy source for colonocytes.[31,32] In addition, short-chain fatty acids promote differentiation and proliferation of colonocytes, stimulate absorption of water and electrolytes, and stimulate contraction of longitudinal muscle. Insoluble fiber greatly adds to fecal volume. Thus, dietary fiber can increase fecal bulk, which increases colonic distension, the major stimulus for normal colonic motility. With increased colonic distension, an improved motility pattern in dogs with FRLBD may result in normal defecation and resolution of clinical signs.

Psyllium comes from the seeds or husks of the plant *Plantago ovata* and consists of approximately 90% soluble fiber. Although there are no studies evaluating the use of soluble fibers in dogs with diarrhea, there are such studies in human beings. Psyllium was beneficial in treating a group of children with idiopathic chronic nonspecific diarrhea.[33] Since the beneficial effects persisted after the withdrawal of fiber supplementation, the authors postulated that psyllium led to an alteration of the colonic flora. In addition, psyllium has also been shown to be beneficial in human adults with nonspecific chronic diarrhea, ulcerative colitis in remission, some patients with IBS, burn patients receiving enteral nutrition, other patients being tube fed, and some patients with other diarrheal disorders.[29]

A highly digestible low-fiber diet supplemented with psyllium hydrophilic mucilloid (Metamucil®; 1–3 tablespoons/day) will benefit many dogs with chronic idiopathic large bowel diarrhea. In the cases reported by the author, the median amount of Metamucil® added to the diet was 1.33 g/kg/day (range: 0.31–4.9 g/kg/day). In some cases, drug therapy for IBS may need to be added to the treatment protocol.

Some dogs can have the amount of supplemented fiber reduced and possibly withdrawn entirely, while others require long-term supplementation. In addition, some dogs can be switched from a highly digestible diet to a regular maintenance diet without relapsing diarrhea.

Prognosis

The prognosis for dogs with FRLBD is very good to excellent for those patients that respond to soluble fiber supplementation. Since no specific clinical findings have been identified that can predict whether an individual dog will respond to fiber therapy, a therapeutic trial is necessary. The prognosis is more guarded for those patients that only partially respond to fiber supplementation and require drug therapy for IBS.

🔑 Key Facts

- The major functions of the large intestine are extraction of water and electrolytes from the ileal effluent, storage of feces, and defecation.
- The most common clinical sign of large intestinal disease is diarrhea, usually characterized by increased frequency of defecation, decreased quantity of stool per defecation, tenesmus, hematochezia, and excess mucus.
- *Trichuris vulpis* infestation is one of the most common causes of acute or chronic large bowel diarrhea in dogs.
- In dogs, irritable bowel syndrome is a diagnosis of exclusion and known causes of large bowel diarrhea must be eliminated before a diagnosis of irritable bowel syndrome can be made.
- A highly digestible low-fiber diet supplemented with psyllium hydrophilic mucilloid at 1–3 tablespoons/day will benefit many dogs with chronic idiopathic large bowel diarrhea.

References

1. Leib MS, Matz ME. Diseases of the large intestine. In: Ettinger SJ, Feldman EC (eds.), *Textbook of Veterinary Internal Medicine*. Philadelphia, WB Saunders, 1995; 1232–1260.
2. Leib M, Matz M. Diseases of the intestines. In: Leib M, Monroe W (eds.), *Practical Small Animal Internal Medicine*. Philadelphia, WB Saunders, 1997; 685–760.
3. Roth L, Walton AM, Leib MS. Plasma cell populations in the colonic mucosa of clinically normal dogs. *J Am Anim Hosp Assoc* 1992; 28: 39–42.
4. German A, Hall E, Kelly D et al. An immunohistochemical study of histiocytic ulcerative colitis in Boxer dogs. *J Comp Pathol* 2000; 122: 163–175.
5. Karaus M, Sarna SK. Giant migrating contractions during defecation in the dog colon. *Gastroenterology* 1987; 92: 925–933.
6. Washabau R, Holt D, Brockman D. Mediation of acetylcholine and substance P induced contractions by myosin light chain phosphorylation in feline colonic smooth muscle. *Am J Vet Res* 2002; 63: 695–702.
7. Washabau R, Stalis I. Alterations in colonic smooth muscle function in cats with idiopathic megacolon. *Am J Vet Res* 1996; 57: 580–587.
8. Snape WJ, Tan ST, Kao HW. Effects of bethanechol and the octapeptide of cholecystokinin on colonic smooth muscle in the cat. *Am J Physiol* 1987; 252: G654–G661.
9. Strombeck DR. Small and large intestine, normal structure and function. In: Strombeck DR, Guilford WG, Center SA, Williams DA (eds.), *Small Animal Gastroenterology*. Philadelphia, WB Saunders, 1996; 318–350.
10. Willard MD. Normal immune function of the gastrointestinal tract. *Sem Vet Med Surg* 1992; 7: 107–111.
11. Cave N. Chronic inflammatory disorders of the gastrointestinal tract of companion animals. *NZ Vet J* 2003; 51: 262–274.
12. Jergens A. Understanding gastrointestinal inflammation – implications for therapy. *J Feline Med Surg* 2002; 4: 179–182.
13. Leib MS, Codner EC, Monroe WE. A diagnostic approach to chronic large bowel diarrhea in dogs. *Vet Med* 1991; 86: 892–899.
14. Campbell BG. Trichuris and other trichinelloid nematodes of dogs and cats in the United States. *Compend Contin Educ Pract Vet* 1991; 13: 769–780.
15. Hendrix CM, Blagburn BL, Lindsay DS. Whipworms and intestinal threadworms. *Vet Clin North Am Small Anim Prac* 1987; 17: 1355–1375.
16. Zajac A, Johnson J, King S. Evaluation of the importance of centrifugation as a component of zinc sulfate fecal flotation examinations. *J Am Anim Hosp Assoc* 2002; 38: 221–224.
17. Leib MS, Codner EC, Monroe WE. Common colonoscopic findings in dogs with chronic large bowel diarrhea. *Vet Med* 1991; 86: 913–921.
18. Lloyd S, Gemmell MA. Efficacy of a drug combination of praziquantel, pyrantel embonate, and febantel against helminth infections in dogs. *Am J Vet Res* 1992; 53: 2272–2273.
19. Zajac AM. Developments in the treatment of gastrointestinal parasites of small animals. *Vet Clin North Am Small Anim Pract* 1993; 23: 671–681.
20. Ewing GO, Gomez JA. Canine ulcerative colitis. *J Am Anim Hosp Assoc* 1973; 9: 395–406.
21. Hall EJ, Rutgers HC, Scholes SFE et al. Histiocytic ulcerative colitis in Boxer dogs in the UK. *J Small Anim Pract* 1994; 35: 509–515.
22. Stokes J, Kruger J, Mullaney T et al. Histiocytic ulcerative colitis in three non-Boxer dogs. *J Am Anim Hosp Assoc* 2001; 37: 461–465.

23. Davies D, O'Hara A, Irwin P et al. Successful management of histiocytic ulcerative colitis with enrofloxacin in two Boxer dogs. *Aust Vet J* 2004; 82: 58–61.

24. Churcher R, Watson A. Canine histiocytic ulcerative colitis. *Aust Vet J* 1997; 75: 710–713.

25. Tams TR. Irritable bowel syndrome. In: Kirk RW, Bonagura JD (eds.), *Current Veterinary Therapy XI.* Philadelphia, WB Saunders, 1992; 604–608.

26. Burrows CF. Medical diseases of the colon. In: Jones BD, Liska WD (eds.), *Canine and Feline Gastroenterology.* Philadelphia, WB Saunders, 1986; 221–256.

27. Horwitz B, Fisher R. The irritable bowel syndrome. *N Engl J Med* 2001; 344: 1846–1850.

28. Johnson SE. Clinical pharmacology of antiemetics and antidiarrheals. *Proc of the Eighth Kal Kan Sym Treat Small Anim Dis,* Columbus, OH, 1984; 7–15.

29. Leib M. Treatment of chronic idiopathic large-bowel diarrhea in dogs with a highly digestible diet and soluble fiber: A retrospective review of 37 cases. *J Am Vet Med Assoc* 2000; 14: 27–32.

30. Dimski DS, Buffington CA. Dietary fiber in small animal therapeutics. *J Am Vet Med Assoc* 1991; 199: 1142–1146.

31. Cranston D, McWhinnie D, Collin J. Dietary fibre and gastrointestinal disease. *Br J Surg* 1988; 75: 508–512.

32. Eastwood MA. The physiological effect of dietary fiber: an update. *Ann Rev Nut* 1992; 12: 19–35.

33. Smalley JR, Klish WJ, Campbell MA et al. Use of psyllium in the management of chronic nonspecific diarrhea of childhood. *J Ped Gastroenterol Nut* 1982; 1: 361–363.

34. Twedt DC. Clostridium perfringens-associated enterotoxicosis in dogs. In: Kirk RW, Bonagura JD (eds.), *Current Veterinary Therapy XI.* Philadelphia, WB Saunders, 1992; 602–604.

35. Kruth SA, Prescott JF, Welch MK et al. Nosocomial diarrhea associated with enterotoxigenic *Clostridium perfringens* infection in dogs. *J Am Vet Med Assoc* 1989; 195: 331–334.

36. Cave N, Marks S, Kass P et al. Evaluation of a routine diagnostic fecal panel for dogs with diarrhea. *J Am Vet Med Assoc* 2002; 221: 52–59.

37. Weese J, Staempfi H, Prescott J et al. The roles of *Clostridium difficile* and enterotoxigenic *Clostridium perfringens* in diarrhea in dogs. *J Vet Intern Med* 2001; 15: 374–378.

38. Marks SL, Melli A, Kass PH et al. Evaluation of methods to diagnose *Clostridium perfringens*-associated diarrhea in dogs. *J Am Vet Med Assoc* 1999; 214: 357–360.

39. Marks S, Kather E, Kass P et al. Genotypic and phenotypic characterization of *Clostridium perfringens* and *Clostridium difficile* in diarrheic and healthy dogs. *J Vet Intern Med* 2002; 16: 533–540.

40. Niilo L. *Clostridium perfringens* in animal disease: A review of current knowledge. *Can Vet J* 1980; 21: 141–148.

41. Marks S, Melli A, Kass P et al. Influence of storage and temperature on endospore and enterotoxin production by *Clostridium perfringens* in dogs. *J Vet Diag Invest* 2000; 12: 63–67.

42. Foster DM, Gookin JL, Poore MF et al. Outcome of cats with diarrhea and *Tritrichomonas foetus* infection. *J Am Vet Med Assoc* 2004; 225: 888–892.

43. Gookin JL, Breitschwerdt EB, Levy MG et al. Diarrhea associated with trichomonosis in cats. *J Am Vet Med Assoc* 1999; 215: 1450–1454.

44. Gookin JL, Stebbins ME, Hunt E et al. Prevalence of and risk factors for feline *Tritrichomonas foetus* and *Giardia* infection. *J Clin Microbiol* 2004; 42: 2707–2710.

45. Gookin JL, Birkenheuer AJ, Breitschwerdt EB, et al. Single-tube nested PCR for detection of *Tritrichomonas foetus* in feline feces. *J Clin Microbiol* 2002; 40: 4126–4130.

46. Gookin JL, Copple CN, Papich MG, et al. Efficacy of ronidazole for treatment of feline *Tritrichomonas foetus* infection. *J Vet Intern Med* 2006; 20: 536–543.

6.4.5 Feline megacolon

Robert J. Washabau

Etiology

The etiopathogenesis of idiopathic megacolon in the cat is still incompletely understood. Several reviews have emphasized the importance of considering an extensive list of differential diagnoses (e.g., neuromuscular, mechanical, inflammatory, metabolic/endocrine, pharmacological, environmental, and behavioral causes) for the obstipated cat (Table 6.1).[1] A review of published cases suggests that 96% of cases of obstipation are accounted for by idiopathic megacolon (62%), pelvic canal stenosis (23%), nerve injury (6%), or Manx sacral spinal cord deformity (5%).[2] It is important to consider an extensive list of differential diagnoses in an individual animal, but it should be kept in mind that most cases are idiopathic, orthopedic, or neurological in origin.

Pathophysiology

Megacolon develops through two pathological mechanisms: dilation and hypertrophy. Dilated megacolon is the end stage of colonic dysfunction in idiopathic cases. Cats affected with idiopathic dilated megacolon have a permanent loss of colonic structure and function. Medical therapy may be attempted in such cases, but most affected cats eventually require colectomy. Hypertrophic megacolon, on the other hand, develops as a consequence of obstructive lesions (e.g., malunion of pelvic fractures, tumors, or foreign bodies). Hypertrophic megacolon may be reversible with early pelvic osteotomy or it may progress to irreversible dilated megacolon if appropriate therapy is not instituted.

Constipation and obstipation are earlier manifestations of the same problem.[3] Constipation is defined as the infrequent or difficult evacuation of feces, but does not necessarily imply a permanent loss of function. Many cats suffer from one or two episodes of constipation without further progression. Intracta-

Table 6.1: Differential diagnoses for constipation in the cat

Neuromuscular dysfunction
- Colonic smooth muscle: idiopathic megacolon, aging
- Spinal cord disease: lumbosacral disease, cauda equina syndrome, sacral spinal cord deformities (Manx cat)
- Hypogastric or pelvic nerve disorders: traumatic injury, malignancy, dysautonomia
- Submucosal or myenteric plexus neuropathy: dysautonomia, aging

Mechanical obstruction
- Intraluminal: foreign material (bones, plant material, hair), neoplasia, rectal diverticula, perineal hernia, anorectal strictures
- Intramural: neoplasia
- Extraluminal: pelvic fractures, neoplasia

Inflammation
- Perianal fistula, proctitis, anal sac abscess, anorectal foreign bodies, perianal bite wounds

Metabolic and endocrine
- Metabolic: dehydration, hypokalemia, hypercalcemia
- Endocrine: hypothyroidism, obesity, nutritional secondary hyperparathyroidism

Pharmacological
- Opioid agonists, cholinergic antagonists, diuretics, barium sulfate, phenothiazines

Environmental and behavioral
- Soiled litter box, inactivity, hospitalization, change in environment

ble constipation that has become refractory to control is referred to as obstipation and implies a permanent loss of function. A cat is assumed to be obstipated only after several consecutive treatments have failed. Recurring episodes of constipation or obstipation may culminate in the syndrome of megacolon.

The pathogenesis of idiopathic dilated megacolon appears to involve the functional disturbance of colonic smooth muscle. In-vitro isometric stress measurements have been performed on colonic smooth muscle obtained from cats with idiopathic dilated megacolon.[4,5] These studies initially suggested that the disorder of feline idiopathic megacolon is a generalized dysfunction of colonic smooth muscle, and that treatments aimed at stimulating colonic smooth muscle contraction might improve colonic motility. More recent studies suggest that the lesion may begin in the descending colon and progress to involve the ascending colon over time.[6]

Clinical history

Constipation, obstipation, and megacolon may be observed in cats of any age, sex, or breed; however, most cases are observed in middle-aged (mean = 5.8 years), male cats (70% male, 30% female) of DSH (46%), Domestic Longhair (15%), or Siamese (12%) breeding.[2] Affected cats are usually presented for reduced, absent, or painful defecation for a period of time ranging from days to weeks or months. Some cats are observed making multiple, unproductive attempts to defecate in the litter box, while other cats may sit in the litter box for prolonged periods of time without assuming a defecation posture. Dry, hardened feces are observed inside and outside of the litter box. Occasionally, chronically constipated cats have intermittent episodes of hematochezia or diarrhea due to mucosal irritation caused by fecal concretions. This may give the pet owner the erroneous impression that diarrhea is the primary problem. Prolonged inability to defecate may result in other systemic signs, including anorexia, lethargy, weight loss, and vomiting.

Clinical presentation

Colonic impaction is a consistent physical examination finding in affected cats. Other findings will depend on the severity and pathogenesis of constipation. Dehydration, weight loss, debilitation, abdominal pain, and mild to moderate mesenteric lymphadenopathy may also be observed in cats with severe idiopathic megacolon. Colonic impaction may be so severe as to render it difficult to differentiate impaction from colonic, mesenteric, or other abdominal neoplasia. Cats with constipation due to dysautonomia may have other signs of autonomic nervous system failure, such as urinary and fecal incontinence, regurgitation due to megaesophagus, mydriasis, decreased lacrimation, prolapse of the nictitating membrane, and bradycardia.

Diagnosis

Digital rectal examination should be carefully performed with sedation or anesthesia in all cats. Pelvic fracture malunion may be detected on rectal examination in cats with pelvic trauma. Rectal examination might also identify other unusual causes of constipation, such as foreign bodies, rectal diverticula, strictures, inflammation, or neoplasia. Chronic tenesmus may be associated with perineal herniation in some cases. A complete neurological examination with special emphasis on caudal spinal cord function should be performed to identify neurological causes of constipation, e.g. spinal cord injury, pelvic nerve trauma, and Manx sacral spinal cord deformity.

6

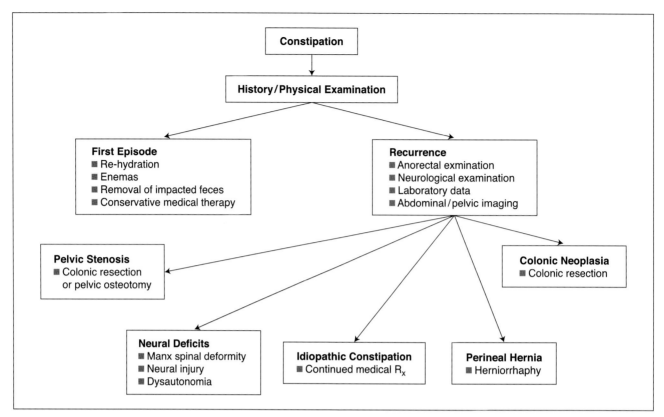

Figure 6.10:
Constipation. This figure shows a systematic work-up for a cat presented for constipation.

While most patients with obstipation and megacolon are unlikely to have significant changes in laboratory data (e.g., CBC, serum chemistry, and urinalysis), these tests should nonetheless be performed in all cats presented for constipation (Figure 6.10). Metabolic causes of constipation, such as dehydration, hypokalemia, and hypercalcemia may be detected in some cases. Though hypothyroidism is a rare cause of constipation in cats, basal serum T4 concentration and other thyroid function tests should also be considered in cats with additional signs consistent with hypothyroidism. Constipation could theoretically also develop following successful treatment of feline hyperthyroidism.

Abdominal radiography should be performed in all constipated cats to characterize the severity of colonic impaction, and to identify predisposing factors such as intraluminal radio-opaque foreign material (e.g., bone chips), intraluminal or extraluminal mass lesions, pelvic fractures, and spinal cord abnormalities. The radiographic findings of colonic impaction cannot be used to distinguish between constipation, obstipation, and megacolon in idiopathic cases. The first or second episodes of constipation in some cats may be severe and generalized but may still resolve with appropriate treatment.

Ancillary studies may be indicated in some cases. Extraluminal mass lesions may be further evaluated by abdominal ultrasonography and ultrasound-guided biopsy, whereas intraluminal mass lesions are best evaluated by endoscopy. Colonoscopy may also be used to evaluate the colon and anorectum for suspected inflammatory lesions, strictures, sacculations, and diverticula. Barium enema contrast radiography may be used if colonoscopy is not possible. Both colonoscopy and barium enema contrast radiography will require general anesthesia and evacuation of impacted feces. Cerebrospinal fluid analysis, CT or MRI, and electrophysiological studies should be considered in animals with evidence of neurological impairment. Finally, colonic biopsy or anorectal manometry will be necessary to diagnose suspected cases of aganglionic megacolon.

Treatment

The specific therapeutic plan will depend upon the severity of constipation and the underlying cause.[1] Medical therapy may not be necessary with first episodes of constipation. First episodes are often transient and resolve without therapy. Mild to moderate or recurrent episodes of constipation, on the other

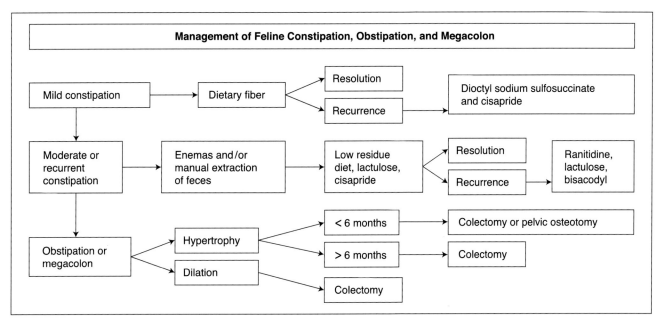

Figure 6.11:
Management of feline obstipation, constipation, and megacolon.

hand, usually require some medical intervention. These cases may be managed, often on an outpatient basis, with dietary modification, water enemas, oral or suppository laxatives, and/ or colonic prokinetic agents. Severe cases of constipation usually require brief periods of hospitalization to correct metabolic abnormalities and to evacuate impacted feces using water enemas, manual extraction of retained feces, or both. Follow-up therapy in such cases is directed at correcting predisposing factors and preventing recurrence. Subtotal colectomy will become necessary in cats suffering from obstipation or idiopathic dilated megacolon. These cats, by definition, are unresponsive to medical therapy. Pelvic osteotomy without colectomy may be sufficient for some cats suffering from pelvic canal stenosis and hypertrophic megacolon.[7] An algorithm for the therapeutic approach to the constipated, obstipated, and megacolonic cat is outlined in Figure 6.11.

Removal of impacted feces

The removal of impacted feces may be accomplished through the use of rectal suppositories, enemas, or manual extraction.

Rectal suppositories. A number of pediatric rectal suppositories are available for the management of mild constipation. These include dioctyl sodium sulfosuccinate (emollient laxative), glycerin (lubricant laxative), and bisacodyl (stimulant laxative).

Table 6.2: Index of pharmaceutical agents for constipation

Drug class	Examples
Rectal Suppositories	■ Bisacodyl (Dulcolax, Boehringer Ingelheim) ■ Dioctyl sodium sulfosuccinate (Colace, Mead Johnson) ■ Glycerine
Enemas	■ Warm tap water ■ Warm isotonic saline ■ Dioctyl sodium sulfosuccinate (Colace, Mead Johnson) ■ Dioctyl sodium sulfosuccinate (Disposaject, PittmanMoore) ■ Lactulose (Cephulac, Merrell Dow; or Duphalac, Reid Rowell) ■ Mineral oil

Oral Laxatives	■ Bulk laxatives
	   – Canned pumpkin
	   – Coarse wheat bran
	   – Psyllium (Metamucil, Searle)
	 ■ Emollient laxatives
	   – Dioctyl calcium sulfosuccinate (Surfax, Hoechst)
	   – Dioctyl sodium sulfosuccinate (Colace, Mead Johnson)
	 ■ Lubricant laxatives
	   – Hyperosmotic laxatives
	   – Lactulose (Cephulac, Merrell Dow; or Duphalac, Reid Rowell)
	   – Mineral oil
	   – Petrolatum (Laxatone; Evsco)
	 ■ Stimulant laxatives
	   – Bisacodyl (Dulcolax; Boehringer Ingelheim)

Prokinetic agents	■ Cisapride (compounding pharmacies)[14] ■ Nizatidine (Axid; Eli Lilly) ■ Ranitidine (Zantac; Glaxo SmithKline)

Enemas. Mild to moderate or recurrent episodes of constipation may require administration of enemas and/or manual extraction of impacted feces. Several types of enema solutions may be administered, such as warm tap water (5–10 mL/kg), warm isotonic saline (5–10 mL/kg), dioctyl sodium sulfosuccinate (5–10 mL/cat), mineral oil (5–10 mL/cat), or lactulose (5–10 mL/cat). Enema solutions should be administered slowly with a well-lubricated 10–12 F rubber catheter or feeding tube. Enemas containing sodium phosphate are contraindicated in cats because of their propensity for inducing severe hypernatremia, hyperphosphatemia, and hypocalcemia in this species.

Manual extraction. Cases unresponsive to enemas may require the manual extraction of impacted feces. Cats should be adequately rehydrated and then anesthetized with an endotracheal tube in place to prevent aspiration should colonic manipulation induce vomiting. Water or saline is infused into the colon while the fecal mass is manually reduced by abdominal palpation. Sponge forceps may also be introduced with caution rectally to break down the fecal mass. It may be advisable to evacuate the fecal mass over a period of several days to reduce the risks of prolonged anesthesia and perforation of a devitalized colon.

Laxative therapy

Laxatives promote evacuation of the bowel through the stimulation of fluid and electrolyte transport or an increase in propulsive motility. They are classified as bulk-forming, emollient, lubricant, hyperosmotic, or stimulant laxatives according to their mechanism of action. There are literally hundreds of products available for the treatment of constipation. Table 6.2 summarizes those products that have been used with some success in cats.

Bulk-forming laxatives. Most of the available bulk-forming laxatives are dietary fiber supplements of poorly digestible polysaccharides and celluloses derived principally from cereal grains, wheat bran, and psyllium.[8] Fiber-supplemented diets are available commercially, or the pet owner may wish to add psyllium (1–4 teaspoons per meal), wheat bran (1–2 tablespoons per meal), or pumpkin (1–4 tablespoons per meal) to canned cat food. Cats should be well hydrated before commencing fiber supplementation to maximize the therapeutic effect. Fiber supplementation is most beneficial in mildly constipated cats, prior to the development of obstipation and megacolon. In obstipated and megacolon cats, fiber may in fact be detrimental and low residue diets may be more beneficial in cats with these conditions.

Emollient laxatives. Emollient laxatives are anionic detergents that increase the miscibility of water and lipid in ingesta, thereby enhancing lipid absorption and impairing water absorption. Dioctyl sodium sulfosuccinate and dioctyl calcium

sulfosuccinate are examples of emollient laxatives available in oral and enema form. Anecdotal experience suggests that dioctyl sodium sulfosuccinate therapy may be most useful in animals with acute but not chronic constipation. As with bulk-forming laxatives, animals should be well-hydrated before emollient laxatives are administered. It should be noted that the clinical efficacy has not been definitively established for emollient laxatives. Dioctyl sodium sulfosuccinate, for example, inhibits water absorption in isolated colonic segments *in vitro*, but it may be impossible to achieve tissue concentrations great enough to inhibit colonic water absorption *in vivo*. Further studies are required to determine the clinical efficacy and therapeutic role of dioctyl sodium sulfosuccinate in the management of the constipated cat.

Lubricant laxatives. Mineral oil and white petrolatum are the two major lubricant laxatives available for the treatment of constipation. The lubricating properties of these agents impede colonic water absorption as well as permit greater ease of fecal passage. These effects are usually moderate, however, and, in general, lubricants are beneficial only in mild cases of constipation. Mineral oil usage should probably be limited to rectal administration because of the risk of aspiration pneumonia with oral administration, especially in depressed or debilitated cats.

Hyperosmotic laxatives. This group of laxatives consists of the poorly absorbed polysaccharides (e.g., lactose or lactulose), the magnesium salts (e.g., magnesium citrate, magnesium hydroxide, or magnesium sulfate), and the polyethylene glycols. Lactose is not effective as a laxative agent in all cats.[12] Lactulose is the most effective agent in this group. The organic acids produced from lactulose fermentation stimulate colonic fluid secretion and propulsive motility. Lactulose administered at a dosage of 0.5 mL/kg body weight PO q 8–12 h fairly consistently produces soft feces in the cat. Many cats with recurrent or chronic constipation have been well managed with this regimen of lactulose. The dosage may have to be tapered in individual cases if flatulence and diarrhea become excessive. Magnesium salts are not currently recommended in the treatment of feline constipation and idiopathic megacolon. Some veterinarians have reported anecdotal successes with the polyethylene glycols.

Stimulant laxatives. The stimulant laxatives (bisacodyl, phenolphthalein, castor oil, cascara, and senna) are a diverse group of agents that have been classified according to their ability to stimulate propulsive motility. Bisacodyl, for example, stimulates nitric oxide-mediated epithelial cell secretion and myenteric neuronal depolarization. Diarrhea results from the combined effect of increased mucosal secretion and colonic propulsion. Bisacodyl, at a dosage of 5 mg per cat PO q 24 h, is the most effective stimulant laxative in the cat. It may be given individually or in combination with fiber supplementation for the long-term management of constipation. Daily administration of bisacodyl should probably be avoided, however, because of injury to the myenteric neurons with chronic usage.

Colonic prokinetic agents

Previous studies of feline colonic smooth muscle function have suggested that stimulation of colonic smooth muscle contraction might improve colonic motility in cats affected with idiopathic dilated megacolon.[4,5,9] Unfortunately, many of the currently available GI prokinetic agents have not proved useful in the therapy of feline constipation, either because of significant side effects (e.g., bethanechol) or because the prokinetic effect is limited to the proximal GI tract (e.g., metoclopramide, domperidone, or erythromycin). The 5-HT$_4$ serotonergic agonists (e.g., cisapride, prucalopride, tegaserod, and mosapride) appear to have the advantage of stimulating motility from the gastroesophageal sphincter to the descending colon with relatively few side effects.[10] Cisapride, for example, increases gastroesophageal sphincter pressure, promotes gastric emptying, and enhances small intestinal and colonic propulsive motility. Cisapride enhances colonic propulsive motility through the activation of colonic neuronal or smooth muscle 5-HT receptors in a number of animal species.[11,12] In vitro studies have shown that cisapride stimulates feline colonic smooth muscle contraction, although it has not yet been conclusively shown that cisapride stimulates feline colonic propulsive motility in vivo.[5,12] A large body of anecdotal experience suggests that cisapride is effective in stimulating colonic propulsive motility in cats affected with mild to moderate idiopathic constipation; cats with long-standing obstipation and megacolon are not likely to show much improvement with cisapride therapy. Cisapride was widely used in the management of canine and feline gastric emptying, intestinal transit, and colonic motility disorders throughout most of the 1990s.[10,13,14] Cisapride was withdrawn from the USA, Canada and certain Western European countries in July of 2000 following reports of untoward cardiac side effects in human patients. Similar cardiac effects have been characterized in experimental dogs, but in vivo effects have not yet been reported in dogs or cats. The withdrawal of cisapride has created a clear need for new GI prokinetic agents, although cisapride continues to be available in several western European countries and from compounding pharmacies throughout the United States.

Prucalopride, a new prokinetic agent currently undergoing drug-development and testing may prove useful in the therapy of GI motility disorders of several animal species.

Misoprostol is a prostaglandin E$_1$ analogue that reduces the incidence of NSAID-induced gastric injury. The main side effects of misoprostol therapy are abdominal discomfort, cramping, and diarrhea. Studies in dogs suggest that prostaglandins may initiate a giant migrating complex pattern and increase colonic propulsive activity. In vitro studies of misoprostol show that it stimulates feline and canine colonic smooth muscle contraction. Given its limited toxicity, misoprostol may be useful in cats (and dogs) with severe refractory constipation.

Ranitidine and nizatidine, classic histamine H$_2$ receptor antagonists, may also stimulate canine and feline colonic motility. These drugs stimulate contraction apparently through the inhibition of tissue acetylcholinesterase and accumulation of acetylcholine at the motor endplate. It is not yet clear how effective these drugs are in vivo, although both drugs stimulate feline colonic smooth muscle contraction in vitro. Cimetidine and famotidine, members of the same class of drug, are without this effect.

Surgery

Colectomy should be considered in cats that are refractory to medical therapy. Cats have a generally favorable prognosis for recovery following colectomy, although mild to moderate diarrhea may persist for weeks to months postoperatively in some cases.[15,16] Pelvic osteotomy without colectomy has been recommended for cats with pelvic fracture malunion and hypertrophic megacolon of less than 6 months duration.[17] Pathological hypertrophy may be reversible with early pelvic osteotomy in such cases. Some surgeons still prefer colectomy in this instance because of the technical difficulty of some pelvic osteotomies.[18]

Prognosis

Many cats have one or two episodes of constipation without further recurrence, although others may progress to complete colonic failure. Cats with mild to moderate constipation generally respond to conservative medical management (e.g., dietary modification, emollient or hyperosmotic laxatives, and colonic prokinetic agents). Early use of colonic prokinetic agents (in addition to one or more laxative agents) is likely to prevent the progression of constipation to obstipation and dilated megacolon in these cats. Some cats may become refractory to these therapies, however, as they progress through moderate or recurrent constipation to obstipation and dilated megacolon; these cats eventually require colectomy. Cats have a generally favorable prognosis for recovery following colectomy, although mild to moderate diarrhea may persist for 4 to 6 weeks post-operatively in some cases.

6

🔑 Key Facts

- ▪ Megacolon is a disorder found most often in male, middle-aged cats, although it may affect cats of any age, gender, or breed.
- ▪ Medical therapy consists of colonic reduction of impacted fecal material, laxative therapy, prokinetic therapy, and surgery.
- ▪ Cats may have transient diarrhea following sub-total colectomy, but most recover normal intestinal function following such surgery.

References

1. Washabau RJ, Holt DE. Pathogenesis, diagnosis, and therapy of feline idiopathic megacolon. *Vet Clin N Am Small Anim Pract* 1999; 29: 589–603.
2. Washabau RJ, Hasler A. Constipation, obstipation, and megacolon. In: JR August (ed.), *Consultations in Feline Internal Medicine, 3rd ed.* Philadelphia, WB Saunders, 1997; 104–112.
3. Washabau RJ, Holt DE. Pathophysiology of gastrointestinal disease. In: Slatter D (ed.), *Textbook of Veterinary Surgery, 3rd ed.* Philadelphia, WB Saunders, 2003; 530–552.
4. Washabau RJ, Stalis I. Alterations in colonic smooth muscle function in cats with idiopathic megacolon. *Am J Vet Res* 1996; 57: 580–587.
5. Hasler AH, Washabau RJ. Cisapride stimulates contraction of feline idiopathic megacolonic smooth muscle. *J Vet Intern Med* 1997; 11: 313–318.
6. Washabau RJ, Holt DE. Segmental colonic dysfunction in cats with idiopathic megacolon. *Proc 15th ACVIM Forum* 1997; 664 (abstract).
7. Schrader SC. Pelvic osteotomy as a treatment for constipation in cats with acquired stenosis of the pelvic canal. *J Am Vet Med Assoc* 1992; 200: 208–213.
8. Rondeau M, Michel K, McManus C et al. Butyrate and propionate stimulate feline longitudinal colonic smooth muscle contraction. *J Feline Med Surg* 2003; 5: 167–173.
9. Washabau RJ. Gastrointestinal motility disorders and gastrointestinal prokinetic therapy. *Vet Clin N Am Small Anim Pract* 2003; 33: 1007–1028.
10. Washabau RJ, Hall JA. Clinical pharmacology of cisapride. *J Am Vet Med Assoc* 1995; 207: 1285–1288.
11. Graf S, Sarna SK. 5-HT-induced colonic contractions: enteric locus of action and receptor subtypes. *Am J Physiol* 1997; 273: G68–G74.
12. Washabau RJ, Sammarco J. Effects of cisapride on feline colonic smooth muscle function. *Am J Vet Res* 1996; 57: 541–546.
13. Washabau RJ, Hall JA. Gastrointestinal prokinetic therapy: serotonergic drugs. *Compend Contin Educ Pract Vet* 1997; 19: 721–737.
14. LeGrange SN, Boothe DM, Herndon S et al. Pharmacokinetics and suggested oral dosing regimen of cisapride: a study in healthy cats. *J Am Anim Hosp Assoc* 1997; 33: 517–523.
15. Rosin E, Walshaw R, Mehlhaff C et al. Subtotal colectomy for treatment of chronic constipation associated with idiopathic megacolon in cats. *J Am Vet Med Assoc* 1988; 193: 850–853.
16. Gregory CR, Guilford WG, Berry CR et al. Enteric function in cats after subtotal colectomy for treatment of megacolon. *Vet Surg* 1990; 19: 216–220.
17. Matthiesen DT, Scavelli TD, Whitney WO. Subtotal colectomy for treatment of obstipation secondary to pelvic fracture malunion in cats. *Vet Surg* 1991; 20: 113–117.
18. Holt DE, Brockman DJ. Large intestine. In: Slatter DH (ed.), *Textbook of Small Animal Surgery, 3rd ed.* Philadelphia, WB Saunders, 2003; 665–682.

6.4.6 Neoplastic diseases of the large intestines

Carolyn J. Henry

Large intestinal cancer is primarily a disease of middle-aged to older dogs, occurring at a median age of 8 years for epithelial tumors and 11 years for mesenchymal masses.[1-4] Adenomatous polyps and carcinoma in situ account for the majority of canine large intestinal neoplastic lesions, but only occur infrequently in the small intestine.[1,5-8] Other canine non-lymphoid large intestinal masses include leiomyomas, leiomyosarcomas, GI stromal tumors, mast cell tumors (MCT), plasmacytomas, rectal ganglioneuromas, neurilemomas, and carcinoids (see 9.4).[2-4,9-16] Of the canine large intestinal malignancies, leiomyosarcomas and GI stromal tumors usually occur in the cecum (Figure 6.12), whereas carcinomas occur more commonly in the rectum and colon.[7,8,15,16] In the dog, adenocarcinomas affect the rectum more commonly than the colon.[8,17,18] In most reports, there has been a slightly higher prevalence of large intestinal cancer in males than in females.[8,17,18] Also, most colorectal tumors occur in purebred dogs, with German Shepherds, West Highland White Terriers, and Collies reportedly being over-represented.[1,2,8,19] However, a true breed predisposition is difficult to discern, given the paucity of reports that are accompanied with population demographics. In two series of visceral MCT, miniature breeds, particularly Maltese, were most frequently affected, but large bowel lesions represented the minority of cases.[9,10]

Previous reports have indicated that feline non-lymphoid cancer is far more common in the small bowel than in the large intestine[20]. However, more recent data suggest that a site predilection for the feline small intestine may no longer exist (personal unpublished data). The mean age of cats with colonic neoplasia is 12.5 years, with adenocarcinoma being the most common tumor.[7,21] Other reported non-lymphoid masses include MCTs, neuroendocrine carcinomas (see 9.4), leiomyosarcomas, fibrosarcomas, and hemangiosarcomas.[7,20–24] This section will focus on the more common non-lymphoid large intestinal masses. The reader is referred to Chapter 9.3 for a discussion of GI lymphoma.

Clinical signs

Dogs with large intestinal tumors are commonly presented because of hematochezia, tenesmus, and dyschezia, or intermittent rectal bleeding that is not associated with defecation.[1,6,25] Colorectal polyps may cause a secondary rectal prolapse.[1,19] Because feline large intestinal masses are more likely to occur in the proximal segments (i.e., in the cecum or colon rather than in the rectum), clinical signs in cats may be less obvious for large bowel disease than they are in dogs.[20] The most commonly reported presenting complaints in cats with non-lymphoid large intestinal neoplasia are weight loss, anorexia, vomiting, and diarrhea.[21,24] Hematochezia and tenesmus are reported less frequently.[6,21] Canine large intestinal leiomyosarcoma, leiomyoma, and GI stromal tumors are most often located in the cecum and generally lack mucosal involvement.[3,16] As such, they are less likely to cause hematochezia, but may be detected due to clinical signs from intestinal obstruction or septic peritonitis secondary to tumor rupture. Paraneoplastic syndromes, including hypoglycemia and erythrocytosis, have been reported with large intestinal smooth muscle tumors.[3,11,26] When paraneoplastic hypoglycemia occurs, dogs can present with central nervous signs, including seizures and ataxia.[3] Paraneoplastic neutrophilic leukocytosis has been reported secondary to canine rectal adenomatous polyps.[25]

Diagnosis

In over half of all affected cats and dogs, rectal examination is useful for identifying colorectal masses.[1,17,21] Most dogs present with solitary masses that tend to be polypoid or annular stenotic lesions, although diffusely infiltrative large bowel adenocarcinoma has been reported in some patients.[1] For animals with non-palpable masses, useful imaging techniques include abdominal radiographs, ultrasonography, CT, rigid proctoscopy, and flexible colonoscopy.[1,21,27] Survey radiographs should be obtained first and may be adequate for the identification of a mass. A case series of dogs with colorectal leiomyoma indicated that contrast studies were required for mass identification in only one of six dogs.[28] The increased availability of ultrasonography in private practice has made this modality an attractive alternative to contrast studies. In one report of cats with intestinal cancer, abdominal ultrasound permitted mass

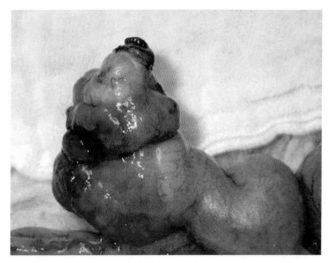

Figure 6.12:
Cecal leiomyosarcoma. Although cecal malignancies are uncommon in dogs, this is the most common site for leiomyosarcomas and gastrointestinal stromal tumors in the canine large intestine.

localization in 84% of imaged cases.[21] Ultimately, diagnosis relies upon biopsy, obtained either surgically or by endoscopy. Caution is advised when relying on endoscopic biopsy for definitive diagnosis, as one report indicated discordant results between surgical and endoscopic biopsy specimens in three of ten dogs. In all three cases, the diagnosis determined from the surgical biopsy specimen was more severe than that noted on the original endoscopic biopsy.[1] The appearance of lesions on endoscopy or at surgery may help to predict the prognosis. In one report of dogs with colorectal adenocarcinoma, those patients with single, pedunculated polypoid masses had the longest mean survival time (32 months), compared to dogs with masses with a nodular or cobble-stone appearance (12 months), or those with annular masses causing strictures (1.6 months).[17]

As with small intestinal tumors, immunohistochemistry may aid in differentiating intestinal tumor types. Recent data suggests that most tumors previously reported as canine GI leiomyosarcomas were, in fact, GI stromal tumors.[16] In one report of 50 canine GI tumors originally diagnosed as leiomyomas, leiomyosarcomas, or spindle cell sarcoma, 21 (42%) were reclassified as GI stromal tumors on the basis of histological review and immunohistochemistry. Ten of these occurred in the large intestine, with seven in the cecum.[16] The use of immunohistochemistry to detect desmin, smooth muscle actin, and KIT (CD117) helps to differentiate true smooth muscle tumors from GI stromal tumors.

6

Staging

Colonoscopy and proctoscopy are essential for complete tumor staging in dogs with colorectal cancer.[17] In one report, four dogs that were treated by local excision without presurgical endoscopy were later found to have lesions proximal to the surgical site.[17] In addition to assessment of local disease extent, full staging to rule out metastatic disease is warranted. Metastases occurred in 16 of 19 cats with non-lymphoid large intestinal masses in one study, with metastatic sites including colonic and mesenteric lymph nodes, liver, omentum, peritoneum, spleen, bladder, urethra, mesocolon, lungs, and duodenum.[21] Reported metastatic rates for canine rectal carcinoma vary widely. Two large series of cases dating back to 1975 or earlier reported metastatic rates of 64% or greater, whereas no metastases were noted in a series of 78 dogs diagnosed with colorectal adenocarcinoma between 1973 and 1984.[14,17,18] When metastasis occurs, the common sites include the regional lymph nodes, lungs, liver, and spleen.[14,18] Metastasis via presumed tumor cell implantation has also been reported with colorectal carcinoma, resulting in lesions in the periproctal area.[18,27] As in humans, canine GI stromal tumors tend to metastasize within the abdominal cavity, with sites including the liver, spleen, mesentery, serosa, and mesenteric lymph nodes. The metastatic rate in dogs in one report was 29%.[16]

Treatment

Surgery is the treatment of choice for most large intestinal masses and may provide excellent long-term outcome for patients with solitary masses.[29] The surgical approach chosen depends on tumor location, but may entail local resection after eversion of the mass through the anus, anal pull-out, or abdominoanal pull-through procedures. Alternatively, laparotomy or sagittal pubic osteotomy approaches may be necessary. The latter has been described for treatment of various inaccessible intrapelvic masses in 24 dogs.[29] This approach facilitated surgical exploration of the affected region in a report with seven dogs with masses involving the colon or rectum. Excision was attempted only in cases where regional metastatic disease was not identified. Alternatively, treatment of benign or inaccessible rectal masses using transanal endoscopic excision and cautery has been reported for six dogs and resulted in a cure in three dogs and a significant improvement in two.[30] Rectal perforation is, however, a potential complication of this and other colonic surgical procedures.

Dogs undergoing excision or cryosurgery for colorectal adenocarcinoma live significantly longer (by an average of 7 to 9 months) than those undergoing biopsy alone.[17] Mass excision, along with margins of 4 to 8 cm of normal surrounding intestinal tissue is recommended to ensure complete tumor removal.[25] The mean post-surgical survival in 57 dogs with colorectal tumors was 20.6 months and was influenced by tumor type and surgical margins. Dogs with an adenoma or carcinoma in situ survived significantly longer than those with an invasive carcinoma. Also, dogs with clean surgical margins lived significantly longer than those with tumor cells within the surgical margins.[8]

In cats, aggressive surgery provides for longer survival times than do more limited procedures. Subtotal colectomy resulted in a median survival time of 138 days, compared to 68 days for cats that received a lesser resection and only 10 days for cats that only had a biopsy taken.[21] A thorough surgical exploration of the abdomen is advised, as metastatic disease warrants a poor prognosis. In one study, cats with metastasis to the lymph nodes or abdominal organs at the time of surgery had a median survival time of 49 days, compared to 259 days for those without metastasis.[21]

The use of colostomy has been reported infrequently for dogs with colorectal tumors.[27,31] In one report, an incontinent end-on colostomy was used after resection of an annular rectal adenocarcinoma. The device required twice daily management by the owner, but the management was reported to be relatively simple and not associated with any complications.[27]

Reports of chemotherapy for the treatment of canine and feline large intestinal cancer are sparse. One dog treated with cyclophosphamide and 5-fluorouracil after surgery for diffuse colonic adenocarcinoma had persistence of clinical signs and died within three months.[32] More promising results have been reported for a limited number of cats treated with chemotherapy. The reported median survival time for four cats receiving adjuvant doxorubicin for colonic carcinoma was 280 days, compared to 56 days for 12 cats that did not receive chemotherapy.[21] Adjuvant therapy that has been investigated for treatment of large intestinal cancer in dogs and humans includes NSAIDs in an attempt to capitalize on their anti-inflammatory and putative anti-neoplastic properties and to target COX-2 receptors, which are up-regulated in the majority of canine patients with colorectal neoplasms.[33,34] In a report of eight dogs with tubulopapillary rectal polyps, all but one dog treated with piroxicam (dose equivalent: 0.24–0.46 mg/kg/day administered per rectum q 3 days or 0.34 mg/kg PO on alternate days) demonstrated symptomatic improvement including reduction in hematochezia and tenesmus.[33] This therapy has not yet been evaluated in cats with large intestinal neoplasia. Targeted therapy of GI stromal tumors using receptor tyrosine kinase inhibitors has shown promise in human oncology, but awaits further evaluation in companion animals.

Follow-up and prognosis

Recommended follow-up procedures for dogs undergoing removal of colorectal masses include a rectal examination every three months and colonoscopy every six months in order to allow for early detection of recurrent or new lesions.[1,35] Recurrence of clinical signs is not uncommon, having been reported in 75% of dogs with multiple masses at surgery and all dogs with diffuse lesions in one case series.[1] For dogs with carcinoma in situ or solitary masses, recurrence of clinical signs is less common. When recurrence occurs, it generally does so within the first year after surgery (270 to 365 days post surgery).[1]

Malignant transformation of benign lesions (adenomatous polyp) to more aggressive ones (carcinoma in situ or invasive carcinoma) is a concern in human patients and is the basis for regular follow-up examinations. A similar progression has been reported in a small percentage (18%) of dogs in one report, although the mechanisms underlying this progression are unclear.[1]

The overall survival time for dogs with colorectal tumors varies by tumor type and location. The best prognoses are offered for dogs with rectal polyps or smooth muscle tumors and the worst (11 days or less) are reported for patients with MCT.[10] Although the reported median survival times for cats with large intestinal cancer are poor (< 3.5 months), individual survival times of up to 28 months have been reported.[6,25,32] Attempts to identify appropriate biological markers to predict tumor behavior have not yielded clinically useful options to date. The detection of p53 overexpression in tumor tissue is not of prognostic significance for canine epithelial colorectal tumors or gastrointestinal MCT.[8,9] Pending the discovery of more accurate markers for tumor behavior, histological type, tumor staging, and surgical margin assessment are the most reliable tools for prognostication and should be used in conjunction with clinical patient reassessment to develop a sound plan for case management.

6

🔑 Key Facts

- Adenomatous polyps and carcinoma in situ are the most common large intestinal tumors in dogs, whereas adenocarcinomas predominate in cats.
- Many canine gastrointestinal mesenchymal tumors that were once classified as leiomyomas or leiomyosarcomas have more recently been correctly classified as gastrointestinal stromal tumors.
- Hematochezia, tenesmus, and dyschezia are clinical signs typically noted in dogs with large intestinal tumors.
- Because large intestinal tumors in cats tend to occur in the more proximal segments, clinical signs may be less obvious than in dogs, where large intestinal masses occur more commonly in the rectum.
- Colonoscopy and proctoscopy are advised as part of tumor staging to rule out additional lesions prior to surgery.

References

1. Valerius KD, Powers BE, McPherron MA et al. Adenomatous polyps and carcinoma in situ of the canine colon and rectum: 34 cases (1982–1994). *J Am Anim Hosp Assoc* 1997; 33: 156–160.
2. Holt PE, Lucke VM. Rectal neoplasia in the dog: a clinicopathologic review of 31 cases. *Vet Rec* 1985; 116: 400–405.
3. Kapatkin AS, Mullen HS, Matthiesen DT et al. Leiomysarcoma in dogs: 44 cases (1983–1988). *J Am Anim Hosp Assoc* 1991; 201 (7): 1077–1079.
4. ter Haar G, van der Gaag I, Kirpensteijn J. Canine intestinal leiomyosarcoma. *Vet Quart* 1998; 20 Suppl 1: S111–S112.
5. White RAS, Gorman NT. The clinical diagnosis and management of rectal and pararectal tumors in the dogs. *J Small Anim Pract* 1987; 28: 87–107.
6. Birchard SJ, Couto CG, Johnson S. Nonlymphoid intestinal neoplasia in 32 dogs and 14 cats. *J Am Anim Hosp Assoc* 1986; 22: 533–537.
7. Head KW, Else RW, Dubielzig RR. Tumors of the alimentary tract. In: Meuten DJ (ed), *Tumors in Domestic Animals, 4th ed.* Ames, Iowa State Press 2002; 401–481

8. Wolf JC, Ginn PE, Homer B et al. Immunohistochemical detection of p53 tumor suppressor gene protein in canine epithelial colorectal tumors. *Vet Pathol* 1997; 34: 393–404.
9. Ozaki K, Yamagami T, Nomura K et al. Mast cell tumors of the gastrointestinal tract in 39 dogs. *Vet Pathol* 2002; 39: 557–564.
10. Takahashi T, Kadosawa T, Nagase M et al. Visceral mast cell tumors in dogs: 10 cases (1982–1997) *J Am Vet Med Assoc* 2000; 216: 222–226.
11. Cohen M, Post GS, Wright JC. Gastrointestinal leiomyosarcoma in 14 dogs. *J Vet Intern Med* 2003; 17: 107–110.
12. Reimer ME, Reimer MS, Saunders GK et al. Rectal ganglioneuroma in a dog. *J Am Anim Hosp Assoc* 1999; 35: 107–110.
13. Singleton WB. An unusual neoplasm in a dog (a probable neurilemoma of the caecum). *Vet Rec* 1956; 68: 1046.
14. Patnaik AK, Hurvitz AI, Johnson GF. Canine intestinal adenocarcinoma and carcinoid. *Vet Pathol* 1980; 17: 149–163.
15. Gibbons GC, Murtaugh RJ. Cecal smooth muscle neoplasia in the dog: report of 11 cases and literature review. *J Am Anim Hosp Assoc* 1989; 25: 191–197.

6

16. Frost D, Lasota J, Miettinen M. Gastrointestinal stromal tumors and leiomyomas in the dog: A histopathological, immunohistochemical, and molecular genetic study of 50 cases. *Vet Pathol* 2003; 40: 42–54.

17. Church EM, Mehlhaff CJ, Patnaik AK. Colorectal adenocarcinoma in dogs: 78 cases (1973–1984). *J Am Vet Med Assoc* 1987; 191: 727–730.

18. Schaffer E, Schiefer B. Incidence of canine rectal carcinomas. *J Small Anim Pract* 1968; 9: 491–496.

19. Sieler RJ. Colorectal polyps of the dog: a clinicopathologic study of 17 cases. *J Am Vet Med Assoc* 1979; 174: 72–75.

20. Turk MAM, Gallina AM, Russell TS. Nonhematopoietic gastrointestinal neoplasia in cats: a retrospective study of 44 cases. *Vet Pathol* 1981; 18: 614–620.

21. Slawienski MJ, Mauldin GE, Mauldin GN et al. Malignant colonic neoplasia in cats: 46 cases (1990–1996). *J Am Vet Med Assoc* 1997; 211: 878–881.

22. Barrand KR, Scudamore CL. Intestinal leiomyosarcoma in a cat. *J Small Anim Pract* 1999; 40: 216–219.

23. Patnaik AK, Liu SK, Johnson GF. Feline intestinal adenocarcinoma: a clinicopathologic study of 22 cases. *Vet Pathol* 1976; 13: 1–10.

24. Cribb AE. Feline gastrointestinal adenocarcinoma: a review and retrospective study. *Can Vet J* 1988; 29: 709–712.

25. Phillips BS. Tumors of the intestinal tract. In: Withrow SJ, MacEwen EG (eds.), *Small Animal Clinical Oncology, 3rd ed.* Philadelphia, WB Saunders, 2001; 335–346.

26. Sato K, Hikasa Y, Takehito M et al. Secondary erythrocytosis associated with high plasma erythropoeitin concentrations in a dog with cecal leiomyosarcoma. *J Am Vet Med Assoc* 2002; 220: 486–490.

27. Kumagai D, Shimada T, Yamate J et al. Use of an incontinent end-on colostomy in a dog with annular rectal adenocarcinoma. *J Small Anim Pract* 2003; 44: 363–366.

28. McPherron MA, Withrow SJ, Seim HB et al. Colorectal leiomyomas in seven dogs. *J Am Anim Hosp Assoc* 1992; 28: 43–46.

29. Davies JV, Read HM. Sagittal pubic osteotomy in the investigation and treatment of intrapelvic neoplasia in the dog. *J Small Anim Pract* 1990; 31: 123–130.

30. Holt PE, Durdey P. Transanal endoscopic treatment of benign canine rectal tumors: preliminary results in six cases (1992 to 1996). *J Small Anim Pract* 1999; 40: 423–427.

31. Hardie EM, Gilson SD. Use of colostomy to manage rectal disease in dogs. *Vet Surg* 1997; 26: 270–274.

32. Feeney DA, Klausner JS, Johnston GR. Chronic bowel obstruction caused by primary intestinal neoplasia: a report of five cases. *J Am Anim Hosp Assoc* 1982; 18: 67–77.

33. Knottenbelt CM, Simpson JW, Tasker S et al Preliminary clinical observations on the use of piroxicam in the management of rectal tubulopapillary polyps. *J Small Anim Pract* 2000; 41: 393–397.

34. McEntee MF, Cates JM, Neilsen N. Cyclooxygenase-2 expression in spontaneous intestinal neoplasia of domestic dogs. *Vet Pathol* 2002; 39: 428–436.

35. Leib MS, Campbell S, Martin RA. Endoscopy case of the month: rectal bleeding in a dog. *Vet Med* 1992; 526–532.

7   Liver

Jan Rothuizen

7.1   Anatomy

The liver is one of the largest organs in the body. It weighs approximately 3% of the total body weight in adult dogs and cats. In very young growing animals, it accounts for 5% of the body weight. The shape of the liver in dogs and cats is different from that of most other mammals such as cattle, horses, and humans. The domesticated carnivores have deeply incised lobes, which are individually recognizable, whereas they are largely fused in other species. This may be due to the concave shape of the diaphragm in the dog and cat, which leads to relatively large excursions during in- and expiration, so that the liver needs to be able to fold and unfold while following the diaphragm. The deeply separated lobes, which connect at the hilus of the liver, make it relatively easy to resect an entire liver lobe in dogs and cats. By far the largest liver lobe is the left lateral lobe, which encompasses 30–40% of the entire liver mass. This large lobe is therefore the easiest one to approach for the collection of liver biopsies. The peripheral part of the left lateral lobe is far away from critical structures such as large veins, arteries, or bile ducts. From a dorsoventral perspective, the position of the liver is somewhat turned to the right. The gall bladder, large bile ducts, and blood vessels of the liver enter the organ at the hilus in the right upper abdominal quadrant. The liver follows the contours of the diaphragm and the abdominal section of the rib cage.

In dogs, the liver lies entirely within the rib cage and, therefore, is normally not palpable. Depending on the shape of the rib cage, the liver lies more or less hidden within it. In brachycephalic dogs, which have a wide rib cage and a more flattened diaphragm, any enlargement will result in the liver being palpable. In contrast, in racing hounds with a deep rib cage, the liver may only become palpable behind the last rib when it is severely enlarged. In healthy cats, the ventral border of the liver can often be palpated and the feline liver is always palpable when enlarged. Since feline hepatobiliary diseases are usually associated with hepatomegaly, abdominal palpation is often informative in cats with liver disease.

The stomach is in contact with the visceral surface of the liver. As a result, changes in size or shape of the liver cause displacement of the stomach. This is one possible explanation why vomiting is often a major clinical sign in patients with liver disease.

The peritoneal capsule of the liver forms ligaments, which fixate the organ in its position while maintaining a degree of movability. The falciform ligament is located in the midline and attaches the liver to the ventral abdominal wall and also contains the abdominal retroperitoneal fat mass. The other fixation points of the liver are the left and right triangular ligaments and the short coronary ligament, which connect the liver with the diaphragm laterally and in the midline, respectively. Finally, the right hepatorenal ligament connects the liver with the right kidney.

7.1.1   Biliary system

One of the main functions of the liver is the detoxification or catabolism of many exogenous and endogenous compounds. Many compounds undergo biotransformation in the hepatocytes. Larger molecules (i.e., molecular weight > 300), such as steroid hormones, bilirubin, bile salts, and many toxins are excreted by the biliary system. In contrast, smaller exogenous or endogenous molecules (i.e., urea or allantoin) are excreted via the urine.

The biliary system is a branched tree, which serves as a collection system for bile from each individual hepatic cell. In each hepatic lobule, the hepatocytes are organized in liver cell plates, which radiate around a central vein. These hepatocyte plates connect the central vein with several portal areas. Blood flows from the portal areas to the central vein, while bile flows from the central areas to the portal areas and the common bile duct. An alternative view (formulated by Rappaport) sees the portal tract in the center of the hepatic lobule and the region supplied by blood vessels originating in this portal tract of the lobule. According to this view, the central veins lie in the periphery of the lobule and are called terminal hepatic veins (THV). However, there is a tendency to return back to using the old nomenclature (central vein), but the terms central vein and THV are often used interchangeably.

The lateral membranes connecting adjacent liver cells contain a specialized region, the canalicular membrane. The space between the canalicular membranes of adjacent cells is sealed by tight junctions and forms the smallest branches of the biliary system, the canaliculi. This excretory region of the hepatocyte membrane constitutes 15% of the hepatocellular surface. Most molecules are excreted across this membrane by their own specialized transporters, which can actively excrete against a very high concentration gradient. Thus, the canalicular membrane is a highly specialized section of the hepatocellular membrane.

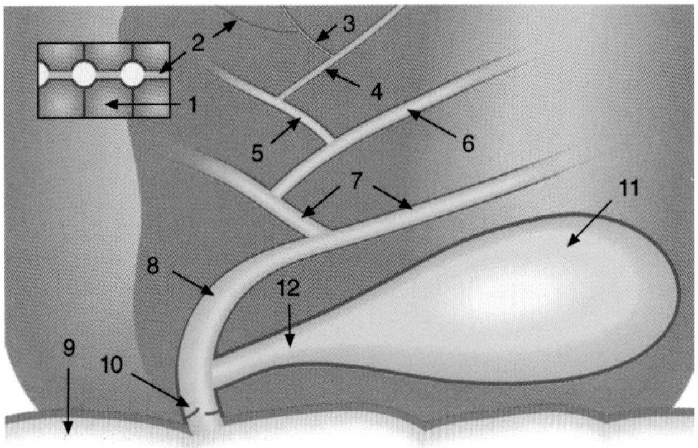

7

Figure 7.1:
Bile flow. This figure shows a schematic representation of bile flow in dogs and cats. Bile is produced by the transport of a large number of molecules across the canalicular membranes of the hepatocytes (1) into the canaliculi (2). The canaliculi drain into the canals of Hering (3), which drain into the intrahepatic bile ductules (4). These then drain into the interlobular ducts (5), septal ducts (6), and hilar ducts (7), which collect all the bile from one liver lobe. The hilar ducts merge to form the common bile duct (ductus choledochus; 8), which opens into the duodenum (9) on Vater's papilla and is protected against the reflux of duodenal contents by the muscular sphincter of Oddi (10). The gall bladder (11) is connected to the common bile duct by the cystic duct (12).

Bile is excreted by hepatocytes into the canaliculi, which then transport the bile to the portal tracts where they enter the canals of Hering (Figure 7.1). These short connecting ducts are in part lined by hepatocytes, in part by cuboidal cholangiocytes.[2] Some of the cells of the canal of Hering are the stem cells of the liver, which can differentiate into hepatocytes as well as cholangiocytes, and thus function as stem cells for all the main cell types of the liver. These hepatic progenitor or stem cells are also called oval cells. All hepatocytes have an enormous capacity to divide and thus allow for regeneration of the liver mass after loss due to damage. Therefore, all hepatocytes have stem-cell-like characteristics. However, many biliary epithelial cells can only be replenished by oval stem cells.

The canals of Hering drain into the smallest branches of the intrahepatic bile ducts, which are completely lined by cholangiocytes. From the smallest bile ductules, the bile flows to the interlobular ducts, the septal ducts, and via the hilar ducts of each liver lobe into the common bile duct (ductus choledochus). The ductus choledochus is only 2–3 mm in diameter in dogs and cats, and may be difficult to find with ultrasonography. However, in patients with a common bile duct obstruction, dilation of the common bile duct is easily visible ultrasonographically and serves as the hallmark feature of common bile duct obstruction. The common bile duct runs to the duodenum and enters the major duodenal papilla some 3–6 cm caudal to the pylorus, depending on the size of the animal. The junction of the common bile duct and the duodenum, Vater's papilla, is located close to the head of the pancreas and is surrounded by the muscular sphincter of Oddi. In cats, the pancreatic duct and the common bile duct merge and enter the duodenum together on the major duodenal papilla. This may explain why in cats concurrent pancreatitis and cholangiohepatitis / cholangitis occur quite frequently. In contrast to cats, the bile duct and the pancreatic duct usually end separately in dogs. The gallbladder is connected with the common bile duct via the short cystic duct.

The gall bladder provides the main storage facility for bile and concentrates the bile approximately tenfold. Bile is also concentrated in the larger bile ducts. In healthy dogs and cats, a completely filled gallbladder contains around 1 ml of bile/kg body weight. Less than half of the bile produced is stored and concentrated. The remainder is immediately transported into the duodenum via the common bile duct. Stimulation of the muscular wall of the gall bladder to contract (by cholecystokinin released from the duodenal mucosa) produces a gradual release of bile that lasts for several hours. The bile then enters the duodenum by rhythmic relaxations of the sphincter of Oddi. Emptying of the gall bladder is very variable and almost never complete.[3] An empty gall bladder during ultrasonography is an abnormal finding. Opioid drugs can cause complete closure of the sphincter of Oddi, so that during anesthesia the gall bladder may appear dilated; this usually resolves after anesthesia. Dilation of the larger bile ducts and / or the common bile duct indicates abnormalities such as cholangitis or bile duct obstruction.

7.1.2 Blood supply

The blood supply of the liver is both arterial and venous. Arterial blood comes from the hepatic artery, while venous blood is supplied through the portal vein. The outflowing blood is collected by a number of hepatic veins that enter into the inferior vena cava near the diaphragm. The total blood flow to the liver accounts for about 20–25% of the cardiac output (100–130 ml/min/100 g liver tissue). The portal vein accounts for 70% of the total blood flow to the liver and separates into two main branches entering the liver at the hilus. The right branch of the portal vein supplies the right side of the liver, while the bigger and longer left branch supplies the left and central portions of the liver. The intrahepatic portal vein divides into smaller branches, with the smallest branches ending in the portal areas. Histologically, the terminal branches of the portal vein are the largest structures of the portal areas. These terminal branches end in inlet venules, which penetrate the periportal cell layer, the so-called limiting plate, where it distributes the portal blood to the sinusoids. The hepatic artery also enters the liver at the hepatic hilus. Its branches accompany the portal vein. Terminal arterial branches end into the periportal sinusoids and connect with the venous and sinusoidal system. The biliary system of the liver is only supplied with arterial blood, while the parenchyma receives both portal and arterial blood. The sinusoidal blood enters the central veins, also known as terminal hepatic veins, in the liver lobule. The central veins then drain into branches of the hepatic vein. Finally, several branches of the hepatic vein enter into the caudal vena cava.[4]

The ratio between portal and arterial blood supply is not constant but varies with both physiological and pathological conditions. Portal blood flow increases following food ingestion, whereas the arterial blood supply increases when the portal blood flow is insufficient and decreases in the case of hepatic venous congestion. In patients with diseases that are associated with a severely decreased or total lack of portal blood flow (i.e., congenital portosystemic shunts, portal vein thrombosis), the arterial blood flow may increase by 100%, but even then the total hepatic blood flow remains subnormal. However, without this compensatory arterial blood flow the liver would not be able to survive. Histologically, the arterialization of the liver becomes visible after about 2 weeks. The hepatic arteries respond to the hypoperfusion of the liver and increase their blood flow. In addition, the arterial branches become tortuous and hypertrophic. Histologically, this can be recognized as an increased number of arterial sections in the portal areas. In the parenchyma, portal hypoperfusion causes hepatocellular atrophy.

In comparison, changes in arterial blood flow do not affect portal blood flow.[4] During periods of fasting, the hepatic artery and the portal vein each supply approximately 50% of the hepatic oxygen requirement. In the case of hypoxia, which can occur in patients with anemia, the hepatic blood supply remains unchanged. When the oxygenation of the liver becomes deficient, either due to reduced erythrocyte oxygen binding or due to decreased perfusion, the liver adapts by an increased efficiency of oxygen uptake from approximately 40% up to nearly 100%. Hypoxia does not affect the total perfusion of the liver or the ratio between arterial and portal blood supply. Due to the large volume and the compliance of the hepatic vascular bed approximately 10–15% of the total blood volume is contained in the liver. This may increase by 100% in patients with severe congestive heart disease. Also, the large hepatic blood reservoir plays a role in compensating for acute blood loss.

It is important to note that, at the histological level, the liver consists of functional hemodynamic units or acini that are different from the lobules that are mere anatomically descriptive units. The acinar concept, which was proposed by Rappaport, places the portal vein at the center of the acinus

with several central veins, also known as terminal hepatic veins (THV), at the periphery. The arteries and portal vein branches enter the liver via the portal areas. Portal blood is distributed from the larger portal veins throughout the acinus and drains into the sinusoids via short perpendicular inlet venules, which have a sphincter function and regulate the portal blood flow into the capillary bed. The THV collect blood at the outlet side of the sinusoids. Small tributaries of the hepatic artery enter the sinusoidal system at different places. Their blood flow is also controlled by a sphincter, which intermittently allows the flow of arterial blood, thus regulating the difference in pressure between the arterial system (100–110 mmHg) and the portal (0–5 mmHg) and sinusoidal (5–10 mmHg) systems.

According to the acinar concept, the liver circulatory units are divided into three zones, with the closest (Zone 1) around the portal area receiving blood with the highest contents of oxygen, growth factors, and nutrients, and Zone 3, which is farthest away from the portal area, and thus receives blood with the lowest concentrations of these compounds. In the case of sudden hypoxia or shock, when there is not sufficient time for compensation by increasing the oxygen binding of red blood cells or a more efficient oxygen uptake by the liver, the hepatocytes located in Zone 3 become necrotic. This results in centrolobular (Zone 3) hepatocellular necrosis. Such conditions are usually associated with increases in serum hepatic enzyme activities.

7.1.3 Microanatomy

The predominant cell type of the liver is the epithelial cell or hepatocyte. Hepatocytes make up 60% of the all the cells in the liver and since they are also the largest cell type found in the liver, they make up 80% of the liver volume (approximately 200,000 cells per mg hepatic tissue). Altogether, the liver contains about 100 billion hepatocytes. Other cell types that are present in the liver are endothelial cells, bile duct epithelial cells, Kupffer cells, and fat-storing cells. The latter cell type is also known as stellate cells.[5]

The hepatocytes are arranged in cell plates that are only one layer thick, radiating around the THVs. The free outer membranes on both sides of the hepatocyte are in contact with the sinusoids. Due to the numerous microvilli of that part of the membrane, the sinusoidal membrane occupies 70% of the overall hepatic cell surface area. A portion of the lateral membranes of adjacent cells form the bile canaliculi that are surrounded by tight junctions, which connect the hepatocytes on either side of the canaliculi. The canalicular membrane comprises approximately 15% of the hepatocyte membrane, and has a specialized excretory function. The sinusoidal membrane is separated from the sinusoids by one cell layer of sinusoidal

7

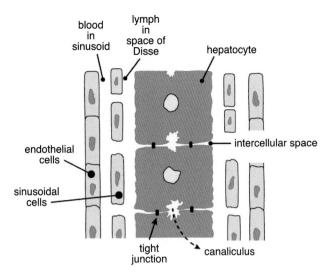

Figure 7.2:
Arrangement of cell types in the liver. This diagram shows the arrangement of endothelial cells, sinusoidal cells, and hepatocytes, which respectively form the conduits for blood, lymph, and bile flow. Hepatocellular necrosis leads to a direct connection between the canaliculi (i.e., the space of bile flow) and the space of Disse, resulting in a leakage of bile into the circulation (intrahepatic cholestasis).

Table 7.1: Hepatocyte functions in the different sublobular regions
Note that both lipid and protein metabolism are functions that are not localized to one region.

Zone 1: periportal area	Zone 3: centrolobular area
Bilirubin excretion	Copper excretion
Bile acid excretion, bile-salt-dependent bile production	Bile-salt-independent bile production
Gluconeogenesis, glycogenolysis → glucose production	Glycolysis, glyconeogenesis → glucose clearance
Ammonia detoxification through urea cycle enzymes	Ammonia detoxification through glutamine formation
Glutathione production → protection against oxidative stress	Biotransformation; cytochrome p450 enzyme-dependant detoxification; conjugation reactions

cells (about 7% of the liver cells). Between the hepatocytes and the sinusoidal cell layers is the perisinusoidal space of Disse (Figure 7.2). The endothelial cell lining is fenestrated, and these openings permit even large molecules to be exchanged between the sinusoidal blood and the space of Disse. However, cells cannot pass through the fenestrations and remain in the circulation.

The perisinusoidal space represents the beginning of the hepatic lymphatic system and leads lymph in a direction opposite to that of the blood flow, but in conjunction with the bile flow. The sinusoidal cells (endothelial and Kupffer cells) are very efficient in removing endotoxins and particles, such as bacteria. This, together with the many detoxifying metabolic functions of the hepatocytes and the biliary excretion of toxic substances, make the liver an important guardian against toxic substances entering the body from the GI tract. The bile in the canaliculi flows opposite to the blood flow into short collecting ducts (canals of Hering), which drain bile from the acini into bile ductules of the portal area. The luminal surface of these ductuli and the larger bile ducts are covered with cuboidal biliary epithelium.

Although hepatocytes are generally uniform and thus capable of performing most metabolic functions, there is some heterogeneity with respect to some functions. For example, enzymes that are part of the urea cycle are predominantly found in the hepatocytes of Zone 1 around the portal area. Also, the incorporation of ammonia in glutamine, which is regulated by glutamine synthetase, occurs exclusively in the hepatocytes around the central vein (THV). Carbohydrate metabolism also shows some degree of zonal organization, although it is not as strict as that of ammonia metabolism. Lipid and protein metabolism are not restricted to one particular zone. Drug metabolism via the cytochrome p450 mixed function oxidase system appears to be primarily located around the central veins. Copper accumulation in patients with copper storage disease mostly affects cells in Zone 3 in all dog breeds (Table 7.1).

7.2 Physiology

The liver has an enormous reserve capacity and removal of up to 70% of the normal liver can be sustained without any clinical effect. The liver also has a huge regenerative capacity following the loss of hepatocytes. Liver cells can divide more than 40 times, so that the organ theoretically has the capacity to completely renew itself a number of times. However, when diseased, the regenerative capacity decreases and, at the same time, there is a tendency to produce more non-functional matrix (i.e., hepatic fibrosis). Hepatic growth and regeneration are regulated by growth factors of which hepatocyte growth factor (HGF) is the most important one. HGF is produced in the fat-storing cells (also known as Ito or stellate cells) upon stimulation by stimulation factors, such as insulin-like growth factor (IGF), insulin, and others, that reach the liver with the portal blood supply. Therefore, the supply of portal blood is essential for maintaining hepatic functional mass and regeneration. In turn, animals with congenital portosystemic shunts experience a reduced hepatic growth resulting in an undersized and hypofunctional liver, which usually grows to its normal size and weight within two weeks after surgical ligation of the shunt. Another feature making the liver highly flexible in facing changing demands is the fact that its metabolic and transport processes follow the Michaelis-Menten kinetic curve. These processes are therefore capable of adapting to changing substrate concentrations; however, they are also saturable and adaptation is, thus, not unlimited. The liver plays a key role in many metabolic processes and in homeostasis. In general, the organ detects the metabolic requirements of the extrahepatic tissues and responds by metabolic adaptation.

The plasma concentrations of glucose and many proteins are regulated by the liver, and may be reduced in patients with hepatic dysfunction. In order to be able to be transported through the vascular system, triglycerides from adipose tissue or intestinal chylomicrons are converted into lipoproteins by the liver. Other metabolic functions of the liver include the biotransformation of endogenous products varying from ammonia to steroid hormones and the removal of exogenous toxic products (e.g., toxic chemicals and endotoxins from intestinal bacteria). A number of toxic substances are directly excreted by the liver (e.g., heavy metals), while others are modified by the liver and then released into the circulation in a form that can be excreted by the kidneys (e.g., uric acid is converted to allantoin, ammonia to urea, and steroids are transformed and conjugated). Large molecules with molecular masses above 300 Da are preferentially excreted into the bile after being conjugated to make them more hydrophilic. Another important metabolic function of the liver is the production of primary bile acids from cholesterol (Figure 7.3).

Apart from all these metabolic functions, the liver also has the capacity to store many substances for future use; examples are glycogen, metal ions, and vitamins. The liver is also capable of producing red blood cells, a function which is physiologically present during embryonic life. Hepatic extramedullary hematopoiesis may be regained and is often found in patients with anemia.

The enormous functional reserve, the exceptional regenerative capacity, and the metabolic flexibility of the liver are responsible for the fact that many liver diseases only cause clinical symptoms when the disease has become chronic and a large portion of its functional and regenerative reserves have been lost. Acute or subacute diseases are often subclinical or only result in mild clinical signs that can easily be overlooked.

Another factor is that the liver is intrinsically involved in the function of many extrahepatic tissues, so that hepatic dysfunction often leads to clinical signs that indicate dysfunction of other organs. Finally, clinical signs encountered in patients with liver disease are commonly nonspecific. Therefore, hepatic diseases are often associated with clinical signs that do not immediately point to the liver, but to a general dysfunc-

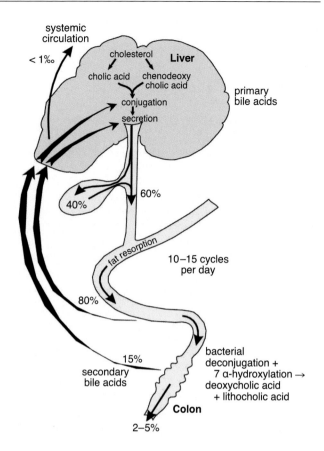

Figure 7.3:
Bile acid metabolism and enterohepatic circulation. Hepatocytes produce bile acids from cholesterol. These primary bile acids are conjugated by the liver and then secreted in the bile. Approximately 40% of primary bile acids get stored in the gall bladder, while 60% reach the small intestine directly. Eighty percent of primary bile acids get re-absorbed in the ileum, while the rest is deconjugated and hydroxylated to secondary bile acids in the large bowel. The majority of these secondary bile acids are reabsorbed, while a small portion is lost in the feces.

tion of vital organs. Also, in most cases, it is not possible to differentiate clinically between different causes of liver disease. However, there is some sublobular specialization of hepatocytes which may aid in diagnosis that is summarized in Table 7.1.

7.3 Diagnostic approach to patients with suspected liver disease

A definitive diagnosis of a disease of the liver, biliary tract, or portal vein usually requires a multi-step approach. The clinical symptoms, which may occur in patients with these diseases, are often nonspecific. A history of symptoms potentially related to hepatic diseases is followed by physical examination, laboratory evaluation, ultrasonography, cytology, histological evaluation of liver biopsies, scintigraphy, or liver function testing.

7.3.1 Prevalence of liver disease

The recognition of hepatic disorders on the basis of history and physical examination is often difficult, because the symptoms are usually nonspecific.[6–8] This nonspecific presentation of patients with liver disease makes accurate statements about prevalence difficult. Liver and biliary tract diseases have been reported to have an incidence of approximately 1–2% of all clinical cases presented to referral practice.[9–12] However, well-documented figures for a first line clinical population are not available. Also, there are breed-specific diseases that need to be taken into account separately. We have investigated the prevalence of inherited portosystemic shunts in several breeds such as the Irish Wolfhound and the Cairn Terrier in the Netherlands and found a prevalence of 4% and 2%, respectively.[9,13,14] In general, the prevalence of portosystemic shunts in commonly affected breeds (around 30 breeds) has been estimated to be around 1–4% of puppies born. Hepatitis is another example of a liver disease, which may be hereditary or be affected by inherited risk factors. The Bedlington Terrier used to have a very high prevalence of copper-associated hepatitis (20–50% of the population) until a mutation in the Murr1 gene was discovered and subclinically diseased animals and carriers could be identified with a DNA test. Copper-associated hepatitis also frequently occurs in Labrador Retrievers (estimated prevalence around 10–15%) and Doberman Pinschers (estimated prevalence around 5%) (see 7.5.1.4). Therefore, it is important to keep breed predispositions in mind when a list of differential diagnoses is being constructed for a specific patient.

7.3.2 Symptoms associated with liver diseases[6]

Because of the lack of specific clinical signs for liver disease, a few factors need to be considered that may help with the interpretation of clinical findings in patients with suspected liver disease. The liver plays an essential role in many metabolic processes. Disturbances in liver function may affect the function of other organ systems, which may point to a disease process of that organ rather than to the liver. Examples of this are hepatic encephalopathy, which may point to a central nervous system disease, or polydipsia, which may point to an endocrine or renal disease. The liver is also often secondarily involved in diseases of other organ systems, so that the same symptoms and abnormal laboratory findings can occur as with primary liver disease. One example is vomiting, which is a frequent symptom in patients with primary liver disease, but at the same time is also a clinical sign in patients with primary GI disorders that could also result in secondary (reactive) hepatitis. In both scenarios, the clinical symptoms are identical and blood biochemical tests would indicate the presence of liver disease, although the primary disease process may not be hepatic in origin. Another example is polyuria and polydipsia, symptoms that are frequently observed in many patients with chronic primary liver disease, but also in patients with several endocrine and paraneoplastic diseases in which the liver is secondarily involved (e.g., Cushing's disease, diabetes mellitus, malignant lymphoma). In all these diseases, the plasma hepatic enzyme activities and serum bile acid concentrations are often increased.

The following symptoms can be observed in different combinations in a variety of liver diseases: apathy, listlessness, reduced appetite, vomiting, weight loss, polydipsia, diarrhea, reduced endurance, ascites, neurological signs, icterus, acholic feces, increased bleeding tendency, painful micturition, frequent micturition, or abdominal pain. Apathy or listlessness is very frequent, as are reduced appetite or vomiting, which may be an indication of nausea. Weight loss occurs frequently in patients with chronic disease. Polydipsia has been reported with a prevalence of 50–60% in patients with chronic liver disease, including cholestatic diseases and portosystemic shunts. Diarrhea occurs infrequently in dogs and cats with liver disease and is usually not a major problem in patients with primary liver disease. As such, dogs and cats presenting only with diarrhea usually do not have primary liver disease as the underlying cause. Ascites occurs only infrequently and only in patients with an extreme loss of hepatic function. Neurological signs (i.e., ataxia and compulsive walking) occur frequently, especially in patients with portosystemic shunting. Such signs of hepatoencephalopathy usually wax and wane. Icterus is infrequent and more than 90% of dogs with liver disease have a normal serum bilirubin concentration. However, cats with hepatopathies have jaundice more frequently. Abnormally lightly colored (i.e., acholic) feces also occur very infrequently and are only seen in patients with bile duct obstruction. Also, an increased bleeding tendency is very infrequent. However, subclinical abnormalities of the coagulation cascade are more frequent. Painful, frequent micturition is also observed infrequently and is only seen in dogs with portosystemic shunts that cannot metabolize uric acid and ammonia, and in turn develop ammonium urate urolithiasis. Abdominal pain is very rare, but is sometimes seen in patients with cholecystitis.

It is important to note that the entire spectrum of symptoms may be observed in different combinations in most hepatobiliary diseases, but that it is usually not possible to relate the symptoms to a specific liver disease. Any combination of the above symptoms should lead to evaluation of the patient for possible liver and/or biliary disease.

7.3.3 Physical examination[6–8]

The most relevant parts of the physical examination are the evaluation of the mucous membranes and sclera, and an abdominal palpation. While mucous membranes are normal in most patients with liver disease, abnormalities may include jaundice, pallor, or spontaneous bleeding. Reduced erythrocyte survival time (increased hemolysis) is very common in patients with hepatobiliary disease. In combination with reduced erythropoietic activity as a consequence of chronic disease in general, the finding of a slight anemia and somewhat pale mucous membranes is very common in patients with chronic hepatobiliary disease. When the mucous membranes are very pale (Htc usually < 15–20%), the underlying cause of the disease is usually hemolytic anemia with secondary hypoxic liver damage. In such cases, a careful search for an underlying cause of the hemolysis is indicated and further evaluation of the liver is not necessary. However, in patients with icterus and moderately pale mucous membranes (Htc > 20%), the primary cause is nearly always hepatic disease and further diagnostic tests should focus on the liver and the biliary system.

Hepatomegaly may be palpable upon abdominal examination, depending on the degree of the enlargement, the depth of the thorax, and the concavity of the diaphragm. Hepatomegaly is uncommon in dogs with liver disease, which more often causes an abnormally small liver in this species. However, hepatomegaly does occur in patients with primary hepatic tumors and diseases with secondary hepatic involvement, such as venous congestion, fatty liver (i.e., secondary to diabetes mellitus), glycogen accumulation (i.e., secondary to hyperadrenocorticism), amyloidosis, lymphosarcoma, or metastatic tumors. In contrast to dogs, cats with hepatobiliary disease often have hepatomegaly. However, when hepatomegaly is present, examination of the circulation is indicated to exclude primary cardiac disease.

Abdominal palpation may also reveal splenomegaly in the case of portal hypertension, but this is also rather nonspecific and not always present in patients with portal hypertension. Ascites may be present and serve as an indication for chronic liver disease with portal hypertension and a reduced capacity to synthesize albumin. Of course, there are many other causes of ascites but an evaluation of serum hepatic enzyme activities, serum bile acids concentrations, and serum albumin concentration is indicated to prove or exclude hepatic involvement.

In most patients with a disease of the hepatobiliary system, the physical examination reveals only nonspecific findings; therefore, a basic laboratory investigation is usually necessary to prove or exclude hepatobiliary disease.

7.3.4 Diagnostic tests for liver disease

A detailed discussion of diagnostic tests for the diagnosis of hepatic disease can be found in chapter 1.4.3. The liver has many different metabolic functions and consists of hepatocytes, the biliary system, Kupffer cells, fat-storing stellate cells, and an arterial and venous blood supply. Although the liver is often considered a homogeneous organ and one tends to speak of hepatic function, there is no single test that adequately identifies hepatic disease or its underlying cause. There are, however, many different tests available by which the presence and nature of liver diseases can be evaluated.[15] Thus, the best approach for diagnosing hepatobiliary diseases is to use screening tests (see 1.4.3) to evaluate hepatobiliary damage and function. If such screening tests indicate the presence of hepatobiliary disease, the diagnosis is made by further diagnostic modalities such as imaging (see 1.3), cytology (see 1.7), and/or histological examination of a liver biopsy (see 1.8). Once a diagnosis has been made, it may be helpful to evaluate specific hepatic functions in order to determine the stage of the disease, which may be important for establishing the prognosis or choosing the most appropriate therapy for a given patient.

It is important to note that some hepatobiliary diseases are characterized by subtle changes in serum enzyme activities, but are associated with severe functional disturbances, while others are associated with severe changes in the serum enzyme activities, yet are not associated with significant hepatic dysfunction. Because of the large reserve capacity of the liver, detection of global hepatic functional impairment by conventional means is not possible until there is at least a 55% loss of hepatic mass. Parameters on a biochemistry profile that are routinely used for assessment of hepatic function include serum and plasma concentrations of albumin, ammonia,[16,17] urea nitrogen, bilirubin, bile acids,[18–20] cholesterol, and glucose. These tests can be used to assess the hepatic capacity to synthesize proteins, detoxify protein degradation products, excrete organic anions and other substances, or maintain euglycemia.

The results of a laboratory evaluation reflect a single point in time in a spectrum of dynamic changes. If the test results are equivocal and the clinical signs are vague, sequential evaluation may be necessary to allow time for the disease to be fully expressed. If the liver is only secondarily involved (such is the case in nonspecific reactive hepatitis), the hepatic changes and concomitant blood test results may normalize within three to four weeks, which makes this a good time span to repeat measurements in the case of equivocal test results as primary hepatic diseases will usually become more apparent, whereas nonspecific changes usually disappear.

7

By using a combination of history, physical examination findings, and the results of screening and hepatobiliary-specific laboratory tests, the clinician should be able to classify the disorder as active or quiescent; characterize the pattern of hepatobiliary disease as primarily hepatocellular, primarily biliary, or mixed hepatobiliary; and estimate the degree of hepatobiliary dysfunction. It is also important to note that results from a serum biochemical profile do not identify the underlying disease process and it is nearly always necessary to collect liver biopsies to reach a definitive diagnosis. In the case of a vascular anomaly (such as inherited portosystemic shunts), specific biochemical tests and ultrasonography and/or scintigraphy are required to arrive at a definitive diagnosis.

7.3.5 Liver biopsy

7.3.5.1 General considerations

As mentioned previously, for many primary hepatobiliary diseases in cats and dogs, a hepatic biopsy is needed to establish a definitive diagnosis and determine a prognosis.[1] In some cases, bile culture is also imperative. Biopsy is indicated 1) to determine the underlying cause of abnormal results of tests of hepatic function and pathology, especially if they persist for longer than one month; 2) to determine the cause of hepatomegaly; 3) to determine hepatic involvement in a systemic illness; 4) to stage a neoplastic disease of the liver; 5) to objectively assess response to therapy in patients with hepatobiliary disease; or 6) to evaluate the progression of a previously diagnosed disease that is not specifically treatable.

Several approaches for the collection of a liver biopsy are available and the choice is dictated by both patient and operator considerations.[1,21,22] All cats and dogs undergoing hepatic biopsy should be fasted for at least 12 hours, regardless of the approach selected. In general, percutaneous needle core biopsy or aspiration (for cytological analysis) of a single cavitary or solid lesion that is highly likely to be a non-lymphoid cancer is avoided unless the owner is unwilling to permit surgery for complete resection. Fine-needle aspiration for cytological analysis is advisable if multiple nodules are noted or if the owner is opposed to treatment of a neoplastic disease even if only a single lesion can be identified. Metastatic cancer may have a similar ultrasonographic appearance to benign hyperplasia or regenerative nodules. Unfortunately, the overall agreement of findings of cytological and histopathological diagnosis was only 44% in one study when evaluating neoplastic lesions of the liver. In patients with an especially small and/or firm fibrotic liver, it can sometimes be difficult to obtain a biopsy specimen by use of a percutaneous needle and this method often results in the collection of small and fragmented specimens that are difficult to interpret. In such cases, a true-cut biopsy usually produces diagnostic samples. The gun device usually leads to sharp, unfragmented slices even in the case of a firm, fibrotic liver. Also, the speed of the device prevents the liver from floating away from the tip of the needle. There is a reported correlation of <40% between findings from an 18-G true-cut needle biopsy and a wedge biopsy for certain hepatobiliary diseases, such as chronic hepatitis, fibrosis, cirrhosis, cholangitis, or portovascular anomaly[17]. If a needle-based biopsy technique is selected, the largest available instrument should used (i.e., preferably 14 G and minimum 16 G) to ensure samples of adequate size for examination. Two good quality 14 G needle biopsy samples are usually sufficient for diagnostic purposes in dogs. In cats, 16 G biopsy needles are usually adequate. It is important to always take at least two biopsy specimens to achieve a good representation of the liver. Samples of this size are representative for an adequate evaluation of most hepatic pathologies. In contrast, samples collected by an 18-G needle are often too small for accurate interpretation.[1]

The animal's coagulation status must be determined before a liver biopsy is performed, regardless of the approach.[23,24] Ideally, a complete coagulation profile is obtained (i.e., one-stage prothrombin time [OSPT or PT]), activated partial thromboplastin time [APTT or PTT], fibrin degradation products, fibrinogen content, and platelet count). Bleeding following ultrasound-guided biopsy is more likely if the platelet count is <40,000 cells/µl, or if the OSPT (dogs) or APTT (cats) is significantly prolonged. However, severely decreased fibrinogen concentrations below 50% of the lower reference range are the strongest contraindication for the collection of a liver biopsy. If possible, von Willebrand's factor should be measured in the serum of susceptible breeds in advance of a liver biopsy because the results of standard coagulation tests are usually normal in affected dogs. A buccal mucosal bleeding time provides an indirect measure of platelet function and should be routinely performed before collecting a hepatic biopsy. In dogs with von Willebrand's disease, desmopressin acetate (DDAVP) should be given (1 mg/kg SC) 30–60 minutes before the procedure to enhance a shift of von Willebrand's factor activity from the endothelial cells into the plasma.

Mild abnormalities in the coagulation parameters do not necessarily preclude a liver biopsy. In fact, the results of routine coagulation tests may not correlate with actual bleeding times at the biopsy site, as was found in one study of human patients.[25] However, the collection of a liver biopsy should be delayed if there is clinical evidence of bleeding or marked abnormalities in the coagulation parameters. Because animals with complete extrahepatic bile duct obstruction (EBDO) may be vitamin K deficient, as manifested by a prolongation of both OSPT and APTT, treatment with vitamin K_1 (5 mg subcutaneously once or twice a day) is indicated for one to two days before biopsy collection. Repeating the OSPT and APTT 24 hours after the administration of vitamin K_1 should demonstrate normal or near-normal results. However, in modern practice, EBDO is mostly an ultrasonographic diagnosis, and a liver biopsy is not required in most of these cases. Some animals with liver disease may have high serum concentrations of proteins induced by vitamin K antagonism (PIVKA), which could suggest potential bleeding tendencies. If there has been a minimal improvement in the coagulation parameters after vitamin K_1 administration, fresh frozen plasma should be administered before the collection of a biopsy. If bleeding is determined to be excessive during biopsy collection or after a biopsy has been collected and if bleeding cannot be controlled locally with direct pressure or application of pro-coagulatory substances, fresh whole blood should be given.

7.3.5.2 Biopsy techniques[1,26,27]

7.3.5.2.1 True-cut biopsy needle

True-cut biopsy needles have an inner needle with a 2-cm long indentation, which is advanced into the hepatic parenchyma, so that the hepatic tissue is pushed into the indentation. Thereafter, the outer sleeve with its cutting edge is advanced over the inner needle, so that the tissue is sliced off, after which the entire instrument is withdrawn. True-cut needles have a sharp tip, which can easily penetrate other structures, and should therefore only be used under ultrasound-guidance or direct visualization, such as during surgery. True-cut needles can be manual, semi-automatic, or for use with a biopsy-gun. The use of semi-automatic needles is advised for cats. The biopsy gun is expensive, but single-use gun needles are cheap. Thus, a biopsy gun is recommended for centers where biopsies are collected frequently. An advantage of the biopsy gun is that the process is very quick and a small firm fibrotic liver that moves relatively freely in a fluid-filled abdominal cavity can be easily biopsied. As mentioned above, true-cut needles should only be used under ultrasound guidance.[1,28,29] However, certain true-cut gun devices have such a strong spring driving the needle that the sudden pressure pulse in the liver parenchyma may cause fatal shock in cats; this has not been observed in dogs. It is extremely important, therefore, to verify that a proper device is being used.

7.3.5.2.2 The Menghini aspiration needle[1]

This type of needle has a tip with a blunt angle, which can penetrate soft tissues, such as the liver, but not the stomach or the intestines. The tip of the needle is used to "palpate" the tissues in order to locate the liver. This needle is usually used blindly, without ultrasound guidance. It does not permit the sampling of focal lesions and is only useful to detect diffuse liver disease, when ultrasound is not available. For population-based studies of a large series of cases, the Menghini technique has many advantages. Interested readers are referred to the WSAVA Standards for Clinical and Histological Diagnosis of Canine and Feline Liver diseases for further information.[1,30]

7.3.5.2.3 Fine needle aspiration[31-34]

Fine-needle aspiration is performed with a 20–22 gauge needle. The aspirate is transferred onto a glass slide and dried before staining with one of several stains, such as May-Grünwald-Giemsa or Diff Quick stain (Harleco, Gibbstown, NJ). Fine-needle aspiration is usually performed under ultrasound guidance in order to sample cells from a focal lesion. However, blind samples can be taken in the area of the 10th intercostal space at the level of the rib to rib-cartilage junction. Hepatic cytology is not suitable for the evaluation of the histological structure of the liver, which is important for the diagnosis of the vast majority of hepatic diseases. However, it is very useful for the detection of tumor cells or hepatic lipidosis. There is no need to test the coagulation status of the patient before a fine-needle aspiration of the liver.

7.3.5.3 Surgical wedge biopsy[35]

Surgical biopsies may provide larger samples than needle or forceps biopsies. In order to avoid taking a sample from an area of nonspecific subcapsular fibrosis, it is important to take wedge samples that are preferably 2 cm deep. In human medicine, multiple deep needle biopsies are considered superior over wedge biopsies, which are more superficial. Percutaneous biopsy techniques should be used in dogs and cats with hepatomegaly and ultrasonographic evidence of diffuse, uniform hepatic parenchymal disease. A fine needle aspirate of the liver for cytological evaluation is often obtained first because evidence for certain disorders such as vacuolar hepatopathy (i.e., hepatic lipidosis or steroid hepatopathy) and lymphoid neoplasia can be presumptively identified by this method.

If the operator is experienced with the biopsy procedure, there is little time involved and only sedation and local anesthesia of the skin and abdominal wall are required in some dogs. The liver itself is not painful upon puncture with large-core needles. However, in cats it is advisable to perform the procedure under general anesthesia.

Visualized percutaneous needle biopsy, either with the aid of ultrasound or modified laparoscopic equipment,[36] allows the selection of the best site or sites and direct or indirect inspection after the biopsy has been collected. In an animal with suspected diffuse or multifocal hepatobiliary disease, multiple biopsy specimens can and should be obtained, which, in general, is considered safe. General anesthesia is required for use of a modified laparoscope. However, ultrasound-guided true-cut needle biopsies are easier to perform and deliver comparable results in most cases.

7

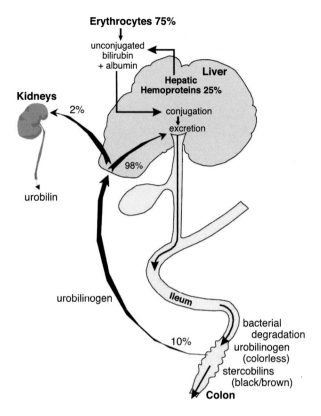

Figure 7.4:
Metabolism of bilirubin. This schematic drawing shows the physiological metabolism of bilirubin. Approximately 75% of unconjugated bilirubin stems from the heme of erythrocytes, while approximately 25% come from hepatic hemoproteins. Bilirubin is conjugated in the hepatocytes and excreted with the bile. In the intestinal lumen, conjugated bilirubin is degraded by bacteria to urobilinogen and stercobilins. Approximately 10% of the urobilinogen is absorbed in the colon, of which 2% is excreted through the kidneys.

As for percutaneous biopsy techniques, liver and / or bile specimens for microbiological culture are aseptically collected first. Then, impression smears for cytological analysis are made by gently touching a specimen to a slide before placing it in fixative. Excess blood is removed by blotting the sample on gauze before the impressions are made. Abnormal populations of cells (e.g., mast cells, lymphoblasts) are readily detectable using rapid stain systems such as Diff Quik. For routine processing and histopathological examination, hepatic tissue specimens are submerged in 10% buffered formalin. Quick fixation is essential and is only possible if the samples are not too thick; therefore, surgical samples should be cut into 2–3 mm thick slices. Samples for copper histochemical staining or tissue quantification are harvested and fixed or preserved according to the specifications of the pathology laboratory selected to do the assays. Other special stains for infectious agents, or fibrous tissue, amyloid, glycogen, or other metabolic products are available and their use must be discussed with the attending pathologist before the tissue specimen is obtained.

7.3.5.4 Gall bladder aspiration

The gall bladder can be safely aspirated under ultrasound guidance using a fine-needle aspiration technique. There is no need to approach the gall bladder transhepatically and any approach is considered safe. Sampling of bile for cytology and culture is especially important in cats, in which infectious cholangitis is one of the most frequent chronic hepatobiliary disorders.

7.4 Complications of liver disease

7.4.1 Ascites

Ascites is abdominal fluid of low protein content and low cellularity, such as can be found in patients with liver disease. Ascites occurs relatively frequently in dogs with chronic liver disease, but is rare in cats. Intrahepatic portal venous hypertension is the most common cause leading to ascites in dogs.[37,38] These patients also commonly show a reduced serum albumin concentration, so that decreased oncotic pressure and portal hypertension both contribute to the formation of ascites.[39] In patients with pre-hepatic causes, such as an arteriovenous fistula or a portal vein thrombosis, the portal blood pressure is usually much higher and the albumin concentration does not decrease as much as it does with intrahepatic causes of ascites, such as chronic hepatitis. Portal vein occlusion may be caused by compression due to masses or a congenital portal vein hypoplasia. Postsinusoidal sphincters have been identified in hepatic veins of dogs and may add to venous outflow resistance. Also, sodium and water retention due to hyperaldosteronism may further enhance the formation of ascites. Extravasation of bile from a ruptured biliary tract or from the gall bladder elicits a strong inflammatory peritonitis with transudation of lymph. In such cases, the peritoneal fluid appears characteristically dark brown or green, and the inflammation causes the fluid to be turbid. Cytological evaluation of this fluid will show that it contains many neutrophils.[40] Bile duct rupture may cause septic peritonitis due to a secondary infection, usually with anaerobic bacteria.

7.4.2 Jaundice

Bilirubin is a waste product of heme degradation (Figure 7.4).[41] Heme mainly stems from the hemoglobin in erythrocytes (65% of all heme production), with a smaller contribution from myoglobin and heme-containing enzyme systems in the liver (30–35%). Bilirubin produced from heme is cleared from the plasma, conjugated by the liver, and excreted into the bile. In the intestinal tract, conjugated bilirubin undergoes bacterial deconjugation and becomes reduced to urobilinogen. Urobilinogen is reabsorbed and then once again cleared by the liver (i.e., enterohepatic circulation). Only a very small amount of it escapes into the systemic circulation and is excreted in the urine. In the colon, urobilinogen is transformed into stercobilin, which gives the feces their normal brown color.

Hepatic handling (i.e., clearance, conjugation, and especially biliary excretion) of bilirubin may become impaired due to hepatic parenchymal and/or biliary diseases. Obstruction of the common bile duct near the duodenum results in impairment of all proximal mechanisms of bilirubin handling (i.e., excretion, conjugation, and clearance), but the resulting mixed conjugated/unconjugated hyperbilirubinemia consists predominantly of the conjugated or direct form. Cholestasis is also associated with increased serum activities of GGT and AP, and with increased serum bile acids concentrations. Biliary tract rupture allows the leakage of bile into the peritoneal cavity. The peritoneum then absorbs the pigments, which in turn leads to severe icterus. Severe hemolysis leads to increased bilirubin production. In addition, the liver develops centrolobular necrosis due to hypoxia. Icterus due to hemolysis is only seen when the hemolysis is acute and severe, resulting in mixed conjugated/unconjugated hyperbilirubinemia due to the combination of hypoxic necrosis and cholestasis with increased production of bilirubin.

The reference ranges for serum total bilirubin concentration in dogs and cats may vary from laboratory to laboratory, but most laboratories agree that concentrations above 0.3 mg/dL in cats and 0.6 mg/dL in dogs are abnormal.

Dogs, especially males, have the necessary renal enzyme systems to produce and conjugate bilirubin, so bilirubinuria may be a normal finding in urine samples from dogs. In contrast, bilirubinuria is an abnormal finding in cats, is associated with hyperbilirubinemia, and is always pathological.

Acholic feces may result from a total absence of pigment in the intestinal tract. Only a small amount of bile pigment is necessary to stain feces to their normal color. Complete EBDO due to cholelithiasis, a tumor of the bile duct, the head of the pancreas, or the duodenal wall may cause such acholic, greasy, gray-colored feces.

Unpigmented, concentrated mucoid bile may develop in patients with chronic severe extrahepatic bile duct obstruction. This "white bile syndrome," may occur in both dogs and cats.

Conjugated bilirubin may easily and irreversibly (covalently) bind to albumin in the circulation.[42] This permanently bound bilirubin is no longer available for normal hepatic clearance from the plasma and therefore stays in the circulation and other tissues until the albumin is degraded. As a consequence, animals may remain icteric for several weeks after the resolution of the cause of the icterus and icteric mucous membranes may not accurately reflect the present situation, but rather be representative of a previous disease state.

7.4.3 Hepatic encephalopathy

Hepatic encephalopathy (HE) is defined as a dysfunction of the brain secondary to hepatic dysfunction. HE occurs frequently in both dogs and cats with severe hepatic dysfunction and represents a complex of neurological symptoms.[43,44] Like icterus, HE is not a diagnosis, as the causes of HE may be quite varied. HE can occur due to two different clinical scenarios, an acute severe total hepatic failure (also called fulminant hepatic failure) or a chronic form, which can be subclinical to severe.

Fulminant hepatic failure can be due to an acute and complete necrosis of the liver and may be caused by infections, such as canine adenovirus 1 or toxins, such as acetaminophen, fungal toxins (e.g., aflatoxicosis), and mushroom toxins (e.g., phalloidin). Fulminant hepatic failure causes severe HE or even hepatic coma. It also causes severe icterus, vomiting, and spontaneous bleeding tendencies due to DIC. The activities of liver enzymes in the serum or plasma are extremely elevated, and many such patients die within a few days. Fortunately, chronic HE is by far the most common form. Chronic HE can be caused by the shunting of portal blood so it bypasses the liver through the portosystemic collateral circulation. Portosystemic shunting may be inherited or acquired, with the latter form being caused by portal hypertension.

In cats, there is another form of HE, which is related to a deficiency of essential amino acids and the development of hepatic lipidosis (see 7.6.1.1). This is the only form of HE that requires amino acid supplementation for successful management; all other forms of HE should be treated by a reduction of dietary protein. Patients with HE may also benefit from the administration of lactulose orally or by enema, in addition to antibiotic therapy with neomycin or another broad-spectrum antibiotic.

In both dogs and cats, chronic HE is most commonly caused by the shunting of portal blood past the liver and is thus also referred to as portosystemic encephalopathy. The great functional reserve of the liver protects animals against HE, even if they have severe liver disease. Even severe portosystemic shunting alone is not sufficient to cause HE in most cases and only leads to HE when present in combination with compromised hepatic function. This situation occurs, for example, in patients with chronic hepatitis leading to portal hypertension and acquired portosystemic collaterals. In dogs and cats with congenital shunts, the hepatic function also becomes increasingly inadequate. Normally, the liver grows due to the expression of

7

Table 7.2: Neurological symptoms in dogs and cats with hepatic encephalopathy (HE)

Neurological symptoms seen in dogs and cats with HE

Stage 1	Apathy, decreased mental alertness, "staring", unawareness of surroundings
Stage 2	Ataxia, circling, head pressing against obstacles, blindness, salivation
Stage 3	Stupor, severe salivation, completely inactive but arouseable
Stage 4	Coma, totally unresponsive

Non-neurological signs associated with liver diseases causing HE

All stages	Polyuria/polydipsia, vomiting, decreased endurance, inactivity, sometimes insufficient growth (e.g., dogs with congenital shunts)
General	Periodic occurrence is very typical

7

growth factors; the expression of which requires the delivery of stimulating factors from the portal circulation. Thus, without these stimulating factors, the liver of animals with congenital shunts lack normal growth as the body grows. This explains why animals with congenital hepatic shunts most commonly develop symptoms when they are six months of age or older.

The clinical symptoms of HE vary and are due to metabolic derangements in the brain. If the underlying disease can be cured, even severe neurological signs disappear completely. Very characteristic is the episodic nature of HE, with fluctuations between grade one and the more advanced stages in the same patient (Table 7.2). Usually one or a few days of severe signs of HE alternate with more ore less normal periods of one or several weeks' duration. Apart from the neurological symptoms of HE, non-neurological signs related to the underlying disease are often seen. Patients with HE rarely have seizures. Seizures without any of the other signs described in Table 7.2 are almost never due to HE.

Essentially, chronic HE is a dysfunction of several neurotransmitter systems. The most important ones involved are the glutamate, the dopamine /noradrenaline, and the gamma-aminobutyric acid and benzodiazepine (GABA / BZ) neurotransmitter systems. For the production and homeostasis of these transmitter systems, the brain utilizes precursors coming from the intestinal tract, which are normally modified by the liver. In patients with portosystemic shunting of blood, the lack of this modification gives these precursors unregulated access to the brain, which cannot adjust to the increased amount of unmodified neurotransmitters.

Glutamate is one of the most important excitatory neurotransmitters in the brain, and is directly influenced by the concentration of ammonia in the circulation (Figure 7.5). Ammonia is mainly produced in the intestinal tract by colonic bacterial degradation of nitrogenous compounds (i.e., proteins, amines, and urea) and also by the intermediary metabolism of glutamine in the mucosa of the entire intestinal tract. The normal liver is extremely efficient in removing ammonia from the portal blood and in one passage of blood through the liver virtually all the ammonia is removed, so that the peripheral concentration is kept very low. Most of the ammonia is converted to urea by enzymes of the urea cycle of the hepatocytes located around the portal areas of the liver lobules; this cycle is exclusive to the liver. The urea is transported by the blood to the kidneys, which in turn excrete it into the urine. Another pathway of ammonia removal utilized by the cells of all tissues (in addition to the liver) is its incorporation in glutamate and glutamine. Glutamine contains two molecules of bound ammonia. Glutamine enters the circulation and becomes metabolized in the intestinal mucosa and the kidneys, where the ammonia is liberated. Intestinal ammonia reenters the cycle, but in the kidneys the ammonia produced in the tubular cells is excreted into the urine. However, in the case of alkalosis, ammonia can easily diffuse back into the renal vein, so that the kidneys then become a contributor to the plasma concentration of ammonia. In patients with portosystemic shunting of portal blood, the efficient removal by the liver largely fails and the plasma concentration of ammonia increases steadily.

Hyperammonemia leads to toxic concentrations of ammonia in the nervous system because the physiological protection by the astrocytes becomes inadequate. The neurons are separated from the blood by a layer of astrocytes, and substances from the circulation have to pass these astrocytes before they can reach the neurons. Under physiological conditions, blood ammonia enters the astrocytes, but then gets scavenged by being incorporated into glutamine by a process that requires ATP and is catalyzed by glutamine synthetase. This enzyme has little functional reserve and cannot handle much more than physiological blood ammonia concentrations (Figure 7.5). The glutamine diffuses into the adjacent neurons where it is converted to glutamate by glutaminase. Glutamate in the neurons is then partly converted to GABA. The excitatory glutamate and inhibitory GABA form a finely tuned equilibrium determining the excitability of postsynaptic neurons. During times of hyperammonemia, the capacity of glutamine synthetase in the astrocytes becomes overloaded and free ammonia diffuses into the neurons. High neuronal ammonia concentrations inhibit glutaminase activity leading to the accumulation of glutamine and depletion of the neurotransmitter glutamate. This disturbed glutamate-glutamine-ammonia shuttle between the astrocytes and neurons is thought to be an important factor in the pathogenesis of HE.

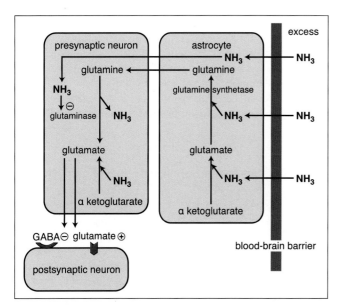

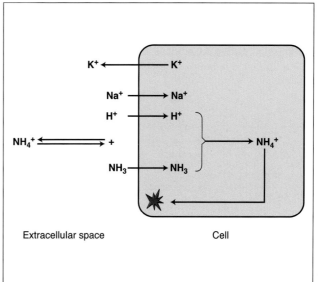

Figure 7.5:
Influence of hyperammonemia on glutaminergic neurotransmitters. Astrocytes are overwhelmed by the amount of ammonia diffusing into them and can no longer incorporate all the ammonia into glutamate and glutamine. The excess ammonia diffuses into the presynaptic neurons and leads to the formation of additional glutamate and the inhibition of glutaminase, which further increases the amount of glutaminergic neurotransmitters in the presynaptic neuron. In turn, this excess of glutaminergic neurotransmitters in the presynaptic neuron leads to overstimulation of the postsynaptic neuron. The minus sign indicates inhibition, while the plus sign indicates activation.

Figure 7.6:
Effect of hypokalemia on intracellular ammonia concentration. Hypokalemia leads to a movement of intracellular potassium into the extracellular space. In return, there is an influx of sodium and hydrogen ions. As a result, extracellular alkalosis ensues and leads to the generation of more ammonia and hydrogen from NH_4^+. Ammonia can easily diffuse into the cell. Within the cell, the excess hydrogen ions and ammonia form NH_4^+ once again. NH_4^+ can not diffuse back out of the cell and gets trapped.

Only the non-ionized form of ammonia, NH_3, can pass through cell membranes, but NH_4^+ cannot. However, inside the neurons both forms are equally toxic. NH_4^+ and NH_3, are both measured when blood ammonia is determined. In extra- and intracellular fluid, there is an equilibrium between NH_4^+ and $NH_3 + H^+$. This equilibrium shifts towards NH_3 during alkalosis and towards NH_4^+ during times of a neutral blood pH or during acidosis. Thus, during alkalosis ammonia has easy access into the neurons, so that the same plasma concentration of ammonia may lead to a more severe encephalopathy than during times of a neutral blood pH or during acidosis. Therefore, alkalosis should be prevented or, if present, corrected. Alkalosis also results in the formation of alkaline urine, from which the non-ionized ammonia is readily reabsorbed, so that the kidneys may spare ammonia instead of excreting it. The most serious form of alkalosis is induced by hypokalemia (Figure 7.6). Low plasma potassium is replenished by an exchange of intracellular potassium against sodium and hydrogen ions. This exchange of hydrogen causes extracellular alkalosis and intracellular acidosis. As a result, ammonia can easily penetrate the cell membrane, but intracellularly it becomes ionized and can no longer leave the cell, so that the neurons further accumulate ammonia. Under these conditions, most of the ammonia pool is intracellular, and relatively moderate elevations in plasma ammonia concentrations may lead to rather severe neurological signs. Such conditions may very well occur in patients with chronic liver disease. The most frequent cause of this situation is portal hypertension, which in turn leads to ascites. The peritoneal fluid originates from the circulatory volume and many animals with ascites are slightly dehydrated, especially during the initial formation of ascites. This slight dehydration in turn activates the renin-angiotensin-aldosterone system, leading to renal sodium retention and potassium loss. In these patients, it is contraindicated to tap much ascitic fluid as the ascitic fluid will reform quickly. For the same reason, it is important to use only potassium-sparing diuretics, especially in anorectic patients that have insufficient potassium intake.

The measurement of blood ammonia concentration is currently the only practical way to diagnose HE.[14,43–46] Mild to moderate hyperammonemia may sometimes be missed in a venous sample. When there is any doubt, an ammonia tolerance test may give more definitive results.[47] This test is also

7

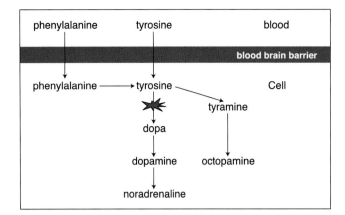

Figure 7.7:
Formation of false transmitters in patients with portosystemic shunts. In patients with portosystemic shunts, aromatic amino acids are not adequately cleared by the liver. As a consequence, more of these aromatic amino acids reach the neurons where they overwhelm the enzymatic capacity to form catecholamines and are instead metabolized to tyramine and octopamine. These "false" transmitters occupy the catecholamine receptors, but are non-functional and thus block monoaminergic neurotransmission.

7

very reliable in diagnosing portosystemic collateral circulation in patients that do not yet have HE. The test is performed by giving a 5% ammonium chloride solution rectally (i.e., by advancing a red-rubber catheter approximately 10–20 cm into the rectum). Only in the case of portosystemic shunting does ammonia bypass the liver and peaks in the peripheral plasma at 20 and 40 min after administration. A distinct increase to above 100 and usually 150 µmol/L is seen in patients with shunting of hepatic blood (reference range <45 µmol/L). The ammonia load given with this test usually does not worsen the encephalopathy and does not pose any risk to the patient. However, it should be avoided in cases in which the basal ammonia concentration is already very high (>150 µmol/L). In approximately 40% of dogs with HE, ammonium biurate crystals can be identified during urinalysis.

In patients with HE, there is also an increased tone of the GABA / BZ receptor system. The underlying mechanism is poorly understood. However, the use of benzodiazepines and barbiturates that activate this receptor system is contraindicated in animals with suspected liver failure.

Additionally, in patients with portosystemic shunting, the aromatic amino acids tyrosine, tryptophane, and phenylalanine, which are absorbed from the intestinal tract, are not adequately cleared by the liver. If abnormally high concentrations of these amino acids reach the brain, an impairment of the catecholamine neurotransmitter system results. Tyrosine is the physiological precursor for the catecholamines (i.e., dopamine and

noradrenaline), but the enzymatic capacity in neurons to utilize tyrosine is limited. In the case of an excess supply of tyrosine to the neurons, they produce alternative metabolites, such as tyramine and octopamine, which in turn occupy the catecholamine receptors, but are not functional (Figure 7.7). As a consequence, increased plasma tyrosine concentrations lead to a blockage of the catecholamine receptors in the central nervous system.

7.4.3.1 Management of hepatic encephalopathy

Mild cases of HE can be treated by feeding a low protein, high carbohydrate diet, which leads to a reduction of the ammonia and amino acid load. It is important to meet the energy requirements of the patient through dietary carbohydrates and fat as catabolism should be avoided in these cases. Cats require about twice as much protein as do dogs, which needs to be taken into account when choosing a diet. More severe cases of HE require treatment with the oral administration of lactulose (1–3 ml/kg/day divided over three doses), which is very efficient. Lactulose is not absorbed in the small intestine and is fermented to volatile free fatty acids by colonic bacteria. The resulting acidification shifts the equilibrium to non-absorbable ionized ammonia, increased colonic motility, and a less ammoniagenic colonic microflora. Also, a non-absorbable antibiotic, such as neomycin, may be useful in treating HE.

7.4.4 Coagulopathies

Because of the integral role of the liver in hemostasis, bleeding tendencies can be one of the presenting signs in cats and dogs with very severe hepatobiliary disease. However, the large functional reserve of the liver prevents clinical hemorrhagic symptoms in nearly all patients with even the most severe cases of liver disease. Most coagulation proteins and inhibitors, except for von Willebrand's factor (vWF) and possibly factor VIII, are synthesized in the liver. An inability to synthesize vitamin K-dependent factors (i.e., factors II, VII, IX, and X) because of a failure of the bile acid-dependent fat absorption that can occur secondary to complete EBDO can cause coagulopathies. Subclinical coagulopathies may occur in diseases of the hepatic parenchyma.[32,33]

The most common cause of a subclinical coagulopathy in patients with hepatobiliary disease is disseminated intravascular coagulation (DIC). This is especially the case in patients with diffuse hepatocellular necrosis, as can occur in patients with hepatitis, lymphosarcoma, or metastatic tumors. Depending on the severity of the disease process (i.e., the amount of thromboplastin released from the necrotic tissue), the coagulopathy may be subclinical or may be clinically apparent. Findings on laboratory tests indicating DIC include a low concentration of fibrinogen, thrombocytopenia, and the presence of fibrin degradation products. Therefore, it is essential to assess the coagulation status in patients with suspected hepatic disease, especially before collecting a liver biopsy. Fibrinogen concentrations below 100 mg/dl (1 g/L) are an absolute contraindication for a liver biopsy.

Although DIC can ultimately lead to blood loss, another mechanism for blood loss in dogs with severe hepatic disease is portal hypertension-induced vascular congestion and fragility. In such cases, blood loss may occur in the stomach or duodenum.

7.4.5 Polyuria and polydipsia

Increased thirst and volume of urination can be seen in patients with severe hepatocellular dysfunction. However, it should be noted that polyuria and polydipsia (PU/PD) is a symptom of liver disease only in dogs, but not in cats. An increased sense of thirst may be a manifestation of HE. Also, excess secretion of ACTH from the intermediate pituitary lobe stimulated by abnormal neurotransmitters can lead to excess cortisol secretion from the adrenal glands and an altered threshold for antidiuretic hormone release in dogs with HE.[44] However, PU/PD also frequently occurs in dogs with liver diseases that are not associated with portosystemic shunting. Although several mechanisms have been proposed, the pathophysiology is still not entirely clear.

7.5 Liver diseases of the dog

7.5.1 Parenchymal liver diseases of the dog

7.5.1.1 Canine hepatitis

Hepatitis is a common liver disease in dogs, but is extremely rare in cats. Therefore, the following discussion on hepatitis is exclusively focused on dogs. The primary inflammatory disease of the hepatobiliary tract in cats is cholangitis, an inflammatory disease of the biliary system, whereas in dogs hepatitis is primarily a parenchymal disease.[5,10]

Any destruction of the hepatic parenchyma either due to apoptosis or necrosis may be followed by an inflammatory reaction, regeneration of the parenchyma, fibrosis, and ductular proliferation. When hepatocellular destruction is limited and the reticulin network remains intact, regeneration with complete restitution of the hepatic structure can occur. However, severe parenchymal destruction with extensive loss of hepatocytes is often followed by ductular proliferation. Many regen-

erative structures contain both hepatic parenchymal and biliary elements and may reflect either a regenerative proliferation of a hepatic stem cell population or the transformation of regenerating hepatocytes into ductular-like structures. These regenerative structures generally are most prominent in the periportal areas. With chronic parenchymal damage or extensive loss of hepatocytes, fibrosis and postnecrotic scarring may occur and may be associated with the formation of intrahepatic portovenous shunts. In such cases, the prolonged regenerative effort will result in regenerative parenchymal nodules.

A definitive diagnosis of hepatitis requires histology of the liver. The histopathological diagnosis should include the type, pattern, and extent of the necrosis and inflammation, the possible cause, and in more chronic cases the presence, pattern, and extent of fibrosis and regeneration. The activity of the inflammatory process is defined by the amount of hepatocellular necrosis and inflammation, while the chronicity is determined by the amount of fibrosis.

7.5.1.1.1 Acute Hepatitis

Etiology

Acute hepatitis can be caused by chemicals (the most common ones are organic solvents such as tetrachloromethane [CCl_4] and phosphorus), drugs (e.g., benzodiazepine in cats, acetaminophen in all mammals, trimethoprim sulfonamide, carprofen, and the antibiotic nalidixate), viral infection (e.g., infectious canine hepatitis), and mycotoxins (especially aflatoxin B1).[10] Hepatitis resulting from sepsis (i.e., reactive hepatitis), leptospirosis, and hemolysis are discussed in other sections below. Drugs containing sulfonamides may induce a severe type of hepatitis, which, however, presents mostly as a chronic disease.

Pathogenesis

Depending on the extent of the hepatocellular necrosis, differing amounts of intracellular enzymes will be released and bile will leak back into the circulation. In an acute hepatitis, all of the serum hepatic enzyme activities are usually elevated. Fever can, but does not always, occur as a result of pyrogens from the necrotic tissue and a reduced removal of endotoxins and bacteria from the portal blood. DIC is also very common. When hepatocellular necrosis is extensive and a significant portion of hepatic function has been lost, the condition is classified as fulminant hepatitis. Fulminant hepatitis leads to the development of HE, DIC, jaundice, and hypoglycemia. The hypoglycemia is due to a lack of glycogen synthesis and glyconeogenesis. Fulminant hepatitis rapidly progresses to coma and death.

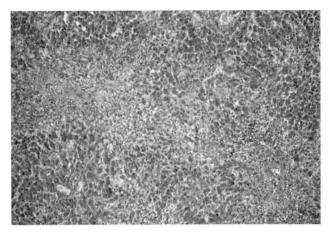

Figure 7.8:
Fulminant hepatitis. This histopathological section from a dog with fulminant hepatitis shows diffuse necrosis of hepatocytes throughout (H&E stain; 40×).

Acute hepatitis is characterized by hepatocellular necrosis that is followed by an inflammatory reaction (Figure 7.8). Depending on the severity of the hepatitis, there may be apoptosis, focal necrosis, and confluent or bridging necrosis. The inflammatory infiltrate consists of round cells and neutrophils. Infection with canine adenovirus-1 is usually characterized by confluent and bridging necrosis in the centrolobular zone and by the presence of intranuclear inclusions in the hepatocytes and Kupffer cells. The virus can be demonstrated in a histological liver section by the presence of intranuclear inclusion bodies or by immunofluorescence. Acute hepatitis may also be caused by various toxins,[49–55] such as mushroom toxins (e.g., *Amanita* spp.), blue-green algae toxins (e.g., Cyanophyceae), idiosyncratic drug toxicities (e.g., sulfonamides, carprofen, or amiodarone), or dose-dependent drug toxicities (e.g., acetaminophen).

Symptoms

Hepatitis is associated with acute illness, apathy, sometimes fever, anorexia, vomiting, dehydration, sometimes icterus, and in severe cases DIC. In its most severe form, fulminant hepatitis, all hepatic functions fail, resulting in rapidly worsening HE, icterus, and bleeding diathesis. The clinical picture, however, is entirely dependent on the severity of the liver damage. Usually, acute hepatitis is a moderately severe disease and most dogs recover completely.

Diagnosis

A serum chemistry profile usually reveals elevations of liver enzyme activities, especially ALT, and sometimes hyperbilirubinemia. The diagnosis is confirmed by percutaneous liver biopsy.

Treatment

As the cause of the hepatitis cannot be identified in most cases, no specific treatment is available or needed. In more severe cases, supportive treatment may include IV fluid administration to correct hypovolemia, shock, acidosis, or alkalosis, hypoglycemia, and electrolyte disturbances. Corticosteroids are contraindicated. In patients with severe liver damage, an antibiotic (e.g., ampicillin) may be a helpful to eliminate bacteremia that can be present due to inadequate hepatic clearance of the portal blood. Phalloidin and acetaminophen intoxication cause oxidative damage and should be treated with silymarin (50 mg/kg/day PO q 24 h for 3–5 days). Silymarin has been reported to be less effective when given a few hours after intoxication. Acetaminophen intoxication may also be treated with the combination of N-acetylcysteine (140 mg/kg PO q 6 h for 3 days), vitamin C (25–35 mg/kg PO q 6 h for 2 days), and cimetidine (5 mg/kg PO q 12 h for 4 days). Dogs with acetaminophen intoxication may have hemolysis and a blood transfusion may be required.

Follow-up

Patients with acute hepatitis recover spontaneously in most cases, but in about 10% of patients the disease progresses to a chronic hepatitis. The chronic disease usually does not lead to clinical signs in the first few months, but often becomes clinically apparent at a much later stage of hepatic dysfunction. It is, therefore, recommended to perform a second liver biopsy four to six weeks after a diagnosis of acute hepatitis to identify patients with chronic hepatitis at an early stage. Early chronic hepatitis is often not associated with abnormal serum liver enzyme activities or bile acids concentrations, and without a control biopsy these cases may be missed.

7.5.1.2 Leptospirosis

Etiology

Leptospira spp. organisms are transmitted with the saliva and urine from infected rats or dogs. Animals may become asymptomatic carriers transmitting the disease without being ill themselves. Experimentally, infection is mostly pathogenic in young dogs and older dogs often remain asymptomatic. After an incubation of one to three weeks, acute illness ensues with uremia and icterus, which is caused by intrahepatic cholestasis. Myositis often causes pain upon palpation and also a painful gait. Without treatment, the resulting renal insufficiency is usually fatal, but depending on the strain of the organism that causes the infection, the hepatic lesions are usually not as severe.

In the liver, leptospirosis causes a nonspecific reactive hepatitis. Bacterial enzymes cause detachment of the tight junctions, which stimulate hepatocyte mitosis. Thus, the most characteristic histological finding is an increased number of mitotic figures in the hepatocytes (Figure 7.9). There is usually extensive intrahepatic cholestasis, and nearly all patients are icteric.

Symptoms

The symptoms of leptospirosis are mainly dominated by renal insufficiency or failure, and include acute illness, malaise, fever, vomiting, icterus, muscle pain and sometimes diarrhea or petechiations due to thrombocytopenia.

Diagnosis

Many patients with leptospirosis have icterus. The serum chemistry profile may reveal uremia and cholestasis with elevated serum bilirubin concentrations, AP activities, and bile acids concentrations. Serum creatinine kinase (CK) activities are often elevated, reflecting the myositis. Many patients also show thrombocytopenia. Urinalysis often reveals indicators of nephritis, such as tubular epithelial cells in the sediment and / or proteinuria.

The histopathology of a liver biopsy mostly shows a nonspecific reactive hepatitis, which may occur with any type of sepsis. A definitive diagnosis can only be made by serology. There is a rapid IgM peak, which reaches a maximum after about 4 days of infection, followed by an IgG peak at least 10 days later. The IgM peak remains for 2–3 weeks, and the specific measurement of IgM in the serum is the only method to confirm the diagnosis in an early stage of the disease. IgG is only indicative for infection in animals that have never been vaccinated, or when serum IgG titers increase over time.

Management

Often, penicillin is initially used until hepatic and renal functions are completely recovered, at which point streptomycin is given on two consecutive days. This prevents the continuing excretion of *Leptospira* in the urine. *Leptospira* excretion stops after two days of penicillin administration and no more *Leptospira* are excreted as long as the penicillin is continued. This is especially important as leptospirosis is an important zoonosis,

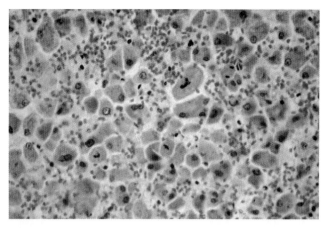

Figure 7.9:
Leptospirosis. This histopathological view shows several mitotic figures of hepatocytes, which is typical for dogs with leptospirosis (H&E stain; 100×).

7

which can lead to morbidity and even acute renal failure in human patients. Alternatively to penicillin and streptomycin, doxycycline at the standard antibiotic dose can be used.

Leptospirosis can be prevented by vaccination, which is important for dogs at risk, such as hunting dogs. However, vaccination only protects from infections due to certain serovars and recently an increasing number of cases have been documented that are due to serovars for which no vaccines are available.

The prognosis depends on the degree of renal damage. Acute illness with jaundice is an indication to examine renal function. Antimicrobial therapy should be started immediately. Despite appropriate therapy, the infection is lethal in many cases. All patients with acute disease associated with jaundice and uremia should be treated as leptospirosis suspects, until leptospirosis has been ruled out.

7.5.1.3 Chronic hepatitis and hepatic cirrhosis

Chronic hepatitis and hepatic cirrhosis are discussed together here because they have the same pathogenesis and their clinical and pathological changes often overlap.[5,10] Chronic hepatitis is characterized by periportal fibrosis, infiltration of the hepatic parenchyma with lymphocytes and plasma cells, and periportal liver cell apoptosis or necrosis. Apoptotic liver cells become smaller and acidophilic, and are also known as acidophilic bodies. Expansion of the inflammation may extend to form porto-portal or porto-central bridging fibrosis. If the fibrosis forms septa connecting the portal and centrolobular areas, the normal functional architecture of the hepatic lobules

7

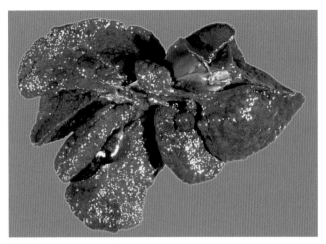

Figure 7.10:
Micronodular cirrhosis. This figure shows a liver from a dog with inherited copper storage disease. The nodules are diffusely dispersed throughout the liver and are generally very small. This finding of micronodular cirrhosis is typical for copper storage disease as opposed to other causes of cirrhosis in dogs.

become permanently disturbed: this is called cirrhosis. The liver has an enormous regenerative capacity, which is more pronounced than that of most other tissues, but in the case of cirrhosis regeneration is non-organized and forms nodules of hyperplasia (Figure 7.10). These nodules embody almost non-functional liver tissue. Cirrhosis represents the end-stage of chronic hepatitis. Macronodular cirrhosis is the most common form of hepatic cirrhosis in dogs, but micronodular cirrhosis can be seen in chronic hepatitis associated with copper storage (Figure 7.10). Chronic hepatitis is associated with fibrosis, and the more fibrosis that occurs, the less capacity the parenchyma has to regenerate. This leads to a permanent loss of hepatocytes and the liver becomes smaller. Fibrosis, especially cirrhosis, also obstructs the normal portal blood flow. Portal blood is required to activate hepatic growth factors, so that decreased portal perfusion also contributes to decreased liver regeneration. Altogether, advanced fibrosis can lead to cirrhosis through a vicious cycle. Therefore, it is crucial that the clinician diagnoses chronic hepatitis during an early stage, permitting intervention. The inflammatory infiltration and the loss of liver cells vary from case to case, depending on the degree of activity of the process. Chronic hepatitis and cirrhosis cause variable degrees of intrahepatic cholestasis, but in most cases there is no icterus.

Etiology

Chronic active hepatitis may be caused by a viral infection.[56] Canine adenovirus-1 (CAV1) is the only known canine hepatitis virus. CAV1 virus infection in non-vaccinated animals leads to fulminant hepatitis. The author has not been able to identify high titers against CAV1 in most dogs with chronic hepatitis. It is also likely that there are other viruses that can cause chronic hepatitis in dogs. However, the lymphocytic and plasmacytic inflammation and the good response to immunosuppressive drugs indicate that a self-perpetuating auto-immune process plays a role in chronic hepatitis.

Chronic hepatitis and cirrhosis may also be due to chemicals or toxins (e.g., aflatoxin). Metabolic alterations in the liver, primarily inherited copper toxicosis, also can lead to damage of hepatocytes with secondary hepatitis and fibrosis. However, in patients with this condition, lesions begin in Zone 3 of the acini instead of in the portal areas. Our group has recently shown that Doberman Pinschers and Labrador Retrievers, which are also frequently affected by hepatitis, have an inherited form of copper storage disease (see 7.5.1.4). In Doberman Pinschers, this form of chronic hepatitis is very aggressive and sex-linked with a predilection for female dogs. Copper-associated hepatitis also occurs frequently in a variety of Spaniel breeds.

Pathogenesis

The gradually progressive hepatocellular necrosis may cause a continuing elevation of all serum liver enzyme activities and serum bile acids concentration. However, in patients where the hepatitis is not very active or in those with end-stage disease that is associated with cirrhosis, the release of hepatic enzymes into the blood stream may be insignificant and in turn the serum enzyme activities may be normal or only slightly elevated. Icterus does not develop consistently.

Chronic hepatitis is always a diffuse process. Hepatic function is diminished due to the loss of functional tissue mass and also reduced portal blood flow. Often the patient shows low serum albumin and fibrinogen concentrations. HE may develop if portosystemic collaterals are formed (Figure 7.11). Patients with end-stage disease usually develop cirrhosis. Hypoalbuminemia and portal hypertension may cause ascites.

Chronic hepatitis may occur at any age. In those breeds that have chronic hepatitis due to abnormal copper metabolism, the gradual accumulation of copper usually leads to onset of clinical signs at an age of 4–7 years. Chronic hepatitis can occur in all breeds, but the most frequently affected ones are Labrador Retrievers (Golden Retrievers are affected to a lesser extent), Doberman Pinschers, all Spaniel breeds, Bedlington Terriers, and West Highland White Terriers (see also 7.5.1.4).

The incidence of chronic hepatitis is relatively high. It is one of the most common liver diseases seen in dogs and accounts for approximately 1% of all cases presented to a referral clinic.

Symptoms

The most frequently observed symptoms in patients with chronic hepatitis are apathy, reduced appetite, vomiting, poor endurance, polydipsia, and sometimes icterus. In advanced cases, there may be ascites and HE.

Diagnosis

Physical examination usually reveals no specific findings. All serum hepatic enzyme activities are more or less increased. In advanced cases there may be hypoalbuminemia. The diagnosis can only be made by the histopathological evaluation of liver biopsies. Ultrasonography prior to biopsy is advised. Cirrhosis may be suspected based on the appearance of a small liver with an irregular surface and structure. Many patients with chronic hepatitis, however, show no abnormalities at all on abdominal ultrasonography.

Management

Prednisolone or prednisone are used as anti-inflammatory (0.5–1.0 mg/kg PO q 12 h) or immunosuppressive (1–2 mg/kg PO q 12 h) agents. If the side effects of the steroids are intolerable, a combination of prednisone (0.5 mg/kg/day PO) and azathioprine (1.0 mg/kg/day PO) can be used. It is important to carefully evaluate the response to treatment by repeat liver biopsies (e.g., every 6 weeks). Corticosteroids themselves cause changes in the liver, therefore, blood work alone is not suitable to evaluate the response to treatment. Medication must be continued until there is complete histological recovery, which is usually after 8–12 weeks.

Without treatment, the disease progresses to cirrhosis. Apart from specific therapy directed at the hepatitis, more advanced cases also require supportive care directed at dehydration and management of the risks of HE. The risk for HE can be predicted by an ammonia tolerance test. Most therapies for hepatitis in dogs have been poorly evaluated. Based on the pathophysiological considerations, one could also treat dogs with hepatitis with ursodeoxycholic acid (ursodiol, 5–15 mg/kg PO q 24 h) and/or S-adenosylmethionine (SAME) at the manufacturer's recommended dose. The clinical effect of these medications has not been proven, but it has become common practice by some clinicians to use a combination of prednisone, ursodiol, and SAME in a polypharmaceutical approach.

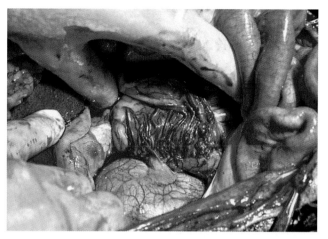

Figure 7.11:
Portosystemic collaterals. Patients with hepatic cirrhosis may develop multiple portosystemic collaterals as the liver can no longer handle physiological portal blood flow. The patient shown here has developed several collaterals near the left kidney.

7

Prognosis

The prognosis for dogs with chronic hepatitis is dependent on the stage of the disease and can be guarded to good. The disease can often be stopped completely. Sometimes there is a recurrence, requiring repeated treatment. In cases of cirrhosis, the prognosis depends on the activity of the ongoing hepatitis and the degree of hepatic regeneration. If the hepatitis is still active, judged by the number of inflammatory cells, significant improvement may be achieved. Even liver perfusion may improve and the portal hypertension may decrease. There is no proven treatment to reduce fibrosis and dogs with chronic forms of hepatitis will have fibrosis even after they have been treated successfully. Depending on the formation of collateral vessels, canine patients with chronic hepatitis may develop portovascular anomalies and require permanent support with a special diet and/or lactulose.

7.5.1.4 Chronic hepatitis due to copper storage in the liver

Etiology

Hepatitis due to copper storage occurs as a result of an inherited defect in the copper metabolism of hepatocytes, resulting in impaired excretion of copper into the bile. Most foods contain an excess of copper, which is absorbed in the small intestine and cleared from the portal blood by the liver. The copper excess is normally excreted into the bile by the hepatocytes and thereby cleared from the body. Copper is an essential ele-

7

ment and, after incorporation into ceruloplasmin by the liver, is distributed throughout the body. The normal metabolic pathways of copper in hepatocytes are only partly known. Intracellular trafficking of copper only occurs in the protein-bound form, since free copper causes oxidative damage to cells. In inherited copper storage disease, the gradual accumulation of copper in the hepatocytes causes oxidative damage and, ultimately, hepatocellular necrosis that induces a secondary inflammatory reaction. The accumulation of copper and inflammation occurs mostly around the central veins, whereas other forms of chronic hepatitis concentrate in and around the portal areas. As with other forms of chronic hepatitis, copper-related hepatitis can also progress to cirrhosis (Figure 7.10). The gradual accumulation of copper leads to the onset of clinical signs at an age of 4–7 years in most breeds. High hepatic copper concentrations ($>1,000\,\mu g/g$ dry liver tissue) indicate an inherited form of copper storage disease. Although copper needs to be excreted with the bile, cholestasis never causes such high copper concentrations in the liver.

Copper storage disease occurs in a variety of breeds: Anatolian Shepherds, Bedlington Terriers, Dalmatians, Doberman Pinschers, Labrador Retrievers, Skye Terriers, all Spaniel breeds, and West Highland White Terriers.[11,57–67] In Doberman Pinchers, the disease affects only females. In other breeds with this disease, both sexes are affected, however, usually with a female overrepresentation. The underlying gene defect has only been discovered in the Bedlington Terrier, where it has been shown to be an autosomal recessive disease. Heterozygote carriers cannot be distinguished phenotypically from homozygote healthy animals. Very recently, a reliable DNA test for the causative deletion in the COMMD1 gene in this breed has been reported (this test is commercially available through VetGen, Ann Arbor, MI).[11] The causative gene is not known for any of the other breeds; therefore, the diagnosis depends on the collection of a liver biopsy, histochemical copper staining, and the quantitative analysis of copper content. The increased copper concentration in the liver of affected dogs can be confirmed only after about 1 year of age, as these dogs may not have stored sufficient copper beforehand.

Pathogenesis

Oxidative damage to cellular organelles causes cell death followed by an inflammatory reaction. A chronic persistent hepatitis develops and as a result the liver loses its regenerative capacity and forms fibrous tissue. In the final stages, cirrhosis may develop.

Bedlington Terriers may develop an acute hemolytic anemia. The hemolysis is probably the result of release of copper from the liver into the blood due to hepatocellular necrosis. Because the liver function is already reduced, this hemolysis usually leads to severe icterus.

Symptoms

The symptoms are the same as those seen in patients with other forms of chronic hepatitis and include apathy, reduced appetite, vomiting, poor endurance, polydipsia, and sometimes icterus.

Diagnosis

Copper hepatotoxicity cannot be differentiated from other forms of chronic hepatitis and hemolysis based on physical examination and blood tests alone. Instead, the diagnosis is based on a histological examination of liver biopsies. The association of the hepatitis with an excessive copper content is based on histochemical copper staining and quantitative copper analysis in a hepatic biopsy. The normal concentration of copper in the dog liver is between 50 and $300\,\mu g/g$ dried hepatic tissue. Bedlington Terriers with copper accumulation have concentrations exceeding $1000\,\mu g/g$ at one year of age, but in other breeds the accumulation seems to progress much slower and even the highest concentrations seen in these breeds are lower than those seen in Bedlington Terriers.

Management

Copper storage disease should be treated with a copper-binding chelating drug.[68] Penicillamine is widely used and is given in two daily doses of 20–35 mg/kg, 30–60 min before each meal. Penicillamine binds copper and the complex is excreted in the urine. Gradual removal of free excessive copper reduces the degree of hepatitis. Female Dobermans, which used to have a poor prognosis when diagnosed with hepatitis, often recover completely when treated with copper-chelating agents.[68] The response to treatment should be evaluated by repeated liver biopsies. For most patients with copper storage disease, a biopsy interval of three months is appropriate.

If the hepatitis appears cured, recurrence should be prevented as the genetic basis for the abnormal copper metabolism remains. Long-term prevention may be achieved with zinc (15 mg/kg PO q 12 h, given with each meal). Zinc induces intestinal metallothionein, which binds copper and prevents copper absorption. Modern low-copper diets are advised for supportive care. There is good evidence from double-blind, randomized and placebo-controlled studies that penicillamine is effective in dogs of different breeds with copper storage disease. There is only limited evidence that trientine, another copper-chelating agent is efficacious in canine patients with copper storage disease and routine use cannot be advised at this point. The beneficial effect of zinc is well proven in different species. Since complete recovery is commonly achieved with penicillamine and zinc there is no need to use other drugs. However, there is no contraindication for the use of ursodiol and SAME in these patients (see 7.5.1.3).

7.5.1.5 Lobular dissecting hepatitis

Etiology

The etiology of lobular dissecting hepatitis is unknown. However, the author has seen this form of hepatitis in kennels where several dogs have had the disease, all at different ages. In the absence of any indication for a toxic cause, this would suggest an, as of yet unknown, infectious etiology.[69]

Pathogenesis

Lobular dissecting hepatitis is a diffuse hepatitis with pericellular fibrosis around all the hepatocytes. The amount of fibrous tissue is excessive and usually leads to severe portal hypertension, which in turn may quickly cause ascites, acquired portosystemic collaterals, and HE. The progression of this disease is usually much more rapid than the regular form of chronic hepatitis and the course of this disease usually takes weeks rather than months. The clinical picture of lobular dissecting hepatitis closely resembles that of hepatic cirrhosis and congenital portal vein hypoplasia. In fact, this condition more appropriately should be termed cirrhosis rather than hepatitis, as this term more appropriately describes the deranged liver lobe architecture. Macroscopically, the liver is small and has a smooth or finely granular surface.

Symptoms

Lobular dissecting hepatitis can be associated with weight loss, vomiting and polyuria, which can be followed by ascites and HE.

Diagnosis

The abdominal fluid from dogs with lobular dissecting hepatitis is usually clear and colorless, but can also be yellow in icteric patients. A serum chemistry profile may or may not show elevated liver enzyme activities, but bile acids concentrations are usually elevated. Plasma ammonia concentration may also be elevated and the ammonia tolerance test is abnormal in most patients.

Liver biopsy is diagnostic for lobular dissecting hepatitis and reveals characteristic histological changes. Percutaneous liver biopsy with a Menghini needle is usually difficult (i.e., these patients have a small, firm liver that "floats" away in the ascites fluid), so that an ultrasound-guided biopsy with a biopsy gun may be necessary.

Management

The management of lobular dissecting hepatitis is similar to that of chronic hepatitis. However, the prognosis of this condition is much worse than that of chronic hepatitis.

7.5.1.6 Nonspecific reactive hepatitis

Pathogenesis

Nonspecific reactive hepatitis describes a condition that is characterized by focal or diffuse hepatic damage with a secondary inflammatory reaction resulting from toxemia or sepsis.[5, 10] Reactive hepatitis can occur in every patient with toxemia, sepsis, inflammation, or a necrotizing process (including tumor necrosis). When such a process is located in the drainage area of the portal vein, all of the toxins are transported to the liver. In addition, generalized sepsis may also cause this form of hepatitis. Reactive hepatitis develops in most cases of gastroenteritis as a result of increased hepatic toxin absorption. It also develops in patients with peritonitis and other inflammatory diseases of organs that are drained by the portal vein.

Dogs with chronic diarrhea as the major clinical sign usually do not have primary liver disease, but rather a primary intestinal disease with a secondary reactive hepatitis. In contrast, vomiting is a common clinical sign in patients with either primary hepatobiliary disease or primary GI disease. It is important, therefore, to carefully take a history, as this may give clues to decide whether the patient has a primary intestinal or hepatic disease.

Circulating toxins, inflammatory mediators, and bacteria cause a proliferation of the reticuloendothelial system and also an infiltration of the liver with neutrophils. Focal hepatic necrosis can also occur. In chronic cases, there is also a component of lymphocytic and plasmacytic infiltration. Reactive hepatitis can also be associated with mild to severe cholestasis of the canaliculi. In some cases that are associated with sepsis, diffuse foci of necrosis, microabscesses, or granulomas can be seen (e.g., *Herpes canis* infection, toxoplasmosis, brucellosis, tuberculosis, *E. coli* infection, or migrating larvae of *Toxocara canis*). Continuous *Toxocara canis* infestation can cause a diffuse granulomatous eosinophilic inflammatory reaction. Hematologically, peripheral eosinophilia may also occur in such cases.

The type of inflammatory cells in patients with secondary nonspecific reactive hepatitis (i.e., predominantly neutrophils and sometimes eosinophils) are different from those in patients with primary chronic active hepatitis (i.e., lymphocytes and plasma cells). Also, the localization of the inflammatory reaction within the liver is different with a diffuse distribution in patients with secondary reactive hepatitis and a portal or periportal distribution with primary chronic hepatitis.

7

7

The clinical symptoms seen in patients with secondary reactive hepatitis are often determined by the primary disorder. Thus, most patients with reactive hepatitis have diarrhea. In patients with sepsis, fever may also be present. Severe reactive hepatitis may also cause icterus.

Diagnosis

A definitive differentiation between primary hepatitis and secondary reactive hepatitis is only possible by the histological examination of liver tissue.

Therapy

As hepatic functions remain well preserved, there is no specific therapy for reactive hepatitis. If reactive hepatitis is diagnosed, the clinician should search for the underlying primary disease process. After the underlying cause of the reactive hepatitis has been successfully treated, the liver will recover spontaneously within a period of about three weeks.

7.5.2 Parenchymal changes of the liver during systemic disease

7.5.2.1 Steroid hepatopathy

Pathogenesis

Cushing's disease and the administration of exogenous corticosteroids cause glycogen accumulation in hepatocytes and vacuolization, also known as ballooning. The liver cells are enlarged leading to hepatomegaly. Steroids cause induction of alkaline phosphatase (AP) activity. However, steroid hepatopathy does not dramatically affect hepatic function, so that the symptoms are usually due to the primary disease process rather than the hepatic changes.[5,70,71]

Symptoms

The symptoms seen with steroid hepatopathy are those of hyperadrenocorticism.

Diagnosis

The diagnosis of steroid hepatopathy is made by liver histology or cytology. The steroid-induced AP can be differentiated from other sources of AP as it remains active after heating the plasma to 65°C for 2 min. However, later on in the disease process, both the steroid-induced as well as hepatic AP may be increased.

Management

The glucocorticoid-induced changes of the liver disappear spontaneously within 4–12 weeks after the discontinuation of steroid administration or successful therapy of hyperadrenocorticism.

7.5.2.2 Hepatic steatosis in diabetes mellitus

Pathogenesis

In patients with diabetes mellitus, lipolysis in the adipose tissue is increased leading to an increased delivery of fatty acids to the liver. In addition, the production of triglycerides is also increased. As a result, fat accumulates in the hepatocytes and causes microvesicular, and in advanced cases, macrovesicular steatosis (lipidosis).[5]

Symptoms

Hepatic steatosis is mostly subclinical, and patients usually present with clinical signs due to the underlying diabetes mellitus, such as PU/PD and weight gain.

Diagnosis

Serum hepatic enzyme activities and bile acids concentrations can be slightly to moderately increased in patients with hepatic steatosis. The histological or cytological demonstration of steatosis in combination with persistent hyperglycemia is diagnostic. Indeed, the cytological evaluation of smears from fine needle aspirates is diagnostic in most cases.

Management

Specific treatment of the fatty change of the liver is not necessary, as it gradually disappears with regulation of the diabetes mellitus. There are idiopathic forms of hepatic steatosis, which may be chronic, but do not cause considerable hepatic dysfunction. There is no known treatment for these cases.

7.5.2.3 Hypoxic liver damage

Pathogenesis

Hepatic degeneration or necrosis can occur due to hypoxia of the liver. The usual causes of hepatic hypoxia are severe hemolysis and shock. Hepatic hypoxia leads to centrolobular necrosis, followed by a secondary inflammatory reaction of polymorphonuclear cells and intrahepatic cholestasis.[5,41]

Symptoms

Hypoxic liver damage normally does not lead to recognizable clinical signs as the patient usually displays pronounced clinical signs of the underlying hemolysis or shock.

Diagnosis

Hepatic changes due to hypoxia are specific, but they can only be confirmed by histopathology. However, in most patients with severe hemolysis or shock, the secondary hepatic changes are not of primary interest and instead the diagnostic effort is directed at identifying the underlying cause of the hemolysis or shock. It is important to note that patients with primary liver diseases also often show icterus in combination with anemia, but in patients with hypoxic liver damage, the anemia is much less pronounced than in patients with primary hemolytic anemia.

Management

Management involves treatment of the underlying cause. The liver usually recovers spontaneously.

7.5.2.4 Amyloidosis

Pathogenesis

Amyloidosis of the liver is very rare in dogs and is most commonly seen in Shar Peis. It occurs more commonly in Siamese cats. Deposits of amyloid in the liver are visible as amorphous hyaline and eosinophilic material in the space of Disse. Depending on the amount of amyloid deposit, the liver may be enlarged on abdominal palpation. Hepatic enzyme activities and bile acids concentrations in serum or plasma are usually increased. Amyloidosis usually causes concurrent glomerular damage and proteinuria. The liver becomes severely enlarged and fragile. Many patients die suddenly due to spontaneous hepatic rupture.

Symptoms

Sudden death due to hepatic rupture and abdominal blood loss may occur. Renal lesions are usually present and may cause proteinuria and nephrotic syndrome.

Diagnosis

Amyloidosis is diagnosed by cytological examination of a hepatic aspirate.

Management

There is no know treatment for this disease and it is usually lethal.

7.5.3 Vascular diseases of the liver

7.5.3.1 Congenital portosystemic vascular anomalies

Pathogenesis

Congenital portosystemic vascular anomalies or shunts (PSS) are congenital vessels that connect the portal vein and a large vein outside the splanchnic venous system; usually the vena cava or the azygos vein.[4] Portosystemic shunts occur in many different dog breeds. Cairn and Yorkshire Terriers, Maltese Terriers, Dachshunds, Labrador Retrievers, Bernese Mountain dogs, Hovawarts, and Irish Wolfhounds are frequently affected.[72] In a number of breeds, the incidence reported is between 1–5% of dogs born and it is likely that this number applies to most affected breeds.[9,13–14] Small dog breeds commonly have extrahepatic shunts, while large breeds more frequently have intrahepatic shunts, but presumably they are inherited in all dog breeds. Shunts also occur in cats (see 7.6.2.1). In both dogs and cats, PSS affect both females and males.

Portosystemic vascular shunts are large-diameter vessels leading to a preferential flow of portal blood through the shunt, thereby bypassing the liver. Quantitative measurements have revealed that, in most cases, >95% of the portal blood bypasses the liver. This is in part compensated for by an increased arterial blood supply to the liver. The oxygen supply for the hepatic parenchyma is therefore maintained. However, toxic compounds such as ammonia are not cleared adequately from the portal blood, which results essentially in autointoxication, in turn leading to neurological signs, as the brain is most sensitive to this autointoxication. In addition, endotoxins that are not cleared by the liver can cause vomiting. Portal blood also contains hormones and growth factors that induce the pro-

7

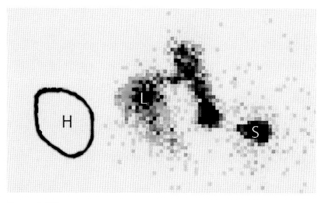

Figure 7.12:
Splenic scintigraphy – normal dog. A small amount (2 mCi) of ^{99m}Tc was injected into the splenic pulp (S) of this dog under ultrasound guidance and the patient was imaged for a period of 4 minutes. This image is a reformatted image of the first 7 seconds of the study. The heart (H) has been drawn into the image. Note that all of the radioactivity reaches the liver (L) and none the heart (H), demonstrating normal portal blood flow. (Image courtesy of Dr. Robert C. Cole, Texas A&M University.)

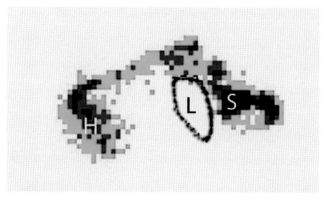

Figure 7.13:
Scintigraphy – portoazygos shunt. A small amount (2 mCi) of ^{99m}Tc was injected into the splenic pulp (S) of this dog under ultrasound guidance and the patient was imaged for a period of 4 minutes. This image is a reformatted image of the first 7 seconds of the study. The liver (L) has been drawn into the image. Note that the radioactivity bypasses the liver and appears first within the heart (H), indicating the presence of a portosystemic shunt. With this type of study, it is possible to determine whether a single shunt vessel or multiple shunt vessels are present and also whether the shunt vessel or vessels drain into the caudal vena cava or the azygos vein. In this case, a portoazygos shunt was suspected and confirmed during surgery. (Image courtesy of Dr. Robert C. Cole, Texas A&M University.)

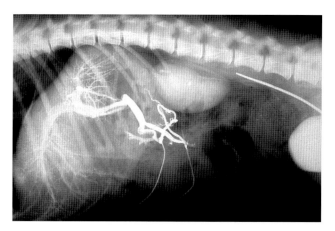

Figure 7.14:
Normal portal blood flow. This figure shows an angiography of the normal portal blood flow in a healthy dog. Note that all the dye injected through the catheter reaches the portal blood directly and evenly distributes throughout the tributaries of the portal vein.

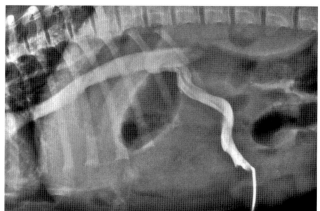

Figure 7.15:
Portocaval shunt. This figure shows an angiogram of a dog with a congenital extrahepatic portocaval shunt. Note that none of the dye injected reaches the liver, but instead immediately reaches the caudal vena cava. In most cases, a diagnosis of a portocaval shunt can be made by abdominal ultrasonography and scintigraphy, and angiography is usually not needed for routine clinical cases.

duction of local hepatocyte growth factor (HGF), which is essential for normal hepatic growth. Impaired regulation of hepatic growth results in poor growth and development of the liver, which stays very much behind as the animal as a whole grows more or less normally. With increasing age, this discrepancy becomes more and more severe, which explains why clinical signs usually do not develop until the patient has reached an age of around 6 months. Histologically, the liver shows signs of hepatocellular atrophy and an increased number of tortuous arterioles in the portal areas. The portal vein branches are so poorly developed that they are usually not histologically distinct. Macroscopically, the portal vein and its branches cranial to the shunting vessel are very narrow.[4]

In many cases of PSS, the kidneys are enlarged and also hyperfunctional. The poor liver function often results in hypoalbuminemia, which, however, is usually not low enough to cause ascites. Poorly soluble ammonium urate crystals are present in the urine in over half of the cases. These crystals can form bladder, kidney, or urethral stones. Such concrements are small, rough, yellow, and radiolucent.

Portosystemic shunts can be localized inside or outside the liver. Intrahepatic shunts usually originate from the left main branch of the portal vein (i.e., persistent ductus venosus), but in some cases they also can originate from the right branch. Intrahepatic shunts occur mostly in large breed dogs. Extrahepatic portocaval shunts are seen in toy or medium-sized breeds, and may originate from the gastroduodenal vein, the gastrosplenic vein, or the mesenteric vein. Most extrahepatic shunts in dogs end in the vena cava just cranial to the right kidney, but others terminate in the azygos or hemiazygos veins. Because the azygos vein is much smaller than the vena cava, the flow through a porta-azygos shunt is much lower and these dogs usually have less severe clinical signs, often becoming apparent at a later age. It is not unusual to be presented with a dog with a porta-azygos shunt that is 5–7 years of age. In rare cases, the portal vein is only connected with a systemic vein, without any normal continuation to the liver cranial to the branch of the shunting vessel.

Symptoms

In almost all cases, the clinical signs include apathy, excessive sleeping, and rapid fatigue. The animal may or may not be underweight, but stunted growth is rarely seen. Polydipsia occurs in many cases (> 50%), as well as occasional vomiting, and a variable appetite. Usually, there are neurologic abnormalities with HE varying between stages 1–4. The symptoms are usually periodic and days with clinical symptoms are followed by gradual improvement and a period without apparent clinical signs, lasting for one to several weeks. The neurological symptoms of HE are discussed in detail in 7.4.3. Some male patients may present with acute dysuria as ammonium urate

stones may lead to urethral obstruction. Although the symptoms usually develop in patients at an age of around 6 months, some patients may develop signs as late as 10 years of age.

Diagnosis

Serum activities of hepatic enzymes and serum concentrations of albumin may or may not be in the abnormal range, but if abnormal the changes are mild. Also, patients with portosystemic shunts never develop icterus. Abdominal radiographs or ultrasound reveal a small liver and large kidneys.[73,74] The measurement of plasma ammonia concentration is the first step to confirm the diagnosis, as it is highly elevated in most cases.[9,16] If there are any doubts as to whether the patient has a PSS, an ammonia tolerance test can be used to confirm the diagnosis. Serum bile acids concentrations, especially postprandial ones, are also increased in most cases,[75] but they have recently been reported to be less sensitive than ammonia.[16] Also, serum bile acids concentrations are nonspecific. There is usually a distinct increase of postprandial serum bile acids concentrations in both dogs and cats with PSS,[75] but such increases can also be seen in patients with cholestatic diseases.[16] In contrast, plasma ammonia concentration is only increased in cases of shunting or with hepatic failure. Also, with the availability of a good table-top analyzer (e.g., blood ammonia checker, Menarini; http://www.menarini.com), ammonia has become a practical parameter to measure. As much as an abnormal plasma ammonia concentration is a useful diagnostic tool for the diagnosis of a PSS, it can not be used to discriminate a single congenital from multiple acquired shunts.[45]

Abdominal ultrasonography may be used to directly visualize the shunt vessel and it is advisable to try to find the localization of the shunt before surgery.[76–81] If ultrasonography is inconclusive, the shunt may be definitively demonstrated by rectal or splenic scintigraphy.[76] Splenic scintigraphy requires a smaller amount of radioactive material than rectal scintigraphy, so that less time is required until the patient can be cleared for surgery (Figures 7.12 and 7.13). Contrast angiography by catheterization of the portal or splenic vein is more invasive and usually not necessary (Figures 7.14 and 7.15). Changes seen with liver histology are not specific for PSS and are similar to those seen with portal vein hypoplasia.[4]

Management

Surgical closure of the shunt is the treatment of choice for patients with PSS. The shunt is closed partially, permitting some portal blood to bypass the liver so that the portal pressure does not suddenly increase too much. There are several techniques such as the traditional method of placing a suture ligature, cellophane banding, or the use of an ameroid constrictor. With all these techniques, the shunt is only closed partially and it then usually closes completely on its own over time (4–8 weeks).[72,82–86] After partial closure of the shunt, more portal blood reaches the liver, so that production of local growth factors commences, followed by rapid growth of the liver, less resistance to portal blood flow, and further improvement of liver perfusion and growth. Such a positive outcome is achieved in about 60% of all cases. Suboptimal results may be due to inadequate development of the portal vein and/or incomplete hepatic growth.[86]

It is important to evaluate blood glucose concentrations before, during, and after surgery, since some of these animals may develop hypoglycemia due to poor liver function. Coagulation should also be checked before surgery and if necessary be corrected by a blood or plasma transfusion.

The surgical results in cats are less optimal than those in dogs.[87] Cats have more problems with the large changes in blood flow and pressure, and often die in the immediate postoperative period.

Especially in small breed dogs, a sudden derangement of brain function (cerebrocortical necrosis) may occur 2–3 days after surgery. The pathogenesis of this complication is unknown, but increased intracranial pressure and cerebral edema is most likely an important cause. In our experience, immediate osmotic diuresis with mannitol may prevent permanent brain damage. The onset of this complication is seen as a sudden mental derangement after an initially good post-operative recovery. If not detected and treated immediately, this complication leads to severe neurological signs very similar to those seen with HE, but without periodic changes and not accompanied by hyperammonemia.

In approximately 20% of patients, incomplete hepatic growth following surgery leads to increased portal pressure, which may initiate the development of acquired portosystemic collaterals. Such patients only show a partial improvement, followed by a recurrence of HE after approximately 6–8 weeks. Even with this complication, such patients usually benefit from surgery. They often need permanent dietary management and lactulose and/or antibiotic therapy, and can often be maintained very well with these measures. Complete recovery usually occurs within 3–4 weeks. Even severe neurological signs are completely reversible in most cases. The prognosis of surgical intervention depends on the type of the shunt.

Some owners opt not to pursue surgical therapy and supportive care may consist of a low protein diet, lactulose, and/or antibiotic therapy with a poorly absorbable antibiotic (i.e., neomycin, see 7.4.3).[44,73,88] The long-term prognosis for conservatively managed patients has not been studied in detail, but it is generally assumed that conservative management is less than ideal.

7.5.3.2 Hepatic congestion

Pathogenesis

Hepatic congestion is usually caused by congestive heart disease such as atrial fibrillation or pericardial effusion. An obstruction of the thoracic part of the caudal vena cava by a tumor or thrombus can also cause hepatic congestion. Ascites caused by hepatic congestion is always hemorrhagic, because erythrocytes escape from the congested capillary bed. In contrast, ascites due to primary liver disease is usually clear and colorless.

Hepatic congestion has no important functional consequences for the liver.[4] Hepatic enzymes, bile acids, and albumin are usually not or only mildly abnormal.

The congested liver is enlarged, darkly colored, and usually has a layer of fibrin attached to the capsule. In chronic cases, the capsule becomes thick and fibrotic. There is no formation of portosystemic collaterals because there is no pressure gradient between the portal vein and the systemic circulation.

Symptoms

The symptoms of hepatic congestion are those of the underlying disease process. As the liver functions remain largely unchanged, there are generally no signs of liver disease or failure.

Diagnosis

Ultrasonographic changes are typical of hepatic congestion and reveal congested branches of the hepatic vein. A severely congested liver should not be biopsied because of the increased risk of hemorrhage.

Management

No treatment for hepatic congestion is required, but hepatic congestion resolves when the underlying disease process is treated.

7.5.3.3 Primary portal vein hypoplasia

Pathogenesis

There has been much confusion about this condition in the literature, mainly because different names have been used for it, including microvascular dysplasia and congenital liver fibrosis.[4,45,89–93] However, the name primary portal vein hypoplasia has recently been adopted by the WSAVA standardization panel for hepatic diseases and should thus be used exclusively. Primary portal vein hypoplasia is characterized by an insufficient development of the terminal intrahepatic branches of the portal vein. Consequently, portal blood does not reach the hepatocytes. This disease may vary from a slight reduction of the number of terminal portal branches to a complete absence of them. In the latter case, there is usually also an abnormal extrahepatic portal vein, which may have a very thick fibrotic wall. There is a tendency for the formation of portal fibrosis, the degree of which may also vary from virtually absent to severe. There are many subclinical cases that may only be identified by chance after blood work reveals increased serum bile acids or plasma ammonia concentrations. More severe cases may present for ascites and HE, and may reveal acquired portosystemic collaterals upon abdominal ultrasound examination. Severe cases are usually presented at a young age, most often within the first year of life. There is reduced portal blood flow to the liver, which, depending on the severity of the condition, does not increase adequately as the patient is growing. In contrast to dogs with PSS, the kidneys are not enlarged in dogs with primary portal vein hypoplasia. Primary portal vein hypoplasia is congenital and is not progressive.

Histologically, there is hypoplasia of the terminal branches of the portal vein, and arteriolar hyperplasia. There may also be a variable amount of portal fibrosis. These changes are, however, not specific and may also be present in dogs with PSS or arteriovenous fistulas.

Symptoms

Patients with primary portal vein hypoplasia can present with ascites, HE, polydipsia, and occasionally vomiting. Symptoms may be mild or absent in less severe or subclinical cases, respectively.

Diagnosis

Blood work may show hypoalbuminemia, increased serum bile acids and plasma ammonia concentrations, and an abnormal ammonia tolerance test. Elevation of liver enzyme activities may or may not be present. The differentiation of primary portal vein hypoplasia from chronic hepatitis/cirrhosis can only be made by a histological examination of a liver biopsy. In cases with portal vein hypoplasia, the histological findings are identical to that of PSS. Therefore, the differentiation from PSS is based on the histological interpretation in combination with ultrasonography and/or scintigraphy. Dogs with severe portal vein hypoplasia show hepatofugal flow (i.e., flow in the portal vein that is directed away from the liver; Figure 7.16) when examined by Doppler ultrasonography. Ultrasonographic exclusion of PSS is part of the diagnosis; which, there-

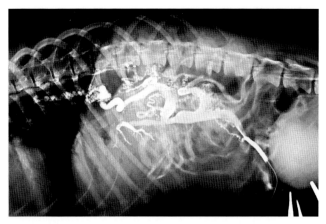

Figure 7.16:
Primary portal vein hypoplasia. This figure shows an angiogram in a dog with primary portal vein hypoplasia. Note that none of the injected dye appears to reach the liver but instead is shunted away from the liver. Such hepatofugal blood flow can also be documented by abdominal ultrasound.

fore, also depends on the experience of the ultrasonographer. Ascites may be present in dogs with portal vein hypoplasia (colorless), arteriovenous fistula (colorless), hepatic congestion (hemorrhagic), and portal vein thrombosis (hemorrhagic), but not in dogs with congenital shunts.

Management

There is no specific therapy for primary portal vein hypoplasia and recovery is not possible. Only symptomatic treatment can be employed to reduce HE (i.e., diet, lactulose, and/or neomycin) and limit the formation of ascites (i.e., potassium-sparing diuretics).

7.5.3.4 Portal vein thrombosis

Pathogenesis

Thrombosis of the portal vein is a rare disease, seen in patients that are hypercoagulable, as occurs in patients with nephrotic syndrome or in those with an abnormal intima of the portal vein.[4,38] In some cases, it is associated with pancreatitis or with chronic exposure to corticosteroids (endogenous or exogenous). Depending on the degree of obstruction of the portal vein, portal vein thrombosis can lead to acute portal hypertension if the obstruction occurs suddenly or portal hypertension and formation of collaterals when there is gradual occlusion. Thrombosis may occur in the left or the right main branch of the portal vein. This may lead to a one-sided atrophy of the liver and compensatory hyperplasia of the other side, which in turn may result in dislocation of the stomach. The liver, which is deprived of portal blood, develops atrophy of the portal venous branches and concurrently compensatory hypertrophy of the arterioles. This histological picture is usually indistinguishable from that seen in patients with congenital shunts, primary portal vein hypoplasia, or an arteriovenous fistula.

Hemorrhagic ascites is only seen in patients with portal vein thrombosis and hepatic congestion. Patients with chronic portal vein thrombosis may develop portosystemic collaterals and may show clinical signs of HE.

Symptoms

Many patients with portal vein thrombosis have hemorrhagic ascites. In chronic cases there may also be signs of HE. In the acute phase, there is general malaise and apathy, and often also nausea and vomiting.

Diagnosis

Blood work often reveals increased serum liver enzyme activities and serum bile acids concentrations. In chronic cases with portosystemic collateral formation, hyperammonemia may also be present. The diagnosis can be made during abdominal ultrasonography by direct visualization of the thrombus. Doppler examination reveals a reduced portal blood flow, which may be hepatofugal in chronic cases. One-sided thrombosis of a main branch of the portal vein is usually accompanied by an asymmetric liver.

Management

Therapy depends on the underlying disorder (e.g., nephrotic syndrome). Acute thrombosis may be relieved surgically. Platelet inactivation by aspirin (0.5 mg/kg PO q 12 h) has been advised, but a beneficial effect has not yet been documented. Patients with a one-sided thrombosis of a main branch usually recover spontaneously when the perfused side of the liver hypertrophies in compensation and normal liver function is restored. In chronic cases with HE, symptomatic therapy for HE may be required.

7.5.3.5 Arteriovenous fistulas

Pathogenesis

Arteriovenous fistulas are shunts between the hepatic artery and the portal venous system and represent a rather uncommon congenital disorder.[4,94] Arteriovenous fistulas will lead to an abnormally high arterial pressure in the portal system, thus leading to portal hypertension. The fistulas are usually located within a liver lobe and consist of multiple tortuous, pulsatile vessels, which may be recognized during abdominal ultrasonography. Dogs with this disease often also have portal vein hypoplasia, which is associated with a guarded prognosis for surgical correction, but hepatic lobectomy may be sufficient to remove the fistula. Portal hypertension leads to the formation of multiple portosystemic collaterals and ascites. Intrahepatic fistulas cause a reversal of blood flow in the portal system, also known as hepatofugal blood flow (i.e., blood flow away from the liver). Hepatofugal blood flow can be diagnosed by Doppler ultrasonography. It can also be seen in patients with primary portal vein hypoplasia and in some patients with portal vein thrombosis.

Patients with arteriovenous fistulas usually have multiple fistulas that are distinctly visible as wide, tortuous, and pulsatile vessels. Intrahepatic fistulas result in an enlarged liver lobe that contains many cavernous vessels. Histologically, the portal areas show many arterioles and hypoplastic portal veins.

Symptoms

Patients with arteriovenous fistulas present with the same clinical symptoms as those with portal hypertension, including HE, ascites, depression, anorexia, and vomiting.

Diagnosis

The laboratory evaluation of patients with arteriovenous fistulas shows increased serum bile acids concentrations and usually also an increased plasma ammonia concentration that is due to the formation of the portosystemic collaterals. Ultrasonography reveals wide tortuous pulsatile vessels.

Management

Surgical removal of the affected liver lobe or the extrahepatic fistula has been found to be beneficial. However, if the patient also has congenital portal vein hypoplasia, lobectomy may only lead to a partial improvement and these patients will need permanent management with a low protein diet, lactulose, and / or antibiotic therapy. Appropriately managed dogs can be well maintained for many years.

7.5.4 Diseases of the biliary tract

7.5.4.1 Cholecystitis

Pathogenesis

Cholecystitis and biliary mucocele are rare diseases in the dog.[95] Infection of the common bile duct through reflux from the duodenum is possible, though infection can also be hematogenous.[2] The infectious agents often cultured in these patients are *E. coli* and sometimes streptococci or staphylococci. *Clostridia* spp. may reside in the bile without causing disease, but they may also become pathogenic. Predisposing factors for cholecystitis are gallstones, which only occur rarely in dogs, and extrahepatic cholestasis. In some cases, an acute emphysematous cholecystitis develops. In addition, spontaneous perforation of the gallbladder may sometimes occur, causing ascites and aseptic peritonitis. Dogs with a biliary mucocele may also develop cholecystitis. In these cases, there is a typical radiating structure of the abnormal, thick gall bladder contents seen ultrasonographically, which has been described as an orange- or kiwi-fruit structure.

Symptoms

The most common symptoms of dogs with cholecystitis are upper abdominal pain, vomiting, and sometimes fever. Not all cases are associated with icterus. There may be occult blood loss from an affected blood vessel in the gallbladder causing anemia. In the case of gallbladder rupture, severe jaundice and ascites with general malaise due to peritonitis is seen.

Diagnosis

The common findings in patients with cholecystitis, such as jaundice, increased AP and GGT activities, and raised bile acids concentration, are not specific for this disease. There is usually leukocytosis. Liver histology reveals a nonspecific reactive hepatitis and is, thus, usually not diagnostic. Ultrasonography demonstrates possible gall stones, which are often radiolucent. A mucocele has a very specific ultrasonographic appearance. The diagnosis is made by fine-needle aspiration of the gall bladder under ultrasound guidance, for which no anesthesia is required. Cytology and culture of the bile reveal inflammatory cells and bacteria.

Management

Antibiotic management is the treatment of choice for dogs with cholecystitis. Antibiotics that are effectively excreted in the bile (i.e., ampicillin or chloramphenicol) should be administered for 3–4 weeks. Ampicillin is usually very effective (15 mg/kg IV q 8 h for 4 weeks). In cases of biliary calculi, gallbladder bleeding, biliary mucocele, or gall bladder rupture, a cholecystectomy should be performed.

7.5.4.2 Biliary duct or gall bladder rupture

Pathogenesis

Bile duct rupture is the tearing of the bile duct from the rest of the biliary system. This is usually caused by trauma and leads to leakage of bile from the affected lobe into the peritoneal cavity. Leakage of a large amount of unconcentrated bile (the bile is concentrated more distally, in the gallbladder), causes clinically detectable ascites. The resorption of bilirubin from the peritoneal cavity causes severe icterus. The high concentration of bile acids from the leaking bile causes chemical peritonitis, resulting in general illness and vomiting. Occasionally, spontaneous rupture of the gallbladder occurs as a result of perforating cholecystitis or a biliary mucocele.[95]

Symptoms

Patients with a rupture of the biliary system develop severe icterus and ascites within a few days. Vomiting is also common and there is general malaise and anorexia.

Diagnosis

A history of recent trauma in a patient with icterus and ascites may be a strong indication of a biliary system rupture. Aspiration of the ascitic fluid reveals free bile in the abdominal cavity, which is diagnostic. Due to the resulting bile peritonitis, the fluid is a mixture of bile with erythrocytes and inflammatory cells, resulting in a brown turbid fluid.

Therapy

The therapy of biliary system rupture is surgical and depends on the exact location of the rupture. The prognosis is usually good.

7.5.4.3 Cystic liver disease

There are different types of cysts in the liver that are all usually subclinical.[2,96,97] Such cysts are quite rare and are due to a variety of congenital developmental abnormalities of the intra- and/or extrahepatic bile ducts. Some cystic processes (e.g., Caroli's disease) are also associated with renal cystic disease and fibrosis. The cystic structures are usually visible during ultrasonography, but histological evaluation of hepatic biopsies

7

is required to further classify the lesion. Severe forms of cystic liver disease can cause hepatic dysfunction. There is no treatment for these rare conditions.

7.5.4.4 Extrahepatic bile duct obstruction (EBDO)[2,98]

Extrahepatic bile duct obstruction is an obstruction of the common bile duct due to extraluminal compression or intraluminal obstructive lesions.[98] Most frequently, EBDO is caused by tumors arising from the pancreas or the proximal duodenum. Biliary tumors are rare in both dogs and cats. Severe inflammatory conditions of the pancreas, duodenum, or common bile duct may also cause an obstruction. Cholelithiasis can cause EBDO in both dogs and cats. EBDO is more common in dogs than in cats.

Clinical features

Clinical signs, clinicopathological findings, and ultrasonographic changes in dogs and cats with EBDO, are not distinguishable from those of lymphocytic cholangitis (i.e., anorexia, depression, vomiting, jaundice, and/or hepatomegaly).

Diagnosis

Dogs and cats with complete EBDO show elevated serum AP and ALT activities. Fasting serum bile acids and bilirubin concentrations are also highly elevated. An elevated serum GGT activity is also indicative for severe cholestasis. Acholic feces and vitamin K-responsive coagulopathy are rare but important indicators.[99] Ultrasonography may reveal changes consistent with EBDO and biliary scintigraphy may also provide supportive findings.[100] Because bile flow into the intestine is obstructed, the large bile ducts proximal to the obstruction become distended and tortuous. These findings are identical to those of lymphocytic cholangitis. Histological examination of a liver biopsy is thus the only method to discriminate EBDO from chronic cholangitis. Secondary hepatic consequences of an unrelieved EBDO may include bile canalicular plugs, biliary epithelial hyperplasia, bile ductule multiplication, periportal fibrosis, and variable degrees of neutrophilic inflammation and necrosis.

Treatment

A combined surgical and medical therapeutic approach is usually needed for the treatment of dogs and cats with EBDO.[101] After the animal is stabilized (i.e., normalized fluid and electrolyte status, vitamin K supplementation), surgery is required to relieve the obstruction. It is usually impossible to identify the precise cause of EBDO with ultrasonography and an ex-

ploratory surgery may be necessary for definitive diagnosis. If the obstruction cannot be removed, cholecystojejunostomy may need to be performed to re-establish the bile flow. The importance of supportive care postoperatively cannot be overemphasized. Attending to fluid, electrolyte, and nutritional needs is critical to a successful outcome. Biochemical abnormalities associated with EBDO should begin to subside immediately after surgery.

Limited information concerning liver fluke infestation in cats suggests that praziquantel may be effective. Several dosage regimens have been used in the reported clinical cases, although a regimen of 20 mg/kg praziquantel PO or SQ q 24 h for 3 days is currently recommended. Because the use of praziquantel in this situation is an extra-label application, owner consent is recommended.

7.5.5 Neoplastic conditions of the liver

7.5.5.1 Hepatocellular carcinoma and adenoma

Pathogenesis

Epithelial hepatic tumors occur usually only in old dogs (>10 years of age), and less frequently in cats.[102,103] Both adenomas and adenocarcinomas are usually solitary and can become very large. They grow slowly and have little tendency to metastasize. These tumors are usually asymptomatic until the stomach is so severely displaced by the local mass that the dog or cat starts to vomit. Hypoglycemia occurs in about half of the cases due to the production of insulin-like growth factor by the tumor cells. This may cause episodic weakness, especially during exercise. Histologically, these tumors are well-differentiated, so it is not possible to diagnose them by cytological examination of a fine-needle aspirate as it may be difficult to distinguish them from normal liver. In some cases, however, a central necrosis of the mass occurs, which may in turn become infected and may lead to signs of sepsis.

Symptoms

Patients with hepatic epithelial tumors often present with chronic vomiting and sometimes weakness or exercise intolerance. Depending on the size of the tumor, the patient may also present with abdominal distension.

Diagnosis

Abdominal palpation may reveal a cranial abdominal mass. Ultrasonography will confirm the hepatic origin of the mass. The mass may have an echodensity similar or slightly less than that of normal liver. The histology of a liver biopsy is diagnostic. Hepatic enzymes or bile acids may not be elevated. In the case of a single abscess being identified in the liver, it is important to not only puncture the center of the process for cytology and culture, but also to take histological biopsies from the periphery of the abscess, in order not to miss a potential neoplastic lesion that may have led to the abscess.

Management

Surgical removal of the affected liver lobe (lobectomy) is the only definite treatment. This may be successful if the tumor is not localized near the hilus, any large vessels, or the major bile ducts. Peripherally localized carcinomas are usually well resectable. Because many hepatocellular carcinomas secrete insulin-like growth factor, it is important to monitor the blood glucose concentration before and during surgery.

7.5.5.2   Hemangiosarcoma

Hemangiosarcomas are the only common mesenchymal liver tumor. Hemangiosarcomas can originate in the liver or metastasize from the spleen to the liver. In both instances, the tumor is usually spread throughout the liver. This often causes highly elevated serum or plasma liver enzyme activities and serum bile acids concentrations. The cholestasis may also cause jaundice. Hemangiosarcomas usually occur in middle-aged and older patients, and are much more frequent in dogs than in cats.[103,104]

Symptoms

Mesenchymal tumors usually have a severe and rapid course, with anorexia, vomiting, weight loss, and sometimes icterus. Some patients may present for acute onset of hemorrhagic ascites due to rupture of the tumor.

Diagnosis

Patients with hemangiosarcoma may a have palpable liver mass and icterus. Serum chemistry often reveals elevated liver enzyme activities and bile acids concentrations, but this is not specific. The mass can usually be visualized by abdominal ultrasonography and a fine-needle aspirate or biopsy can be collected under ultrasound-guidance. Histology is preferable to cytology for the definitive diagnosis of this tumor.

Therapy

Mesenchymal tumors are usually inoperable and rapidly progressive. Survival times are usually not more than a few weeks.

7.5.5.3   Malignant lymphoma

Pathogenesis

The liver is often affected by various types of lymphoma. Infiltration of tumor cells causes hepatomegaly and, in some cases, intrahepatic cholestasis can also occur. Because hepatic damage is diffuse and widespread, hepatic lymphoma is often associated with severe liver dysfunction. Usually, the tumor cell infiltration is most severe in the portal areas and around the central veins. In very rare cases, this may cause portal hypertension, leading to the formation of ascites and portosystemic collaterals. While the liver is only one of multiple sites affected by lymphoma, it is often one of the easiest sites to sample tissue for diagnosis. Cytology is adequate for diagnosis in most cases.

Symptoms

The clinical signs of lymphoma are highly variable and are dependant on the other organ systems that are involved. Hepatic involvement may cause icterus, malaise, anorexia, and vomiting. Hepatomegaly and splenomegaly may cause abdominal distension.

Diagnosis

A diagnosis of hepatic lymphoma is made by cytology or histology of the liver. Blood coagulation is often abnormal. However, this does not preclude the clinician from taking a fine-needle aspirate, but an abnormal coagulation profile is a contraindication for the collection of biopsies.

Therapy

Chemotherapy may be considered, but when the liver is involved the results are less favorable than with other forms of lymphoma.

7

7.5.5.4 Bile duct carcinoma

Pathogenesis

A bile duct carcinoma is a tumor of the biliary epithelium and occurs infrequently.[104,105] Bile duct carcinomas usually metastasize quickly throughout the liver via the lymphatics and the biliary tree. This can cause severe cholestasis and icterus.

Symptoms

Many patients with bile duct carcinoma have severe icterus, general malaise, and often vomiting. The liver is often enlarged and palpable.

Diagnosis

Physical examination and laboratory evaluation indicate cholestasis. The tumor is usually detectable by ultrasonography and the diagnosis is made by ultrasound-guided biopsy. Both fine-needle aspiration and histological biopsies are diagnostic.

Management

As bile duct carcinomas spread quickly, there is no treatment and the disease is fatal.

7.6 Liver diseases in the cat

7.6.1 Parenchymal liver diseases in cats

7.6.1.1 Hepatic lipidosis

Pathogenesis

Diabetes mellitus can lead to fat accumulation in the liver in all species. However, in cats, the most common form of hepatic lipidosis is idiopathic hepatic lipidosis (steatosis). Idiopathic hepatic lipidosis used to be the most common hepatic disease of cats in North America and Europe. In the recent past, there has been a dramatic decrease in the incidence of this disease. Adipose cats seem to be predisposed, but the trigger of the disease is catabolism and cats can develop hepatic lipidosis when they consume insufficient amounts of calories or do not eat at all due to any cause. In cats with experimentally induced hepatic lipidosis, deficiency of certain essential amino acids, such as arginine and methionine, may play a role in hepatic lipid accumulation. Also, an amount of carbohydrates less than what is needed for maintenance stimulates the mobilization of fatty acids from the body fat. The fatty acids released into the

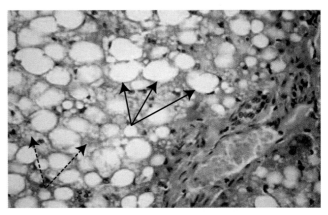

Figure 7.17:
Hepatic lipidosis – histopathology. This figure shows a histopathological image of a liver biopsy from a cat with hepatic lipidosis. The image shows both macro- (solid arrows) and microvesicular (dotted arrows) steatosis. (H&E stain, 40×).

blood in the periphery are then cleared by the liver and fat accumulates in the liver, causing lipidosis. The utilization of triglycerides as an energy source in different tissues depends on the presentation of fats as lipoproteins, such as VLDLs. There is some suggestion that the lipoprotein metabolism is not normal in cats that develop lipidosis.[106,107] Fasting cats may not be able to supply the essential amino acids, which are required for the production of the apoprotein moiety of lipoproteins. Arginine is an essential intermediate in the urea cycle and a lack of arginine causes reduced function of the hepatic urea cycle. It is very common to find high plasma ammonia concentrations in cats with severe lipidosis of the liver. These cats often develop signs of HE and, as a result, eat even less and enter a vicious cycle, which is fatal without intervention.

Many cats with hepatic lipidosis show mild to moderate hyperglycemia. This is not believed to be due to stress secondary to chronic disease, since these cats also have an impaired glucose tolerance. The exact underlying mechanism for this insulin resistance is not known. Whatever the cause, hyperglycemia is another possible factor that can further contribute to the accumulation of triglycerides in the liver. Hepatic lipidosis causes cell swelling, hepatomegaly, and intrahepatic cholestasis. Most cats with hepatic lipidosis are icteric.

Symptoms

Cats with hepatic lipidosis are usually presented with a history of anorexia, malaise, and icterus. HE may occur, with apathy, ptyalism, and ataxia.

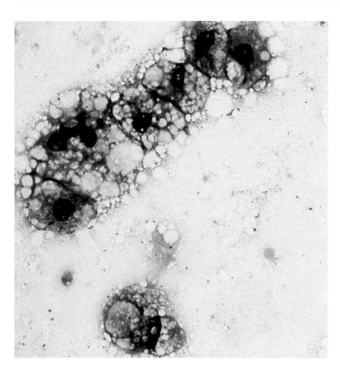

Figure 7.18:
Hepatic lipidosis – cytology. This cytological picture shows a smear from a fine-needle aspirate of the liver. There are only a few hepatocytes, most of which show a grossly distended cytoplasm with many clear vacuoles. This finding of fatty infiltration of hepatocytes in a cat is consistent with a diagnosis of hepatic lipidosis. (Diff Quick stain, magnification 150×; image courtesy of Dr. A. Rick Alleman, University of Florida, Gainesville, FL.)

Diagnosis

A physical examination of cats with hepatic lipidosis usually reveals icterus and hepatomegaly. The clinicopathological findings are usually consistent with cholestasis with total bilirubin concentrations ranging up to 20 mg/dl and/or mild to moderate non-regenerative anemia. Normal to high (i.e. 3- to 5-fold increase) ALT activities and high (i.e. 10- to 15-fold increase) AP activities are usually present. There is often mild to moderate hyperglycemia and, in severe cases, hyperammonemia. Hepatomegaly can be confirmed by abdominal ultrasonography, which also often shows generalized hyperechogenicity. However, cats with hepatic lipidosis do not have any evidence of localized structural disease, such as mass lesions, or a dilated gallbladder and/or bile ducts. A diagnosis of hepatic lipidosis can only be made by the evaluation of hepatic cells (Figure 7.17). A cytological smear of a fine-needle aspirate is diagnostic in most cases. Sudan III can be applied to unstained smears to confirm lipid vacuolation of the hepatocytes (Figure 7.18).

Management

The most important goal of the management of feline patients with hepatic lipidosis is to get them out of their catabolic state and to supply the amino acids essential to prevent further fat accumulation and development of HE. Complete nutritional support along with treatment of known concurrent and possibly precipitating conditions are the corner stones to allow recovery.[108,109] Feeding via a nasoesophageal or gastric tube is necessary if the cat is unable to be fed orally. It is essential to choose a high protein diet as cats with hepatic lipidosis cannot metabolize fat or carbohydrates efficiently. Severely affected cats are first stabilized by attending to their fluid and electrolyte needs (i.e., potassium is usually low, and hypokalemia is a risk factor for HE). During this time, nutritional support can be provided via a nasoesophageal or nasogastric tube with a liquid enteral diet, such as CliniCare Feline Liquid Diet (Abbott Laboratories, North Chicago, IL). The use of a large bore Pezzer mushroom-tip tube (Bard urological catheter, Bard Urological Division, Covington, GA; 16 or 18 Fr; a Foley catheter should not be used) allows the use of blenderized diets (Feline p/d or k/d, Hill's Pet Products, Topeka, KS; a mixture of one can with 11/2 cups water yields a slurry with 0.9 kcal/ml) for administration at home. Feline k/d or Veterinary Diet NF (Nestlé Purina Company, St. Louis, MO) is preferred for the initial treatment of cats with HE. These diets are then gradually switched to a higher protein diet when the signs of encephalopathy have subsided. Several other diets are made to be used undiluted (i.e., feline a/d, Hill's Pet Products, Topeka, KS [1.3 kcal/ml] and Maximum-Calorie, Eukanuba Veterinary Diets, The Iams Company, Dayton, Ohio [2.1 kcal/ml]), making home feeding for the first 1–2 weeks even easier. It is not known whether supplementation with taurine, carnitine, or arginine hastens recovery.

Cats that cannot tolerate full feeding because of gastroparesis, as indicated by vomiting during feeding or repeated retrieval of a residual gastric fluid volume of more than 10 ml of food or fluid before the next feeding, may benefit from potassium supplementation if they are hypokalemic, or from the administration of a prokinetic agent such as metoclopramide (0.2 to 0.5 mg/kg SC q 6–8 h, or via feeding tube 15–20 minutes before feeding). Cisapride (0.5 mg/kg PO q 8–12 h) is a potent prokinetic agent, but can only be obtained from veterinary compounding pharmacies. Hypophosphatemia may develop during re-feeding and, if severe, can lead to hemolytic anemia. For cats with a coagulopathy, vitamin K_1 (0.5 mg/kg SC q 12 h) is recommended.

Results of recent studies of experimentally induced hepatic lipidosis in cats indicate that a high-protein diet may hasten recovery. This is the only condition in which HE should be treated with a high protein diet. Also, it is not recommended to administer insulin, because this may induce severe hypoglycemia.

7

The dietary measures often have to be continued for a long period, which the owner can do at home. Cats that are susceptible to developing hepatic lipidosis will often develop another episode later in their life. An average of 60–70% of cats hospitalized for the treatment of hepatic lipidosis do recover. However, it is important to make the owner aware of any susceptibility so that future episodes of hepatic lipidosis can be prevented.

7.6.1.2 Acute toxic hepatopathy

Pathogenesis

Diazepam and stanozolol have been reported to be hepatotoxic in some cats.[52–54] Potentially, tetracycline can also be hepatotoxic in cats, but this relationship needs to be further evaluated. While toxic effects of these drugs do occur, all three drugs have been used extensively and toxic reactions are considered to be rare. Adverse reactions of the liver to tetracycline have been found not to be lethal, and the liver lesions observed were relatively mild.[55] Diazepam toxicity is usually fatal and the liver of cats with diazepam toxicity shows massive centrilobular necrosis and exudative cholangitis. Although this seems to be a rare complication, the hepatic necrosis is so severe that one should consider alternative treatments to diazepam. Cats with stanozolol toxicity show severe centrilobular lipidosis and pronounced intrahepatic cholestasis. Stanozolol toxicity is fatal in the majority of affected cats, but most of these patients do have a pre-existent kidney dysfunction. Like dogs, cats may also have a severe dose-dependent hepatic necrosis after high doses of acetaminophen (see acute hepatitis in dogs, 7.5.1.1.1).[10,48,49] All these toxic reactions are characterized by severe hepatocellular damage and these patients usually have very high serum activities of liver enzymes and are often icteric.

Diagnosis

It is important to ask the owner of feline patients with acute hepatopathies for any possible exposure to known hepatotoxins in the recent history. The liver of cats with a hepatotoxicity is usually enlarged, but this is true for most liver diseases of cats. Serum ALT and AST activities and serum bilirubin concentration are often highly elevated. Histological examination of liver biopsies shows nonspecific changes. Therefore, the diagnosis is often based on a combination of history, disease course (acute), very high serum ALT and/or AST activities, and histopathological findings.

Treatment

In cats with suspected acute hepatotoxicity, general supportive care is given. Prevention of further exposure, management of fluid and electrolyte disturbances, anti-emetic therapy, and other symptomatic and supportive measures as indicated in the individual case are required. There is no specific therapy for most hepatotoxicities. For acetaminophen intoxication: see acute hepatitis in dogs (7.5.1.1.1)

7.6.1.3 Hepatopathy due to infectious peritonitis (FIP)

Pathogenesis

Manifestations of FIP are chronic and may vary depending on the organs involved. Ascites or pleural effusion may or may not be present. The liver is often affected in patients with FIP, exhibiting a granulomatous inflammatory reaction.[10,110]

Diagnosis

Cats with FIP commonly have a hypergammaglobulinemia, however, so do cats with lymphocytic cholangitis.[10] Hepatic granulomas due to FIP are too small to be detected by ultrasonography, but they are microscopically visible upon the evaluation of a liver biopsy. Although these granulomas are not entirely specific for FIP, they allow a very strong suspicion of a diagnosis of FIP.

Management

There is no known therapy for FIP that is efficacious.

7.6.1.4 Hepatic changes due to hyperthyroidism

Hyperthyroidism causes fatty infiltration of hepatocytes. This fatty infiltration of the liver does not cause clinical signs of hepatic dysfunction, but in many cases the serum activities of the liver enzymes and serum concentrations of bile acids are abnormally high.[5,111] The fatty changes of the liver are not severe and there is usually no hepatic enlargement. A number of symptoms associated with hyperthyroidism mimic those of primary hepatic disease: polyuria, vomiting, diarrhea, and weight loss. Hence, these clinical findings may prompt the clinician to measure serum activities of liver enzymes and serum bile acids concentrations. A subsequent liver biopsy may reveal histological changes suggestive of hyperthyroidism. In most patients, treatment of hyperthyroidism will lead to a resolution of hepatic changes.

7.6.1.5 Nonspecific reactive hepatitis and amyloidosis

See 7.5.1.6 and 7.5.2.4 for a discussion of these diseases in the dog.

7.6.2 Vascular liver diseases in cats

7.6.2.1 Congenital portosystemic shunt

In contrast to dogs, which are affected by multiple vascular liver diseases, the only vascular anomaly of significance in cats is congenital portosystemic vascular anomaly, also known as congenital portosystemic shunt (CPSS).[87,91]

Cats are affected by a wide variety of shunts, which are usually localized outside the hepatic parenchyma. Such extrahepatic shunts can be located between the liver and the diaphragm, but also as far back as the pelvic canal. However, as in dogs, CPSS can sometimes also be intrahepatic.[87] There is no breed or sex predisposition for CPSS in cats and the incidence of CPSS is much lower in cats than it is in dogs. In cats, it is not only important to monitor the serum blood glucose concentration during and following surgical correction of the shunts, but also the clinician should be aware of the risk of an insufficient intake of essential amino acids. Supplementation of these amino acids may be administered intravenously or orally. Congenital shunts are the only condition in cats that is associated with microhepatica.

Symptoms

Obvious behavioral and neurological abnormalities (e.g., dementia, ataxia) are commonly seen in cats with CPSS. Also, intermittent ptyalism is a much more frequent manifestation of HE in cats than it is in dogs.

Diagnosis

It is the author's opinion that, as in dogs, the most accurate modality to diagnose portosystemic shunting is by measuring the plasma ammonia concentration. In cases where a single plasma ammonia concentration does not provide a definitive answer, an ammonia tolerance test may be diagnostic. Serum bile acids concentrations may also be indicative of a portosystemic shunt, but they are nonspecific. As in dogs with PSS, hypoalbuminemia and ammonium biurate crystalluria may also be present in affected cats.

A diagnosis of CPSS in cats can be confirmed by ultrasonography, transcolonic or splenic portal scintigraphy, or contrast portal venography. The liver size in affected cats is usually smaller than normal. A hepatic biopsy specimen should always be obtained to ensure that the hepatic histological changes that are characteristic of CPSS are present: lobular hepatocellular atrophy, inconspicuous portal vein tributaries, arteriolar duplication, and, occasionally, mild lipidosis and vacuolar changes. In Persian cats, the co-existence of cystic kidney and liver disease that is associated with hepatic fibrosis is a contraindication for surgery.

Treatment

The definitive treatment for CPSS in cats is the surgical ligation of the anomalous vessel, assuming there is adequate intrahepatic portal venous vasculature to accept the redirected blood flow. This surgical procedure is best performed at referral centers or veterinary colleges. Older cats (>5 years of age) or cats with pre-existing neurological signs may be at greater risk of a poor outcome following surgical treatment of CPSS. The author recommends to treat cats that undergo surgery for CPSS symptomatically (i.e., diet, lactulose) before surgery, and to continue treatment for 1 month after surgery.

The success rate of surgery for CPSS in cats is lower than that in dogs and only 40–50% of cats recover. Cerebrocortical necrosis is a relatively frequent postoperative complication in cats and causes irreversible brain damage.

7.6.3 Diseases of the biliary system in cats

Hepatitis is a rare disease in cats. However, cholangitis, an inflammatory disease of the hepatobiliary system, is common in cats.[2] In a recent retrospective study of inflammatory liver diseases in 78 cats, more than 80% of cats with cholangiohepatitis also had histological evidence of IBD, and about half had changes consistent with mild pancreatitis, implying that there is a relationship between inflammatory diseases of the abdominal organs.[112] However, this relationship needs further clarification.

Cats may have different forms of cholangitis, which have been referred to by different names in the literature. However, overall, there are three different forms of cholangitis in cats: neutrophilic cholangitis, lymphocytic cholangitis, and cholangitis due to liver flukes (see 7.6.3.1–7.6.3.3 below).

7

7

7.6.3.1 Neutrophilic cholangitis

Pathogenesis

Neutrophilic cholangitis is due to an ascending infection of the biliary tree from the intestinal tract. Histologically, neutrophilic cholangitis is characterized by neutrophils in the lumen of the bile ducts and in the epithelium of the walls of the biliary tree. There may also be a neutrophilic inflammatory reaction around the bile ducts in the portal area. Neutrophilic cholangitis is usually an acute disease, but when it becomes more chronic, the inflammatory infiltrate may show a mixture of neutrophils, lymphocytes, and plasma cells. The associated diffuse inflammation of the entire biliary tree often causes cholestasis. Most of these cats, but not all, are distinctly icteric. However, there is no obstruction at the opening of the common bile duct into the duodenum and hence, there is no distension of the bile ducts.[112,113]

Symptoms

The clinical signs of patients with neutrophilic cholangitis are those of acute or subacute (1–3 weeks) inflammation with general illness, often with fever and icterus. However, the degree of icterus is variable.

Diagnosis

Serum bile acids concentrations and, in many cases, serum activities of ALT are increased, but these findings are nonspecific.[75] Serum liver enzyme activities are usually typical of a mixed pattern of parenchymal and biliary injury, with normal to twofold elevations of AP activity and as high as tenfold elevations of ALT activity. Ultrasonography usually reveals no changes, but there may be thickening of the gall bladder wall.

A diagnosis of neutrophilic cholangitis can only be made by examining the bile. Gall bladder puncture with a thin needle should be performed under ultrasonographic guidance. Bile should be evaluated cytologically and by bacterial culture, which also permits the determination of the sensitivity of the cultured organism. Bacterial culture most often yields enteric organisms, such as *E. coli*, or in some cases *Pseudomonas* spp., or *Enterococcus* spp. Histological evaluation of a liver biopsy is helpful, but examination of the bile is essential.

Management

The routine treatment for neutrophilic cholangitis is the administration of antibiotics that are excreted well into the bile. The author prefers a treatment period of 3–4 weeks with amoxicillin and clavulanic acid. It is advisable to objectively evaluate the therapy by re-examination of the bile after completion of the antibiotic treatment course. The prognosis of feline patients with neutrophilic cholangitis is usually very good if a diagnosis is made early in the disease process.

7.6.3.2 Lymphocytic cholangitis

Pathogenesis

The pathogenesis of the lymphocytic form of cholangitis is very different than that of the neutrophilic form. Lymphocytic cholangitis is a chronic disease that progresses slowly over many months or even years. The inflammatory cells involved in this disease process are lymphocytes and plasma cells. The inflammatory cells can be found in the lumen of the bile ducts and in the bile duct epithelium, but they also progress to around the bile ducts in the portal areas (Figure 7.19).[2,113–116] The inflammatory response of this condition causes portal fibrosis, and in very chronic cases, bridging fibrosis between the portal areas of different lobules leading to severe fibrotic changes. The chronic inflammation of the bile ducts causes irregular distension of the bile ducts in and outside the liver. Abdominal ultrasonography shows dilated bile ducts (Figure 7.20) and thickened walls of the bile ducts that are usually readily detectable during ultrasonography.[101,113]

The differential diagnosis for a lymphocytic cholangitis is an extrahepatic bile duct obstruction. The latter condition is rare, whereas lymphocytic cholangitis occurs quite frequently in cats. Histologically, the two diseases appear distinctly different. Because most affected cats have hyperglobulinemia and in some cases abdominal effusion, they can easily be misdiagnosed as having the effusive form of FIP; therefore, a liver biopsy is essential in differentiating these two conditions. The lymphocytic inflammation suggests an autoimmune-mediated disease process. At the same time, there is some evidence that this condition may be associated with a chronic bacterial infection with spirochetal bacteria (i.e., *Helicobacter*-like organisms).[115] The most prominent finding on blood work is an elevated gamma globulin concentration, similarly to what is usually seen in cats with FIP. The liver tends to be enlarged and is therefore palpable in many cases. The diffuse inflammation of the entire biliary tree causes cholestasis and affected cats are often, but not always, icteric.

The chronic deformation of the bile ducts due to inflammatory infiltration makes them prone to secondary infections, such as by intestinal *E. coli*. Such a superimposed infection may cause a more acute exacerbation of the disease. As a result, the typical lymphocytic inflammation may change to an infiltrate with a more mixed inflammatory cell infiltrate.

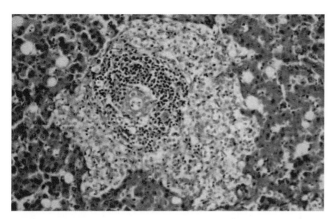

Figure 7.19:
Lymphocytic cholangitis. Histopathological image of a liver biopsy from a cat with lymphocytic cholangitis. The image is centered on a portal area and shows a large number of lymphocytes in and around the portal bile duct. (H&E stain, 100×)

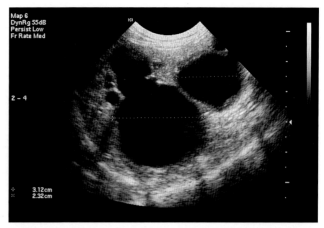

Figure 7.20:
Lymphocytic cholangitis. This figure shows an ultrasonographic image captured in a cat with lymphocytic cholangitis. Note the multiple dilated intra- and extrahepatic bile ducts.

7

Symptoms

As with other biliary diseases, the main clinical symptoms in cats with cholangitis are caused by nausea: decreased appetite, irregular eating, occasional vomiting, and chronic weight loss. Cholestasis may lead to icterus, which is present in most, but not all, cases of cholangitis.

Diagnosis

Lymphocytic cholangitis may be associated with a palpable enlargement of the liver. Blood work may reveal high serum bile acids concentrations with variable increases in serum ALT activity. The most consistent abnormal finding on blood work is an elevated serum gamma globulin concentration. Abdominal ultrasonography usually indicates a diffusely enlarged liver, often with an increased echodensity, which is, however, not specific either. In chronic cases, both intra- and extrahepatic bile ducts are irregularly distended. These ultrasonographic changes, in association with the typical histological findings of a liver biopsy, allow for a diagnosis.

Hepatic fluke infestation (i.e., *Platynosomum concinnum*), which is rather uncommon in cats, can also lead to cholangitis.[116] However, the two diseases of the biliary system can be distinguished based on the clinical history and the type of inflammatory cells present.

Management

Lymphocytic cholangitis responds well to medication with ursodiol (ursodeoxycholic acid at 10–15 mg/kg PO q 24 h; can be divided into two doses),[112–115] which suppresses the inflammatory response. Long-term treatment is mandatory at the same dosage. It is important to evaluate the response to therapy by repeat liver biopsy after 8 weeks of treatment. Medication must be continued until a complete resolution of the inflammation can be seen histologically. It is advisable to concurrently treat these cats during the first four weeks of therapy with amoxicillin and clavulanic acid to treat any possible superimposed infections. Corticosteroids have often been recommended for the treatment of lymphocytic cholangitis, but evaluation of a series of cases seen at the University of Utrecht has revealed no beneficial effect for steroid administration.

Nutritional support is an important component of medical therapy for cats with cholangiohepatitis. A balanced high-protein (i.e., 30% to 40% protein on a dry matter basis) maintenance diet is fed to cats that do not have signs of HE (see 7.6.1.1; recommendations for dietary management of hepatic lipidosis). Most cats that survive the initial period of treatment of 1 to 2 months have a good chance for cure and long-term survival. Cats with lymphocytic cholangiohepatitis appear to live comfortably for months to years. However, the dilation and fibrosis of the biliary system is permanent and these cats are predisposed to developing secondary bacterial infections (e.g., *E. coli*) of their abnormal bile ducts.

7.6.3.3 Extrahepatic bile duct obstruction (EBDO)

See 7.5.4.4 in the section on canine liver disease.

Extrahepatic bile duct obstruction in cats can be caused by infestation with liver flukes (e.g., *Platynosomum* spp., *Amphimerus pseudofelineus, Metametorchis intermedius*).[117,118] Hepatic fluke infestation has been reported most commonly in cats from areas with a warm, humid climate. Most cats are sub-clinical but hepatic fluke infestation may be responsible for EBDO in severely affected cats. Cats can acquire the infection by ingesting infected snails and lizards or freshwater fish. Histopathological changes of the hepatobiliary system induced by liver fluke infestation are mostly nonspecific. However, cross-sections of flukes within bile ducts are occasionally seen histologically. The diagnosis is made by finding fluke ova in the feces of cats with compatible clinicopathological findings at abdominal exploratory.

Limited information concerning liver fluke infestation in cats suggests that praziquantel may be effective. Several dosage regimens have been used in reported clinical cases, although a regimen of 20 mg/kg praziquantel PO or SC q 24 h for 3 days is currently recommended. Because the use of praziquantel in this situation is an extra-label application, owner consent is recommended.

7.6.4 Neoplasia

Primary hepatobiliary neoplasia is rare in cats, but bile duct carcinoma and hepatocellular carcinoma are reported most often.[105]

The systemic tumor most commonly affecting the liver of cats is lymphoma and related myeloproliferative diseases. Hepatic metastases from malignancies of the mammary gland, pancreas, kidney, and GI tract have also been observed in cats.

Clinical features

Clinical signs of hepatic neoplasia in cats are variable and are dependant on the tumor type and extension. Tumors of the hepatic parenchyma commonly cause hepatomegaly, while icterus is a rare finding seen in patients with other tumors, such as bile duct carcinomas.

Diagnosis

Abdominal ultrasonography may reveal generalized or focal lesions of the liver. Abnormal hepatic enzyme activities are common, but are nonspecific. The diagnosis should be confirmed with histological or cytological examination of a liver biopsy.

Treatment

Surgical resection of a primary hepatobiliary neoplasm that is confined to one liver lobe and has not metastasized may result in prolonged survival. The size of the neoplasm is less important in determining the prognosis than the degree of invasiveness and the presence of regional or distant metastases. The prognosis for cats with benign hepatocellular or biliary tumors after resection is good.

⚷ Key Facts

- The diagnostic accuracy of histopathology is adequate if it is based on 2–3 biopsy specimens collected with a true-cut or Menghini biopsy needle. The recommended size of the biopsy instrument used is 14G in medium and large dogs and 16G in cats and small dogs.
- In cats, hepatic encephalopathy may be due to portosystemic shunting or hepatic lipidosis. Hepatic encephalopathy in cats with hepatic lipidosis does not require dietary protein restriction.
- Acute hepatitis in dogs may develop into chronic hepatitis, therefore re-evaluation of a liver biopsy 4–6 weeks after an acute episode of hepatitis is indicated.
- Evaluation of the course of most liver diseases requires repeated sampling of liver biopsies as results of blood tests do not provide adequate information.
- Centrolobular copper accumulation in dogs is always due to a primary (genetic) copper storage disease and is not a result of cholestasis.
- Feline neutrophilic cholangitis can only be definitively diagnosed by bile analysis. Gall bladder puncture should be performed routinely in suspected cases.
- Treatment with corticosteroids has no long-term beneficial effects in cats with lymphocytic cholangitis.
- The effect of most therapeutic strategies for hepatic and biliary diseases of dogs and cats are empirical and are not supported by relevant research.

References

1. Rothuizen J, Desmet VJ, van den Ingh T et al. Sampling and handling of liver tissue. In: *WSAVA Standards for Clinical and Histological Diagnosis of Canine and Feline Liver Diseases*. Edinburgh, Churchill Livingstone, 2006; 5–14.
2. van den Ingh T, Cullen JM, Twedt DC et al. Morphological classification of biliary disorders of the canine and feline liver. In: *WSAVA Standards for Clinical and Histological Diagnosis of Canine and Feline Liver Diseases*. Edinburgh, Churchill Livingstone, 2006; 61–76.
3. Bosje JT, Bunch SE, van den Brom W et al. Plasma ^{14}C-cholic acid clearance in healthy dogs and dogs with cholestasis or a congenital portosystemic shunt. *Vet Rec* 2005; 23: 109–112.
4. Cullen JM, van den Ingh T, Bunch SE et al. Morphological classification of circulatory disorders of the canine and feline liver. In: *WSAVA Standards for Clinical and Histological Diagnosis of Canine and Feline Liver Diseases*. Edinburgh, Churchill Livingstone, 2006; 41–59.
5. Cullen JM, van den Ingh T, van Winkle T et al. Morphological classification of parenchymal disorders of the canine and feline liver; reversible hepatic injury and amyloidosis. In: *WSAVA Standards for Clinical and Histological Diagnosis of Canine and Feline Liver Diseases*. Edinburgh, Churchill Livingstone, 2006; 77–84.
6. Rothuizen J, Meyer HP. History, physical examination, and signs of liver disease. In: Ettinger SJ, Feldman EC (eds.) *Textbook of Veterinary Internal Medicine*, 5th ed. Philadelphia, WB Saunders, 2000; 1272–1277.
7. Hughes D, King LG. The diagnosis and management of acute liver failure in dogs and cats. *Vet Clin North Am Small Anim Pract* 1995; 25: 437–460.
8. Hess PR, Bunch SE. Diagnostic approach to hepatobiliary disease. In: Bonagura JD (ed.) *Kirk's current veterinary therapy XIII*. Philadelphia, WB Saunders, 2000; 659–664.
9. Meyer HP, Rothuizen J, Ubbink GJ et al. Increasing incidence of hereditary intrahepatic portosystemic shunts in Irish Wolfhounds in the Netherlands (1984 to 1992). *Vet Rec* 1995; 136: 13–16.
10. van den Ingh T, Van Winkle T, Cullen JM et al. Morphological classification of parenchymal disorders of the canine and feline liver; hepatocellular death, hepatitis and cirrhosis. In: *WSAVA Standards for Clinical and Histological Diagnosis of Canine and Feline Liver Diseases*. Edinburgh, Churchill Livingstone, 2006; 85–102.
11. Wijmenga C, Klomp LW. Molecular regulation of copper excretion in the liver. *Proc Nutr Soc* 2004; 63: 31–39.
12. Andersson M, Sevelius E. Breed, sex, and age distribution in dogs with chronic liver disease: a demographic study. *J Small Anim Pract* 1991; 32: 1–5.
13. van Straten G, Leegwater PA, de Vries M et al. Inherited congenital extrahepatic portosystemic shunts in Cairn Terriers. *J Vet Intern Med* 2005; 19: 321–324.
14. Ubbink GJ, van de Broek J, Meyer HP et al. Prediction of inherited portosystemic shunts in Irish Wolfhounds on the basis of pedigree analysis. *Am J Vet Res* 1998; 59: 1553–1556.
15. Sutherland RJ. Biochemical evaluation of the hepatobiliary system in dogs and cats. *Vet Clin North Am Small Anim Pract* 1989; 19: 899–927.
16. Gerritzen-Bruning MJ, van den Ingh T, Rothuizen J. Diagnostic value of fasting plasma ammonia and bile acid concentrations in the identification of portosystemic shunting in dogs. *J Vet Intern Med* 2006; 20: 13–19.
17. Sterczer A, Meyer HP, Boswijk HC et al. Evaluation of ammonia measurements in dogs with two analyzers for use in veterinary practice. *Vet Rec* 1999; 144: 523–526.
18. Center SA. Serum bile acids in companion animal medicine. *Vet Clin North Am Small Anim Pract* 1993; 23: 625–657.
19. Trainor D, Center SA, Randolph F et al. Urine sulfated and nonsulfated bile acids as a diagnostic test for liver disease in cats. *J Vet Intern Med* 2003; 17: 145–153.
20. Center SA, Manwarren T, Slater MR et al. Evaluation of twelve-hour preprandial and two-hour postprandial serum bile acids concentrations for diagnosis of hepatobiliary disease in dogs. *J Am Vet Med Assoc* 1991; 199: 217–226.
21. Gagne JM, Weiss DJ, Armstrong PJ. Histopathologic evaluation of feline inflammatory liver disease. *Vet Pathol* 1996; 33: 521–526.
22. Roth L, Meyer DJ. Interpretation of liver biopsies. *Vet Clin North Am Small Anim Pract* 1995; 25: 293–303.
23. Badylak SF. Coagulation disorders and liver disease. *Vet Clin North Am Small Anim Pract* 1988; 18: 87–92.
24. Bigge LA, Brown DJ, Penninck DG. Correlation between coagulation profile findings and bleeding complications after ultrasound-guided biopsies: 434 cases (1993–1996). *J Am Anim Hosp Assoc* 2001; 37: 228–233.
25. Dillon JF, Simpson KJ, Hayes PC. Liver biopsy bleeding time: an unpredictable event. *J Gastroenterol Hepatol* 1994; 9: 269–271.
26. Cole T, Center SA, Flood SN et al. Diagnostic comparison of needle biopsy and wedge biopsy specimens of the liver in dogs and cats. *J Am Vet Med Assoc* 2002; 220: 1483–1490.
27. Léveillé R, Partington BP, Biller DS et al. Complications after ultrasound-guided biopsy of abdominal structures in dogs and cats: 246 cases (1984–1991). *J Am Vet Med Assoc* 1993; 203: 413–415.
28. Partington BP, Biller DS. Hepatic imaging with radiology and ultrasound. *Vet Clin North Am Small Anim Pract* 1995; 25: 305–335.
29. Pechman RD. The liver and spleen. In: Thrall DR (ed.) *Textbook of Veterinary Diagnostic Radiology*. Philadelphia, W.B. Saunders, 1986; 391–400.
30. Rothuizen J. Seeking global standardization on liver disease. *J Small Anim Pract* 2001; 42: 424–425.
31. Cole TL, Center SA, Flood SN et al. Diagnostic comparison of needle and wedge biopsy specimens of the liver in dogs and cats. *J Am Vet Med Assoc* 2002; 220: 1483–1490.
32. Stockhaus C, van den Ingh T, Rothuizen J et al. A multistep approach in the cytologic evaluation of liver biopsy samples of dogs with hepatic diseases. *Vet Pathol* 2004; 41: 461–470.
33. Cohen M, Bohling MW, Wright JC et al. Evaluation of sensitivity and specificity of cytologic examination: 269 cases (1999–2000). *J Am Vet Med Assoc* 2003; 222: 964–967.
34. Stockhaus C, Teske E, van den Ingh T et al. The influence of age on the cytology of the liver in healthy dogs. *Vet Pathol* 2002; 39: 154–158.
35. Cole TL, Center SA, Flood SN et al. Diagnostic comparison of needle and wedge biopsy specimens of the liver in dogs and cats. *J Am Vet Med Assoc* 2002; 220: 1483–1490.
36. Richter KP. Laparoscopy in dogs and cats. *Vet Clin North Am Small Anim Pract* 2001; 31: 707–727.
37. Hess PR, Bunch SE. Management of portal hypertension and its consequences. *Vet Clin North Am Small Anim Pract* 1995; 25: 461–483.
38. Johnson SE. Portal hypertension. Part I. Pathophysiology and clinical consequences. *Comp Cont Edu Pract Vet* 1987; 9: 741–748.
39. Johnson SE: Portal hypertension. Part II. Clinical assessment and treatment. *Comp Cont Edu Pract Vet* 1987; 9: 917–928.
40. Steyn PF, Wittum TE. Radiographic, epidemiologic, and clinical aspects of simultaneous pleural and peritoneal effusions in dogs and cats: 48 cases (1982–1991). *J Am Vet Med Assoc* 1993; 202: 307–312.
41. Rothuizen J, van den Brom WE. Bilirubin metabolism in canine hepatobiliary and haemolytic disease. *Vet Q* 1987; 9: 235–240.
42. Rothuizen J, van den Ingh T. Covalently protein-bound bilirubin conjugates in cholestatic disease of dogs. *Am J Vet Res* 1988; 49: 702–704.

7

43. Rothuizen J, van den Ingh T. Arterial and venous ammonia concentrations in the diagnosis of canine hepato-encephalopathy. *Res Vet Sci* 1982; 33: 17–21.

44. Maddison JE. Newest insights into hepatic encephalopathy. *Eur J Comp Gastroenterol* 2000; 5: 17–21.

45. Szatmari V, Rothuizen J, van den Ingh TS et al. Ultrasonographic findings in dogs with hyperammonemia: 90 cases (2000–2002). *J Am Vet Med Assoc* 2004; 224: 717–727.

46. Meyer HP, Rothuizen J, Tiemessen I et al. Transient metabolic hyperammonaemia in young Irish Wolfhounds. *Vet Rec* 1996; 138: 105–107.

47. Rothuizen J, van den Ingh TS. Rectal ammonia tolerance test in the evaluation of portal circulation in dogs with liver disease. *Res Vet Sci* 1982; 33: 22–25.

48. Rothuizen J, Biewenga WJ, Mol JA. Chronic glucocorticoid excess and impaired osmoregulation of vasopressin release in dogs with hepatic encephalopathy. *Domest Anim Endocrinol* 1995; 12: 13–24.

49. Aronson LR, Drobatz K. Acetaminophen toxicosis in 17 cats. *J Vet Emerg Crit Care* 1996; 6: 65–69.

50. MacNaughton SM. Acetaminophen toxicosis in a Dalmatian. *Can Vet J* 2003; 44: 142–144.

51. Beasley VR. Toxicology of selected pesticides, drugs, and chemicals. *Vet Clin North Am Small Anim Pract* 1990; 20: 545–564.

52. Center SA, Elston TH, Rowland PH et al: Fulminant hepatic failure associated with oral administration of diazepam in 11 cats. *J Am Vet Med Assoc* 1996; 209: 618–625.

53. Hughs D, Moreau RE, Overall KL et al. Acute hepatic necrosis and liver failure associated with benzodiazepine therapy in six cats, 1986–1995. *J Vet Emerg Crit Care* 1996; 6: 13–20.

54. Harkin KR, Cowan LA, Andrews GA et al. Hepatotoxicity of stanozolol in cats. *J Am Vet Med Assoc* 2000; 217: 681–684.

55. Kaufman AC, Greene CE. Increased alanine transaminase activity associated with tetracycline administration in a cat. *J Am Vet Med Assoc* 1993; 202: 628–630.

56. Boomkens SY, Penning LC, Egberink HF et al. Hepatitis with special reference to dogs. A review on the pathogenesis and infectious etiologies, including unpublished results of recent own studies. *Vet Q* 2004; 26: 107–114.

57. Mandigers PJ, van den Ingh TS, Spee B et al. Chronic hepatitis in Doberman pinschers. A review. *Vet Q* 2004; 26: 98–106.

58. Mandigers PJ, van den Ingh TS, Bode P et al. Association between liver copper concentration and subclinical hepatitis in Doberman Pinschers. *J Vet Intern Med* 2004; 18: 647–650.

59. Speeti M, Stahls A, Meri S et al. Upregulation of major histocompatibility complex class II antigens in hepatocytes in Doberman hepatitis. *Vet Immunol Immunopathol* 2003; 96: 1–12. Erratum in: *Vet Immunol Immunopathol* 2005; 103: 295.

60. Spee B, Mandigers PJ, Arends B et al. Differential expression of copper-associated and oxidative stress related proteins in a new variant of copper toxicosis in Doberman pinschers. *Comp Hepatol* 2005; 4 (3): 1–13.

61. Webb CB, Twedt DC, Meyer DJ. Copper-associated liver disease in Dalmatians: a review of 10 dogs (1998–2001). *J Vet Intern Med* 2002; 16: 665–668.

62. Schultheiss PC, Bedwell CL, Hamar DW et al. Canine liver iron, copper, and zinc concentrations and association with histologic lesions. *J Vet Diagn Invest* 2002; 14: 396–402.

63. Kawamura M, Takahashi I, Kaneko JJ. Ultrastructural and kinetic studies of copper metabolism in Bedlington Terrier dogs. *Vet Pathol* 2002; 39: 747–750.

64. Favier RP, Spee B, Penning LC et al. Quantitative PCR method to detect a 13-kb deletion in the MURR1 gene associated with copper toxicosis and HIV-1 replication. *Mamm Genome* 2005; 16: 460–463.

65. Ubbink GJ, Van den Ingh TS, Yuzbasiyan-Gurkan V et al. Population dynamics of inherited copper toxicosis in Dutch Bedlington Terriers (1977–1997). *J Vet Intern Med* 2000; 14: 172–176.

66. Rothuizen J, Ubbink GJ, van Zon P et al. Diagnostic value of a microsatellite DNA marker for copper toxicosis in West-European Bedlington Terriers and incidence of the disease. *Anim Genet* 1999; 30: 190–194.

67. Bosje JT, van den Ingh TS, Fennema A et al. Copper-induced hepatitis in an Anatolian Shepherd dog. *Vet Rec* 2003; 152: 84–85

68. Mandigers PJ, van den Ingh TS, Bode P et al. Improvement in liver pathology after 4 months of D-penicillamine in 5 Doberman Pinschers with subclinical hepatitis. *J Vet Intern Med* 2005; 19: 40–43.

69. van den Ingh TS, Rothuizen J. Lobular dissecting hepatitis in juvenile and young adult dogs. *J Vet Intern Med* 1994; 8: 217–220.

70. Wiedmeyer CE, Solter PE, Hoffmann WE. Alkaline phosphatase expression in tissues from glucocorticoid-treated dogs. *Am J Vet Res* 2002; 63: 1083–1088.

71. Wiedmeyer CE, Solter PE, Hoffmann WE. Kinetics of mRNA expression of alkaline phosphatase isoenzymes in hepatic tissues from glucocorticoid-treated dogs. *Am J Vet Res* 2002; 63: 1089–1095.

72. Hunt GB. Effect of breed on anatomy of portosystemic shunts resulting from congenital diseases in dogs and cats: a review of 242 cases. *Aust Vet J* 2004; 82: 746–749.

73. Winkler JT, Bohling MW, Tillson DM et al. Portosystemic shunts: diagnosis, prognosis, and treatment of 64 cases (1993–2001). *J Am Anim Hosp Assoc* 2003; 39: 169–185.

74. Washizu M, Katagi M, Washizu T et al. An evaluation of radiographic hepatic size in dogs with portosystemic shunt. *J Vet Med Sci* 2004; 66: 977–978.

75. Center SA, Baldwin BH, Erb H et al. Bile acid concentrations in the diagnosis of hepatobiliary disease in the cat. *J Am Vet Med Assoc* 1986; 189: 891–896.

76. Szatmari V, Rothuizen J, Voorhout G. Standard planes for ultrasonographic examination of the portal system in dogs. *J Am Vet Med Assoc* 2004; 224: 698–699, 713–716.

77. Szatmári V, Rothuizen J. Ultrasonographic identification and characterization of congenital portosystemic shunts and portal hypertensive disorders. In: *WSAVA Standards for Clinical and Histological Diagnosis of Canine and Feline Liver Diseases.* Edinburgh, Churchill Livingstone, 2006; 15–40.

78. Lamb CR, Burton CA. Doppler ultrasonographic assessment of closure of the ductus venosus in neonatal Irish Wolfhounds. *Vet Rec* 2004; 155: 699–701.

79. Szatmari V, Rothuizen J, van Sluijs FJ et al. Ultrasonographic evaluation of partially attenuated congenital extrahepatic portosystemic shunts in 14 dogs. *Vet Rec* 2004; 155: 448–456.

80. d'Anjou MA, Penninck D, Cornejo L et al. Ultrasonographic diagnosis of portosystemic shunting in dogs and cats. *Vet Radiol Ultrasound* 2004; 45: 424–437.

81. Santilli RA, Gerboni G. Diagnostic imaging of congenital portosystemic shunts in dogs and cats: a review. *Vet J* 2003; 166: 7–18.

82. Havig M, Tobias KM. Outcome of ameroid constrictor occlusion of single congenital extrahepatic portosystemic shunts in cats: 12 cases (1993–2000). *J Am Vet Med Assoc* 2002; 220: 337–341.

83. Koblik PD, Hornof WJ. Transcolonic sodium pertechnetate Tc 99m scintigraphy for diagnosis of macrovascular portosystemic shunts in dogs, cats, and pot-bellied pigs: 176 cases (1988–1992). *J Am Vet Med Assoc* 1995; 207: 729–733.

84. Meyer HP, Rothuizen J, van Sluijs FJ et al. Progressive remission of portosystemic shunting in 23 dogs after partial closure of congenital portosystemic shunts. *Vet Rec* 1999; 144: 333–337.

85. Wolschrijn CF, Mahapokai W, Rothuizen J et al. Gauged attenuation of congenital portosystemic shunts: results in 160 dogs and 15 cats. *Vet Q* 2000; 22: 94–98.

86. Kummeling A, Van Sluijs FJ, Rothuizen J. Prognostic implications of the degree of shunt narrowing and of the portal vein diameter in dogs with congenital portosystemic shunts. *Vet Surg* 2004; 33: 17–24.

87. Levy JK, Bunch SE, Komtebedde J. Feline portosystemic vascular shunts. In: Bonagura JD, Kirk RW (eds.) *Kirk's Current Veterinary Therapy XII: Small Animal Practice.* Philadelphia, WB Saunders, 1995; 743–749.

88. Meyer HP, Chamuleau RA, Legemate DA et al. Effects of a branched-chain amino acid-enriched diet on chronic hepatic encephalopathy in dogs. *Metab Brain Dis* 1999; 14: 103–15.

89. Szatmari V, van den Ingh TS, Fenyves B et al. Portal hypertension in a dog due to circumscribed fibrosis of the wall of the extrahepatic portal vein. *Vet Rec* 2002; 150: 602–605.

90. Spee B, Penning LC, van den Ingh TS et al. Regenerative and fibrotic pathways in canine hepatic portosystemic shunt and portal vein hypoplasia, new models for clinical hepatocyte growth factor treatment. *Comp Hepatol* 2005; 4 (7): 1–11.

91. Zandvliet MM, Szatmari V, van den Ingh T et al. Acquired portosystemic shunting in 2 cats secondary to congenital hepatic fibrosis. *J Vet Intern Med* 2005; 19: 765–767.

92. van den Ingh TS, Rothuizen J, Meyer HP. Portal hypertension associated with primary hypoplasia of the hepatic portal vein in dogs. *Vet Rec* 1995; 137: 424–427.

93. Schermerhorn T, Center SA, Dykes NL et al. Characterization of hepatoportal microvascular dysplasia in a kindred of Cairn Terriers. *J Vet Intern Med* 1996; 10: 219–230.

94. Schaeffer IG, Kirpensteijn J, Wolvekamp WT et al. Hepatic arteriovenous fistulae and portal vein hypoplasia in a Labrador Retriever. *J Small Anim Pract* 2001; 42: 146–150.

95. Pike FS, Berg J, King NW et al. Gallbladder mucocele in dogs: 30 cases (2000–2002). *J Am Vet Med Assoc* 2004; 224: 1615–1622.

96. Gorlinger S, Rothuizen J, Bunch S et al. Congenital dilatation of the bile ducts (Caroli's disease) in young dogs. *J Vet Intern Med* 2003; 17: 28–32.

97. van den Ingh TS, Rothuizen J. Congenital cystic disease of the liver in seven dogs. *J Comp Pathol* 1985; 95: 405–414.

98. Schulze C, Rothuizen J, van Sluijs FJ et al. Extrahepatic biliary atresia in a Border Collie. *J Small Anim Pract* 2000; 41: 27–30.

99. van den Ingh TS, Rothuizen J, van den Brom WE. Extrahepatic cholestasis in the dog and the differentiation of extrahepatic and intrahepatic cholestasis. *Vet Q* 1986; 8: 150–157.

100. Boothe HW, Boothe DM, Komkov A et al. Use of hepatobiliary scintigraphy in the diagnosis of extrahepatic biliary obstruction in dogs and cats: 25 cases (1982–1989). *J Am Vet Med Assoc* 1992; 201: 134–141.

101. Buote NJ, Webster CRL, Freeman L et al. Cholecystoenterostomy in cats – etiology and prognosis: 22 cases (1994–2003). *J Vet Intern Med* 2004; 18: 246.

102. Liptak JM, Dernell WS, Monnet E et al. Massive hepatocellular carcinoma in dogs: 48 cases (1992–2002). *J Am Vet Med Assoc* 2004; 225: 1225–1230.

103. Carpenter JL, Andrews LK, Holzworth J. Tumors and tumor-like lesions. In: Holzworth J (ed.) *Diseases of the Cat: Medicine and Surgery.* Philadelphia, WB Saunders, 1987; 500–505.

104. Thamm DH. Hepatobiliary tumors. In: Withrow RG, MacEwen EG (eds.), *Small Animal Clinical Oncology,* 3rd edition. Philadelphia, WB Saunders, 2001; 327–334.

105. Charles JA, Cullen JM, van den Ingh T et al. Morphological classification of neoplastic disorders of the canine and feline liver. In: *WSAVA Standards for Clinical and Histological Diagnosis of Canine and Feline Liver Diseases.* Edinburgh, Churchill Livingstone, 2006; 117–124.

106. Biourge VC, Massat B, Groff JM et al. Effects of protein, lipid, or carbohydrate supplementation on hepatic lipid accumulation during rapid weight loss in obese cats. *Am J Vet Res* 1994; 55: 1406–1415.

107. Center SA, Crawford MA, Guida L et al. A retrospective study of 77 cats with severe hepatic lipidosis: 1975–1990. *J Vet Intern Med* 1993; 7: 349–359.

108. Armstrong PJ, Hardie EM. Percutaneous endoscopic gastrostomy: a retrospective study of 54 clinical cases in dogs and cats. *J Vet Intern Med* 1990; 4: 202–206.

109. Armstrong PJ, Hand MS, Frederick GS. Enteral nutrition by tube. *Vet Clin North Am Small Anim Pract* 1990; 20: 237–275.

110. Sparkes AH, Gruffyd-Jones TJ, Harbour DA. Feline infectious peritonitis: a review of clinicopathological changes in 65 cases and a critical assessment of their diagnostic value. *Vet Rec* 1991; 129: 209–212.

111. Broussard JD, Peterson ME, Fox PR. Changes in clinical and laboratory findings in cats with hyperthyroidism from 1983 to 1993. *J Am Vet Med Assoc* 195; 206: 302–305.

112. Weiss DJ, Gagne JM, Armstrong PJ. Relationship between feline inflammatory liver disease and inflammatory bowel disease, pancreatitis, and nephritis in cats. *J Am Vet Med Assoc* 1996; 209: 1114–1116.

113. Gagne JM, Armstrong PJ, Weiss DJ et al. Clinical features of inflammatory liver disease in cats: 41 cases (1983–1993). *J Am Vet Med Assoc* 1999; 214: 513–516.

114. Lucke VM, Davies JD. Progressive lymphocytic cholangitis in the cat. *J Small Anim Pract* 1984; 25: 249–260.

115. Boomkens SY, de Rave S, Pot RG et al. The role of *Helicobacter* spp. in the pathogenesis of primary biliary cirrhosis and primary sclerosing cholangitis. *FEMS Immunol Med Microbiol* 2005; 44: 221–225.

116. Day MJ. Immunohistochemical characterization of the lesions of feline progressive lymphocytic cholangitis/cholangiohepatitis. *J Comp Path* 1998; 119: 135–147.

117. Bielsa LM, Greiner EC. Liver flukes (*Platynosomum concinnum*) in cats. *J Am Anim Hosp Assoc* 1985; 21: 269–274.

118. Lewis DT, Malone JB, Taboada J et al. Cholangiohepatitis and choledochectasia associated with *Amphimerus pseudofelineus* in a cat. *J Am Anim Hosp Assoc* 1991; 27: 156–161.

7

8   Exocrine Pancreas

Jörg M. Steiner

8.1   Anatomy

The pancreas in dogs and cats is a long narrow structure that can be divided into a right and a left limb. In between these two limbs is the head of the pancreas, which, in contrast to humans, is not an easily discernible structure in dogs (Figure 8.1) and cats. The right limb of the pancreas lies directly next to the duodenum, while the left limb is situated next to the spleen. The pancreas is made up of lobules of pancreatic tissue, which in turn are made up of acinar cells (Figure 8.2). In between the lobules there are the islets of Langerhans (Figure 8.2), which are collections of neuroendocrine cells. These neuroendocrine cells make up the endocrine portion of the pancreas and synthesize and secrete a variety of regulatory polypeptides, most importantly insulin and glucagon. The acinar cells produce digestive enzymes and zymogens, which are released into the duct system that leads to the duodenum.

Dogs usually have two pancreatic ducts. The main pancreatic duct, ductus pancreaticus, empties into the duodenum on the major duodenal papilla together with the common bile duct. The lumen of the pancreatic duct is separated from the duodenum by the sphincter of Oddi, which is a muscular sphincter that is essential in preventing duodenal contents from entering the pancreatic duct. Dogs and approximately 20% of cats have a second pancreatic duct, the accessory pancreatic duct (ductus pancreaticus accessorius) that empties on the minor duodenal papilla, approximately 1–3 cm distal to the major duodenal papilla into the duodenum.[1]

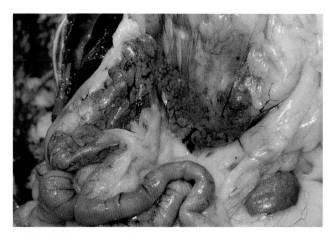

Figure 8.1:
Normal canine pancreas. This figure shows a normal canine pancreas collected during necropsy. Note the right and left limbs on either side of the head of the pancreas. In dogs and cats, the head of the pancreas is not as clearly demarcated as is the case in humans, but it can be identified by the pancreatic artery, vein, and duct that enter the pancreas in this area. (Image courtesy of Dr. Shelley Newman, University of Tennessee, USA.)

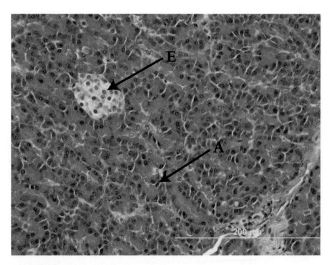

Figure 8.2:
Histological view of the pancreas. This figure shows a histological view of a normal dog pancreas. The majority of the cells are exocrine pancreatic cells (A) arranged in acini that subsequently form the pancreatic lobules. The islets of Langerhans are composed of clusters of endocrine cells (E), which have smaller nuclei and a more vacuolated cytoplasm. (H&E stain, 40×; image courtesy of Dr. Shelley Newman, University of Tennessee, USA.)

Table 8.1: Secretory products of the exocrine pancreas
This table shows a list of secretory products of the exocrine pancreas and their main functions. There are three types of secretory products: zymogens of pancreatic digestive enzymes, pancreatic enzymes, and other molecules that are neither.

Enzymes secreted as zymogens	Enzymes secreted in an active form	Other secretory products
trypsinogen	lipase	water
chymotrypsinogen	amylase	bicarbonate
proelastase	carboxylesterase	procolipase
prophospholipase	desoxyribonuclease	intrinsic factor
kallikreinogen	ribonuclease	antimicrobial factors
procarboxypeptidase		pancreatic secretory trypsin inhibitor (PSTI)
		trophic factors for the intestinal tract

8.2 Physiology

The exocrine pancreas has several important functions. Most importantly, the acinar cells, which make up the bulk of the exocrine pancreas, synthesize and secrete many digestive enzymes and zymogens of digestive enzymes (Table 8.1).[2] These digestive enzymes produced by the pancreas are required for digestion of the diet. While the digestive tract is characterized by redundancy (i.e., the digestion of each dietary component is facilitated by more than one process), most dogs and cats require at least some pancreatic function for digestion. However, there are isolated cases of patients that have virtually no residual exocrine pancreatic function and which do not have any clinical signs of maldigestion. In addition to the synthesis and secretion of pancreatic digestive zymogens and enzymes, the exocrine pancreas also synthesizes and secretes a variety of other molecules (Table 8.1), such as intrinsic factor, which is crucial for cobalamin absorption; colipase, which is needed to reverse the inhibition of pancreatic lipase by bile salts; a trypsin inhibitor; antibacterial factors; and probably certain trophic factors that have been hypothesized to affect intestinal mucosal thickness.[2,3]

Some digestive enzymes are synthesized and secreted as active enzymes, while others are synthesized and secreted as inactive proforms or zymogens.[2] In general, any enzyme that is capable of digesting components of the cellular membrane, such as proteins and phospholipids are secreted as zymogens, while those enzymes that digest components that are normally located inside of organelles or the nucleus are secreted as active enzymes. Examples of enzymes that are secreted as zymogens (Table 8.1) are trypsin (i.e., trypsinogen), chymotrypsin (i.e., chymotrypsinogen), elastase (i.e., proelastase), and phospholipase (i.e., prophospholipase).[2] In contrast, examples of enzymes that are secreted as active enzymes (Table 8.1) are lipase, amylase, desoxyribonuclease, or ribunuclease.[2]

Pancreatic enzymes and zymogens of pancreatic enzymes are synthesized by protein synthesis; that is, DNA is transcribed to mRNA in the nucleus of the acinar cells, and the mRNA in turn is read at the ribosomes to be translated into a polypeptide strand, the pre-pro-enzyme or pre-enzyme (in the case of enzymes that are secreted as active enzymes). The pre-enzymes and pre-pro-enzymes are then internalized into the rough endoplasmic reticulum. During the process of internalization, a small signal peptide is removed, leaving the pro-enzyme or enzyme. The zymogens and enzymes are then processed by the Golgi apparatus, where they undergo glycosylation and other post-translational changes. At the distal end of the Golgi apparatus, the zymogens and enzymes are then packaged into zymogen granules. These zymogen granules are then released into the duct lumen by exocytosis.

Peptides, amino acids, and fatty acids containing eight or more carbon atoms or their monoglycerides are the most important stimuli of CCK release from the neuroendocrine cells in the duodenum and jejunum. CCK stimulates gall bladder contraction and also leads to the secretion of zymogen granules from the acinar cells into the pancreatic duct system. A small amount of zymogen granules are also released into the vascular space.

Activation of pancreatic trypsinogen to trypsin is by hydrolysis, which is catalyzed by enteropeptidase, another serine protease that is secreted by the duodenal mucosa. In turn, activated trypsin then activates more trypsinogen molecules and other zymogens.[2] Pancreatic digestive enzymes are crucial for the digestion of most dietary components, but oral, gastric, and brush border enzymes also contribute to this process. This contribution can be quite significant; for example, under physiological conditions, a significant portion of dietary fat is digested by gastric lipase.[4]

As said before, the main function of the exocrine pancreas is to digest dietary components. One important dietary component in carnivores and omnivores is meat, which includes pancreatic tissue; thus, the pancreas is always in danger of digesting itself. However, there are several mechanisms in place to prevent such autodigestion.[5] First of all, the pancreas synthesizes and secretes all the enzymes that can be dangerous to itself as inactive preforms or zymogens. Secondly, these zymogens are stored in zymogen granules within the acinar cells and are kept strictly separate from the lysosomes as lysosomal enzymes are capable of activating zymogens and so such strict separation is important to prevent pancreatic autodigestion.[5] Thirdly, pancreatic zymogens are inhibited from autoactivation by the adverse conditions (e.g., pH) within the zymogen granules. This may not completely abolish autoactivation, but certainly decreases its likelihood. Fourthly, there is a small inhibitory molecule, pancreatic secretory trypsin inhibitor (PSTI), that is co-synthesized, co-transported, and co-stored with the pancreatic zymogens. PSTI inhibits any prematurely activated trypsin molecules, thereby preventing the cascade of pancreatic enzyme activation. PSTI probably plays a crucial role in preventing pancreatitis in normal individuals. In humans, hereditary pancreatitis is caused by mutations of the genes encoding PSTI (i.e., SPINK gene) or trypsinogen.[6] These mutations either lead to the production of non-functional PSTI or of a trypsin that is not effectively inhibited by PSTI. Recently, mutations have also been identified in the SPINK gene of Miniature Schnauzers with pancreatitis.[7] Fifthly, there is a unidirectional flow of pancreatic juice in the pancreatic duct. Pancreatic zymogens are activated in the small intestine and it is crucial that these activated enzymes cannot return to the pancreas where they could lead to pancreatic autodigestion and pancreatitis. Sixthly, and finally, if all of these safety mechanisms are overcome and activated pancreatic enzymes escape into the vascular space, they are quite effectively removed by proteinase inhibitors, such as α_1-proteinase inhibitor (α_1-PI) and α_2-macroglobulin.[8] Trypsin bound to α_1-PI is quickly transferred to α_2-macroglobulin, which is then trapped in the reticuloendothelial system of the spleen and thus removed

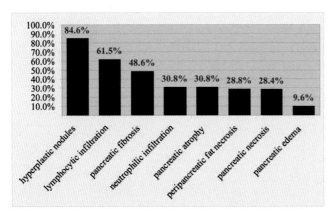

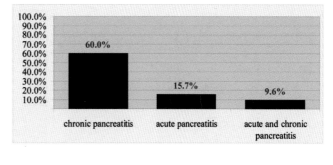

Figure 8.3:
Frequency of histopathological lesions in dogs. This figure shows the frequencies of histopathological lesions of the pancreas of 73 dogs presented for necropsy to the Department of Pathology at the Animal Medical Center in New York. The dogs evaluated were affected by a wide variety of diseases and died of various causes. Each pancreas was sectioned every 2 cm and each section was evaluated for neutrophilic infiltration, lymphocytic infiltration, pancreatic necrosis, peripancreatic fat necrosis, edema, pancreatic fibrosis, pancreatic atrophy, and pancreatic hyperplastic nodules. With the exception of hyperplastic nodules, all the other lesions can be considered as evidence of previous or current pancreatic inflammation.

Figure 8.4:
Frequency of histopathological lesions in cats. This figure shows the frequencies of histopathological lesions of the pancreas of 115 cats presented for necropsy to the Department of Pathology at the University of California, Davis. The cats were affected by a wide variety of diseases and died of various causes. Three biopsies were taken from each pancreas (left limb, right limb, and pancreatic head) and each section was evaluated separately for evidence of either acute or chronic pancreatitis. Lesions that were considered to be suggestive of acute pancreatitis were interstitial edema and/or necrosis of mesenteric fat or neutrophilic infiltration of the pancreas. Lesions that were considered to be suggestive of chronic pancreatitis were lymphocytic infiltration, interstitial fibrosis, and cystic acinar degeneration.[13]

from the circulation. There may be other protective mechanisms that are as yet unknown, but it is still quite impressive how many protective mechanisms are in place to prevent the pancreas from damaging itself.

8.3   Diseases of the exocrine pancreas

The true incidence of exocrine pancreatic disease in dogs and cats is unknown. However, one study of necropsy findings reported that 1.7% of 9,342 canine pancreata and 1.3% of 6,504 feline pancreata showed significant pathological lesions at necropsy.[9] Roughly 50% of these lesions were classified as pancreatitis in both species, making pancreatitis the most common exocrine pancreatic disease in both dogs and cats.

8.3.1   Pancreatitis

Introduction and definitions

Pancreatitis describes pancreatic inflammation. It is the most common exocrine pancreatic disease in both dogs and cats. In an older study from Europe, histopathological evidence of

pancreatitis was found in 1.0% of 9,342 canine pancreata and 0.6% of 6,504 feline pancreata.[9] However, recently, it has been suggested that the true prevalence of pancreatitis is by far greater. In one study, more than 21% of 73 dogs undergoing necropsy at the Animal Medical Center in New York City had macroscopic lesions suggesting pancreatitis.[10] Pancreata from all 208 dogs were sectioned every 2 cm and a total of 64% had histological lesions of acute and/or chronic pancreatitis (Figure 8.3).[11] In another study, 25.6% of 200 unselected dogs submitted to necropsy through a group of first-opinion practices in the UK showed evidence of chronic pancreatitis and 2.0% showed evidence of acute pancreatitis.[12] These data suggest that pancreatitis is far more common in dogs than previously suspected. However, the data also suggest that infiltration of the pancreas with inflammatory cells is not necessarily clinically significant and more research is needed to characterize clinically significant disease better.

Similar data have recently been reported for cats.[13] In a study of 115 cats submitted for necropsy at the University of California in Davis that had three biopsies collected (one from the left limb, one from the right limb, and one from the body of the pancreas), 67.0% showed lesions suggestive of acute and/or chronic pancreatitis (Figure 8.4).[13] This would suggest that, similarly to dogs, feline pancreatitis is far more common than previously expected, but also that more work is needed to clearly characterize clinically significant disease.

8

8

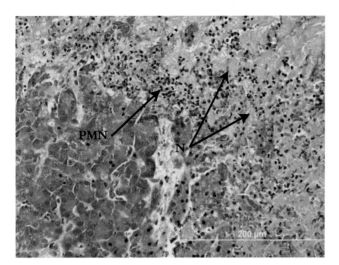

Figure 8.5:
Acute pancreatitis. This image shows a section of pancreas from a dog with acute pancreatitis. Note the marked necrosis (N) of the acinar cells and the infiltration of the pancreatic tissue with neutrophils (PMN). (H&E, 40×; image courtesy of Dr. Shelley Newman, University of Tennessee, USA.)

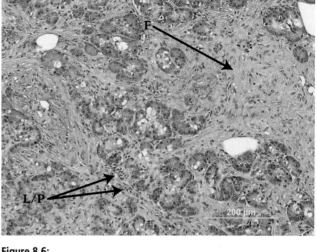

Figure 8.6:
Chronic pancreatitis. This image shows a section of pancreas from a dog with chronic pancreatitis. Notably, there is pancreatic acinar atrophy, evidenced by the lack of pancreatic acinar cells and abundant infiltrative fibrosis (F). Scattered infiltrates of lymphocytes and plasma cells (L/P) are also seen. (H&E, 20×; image courtesy of Dr. Shelley Newman, University of Tennessee, USA.)

As is the case with other organs, pancreatic inflammation can be classified based on different parameters. In human medicine, several international conferences have been held to arrive at an internationally agreed upon multi-disciplinary classification system for pancreatitis.[14] This system was last updated in Atlanta in 1993.[14] Because a similar classification system is not available for veterinary medicine, the author generally adheres to this human classification system. However, it should be pointed out that this classification system sometimes stands in contrast to the definitions used by other authors. In general, pancreatitis is divided into acute and chronic pancreatitis.[14,15] This classification is exclusively based on the histopathological findings, with acute pancreatitis (Figure 8.5) not being associated with permanent histological changes, while chronic pancreatitis is associated with permanent changes, most importantly, pancreatic atrophy and pancreatic fibrosis (Figure 8.6).[15]

Both acute and chronic pancreatitis can be associated with local and systemic complications. Local complications include pancreatic necrosis, pancreatic pseudocyst, and pancreatic abscess. Systemic complications include electrolyte imbalances, acid-base imbalances, DIC, acute renal failure, lung failure, myocarditis, neurological signs (also known as pancreatic encephalopathy), and multi-organ failure. The severity and prognosis of pancreatitis are dependent on the presence of these local and systemic complications.

Etiology

The etiology and pathogenesis of pancreatitis is not clearly understood, but there are many risk factors that have been implicated in causing pancreatitis. Miniature Schnauzers have long been recognized as being at an increased risk for pancreatitis, but only recently has a mutation been identified that may be responsible for this increased risk.[7] Three mutations of the SPINK gene (i.e., the gene encoding the pancreatic secretory trypsin inhibitor, PSTI), have been identified.[7] It is interesting to note that mutations of the SPINK gene, though not the same as the ones that have been identified in the Miniature Schnauzer, are also associated with hereditary pancreatitis in humans.[6] There are some other breeds that have also been suggested to be at an increased risk for pancreatitis, including Boxers, Cavalier King Charles Spaniels, Cocker Spaniels, Collies, and Yorkshire Terriers.[12,16]

Dietary indiscretion, mainly of fatty foods, has anecdotally been blamed for many cases of canine pancreatitis; however, only recently, has a study shown that dietary indiscretion in dogs is in fact associated with a statistically increased risk for pancreatitis in dogs (Foley K, personal communication, 2007). Hyperlipidemia, and more specifically, hypertriglyceridemia, is also considered a risk factor for pancreatitis. In humans, it has been suggested that the risk for pancreatitis is dramatically increased when serum triglyceride concentrations exceed 1,000 mg/dL.[17] In a recent study, an increased serum triglyceride concentration above 900 mg/dL was shown to carry an increased risk for pancreatitis in the dog.[18]

Hypotension and pancreatic hypoperfusion have also been identified as risk factors for pancreatitis and in fact, it has now been speculated that the increased incidence of pancreatitis in human patients undergoing surgery may in fact be caused by pancreatic hypoperfusion, rather than pancreatic trauma.[19] Thus, proper fluid support during anesthetic procedures is crucial in maintaining exocrine pancreatic health. Notwithstanding this, pancreatic trauma (surgical or other) can lead to pancreatitis.[19–21] As a consequence, extreme care should be taken when handling the pancreas during a surgical procedure.[20]

Certain infections have also been implicated in causing pancreatitis; however, such infections are extremely rare in dogs. Anecdotal reports of isolated cases of fungal infiltration of the pancreas leading to pancreatitis are available (Newman SJ, personal communication, 2007). In addition, there are only two reports of a bacterial infection of the pancreas in dogs.[22,23] In the first report, a pancreatic abscess was diagnosed in six dogs. *Klebsiella pneumoniae* was cultured in one of these dogs from the area of the pancreas during surgery and *Pseudomonas aeruginosa* was cultured in a second dog.[22] The bacterial cultures were negative in the remaining four dogs.[22] In the second report, only two of nine dogs with a pancreatic abscess had a positive bacterial culture.[23] Bacterial infections of the pancreas are also extremely rare in cats and have only been associated with a pancreatic abscess in a single cat.[24] However, *Toxoplasma gondii* can infect the feline pancreas. In one study, 38 of 45 cats (84.4%) with toxoplasmosis showed organisms in the pancreas;[25] though, the organisms were limited to the pancreas only in one cat.[25] The hepatic fluke, *Amphimerus pseudofelineus*, can also infest the pancreas of cats and lead to pancreatitis.[26] Other infections, including FIP, feline parvovirus, FIV, and FeLV, have all been implicated in causing pancreatitis, but the evidence is limited. In dogs, infection with *Babesia canis* has been shown to cause pancreatitis.[27]

Drugs can also cause pancreatitis. In humans, approximately 54 drugs and drug classes have been implicated in causing pancreatitis.[19,28] However, demonstration of a cause and effect relationship is difficult and proof of such a relationship has only been demonstrated for a very limited number of agents.[29] In dogs, several agents have been implicated, including calcium, L-asparaginase, potassium bromide, phenobarbital, and antimonial drugs for the treatment of Leishmania.[8,30] In cats, calcium and organophosphates have been implicated as causing pancreatitis.[31] In humans, in comparison, many more drugs have been implicated, including azathioprine, vinca alkaloids, diuretics, and several NSAIDs and antibacterial agents.[19,28] However, steroid administration is currently not considered a risk factor for pancreatitis and the treatment of patients with pancreatitis with steroids is not considered to be contraindicated. Finally, several endocrine disorders, including hyperadrenocorticism, diabetes mellitus, and hypothyroidism have been identified as risk factors for pancreatitis in dogs.[16]

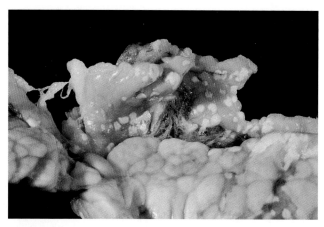

Figure 8.7:
Peripancreatic fat necrosis. This picture shows a canine pancreas with many white raised nodules consistent with peripancreatic fat necrosis. Triglycerides in the tissue surrounding the pancreas are hydrolyzed to fatty acids that then form calcium soaps (saponification). (Image courtesy of Dr. Shelley Newman, University of Tennessee, USA.)

Pathogenesis

Pancreatitis is a complex disease and the pathogenesis is not completely understood. As indicated above, there are many risk factors for pancreatitis. These risk factors ultimately lead to premature activation of the zymogens within the acinar cells, which in turn leads to local damage. Exactly how the enzyme cascade is activated is poorly understood. However, one of the first indicators of ensuing pancreatitis is a decreased secretion of pancreatic enzymes and co-localization of zymogen granules and lysosomes.[32] Co-localization of these cellular compartments leads to a decrease in the pH in the newly formed giant vacuoles compared to the zymogen granules, which favors autoactivation of trypsinogen to trypsin. It is also possible that lysosomal enzymes directly activate trypsinogen. Trypsin, if not immediately scavenged, in turn activates more trypsinogen molecules and other zymogens.[5] The prematurely activated digestive enzymes then lead to local damage. Phospholipase destroys the phospholipid bilayer of the acinar cells, leading to pancreatic necrosis. Lipase hydrolyzes pancreatic and peripancreatic triglycerides to fatty acids, which fall out as calcium soaps and form yellowish nodules in the peripancreatic region (Figure 8.7). Kinins are vasoactive polypeptides that can lead to vasodilation and pancreatic hypoperfusion. Elastase can digest the elastin of the capillaries and lead to bleeding. The local damage then leads to the release of cytokines and recruitment of inflammatory cells. This inflammatory reaction not only leads to further local damage, but also leads to systemic complications, such as hypotension, acid-base abnormalities, DIC, renal failure, lung failure, or multi-organ

8

failure.[33] There is some debate of whether some of these systemic complications could also be due to circulating pancreatic enzymes, but most evidence suggests that these systemic complications are mainly due to the inflammatory reaction instead. One exception may be systemic lipodystrophy, which is characterized by disseminated fat necrosis.[34] There is little doubt that a lipase is involved in this process and it has traditionally been assumed that pancreatic lipase is the causative factor. However, this has not been verified experimentally.

Clinical presentation

In one study of 70 dogs with fatal pancreatitis (i.e., dogs that either died of their disease or were euthanized because of the severity of their disease), the most common clinical signs reported were anorexia (91%), vomiting (90%), weakness (79%), abdominal pain (58%), dehydration (46%), diarrhea (33%), and fever (21%).[35] In comparison, a recent compilation of 159 feline pancreatitis cases reported anorexia (87%), lethargy (81%), dehydration (54%), weight loss (47%), hypothermia (46%), vomiting (46%), icterus (37%), fever (25%), abdominal pain (19%), and diarrhea (12%) as the most common clinical signs.[36] According to these reports, abdominal pain, one of the key clinical signs of pancreatitis in humans, is reported much less frequently in dogs and cats than in humans. While one could stipulate that dogs and cats with pancreatitis are less commonly affected by abdominal pain than are humans, the author believes that it is far more likely that abdominal pain is not accurately identified in small animals. As a consequence, the author strongly believes that abdominal pain should be suspected in all small animal patients diagnosed with pancreatitis. Some patients may not show any obvious evidence of abdominal pain, but others may show classical signs of severe abdominal pain. One such example in dogs is the so-called prayer position (Figure 1.7). Generally, cats appear to have far fewer specific clinical signs than dogs. This may be due to the fact that cats more commonly have mild chronic pancreatitis rather than the more severe forms.

As stated above, diarrhea has been reported to be a fairly common clinical sign in dogs with pancreatitis and has also been observed in some cats with pancreatitis.[35,36] Thus, pancreatitis should be considered as a differential diagnosis in dogs and cats with diarrhea.

Diagnosis

Routine clinical pathology

Routine clinical pathology testing, including CBC, serum chemistry profile, and urinalysis often show mild or nonspecific changes.[31,35] More severe changes can be observed in patients with severe forms of pancreatitis that are affected by systemic complications. Thus findings on routine blood work are not useful for the primary diagnosis of pancreatitis, but should be used as an indicator of the overall health status of the patient.

In a study of 70 dogs with severe pancreatitis, thrombocytopenia was the most common finding on CBC and was reported in 59% of the cases.[35] A neutrophilia with a left shift (55%) and anemia (29%) were also frequently observed. Neutropenia was only rarely observed (3%).[35] In 40 cats with severe pancreatitis, findings on CBC included anemia (26%), hemoconcentration (13%), leukocytosis (30%), and leukopenia (15%).[31]

A routine serum chemistry profile may show mild elevations of hepatic enzymes.[31,35] Electrolyte abnormalities are commonly seen in severe cases and are due to dehydration and severe vomiting. Azotemia can be seen and may be due to dehydration or may be an indicator of acute renal failure secondary to pancreatitis.[31,35] Hypoalbuminemia may also be seen. Hypocalcemia can be seen in severe cases and may be due to hypoalbuminemia or may also be due to the formation of calcium soaps with fatty acids in areas of fat necrosis.

Urinalysis often reveals an elevated urine specific gravity, secondary to dehydration. However, in severe cases, acute renal failure may ensue and the urine specific gravity may drop and casts may be seen in the sediment.

Diagnostic imaging

Abdominal radiographs may show a loss of detail in the cranial abdomen.[31,35,37] In some cases, there may also be a suggestion of a mass in the cranial abdomen. Transposition of abdominal organs can also be seen in some cases and may include a transposition of the duodenum dorsally and laterally, the stomach to the left, and the transverse colon caudally.[31,35,37] However, these findings are rather subjective and a conclusive diagnosis of pancreatitis is not possible on the basis of abdominal radiographs alone.

Thoracic radiographs in patients with pancreatitis are usually normal; however, pleural effusion maybe seen in a small number of severe cases.[35]

In contrast to abdominal radiography, abdominal ultrasonography is highly specific for pancreatitis if stringent criteria are applied (Figure 1.40).[38] Over the last 20 years, abdominal ultrasonography has greatly advanced and is still advancing, leading to an improved resolution of diagnostic images. This progress has made repeated revisions of ultrasonographic diagnostic criteria necessary. When pancreatic ultrasonography in dogs was first introduced more than 20 years ago, the pancreas could not be routinely identified during abdominal ultrasonography and identification of the pancreas was seen as an important indicator for the presence of pancreatitis. With better equipment and more expertise, the pancreas could soon be routinely identified in every dog and cat. However, an enlarged pancreas and/or fluid accumulation around the pancreas were considered highly suggestive of pancreatitis. Further advances led to the recognition that an enlarged pancreas and fluid accumulation around the pancreas alone are not sufficient to make a diagnosis of pancreatitis as pancreatic edema can also be observed with portal hypertension or hypoalbuminemia.[39] While not diagnostic for pancreatitis, various degrees of peripancreatic fluid accumulation are often seen in patients with pancreatitis.[35,40] The pancreas may appear hypoechoic when pancreatic necrosis is present.[35,41] In acute cases, a hypoechoic pancreas is often surrounded by a hyperechoic area that is due to peripancreatic fat necrosis.[35,40] Chronic pancreatitis may be associated with a hyperechoic pancreas indicating the presence of pancreatic fibrosis (Figure 8.8), but this finding is not commonly observed.[42] However, it is important to note that with recent advances in image quality and resolution, echogenicity changes due to pancreatitis must be differentiated from echogenicity changes that are due to pancreatic hyperplastic nodules, which occur extremely frequently in both dogs and cats and is a change associated with age rather than pancreatitis.[43,44] The need for stringent criteria for abdominal ultrasound has been underscored by a recent study, in which two of three cats that were suspected of having pancreatitis, but that did not have any evidence of pancreatitis during exploratory laparotomy or histopathological evaluation of a pancreatic biopsy, were falsely diagnosed with pancreatitis by abdominal ultrasonography.[41] Other, less commonly reported findings in patients with pancreatitis are an enlarged pancreatic papilla and a dilated pancreatic duct. The sensitivity of abdominal ultrasound reported in 70 dogs with severe pancreatitis was 68%.[35] This is higher than the sensitivity reported for cats with pancreatitis, which ranges between 11–35%.[40,45,46] This difference is likely due to the larger size of the organ in the dog.

Contrast-enhanced abdominal CT is the diagnostic tool of choice for human patients suspected of having pancreatitis.[47] This technology is not only highly sensitive for the diagnosis of human pancreatitis, but is also a sensitive tool for the detection of pancreatic necrosis and thus a useful prognostic tool. However, two recent studies showed that contrast-enhanced abdominal CT was inferior to abdominal ultrasonography in cats with suspected pancreatitis.[41,46] A similar study in dogs also failed to show any diagnostic usefulness of this diagnostic tool in dogs suspected of having pancreatitis, though successful use of this technology has been reported in isolated cases.[48,49]

Pancreatitis markers (see also 1.4.4)

Serum amylase and lipase activities are of no clinical value for the diagnosis of pancreatitis in the cat and are of limited clini-

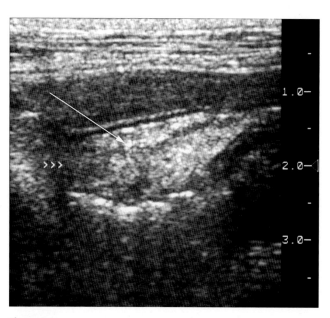

Figure 8.8:
Pancreatic fibrosis. This ultrasonographic image was taken in a cat. The pancreas is markedly hyperechoic (arrow) suggesting pancreatic fibrosis. However, pancreatic fibrosis often is not severe enough to be identified during ultrasound examination. (Image courtesy of Dr. Mark Saunders, Lynks Group, Shelburne, VT, USA.)

8

cal utility in the dog. The specificity of either of these parameters is only approximately 50%, even when stringent criteria are applied.[50] Thus, serum amylase and lipase activities should only be used for the diagnosis of canine pancreatitis until more definitive diagnostic tests can be performed.

Trypsin-like immunoreactivity (TLI) is specific for exocrine pancreatic function. However, the sensitivity of serum TLI concentration for pancreatitis in dogs and cats is only approximately 30–60%, making it a suboptimal diagnostic test for pancreatitis in both species.[41,45,46,51] However, serum TLI concentration remains the diagnostic test of choice for the diagnosis of EPI.

Recently, assays for the measurement of pancreatic lipase immunoreactivity in dogs and cats (cPLI and fPLI, respectively) have been developed and validated.[52,53] Many different cell types in the body synthesize and secrete lipases. In contrast to catalytic assays for the measurement of lipase activity, the use of immunoassays does allow for the specific measurement of lipase originating from the exocrine pancreas.[54]

Serum PLI concentration is specific for exocrine pancreatic function. In one study, serum cPLI concentration was measured in a group of dogs with EPI and the median serum cPLI

8

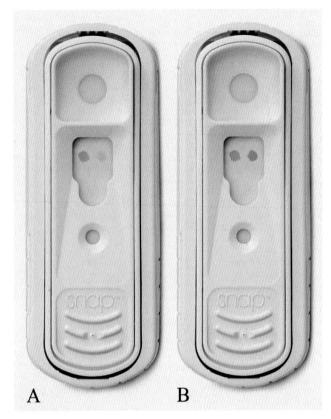

Figure 8.9:
SNAP cPL. This figure illustrates the assay interpretation of the new SNAP cPL test. (a) A test spot that is lighter in color than the control spot indicates a serum Spec cPL concentration within the control range and suggests that pancreatitis is unlikely. (b) A test spot that is darker in color than the control spot suggests that serum Spec cPL is above the control range and pancreatitis may be present.

trol spot suggests that serum Spec cPL is above the control range and that pancreatitis may be present (Figure 8.9b). An abnormal result should always be followed up by the measurement of Spec cPL in the laboratory to confirm the diagnosis and to arrive at a base-line value that can be used to assess the progression of disease.

Pancreatic biopsy

Traditionally, a pancreatic biopsy has been viewed as the most definitive diagnostic tool for pancreatitis. Pancreatic biopsies can be collected during abdominal exploratory or by laparoscopy. The presence of pancreatitis is easily diagnosed by the gross appearance of the pancreas in many cases; however, the absence of pancreatitis can be difficult to prove. In a recent study, histopathological findings in dogs with pancreatitis were evaluated. The pancreata were sectioned every 2 cm.[11] In half of all the dogs with pancreatitis and in two-thirds of dogs with chronic pancreatitis, evidence of pancreatic inflammation was found in less than 25% of all the sections.[11] Thus, even if multiple biopsies are collected, pancreatic inflammation, especially in cases of chronic pancreatitis, may easily be missed. These findings also suggest that laparoscopy is inferior for the collection of a pancreatic biopsy as it is much more difficult to evaluate the entire organ during laparoscopy than during exploratory laparotomy. It should also be noted that while a pancreatic biopsy in itself is not associated with many complications, many patients with pancreatitis are poor anesthetic risks.

Therapy

Treatment of the cause

As with many other diseases, treatment of the underlying cause of pancreatitis should be the primary goal. However, many if not most cases of canine and feline pancreatitis remain idiopathic.[16,31] In a few cases, the cause of the pancreatitis may be obvious (e.g., pancreatitis in a patient after removal of a pancreatic insulinoma). Nevertheless, when the cause of the pancreatitis is not obvious, the patient should be very carefully evaluated for any possible risk factors, such as hypertriglyceridemia, hypercalcemia, history of concurrent conditions, history of dietary indiscretion, anesthetic history, and drug history.[16] When a potential risk factor has been identified, it should be addressed appropriately. For example, if the patient has a history of being treated with potassium bromide and is considered to be in need of antiepileptic therapy, an alternative antiepileptic medication (e.g., zonisamide or levetiracetam) should be chosen.

concentration was significantly decreased compared to healthy dogs and was not detectable in most of the dogs.[55] Serum PLI concentration is also very sensitive for pancreatitis in both dogs and cats.[10,41,51] The sensitivity ranges depending on the study population examined, but is higher than any other diagnostic test currently available. Serum PLI assays are species-specific and separate assays for dogs (Spec cPL™) and cats (fPLI) are available. Currently, the fPLI assay is only available through the Gastrointestinal Laboratory at Texas A&M University (www.cvm.tamu.edu/gilab). In addition, an in-clinic test (SNAP cPL) for the measurement of PLI in dogs has recently been introduced. The assay is semi-quantitative and is evaluated by comparing the color of the test spot with the control spot. A test spot that is lighter in color than the control spot indicates a serum Spec cPL concentration within the control range and suggests that pancreatitis is very unlikely (Figure 8.9a). A test spot that is darker in color than the con-

Identification and management of complications

As mentioned previously, pancreatitis can be associated with a variety of local and systemic complications. It is crucial to carefully monitor the patient for the development of any such local or systemic complications. While some complications, such as dehydration and electrolyte abnormalities may be easily corrected, others, when established, are extremely difficult, if not impossible, to counteract. In human patients, it has been suggested that the presence of organ failure of any major organ as a complication of pancreatitis for a period of more than 24 hours has a dramatic impact on the prognosis. While this may also be the case for veterinary patients, most likely the mere development of any such organ failure should be expected to have a severe negative impact on the overall prognosis. Therefore, patients should be carefully monitored and if any evidence of an impending development of organ failure is identified, aggressive measures should be taken to prevent such complications. For example, dehydration should be treated with aggressive fluid therapy to prevent acute renal failure.

Nutritional considerations

Until recently, it was common practice to hold dogs and cats with acute pancreatitis NPO (nothing per os), in order to "rest" the pancreas. However, there is little evidence that such resting of the pancreas has any beneficial effect and there is mounting evidence that nutritional support is crucial in pancreatitis patients. In human pancreatitis patients, early nutritional support has been shown to have a beneficial effect on outcome and enteral feeding is preferable over parenteral nutrition.[56–58] As a consequence, the author recommends feeding patients with pancreatitis orally if they do not vomit. If the patient does vomit, an antiemetic should be used and the patient should only be held NPO if vomiting cannot be controlled. If the patient has to be held NPO, alternative modes of alimentation, such as a jejunostomy tube, partial parenteral nutrition, or total parenteral nutrition must be considered.[59] Feeding through a jejunostomy tube is preferable from a GI physiology point of view, but requires anesthesia for placement, which may have a negative impact on the overall outcome. Approximately 12 hours after the patient stops vomiting, the patient should be offered a small amount of fresh water. If this does not lead to vomiting, the patient should be offered a small amount of low-fat food, which should be repeated every few hours if the patient does not vomit.

If the patient does not vomit but refuses to eat, an esophagostomy or gastrostomy tube can be used for feeding. However, placement of both of these feeding devices requires general anesthesia and a nasogastric tube may be a better choice in these patients. In humans with acute pancreatitis, nasogastric tubes are commonly used with great success.

Regardless of the route of alimentation, a diet should be chosen that is low in fat. This is especially important in canine patients, where an ultra low-fat diet should be selected.

Analgesia

Abdominal pain or discomfort is one of the key clinical signs in human beings with pancreatitis and has been reported in more than 90% of all human pancreatitis patients.[19] While the reported incidence of abdominal pain in dogs and cats is much lower than this (up to 58% in dogs and up to 25% in cats), the author believes that this difference is not due to an actual difference in the incidence of abdominal pain, but rather due to the inability to correctly identify abdominal discomfort in small animal patients.[31,35] Therefore, the author suggests that every dog and cat with pancreatitis should be suspected of having abdominal pain and should be managed accordingly.[60] Only if analgesic therapy does not appear to have any clinical impact should the analgesic therapy be discontinued.

There are a variety of analgesic options for dogs and cats. Patients that are being treated in a hospital can be treated with meperidine (5–10 mg/kg IM or SC as needed in dogs and 2–5 mg/kg IM or SC as needed in cats), butorphanol (0.2–0.4 mg/kg IV, IM, or SC q 2–4 h), fentanyl (initial dose 4–10 µg/kg IV, then 4–10 µg/kg/h as a constant rate infusion), morphine (0.5–2.0 mg/kg IM or SC q 3–4 h in dogs; 0.05–0.2 mg/kg IM or SC q 3–6 h in cats), lidocaine (2 mg/kg diluted into 50 ml of warm 0.9% NaCl IP q 6–8 h), and a variety of other analgesic drugs.

The selection of analgesic drugs for outpatients is much more limited. Butorphanol (0.55 mg/kg PO in dogs and 0.4 mg/kg PO in cats q 6–12 h) or tramadol (1–4 mg/kg PO q 8–12 hr) can be used orally, while patients with more severe pain can be treated transdermally by use of a fentanyl patch (1/2 to a whole of a 2.5 mg patch [i.e., do not cut patch, but expose half of the membrane] for cats and small dogs [i.e., <5 kg body weight (BW)], a 2.5 mg patch for dogs 5–10 kg BW, a 5.0 mg patch for dogs 10–20 kg BW, a 7.5 mg patch for dogs 20–30 kg BW, and a 10 mg patch for dogs > 30 kg BW); such patches are effective for 3–5 days.

Antiemetic therapy

Antiemetic therapy is very important in the treatment of pancreatitis for two reasons, the importance of providing nutritional support by the enteral route and because vomiting in itself is debilitating to the patient. A variety of antiemetic drugs are available. Dopamine inhibitors, such as metoclopramide, probably are the most commonly used antiemetic agents in small animal practice; however, these agents may not be a good choice in patients with pancreatitis as dopamine is crucial for

8

the regulation of splanchnic perfusion. While the effects of dopamine on pancreatic perfusion have not been evaluated, it seems prudent to use alternative antiemetic agents.

Another class of antiemetics are the HT$_3$-antagonists, such as ondansetron (0.11–0.176 mg/kg IV q 12–24 h in dogs and 0.22 mg/kg IV q 12–24 h in cats) and dolasetron (0.3–0.6 mg/kg IV, SC, or PO q 12–24 h in both dogs and cats). These agents are very effective, but can also be expensive. The advantage of dolasetron is that the intravenous formulation can be used orally, making it a lot more affordable than ondansetron tablets.

Recently, a new antiemetic, maropitant (1 mg/kg SC q 24 h or 2 mg/kg PO q 24 h in dogs; no known dosage for cats), has been licensed for dogs in Europe and the USA. This antiemetic is a NK$_1$-antagonist and is highly effective in inhibiting vomition mediated by both peripheral and central pathways. In Europe, maropitant has been available for about a year and first experiences have shown that it has a high efficacy.[61] Unfortunately, almost no data are available about the off-label use of maropitant in cats.

Protease inhibitors

Based on the pathophysiological evidence that shows that pancreatitis is ultimately caused by the premature activation of digestive pancreatic enzymes, there have been efforts to treat pancreatitis by inhibiting proteases. Aprotinin was one of the first drugs that was evaluated and in the early studies, the progression of experimental canine pancreatitis could be prevented when dogs were treated with aprotinin.[62] In addition, an initial study with another protease inhibitor, gabexate mesylate, in dogs with experimental pancreatitis has shown some promising results.[63] However, studies in human patients with spontaneous pancreatitis have not shown any beneficial effect of any of the protease inhibitors investigated.[64,65] This may have been due to the fact that the dose used in the human patients was much lower than the one used in the dogs with experimental disease. However, it is more likely that the administration of a protease inhibitor in patients with established pancreatitis is simply too late in order to have any beneficial effect. It is possible, on the other hand, that the pretreatment of patients that are in danger of developing pancreatitis may be more useful and patients undergoing endoscopic retrograde cholangiopancreatography (ERCP) may benefit from being treated prior to the procedure.[65] However, the routine use of protease inhibitors in veterinary patients is not indicated at this point in time.

Plasma

Plasma contains a variety of substances, including coagulation factors, proteinase inhibitors (i.e., α_1-PI, α_2-macroglubulin), and albumin, which may all have a beneficial effect in patients with pancreatitis.[66] However, clinical studies in human pancreatitis patients failed to show any beneficial effect of using plasma.[67,68] Despite these findings in human patients, most veterinary clinicians, including the author, believe that plasma has a beneficial effect in dogs with severe forms of pancreatitis. In cats, the benefit of plasma, which is largely unavailable, or any other blood product, is less clear. Also, the appropriate dose of plasma in dogs with severe pancreatitis is unknown. Factors, such as overall severity, systemic complications, and especially serum albumin and antithrombin-III (AT-III) concentrations in the patient should be taken into consideration. However, the goal of plasma therapy in pancreatitis patients is not to normalize the serum albumin or AT-III concentrations.

Antibiotics

Many veterinarians routinely treat dogs and cats with acute or chronic pancreatitis with antibiotics; however, there is little scientific evidence for such practice. For example, the use of antibiotics in humans with acute pancreatitis is still questionable, even though approximately a third of all human pancreatitis patients that die of their disease process die of infectious complications.[69] Although early studies in the 1970s showed no benefit of routine antibiotic use in human pancreatitis patients, studies in the 1990s did show a beneficial effect.[70–72] Several meta-analysis studies have recently been presented on this topic, but their results are contradictory.[73–75] In addition, two recent consensus reports concerning the treatment of severe acute pancreatitis in humans did not recommend the routine use of antibiotics.[56,76] To complicate matters further, dogs and cats with severe pancreatitis are believed to only rarely have infectious complications. In fact, to date, only four dogs and one cat have been reported that had such infectious complications.[22–24] All five of these patients were diagnosed with an infected abscess.[22–24]

In conclusion, the author currently believes that routine therapy of canine and feline pancreatitis patients with antibiotics should be avoided. Instead, antibiotics should only be given if an infectious complication is identified or highly suspected as in patients with a urinary tract infection or aspiration pneumonia.

Anti-inflammatory agents

Non-steroidal anti-inflammatory drugs (NSAIDs) should not be administered to patients with pancreatitis as many of them have been shown to potentially cause pancreatitis. They are all known to cause GI side effects, and they do not appear to have any beneficial effect on pancreatic inflammation.[28]

Glucocorticoids were once believed to cause pancreatitis in both humans and veterinary species.[16,77] However, the scientific basis for this hypothesis is weak and in fact, in humans, glucocorticoids are generally no longer believed to be a risk factor for pancreatitis.[28] It must be borne in mind, however, that patients who receive glucocorticoids generally have diseases that in themselves are considered risk factors for pancreatitis.[28]

About 20 years ago, a new disease entity was described in humans: autoimmune pancreatitis.[78] Since the initial description of the disease, its characterization has been changed and autoimmune pancreatitis is now believed to be an important cause of chronic pancreatitis in humans.[78,79] Autoimmune pancreatitis is characterized by a lymphoplasmacytic infiltration and fibrosis of the pancreas that appears to be mostly distributed in the area around the pancreatic duct system.[78,79] It is interesting to note that most dogs and cats with chronic pancreatitis also have a lymphoplasmacytic inflammation of the pancreas. In addition, many dogs and especially cats with chronic pancreatitis have concurrent inflammatory conditions of other abdominal organs, such as IBD and/or hepatitis/cholangiohepatitis.[80] While not all canine and feline patients with pancreatitis may benefit from glucocorticoid therapy, anecdotal reports have shown that some patients do respond quite favorably. Also, a recent case report has documented the favorable response of a cat with lymphoplasmacytic pancreatitis to prednisolone therapy.[81]

The author recommends evaluating patients with chronic pancreatitis for any potential risk factor or concurrent disease and only treating those patients with glucocorticoids that do not have any identifiable risk factors and/or concurrent conditions that pose a contraindication to the use of corticosteroids (e.g., suppurative cholangiohepatitis). The author measures the PLI concentration (Spec cPL in dogs and fPLI in cats) before treatment is started and rechecks the PLI concentration after 10–14 days of therapy. Treatment should only be continued if the patient has either clinically improved, the serum PLI concentration has decreased, or both.

Dopamine

Dopamine is crucial for splanchnic and pancreatic perfusion and hypotension and pancreatic hypoperfusion can lead to pancreatitis. One study in cats with experimental pancreatitis has shown that the progression of pancreatitis can be halted if patients are treated with dopamine within 12 hours after the induction of pancreatitis.[82] This is obviously not feasible in spontaneous pancreatitis patients. However, treatment of patients at risk for pancreatic hypoperfusion (i.e., patients with pancreatitis that have to undergo general anesthesia) may benefit from dopamine therapy. A low dose (i.e., 2–5 µg/kg/min as a constant rate infusion) should be given, as this dose does not cause peripheral vasoconstriction and so does not negatively affect splanchnic perfusion.

Antioxidants

There is some evidence suggesting that reactive oxygen species (ROS) play a role in the pathogenesis of pancreatitis.[83] Such ROS can lead to tissue damage and also stimulate an inflammatory response. Thus, it has been hypothesized that antioxidants should have a beneficial effect in patients with pancreatitis. Several studies in humans with acute pancreatitis have suggested a beneficial effect.[84–86] However, other, controlled, studies were not able to confirm these effects.[87] A single study in dogs with acute pancreatitis suggested that selenious acid decreased the mortality rate of dogs with acute pancreatitis by 50%.[84] However, the findings of this study are suspect as only historical controls were used, with the control dogs being enrolled in a time period before the period in which the treated dogs were enrolled.[84] In addition, the enrollment occurred over several years and it is, therefore, likely that the dogs enrolled later in the study (i.e., the dogs in the treatment group) would have had less severe disease as the diagnostic modalities for pancreatitis had improved during this period.[84] In conclusion, at this point in time, there is little evidence to suggest that the use of antioxidants in canine and/or feline patients with acute severe pancreatitis would be of benefit.

Recently, it has been speculated that antioxidants may be more efficacious in patients with mild chronic pancreatitis.[88] In a pilot study of five dogs with subclinical pancreatitis, antioxidant administration led to a decrease in median serum cPLI, cTLI, and CRP concentrations, suggesting that further studies would be warranted (Steiner JM, unpublished data, 2007).

8

8

Modulation of inflammatory mediators

Over the last decade it has become clear that pancreatitis is a two-stage disease process with the first stage being caused by premature activation of pancreatic digestive enzymes and the second stage being due to an inflammatory response by the body. In fact, it has been suggested that most systemic complications of pancreatitis are due to the inflammatory response rather than the prematurely activated enzymes. Once the inflammatory reaction has been initiated, proteinase inhibition appears to have little effect on the disease.[64] Therefore, modulation of inflammatory mediators may be a promising method of treatment.

One group of modulators of inflammatory mediators investigated initially were the platelet-activating factor antagonists (PAFANTs) and one of the first compounds in this group investigated was lexipafant. Lexipafant was used in several studies on experimental pancreatitis and also in some small clinical trials in humans with pancreatitis, and all showed a beneficial effect.[89,90] In comparison, a large international multi-center trial with more than 1000 humans with acute pancreatitis failed to show a beneficial effect.[91] However, the results of this study have not yet been published, probably because of commercial constraints and the very disappointing results of the study. Other modulators of inflammatory cytokines are currently being evaluated.

Surgical intervention

A variety of surgical procedures have been suggested for patients with acute and/or chronic pancreatitis, including peritoneal lavage, partial pancreatectomy, and necrosectomy for acute pancreatitis, and partial pancreatectomy and cyst or abscess removal for chronic pancreatitis. There are no studies that have systematically evaluated the effectiveness of pancreatic surgery for either acute or chronic pancreatitis in dogs or cats. The results of such procedures in humans have been rather disappointing and current recommendations for surgical intervention for human pancreatitis patients are rather conservative.[76,92,93] Currently, the only indications for surgery are an infected necrosis, a pancreatic abscess, or a pancreatic pseudocyst that does not regress.[93] There have been isolated reports about surgical intervention in single cases in veterinary patients, but the results are again rather discouraging and it seems prudent to also be conservative when treating dogs and cats with pancreatitis.[22,23]

Prognosis

The prognosis for dogs and cats with pancreatitis is largely dependant on the presence of local and systemic complications. Patients without pancreatic necrosis and no systemic complications have a good prognosis, while patients with extensive pancreatic necrosis and multi-organ failure have a poor prognosis.[94] In dogs and cats, even single organ failure, such as acute renal failure or acute lung failure may not be reversible. In humans with pancreatitis, organ failure in and of itself does not appear to have a major negative effect on outcome, but the presence of any organ failure for more than 24 hours dramatically worsens the prognosis. In comparison, in dogs and cats, the reversal of even single organ failure is not very successful.

In humans, several severity scoring systems (e.g., Ranson's early prognostic signs, the acute physiology and chronic health evaluation II [APACHE II] score, or the sequential organ failure assessment [SOFA] score) are used to evaluate patients on admission.[95,96] This is important because patients may not appear at first to be severely ill clinically, but may develop complications and organ failure shortly after admission. Patients that have a high score on admission must be treated more aggressively to prevent organ failure.[97] Several scoring systems and isolated prognostic factors used in humans have been modified for use in the dog or cat, but none have proven reliable in clinical patients thus far.[94,98]

8.3.2 Exocrine pancreatic insufficiency

Introduction and definition

Exocrine pancreatic insufficiency (EPI), as the name suggests, is a syndrome that is caused by the insufficient synthesis and secretion of pancreatic enzymes. The most common cause of EPI is an absolute lack of pancreatic acinar cells that is due to pancreatic acinar atrophy or chronic pancreatitis (Figure 8.10). In this situation, all the pancreatic digestive enzymes are lacking. In rare cases, a single enzyme may be lacking, but the lack of a single enzyme, even if complete, most likely does not lead to clinical signs. Pancreatic lipase seems to be an exception as pancreatic lipase deficiency has been reported as a cause of clinical signs of EPI in humans and in one dog.[99,100]

Another infrequent cause of EPI is an obstruction of the pancreatic duct by a tumor (Hill S, personal communication, 2007). Such an obstruction, if complete, can lead to a lack of digestive enzymes in the small intestinal lumen, despite normal production of these enzymes. Long-term, an obstructed pancreatic duct can lead to either pancreatitis, pancreatic atrophy, or both, which then can lead to clinical signs of EPI. The most likely cause of an obstruction of the pancreatic duct is a pancreatic adenocarcinoma or another neoplastic condition of the pancreas. Obstructions of the pancreatic duct have been described in humans but have never been conclusively demonstrated in dogs. In cats, there have been reports of pancreatic flukes, *Eurytrema procyonis*, causing pancreatic atrophy.[101]

Pancreatic aplasia and hypoplasia could, in theory, also cause clinical signs of EPI and these conditions are sometimes suspected when EPI is diagnosed at a very early age, but to date no case has been conclusively demonstrated in a puppy or kitten. The definitive diagnosis of this condition would require a diagnosis of EPI at a very young age and the demonstration of a lack of an inflammatory infiltrate and fibrosis upon pancreatic biopsy.

Etiology

The most common cause of EPI in the classical sense, that is the lack of exocrine pancreatic tissue, is pancreatic acinar atrophy (PAA), which is almost exclusively seen in German Shepherd dogs, Rough-coated Collies, and Eurasians.[102,103] Several studies have suggested that PAA is inherited as an autosomal recessive trait in the German Shepherd dog and also the Eurasian.[102,103] However, the search for a genetic marker for this disease has been unsuccessful despite the fact that the entire canine genome has been scanned using a set of microsatellite markers, as no mutations could be identified in several candidate genes.[102] Thus, this condition may not be due to a single gene defect but may instead be multifactorial. While PAA is a hereditary disease, the associated pancreatic atrophy does not appear to be a direct consequence of this genetic disease. Instead, there have been studies to suggest that PAA is ultimately a result of immune-mediated destruction of pancreatic acinar cells.[104,105]

The most common cause of EPI in cats and the second most common cause in dogs is chronic pancreatitis.[106] As with other organs, chronic inflammation can lead to atrophy and fibrosis, which ultimately can lead to the destruction of enough exocrine pancreatic tissue to cause clinical signs of EPI. As previously described, obstruction of the pancreatic duct can also lead to atrophy of the pancreas, but this has only been anecdotally reported in dogs and cats.

Pathogenesis

Pancreatic secretory products, and most importantly, pancreatic enzymes are crucial for the digestion and absorption of food. When pancreatic acinar cells are lacking, regardless of the cause, maldigestion occurs. It is important to note that the GI tract is a highly redundant system and for most pancreatic digestive enzymes there are other enzymes with the same function that are synthesized and secreted by other organs. For example, pancreatic lipase is crucial for fat digestion, but the stomach also synthesizes and secretes a lipase, gastric lipase, which is responsible for a significant portion of normal fat digestion in dogs.[4] Also, the exocrine pancreas has a huge reserve capacity. In humans, it has been estimated that clinical signs of EPI only ensue when more than 90% of exocrine pancreatic function have been lost.[107]

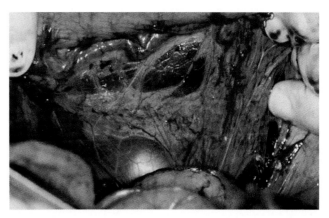

Figure 8.10:
Exocrine pancreatic insufficiency. This picture shows a pancreas in a dog with exocrine pancreatic insufficiency. There is very little pancreatic tissue left and the remaining tissue looks more fibrous than glandular in appearance.

Maldigestion leads to undigested food components in the intestinal lumen, which can lead to diarrhea, proliferation of the small intestinal microflora, and weight loss. It is important to note that these clinical signs are not solely due to maldigestion, but that the lack of functions other than the digestive functions of the exocrine pancreas may also play a role. For example, the pancreas secretes large quantities of bicarbonate, which are necessary to buffer gastric acid. A lack of bicarbonate leads to a decrease in the pH in the duodenum, which can have an effect on brush border and pancreatic enzyme activity or the intestinal microflora. In addition, the pancreas is believed to synthesize and secrete trophic factors that help maintain a normal GI mucosa and a lack of these factors may lead to malabsorption in addition to maldigestion. The exocrine pancreas also is the major source of intrinsic factor in dogs and cats.[3] In sharp contrast to humans, where intrinsic factor is mainly secreted by the gastric mucosa, intrinsic factor in dogs and cats is mainly of exocrine pancreatic origin.[3] In a recent study, 82% of dogs with EPI were shown to have a decreased serum cobalamin concentration with 36% having marked hypocobalaminemia.[108] In another study, 65% of 20 cats with EPI were cobalamin deficient.[109]

Clinical presentation

EPI can be subclinical.[110] In two large series of German Shepherd dogs, severely decreased serum TLI concentrations were identified in several dogs without any clinical signs.[110] Some of these dogs underwent exploratory laparotomy and their pancreatic mass was found to be severely decreased.[110] This once again underscores the overall high degree of redundancy of the GI tract.

The most consistent clinical sign in dogs and cats with EPI is weight loss.[109,111] Loose stools are also commonly observed, but watery diarrhea is rather uncommon.[109,111] Often, affected patients have a poor hair coat and dogs with EPI are commonly reported to have borborygmus and increased flatulence.[111] Many dogs and cats with EPI show an increased appetite and many dogs also show coprophagia, or even pica.[111] In cats, a greasy soiling of the hair coat in the perineal region can be observed (Figure 8.11A). However, in a recent study, only 1 of 20 cats was reported to have such greasy soiling of the haircoat.[109]

Diagnosis

A diagnosis of EPI is made based on the demonstration of a lack of exocrine pancreatic function. Various function tests have been described, including the plasma turbidity test, the PABA (para-aminobenzoic acid) test, the fecal test for undigested starch and muscle fibers, or the fecal proteolytic activity (FPA) test.[112] With the exception of the FPA test, all of these tests are only indirect measures of exocrine pancreatic function, estimating the digestive capacity of the entire GI tract rather than just the function of the exocrine pancreas. The FPA test is slightly different in that the major proteolytic activity of the feces should in fact be based on the presence of two pancreatic enzymes, namely trypsin and chymotrypsin. However, false positive and false negative test results have been observed. Also, there are different methods for testing FPA.[112] The most simple one is the use of a piece of undeveloped radiographic film. In theory, the digestive enzymes in the fecal sample digest the starch in the radiographic film creating a halo. Unfortunately, this method is extremely unreliable and should not be used. Other methods to determine the FPA are more reliable, but are still flawed by many false test results. Thus, FPA can only be recommended for those species in which other, more reliable, diagnostic modalities are not available.

Another approach to estimating exocrine pancreatic function is to measure the amount of pancreatic enzymes or zymogens in the blood or feces. Serum lipase activity was not significantly different between dogs with EPI and healthy dogs.[55] This is most likely due to the fact that many cells from different cellular origins synthesize and secrete lipases, and a lipase activity assay cannot differentiate between these lipases. Serum trypsin-like immunoreactivity (TLI) is the gold standard for the diagnosis of EPI in both dogs and cats.[109,113] The TLI assay is highly species-specific and measures the mass concentration of cationic trypsinogen, cationic trypsin, and some cationic trypsin molecules bound to proteinase inhibitor molecules. Under physiological conditions, only a small amount of the trypsinogen synthesized by pancreatic acinar cells is released into the vascular space. Trypsinogen and trypsin are rather small molecules and thus get quickly excreted by the

kidney. Therefore, only if the pancreas is functioning normally can a small amount of trypsinogen be detected in the serum. In contrast, in patients with EPI, regardless of the cause, the amount of trypsinogen released into the serum, and in turn serum TLI is severely decreased to undetectable. In general, serum TLI is highly sensitive and specific for the diagnosis of EPI in both dogs and cats. There are two special scenarios, however, where serum TLI can be normal despite the patient having EPI. The first scenario is isolated pancreatic lipase deficiency. It has long been recognized that the rate-limiting enzyme of pancreatic digestion is pancreatic lipase. Thus, patients with an isolated lipase deficiency may have clinical signs of EPI but still have a normal serum TLI concentration. Recently, the first dog with such an isolated lipase deficiency has been reported, but such cases are believed to be extremely rare.[100] Another scenario where serum TLI concentration could be normal in a patient with EPI is a patient with an obstructed pancreatic duct. Such cases have not yet been described in the literature, but recently a single dog with this condition has been identified (Hill S, personal communication, 2007). Again, this scenario is believed to be extremely rare.

Recently, assays for the measurement of serum pancreatic lipase immunoreactivity (PLI) in dogs and cats have been developed and validated. The PLI assay is highly species-specific and measures the mass concentration of pancreatic lipase in the serum. Pancreatic lipase is much larger than trypsinogen and is also positively charged. Pancreatic lipase is, thus, repelled from the glomerular membrane and is only very slowly excreted by the kidneys. As a consequence, a larger residual amount of pancreatic lipase remains in the vascular space and the assay is thus less sensitive for EPI. This has recently been demonstrated in a study with 25 dogs with EPI, as the serum cPLI concentrations showed a larger overlap with healthy control dogs than did serum cTLI concentrations.[55] Because PLI assays have been shown to be the superior test for pancreatitis, PLI assays have now been optimized for measurement of normal and increased concentrations and are no longer suited for the measurement of decreased concentrations, as would be seen in patients with EPI.

A fecal assay for the measurement of pancreatic elastase has been developed and is now marketed in Europe. The initial studies showed an acceptable sensitivity and specificity of the assay.[114] However, the estimated positive predictive value was less than 60%.[115] In another study, fecal elastase concentration was shown to be associated with a high number of false positive test results.[116] In this latter study, 6 of 26 dogs with a severely decreased fecal pancreatic elastase concentration were shown to have a normal serum cTLI concentration.[116] It is interesting to note that the dogs with a false positive test result for EPI had a significantly lower serum CCK concentration than did dogs with a true positive test result.[117] This may suggest that patients with chronic small intestinal disease may have fewer neuroendocrine cells in their intestinal mucosa, leading to a decreased stimulation of pancreatic secretion, which may in turn be associated with false positive fecal pancreatic elastase concentrations. A high rate of false positive test results of fecal elastase concentration has also been observed in human patients. Thus, if fecal pancreatic elastase concentration is to be used for the diagnosis of EPI, any positive result must be verified by measurement of a serum cTLI concentration.

Therapy

Digestive enzyme replacement therapy is the mainstay of therapy for EPI.[106,118] Pancreatic enzymes can be replaced by a variety of different options.[119] Dried pancreatic extract from beef or pork pancreas is by far the most common and effective means of pancreatic enzyme replacement. Therapy is started with 1 teaspoon of dried extract per 10 kg body weight and meal. After the patient has responded completely to the therapy, the dose can be slowly decreased until a minimally effective dose has been reached. It is important to note that the content of enzyme activity in the product used may vary from container to container and thus the minimally effective dose may vary slightly over time. Pancreatic enzymes are also available as tablets and capsules but studies in humans and dogs have shown that powder is preferable to other formulations.[119–122] In a recent study, 3 of 25 dogs treated with pancreatic enzyme supplement developed oral bleeding.[123] When this occurs, a coagulation profile should be evaluated to exclude a vitamin K-responsive coagulopathy, which has been reported in a single cat with EPI.[124] In the case of a normal coagulation profile, the dose of pancreatic enzymes should be lowered. Two dogs in the study cited above continued to do well on the lower dose, but in one of the three dogs the clinical signs did return.[123] If a patient refuses to consume the pancreatic powder mixed into their food or in the rare case of a food allergy to the pancreatic powder, fresh raw pancreas from various species can also be used.[119] Beef, pork, sheep, or game pancreas have all been used. Thirty to 90 g (approximately 1–3 ounces) of raw pancreas replace 1 teaspoon of dried pancreatic extract. The pancreas should be divided into portions for one meal each and frozen. The frozen pancreatic tissue maintains its enzymatic activity for long periods of time. Concerns have been raised about the potential threat of infectious contamination of raw frozen pancreas. Theoretically, raw bovine and ovine pancreas carries the risk of BSE transmission and raw porcine pancreas carries the risk of transmission of Aujeszky's disease. However, this risk is more or less academic as dried pancreatic powder would carry exactly the same risk. Game and ovine pancreas can be infested by *Echinococcus* spp. and infestation with this parasite could potentially cause significant disease and even death. These risks should thus be discussed with the owner before initiating therapy. Pre-incubation of the food with the pancreatic extract does not appear to be necessary to achieve a therapeutic response.[120]

Feeding of a low fat diet to EPI patients has been recommended by some authors. However, experimental studies have shown that in dogs treated with pancreatic supplements, fat digestibility does not return to normal, suggesting that fat restriction would increase the risk of deficiencies of fat-soluble vitamins and essential fatty acids.[120] One study did not show any benefit of a fat-restricted diet in dogs with EPI.[108] In addition, two other studies on dogs with EPI did not reveal any significant effect of diet on treatment success.[125,126] As a consequence, the author believes that a high-quality maintenance diet should be used. However, diets with a high fiber content should be avoided as dietary fiber may interfere with fat absorption.

As mentioned above, many patients with EPI are cobalamin deficient and thus every dog and cat with EPI should be evaluated for possible cobalamin deficiency. If cobalamin deficiency is identified, cobalamin supplementation should be added to the management of the patient. Cobalamin is a water-soluble vitamin that must be administered parenterally in deficient patients. The exact dose requirements for dogs and cats are unknown, but over-supplementation with cobalamin is not associated with side effects; thus, relatively high doses of cobalamin are chosen. In cats, a dose of 150–250 µg is given per subcutaneous injection based on the size of the animal. In dogs, a dose of 250–1200 µg SC is given based on the size of the animal. Doses are given weekly for 6 weeks, then every other week for 6 weeks, followed by one more dose after a month and a recheck of serum cobalamin concentration a month later. Most EPI patients that have been treated appropriately will have a normal or even supranormal serum cobalamin concentration at the time of re-evaluation and the cobalamin supplementation can be discontinued.

Serum concentrations of most fat-soluble vitamins have been shown to be decreased in dogs with EPI and can also be assumed to be decreased in cats.[125] However, systematic vitamin supplementation of fat-soluble vitamins has not been investigated in these patients and over-supplementation with these types of vitamins may cause side effects. Anecdotal reports of vitamin E supplementation (400–500 IU PO q 24 h for 1 month) are available, but the beneficial effect of such therapy has not been evaluated.

Many patients with EPI will respond well to enzyme replacement therapy and cobalamin supplementation if indicated. However, a small group of patients does not respond adequately to standard therapy. The potential causes of treatment failure should be evaluated. The type, formulation, and dose of the enzyme supplement should be reviewed and if there is any suspicion that the enzyme replacement may be insufficient, the protocol should be adjusted accordingly. Also, patients should be evaluated for concurrent conditions, such as IBD, diabetes mellitus, or SIBO. Diabetes mellitus can be observed in patients with an underlying chronic pancreatitis as the re-

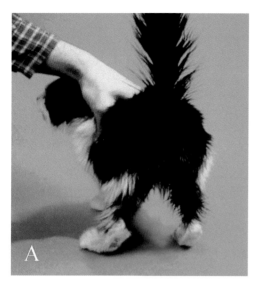
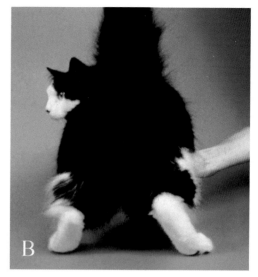

Figure 8.11:
Exocrine pancreatic insufficiency. This picture shows a cat with exocrine pancreatic insufficiency. Panel (A) shows the cat before initiation of therapy. The cat has lost a significant amount of weight and has a poor hair coat. In addition, there is greasy soiling of its hair coat in the perineal region. Panel (B) shows the same cat after treatment with pancreatic enzyme supplementation. (Images courtesy of Dr. David A. Williams, University of Illinois, USA.)

8

sulting atrophy does not spare the pancreatic islet cells. Therapy of the concomitant diabetes mellitus is necessary in such patients.

If there is no evidence of any concurrent disease, a therapeutic trial with an antimicrobial agent can be attempted. It has previously been reported that dogs with EPI commonly also have SIBO and treatment for SIBO is benign.[127] The treatment of choice is tylosin (Tylan powder at 25 mg/kg PO q 12 h for 6 weeks), but other antibiotic agents, such as metronidazole or oxytetracycline can also be used.

If patients still do not respond, antacid therapy can be attempted. A large portion of the orally-administered pancreatic lipase is destroyed by the low pH in the stomach.[128] By increasing the pH in the stomach, this portion may be decreased and the therapeutic response may be improved. However, it also needs to be noted that while an increase in gastric pH will decrease the amount of pancreatic lipase being destroyed during its passage of the stomach, it also will increase the amount of gastric lipase being destroyed and the final result may not lead to a significant change in lipid digestibility. A trial with antacids can be attempted to overcome this problem. H_2 antagonists can initially be tried, but human EPI patients treated with omeprazole showed a superior response over patients treated with H_2 antagonists.[129]

If none of these measures lead to control of the clinical signs, a decrease in the dietary fat may be effective. However, as mentioned above, feeding a low fat diet may be associated with complications and should only be viewed as a last resort.

Prognosis

EPI is usually a life-long condition as pancreatic acinar cells can generally not regenerate. Having said this, there are anecdotal reports of isolated cases of resolving EPI.

Most dogs and cats with EPI can be successfully managed and will have a normal quality of life and a normal life expectancy (Figure 8.11B). A recent study has evaluated the prognostic factors for dogs with EPI.[108] The only factor associated with a poor outcome in this study was the presence of concurrent cobalamin deficiency.[108] As a consequence, the author strongly believes that serum cobalamin concentration should be determined in small animal patients with EPI.

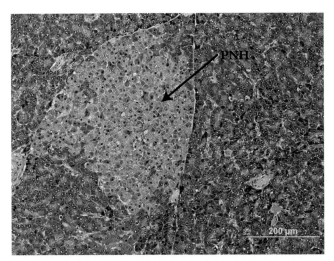

Figure 8.12:
Pancreatic nodular hyperplasia. This figure shows the histopathological appearance of pancreatic nodular hyperplasia (PNH) in a dog. This finding of a proliferation of well-differentiated pancreatic epithelial cells is very common in dogs and cats. In dogs, the presence of pancreatic hyperplastic nodules has been associated with age. (H&E, 20×; image courtesy of Dr. Shelley Newman, University of Tennessee, USA.)

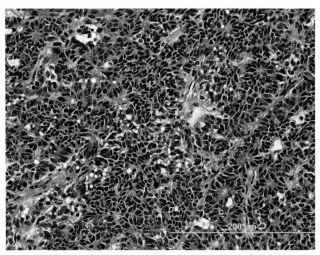

Figure 8.13:
Pancreatic adenocarcinoma. This image shows the histopathological characteristics of an adenocarcinoma in a cat. Please note the disorganized clusters of acinar cells that are characterized by variation in nuclear and cytoplasmic size, prominent nucleoli and occasional mitotic figures. (H&E, 40×; image courtesy of Dr. Shelley Newman, University of Tennessee, USA.)

8

8.3.3   Exocrine pancreatic neoplasia

Neoplastic diseases of the exocrine pancreas can be primary or secondary. Primary neoplastic diseases of the exocrine pancreas can be classified as benign or malignant. Pancreatic adenomas are benign tumors, which are usually singular and can be differentiated from pancreatic nodular hyperplasia (Figure 8.12) by the presence of a capsule. Just as in human beings, pancreatic adenocarcinoma (Figure 8.13) is the most common malignant neoplastic condition of the exocrine pancreas in dogs and cats. But, in contrast to humans, where pancreatic adenocarcinoma is the fourth most common cause of cancer death, it occurs rather infrequently in dogs and cats.[130] Adenocarcinomas are malignant and usually originate from the duct system, but can also originate from acinar tissue.[131] A few cases of pancreatic sarcomas (i.e., spindle cell sarcoma and lymphosarcoma) have also been reported.[131,132] However, it is questionable whether these tumors are primary neoplastic lesions of the exocrine pancreas, metastatic lesions of tumors of other organs, or a localized lesion of a multicentric neoplasia.

Etiology and pathogenesis

As in humans, the etiology of neoplastic conditions of the exocrine pancreas is unknown in dogs and cats. Neoplastic lesions can lead to the transposition of the organs of the cranial abdomen. However, these changes are subclinical in most cases

and the diagnosis is often made as an incidental finding on necropsy examination. In a small number of human patients, the neoplastic growth can actually obstruct the pancreatic duct and cause secondary atrophy of the remaining exocrine pancreas, leading to EPI. Even though such cases have not yet been reported in the cat and have only been anecdotally reported in a single dog, this possibility should be considered and patients presenting with clinical signs compatible with EPI should have their abdomen carefully palpated (Hill S, personal communication, 2007).

In addition to a transposition of abdominal organs, adenocarcinomas can also be associated with tumor necrosis when the tumor outgrows its vascular supply. Tumor necrosis in turn will cause a local inflammatory response, which can lead to the development of clinical signs of pancreatitis. Finally, exocrine pancreatic tumors can also spread to neighboring or distant organs.

Clinical signs and diagnosis

The presentation of canine and feline patients with exocrine pancreatic neoplasia is nonspecific. In a case series of 58 cats, the clinical signs most commonly reported were anorexia (46%), weight loss (37%), lethargy (28%), vomiting (23%), icterus (14%), constipation (9%), and diarrhea (3%).[131] The clinical signs reported in other cases were polyuria, fever, de-

8

hydration, a distended cranial abdomen, and voluminous, pale, soft stools.[132] Polyuria may be a clinical sign of concurrent diabetes mellitus. Obstructive jaundice has also been described in a cat with pancreatic adenocarcinoma.[133] A small number of dogs with multifocal necrotizing steatitis have been described that were ultimately diagnosed with pancreatic adenocarcinoma.[134] Finally, clinical signs related to metastatic lesions have also been reported in some cases of pancreatic adenocarcinoma and may present as lameness, bone pain, or dyspnea. Recently, several cases of paraneoplastic alopecia have been reported in cats with pancreatic adenocarcinoma.[135,136] The reported alopecia consisted of a generalized alopecia of the ventrum, limbs, and face in most cases, with diffuse zones of alopecia in the remaining cats.[135,136]

Neutrophilia, anemia, hypokalemia, bilirubinemia, azotemia, hyperglycemia, and elevations of hepatic enzymes have all been reported in affected patients, but the results of routine blood tests may be unremarkable.[131,132] Elevations of serum hepatic enzyme activities and serum bilirubin concentration are identified most commonly.[137] Hyperglycemia, when present, is related to the concurrent destruction of pancreatic beta cells. Serum activities of lipase and amylase have not been commonly reported in either dogs or cats with pancreatic adenocarcinoma. There are some anecdotal reports indicating that serum lipase activities may be extremely high in dogs with pancreatic adenocarcinoma, but this has not been substantiated in other studies. A single dog with a pancreatic adenocarcinoma and pseudohyperparathyroidism (leading to hypercalcemia) has been described in the literature.[138]

Radiographic findings are also nonspecific in most cases and include a decreased contrast in the cranial abdomen, suggesting peritoneal effusion into this area, transposition of the spleen caudally, and shadowing in the pyloric region.[132] However, in some cases abdominal radiographs can suggest the presence of a mass in the cranial abdomen.[137] Ultrasonographic examination of the abdomen is very helpful and in most cases a soft tissue mass can be identified in the region of the pancreas;[44,137,139] although in many cases, continuation of the mass with pancreatic tissue cannot be conclusively identified.[137] Similarly, neoplastic lesions of the neighboring organs may be falsely presumed to be of pancreatic origin.[44] Also, patients with severe pancreatitis may show an ultrasonographic mass effect in the area of the pancreas that must not be confused with a pancreatic adenocarcinoma.[42,44]

If peritoneal effusion is identified on abdominal ultrasound, a sample should be aspirated and evaluated cytologically. However, in most cases, neoplastic cells do not readily exfoliate into the peritoneal effusion and no neoplastic cells are identified on cytology. Fine needle aspiration or transcutaneous biopsy under ultrasound guidance can be attempted when suspicious masses are identified and has been reported to be successful in approximately 25% of all cases.[137] The low success rate of fine needle aspiration is probably due to the lack of exfoliation of pancreatic adenocarcinoma cells. In other cases, carcinoma cells can be identified but the origin of the cells cannot be determined conclusively.[137] Ultrasound-guided biopsy with histopathological evaluation of biopsy samples has been reported infrequently, but in one study 2 of 2 cases where an ultrasound-guided biopsy of a pancreatic mass was performed a diagnosis of pancreatic adenocarcinoma was made.[137] In 2 of 3 other cases, biopsy of the liver revealed metastatic carcinoma.[137] However, in many cases the diagnosis is made at exploratory laparotomy or even on necropsy examination.

Therapy and prognosis

Pancreatic adenomas are benign and theoretically do not need to be treated unless they cause clinical signs. However, since the final diagnosis of pancreatic adenocarcinoma is often made by way of a surgical biopsy, a partial pancreatectomy should be performed even in cases of suspected pancreatic adenoma. The prognosis in these cases is excellent.

Patients with a pancreatic adenocarcinoma often present at a late stage of the disease. Metastatic disease at the time of diagnosis is common in dogs with this disease and has been reported to occur in 81% of cats.[131,1408] The most common sites of metastatic disease are the liver, abdominal and thoracic lymph nodes, mesentery, intestines, and the lungs; but various other metastatic sites have also been reported.[137] In those few cases where gross metastatic lesions are not identified at the time of diagnosis, surgical resection of the tumor may be attempted, but owners should be forewarned that clean surgical margins are only rarely achieved. Total pancreatectomy and pancreaticoduodenectomy, though theoretically possible, have not been described in dogs and cats with spontaneous disease. However, one report has detailed the management of dogs after experimental total pancreatectomy.[141] Also, extrapolation from human patients suggests a high morbidity and mortality for these procedures. The complicated post-surgical lifelong management of EPI and diabetes mellitus, make total pancreatectomy less than desirable.[142] In human patients, the use of pancreatic surgery for the treatment of pancreatic adenocarcinoma is highly controversial and some surgeons recommend that this procedure only be undertaken by teams that perform at least 50 of these procedures per year. Chemotherapy or radiation therapy have shown little success in human or veterinary patients with pancreatic adenocarcinomas.[142] Overall, the prognosis for dogs and cats with pancreatic adenocarcinoma is grave.[140,142]

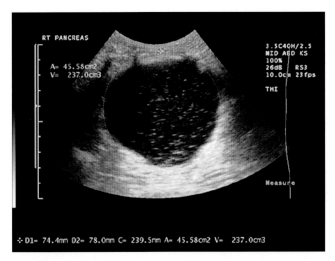

Figure 8.14.
Pancreatic pseudocyst. This image shows the ultrasonographic image of a pancreatic pseudocyst in a dog. The pseudocyst is characterized by a large almost completely anechoic structure that is associated with the pancreas. In this patient, the volume of the pseudocyst was estimated at 237 ml. (Image courtesy of Dr. Kathy Spaulding, Texas A&M University, USA.)

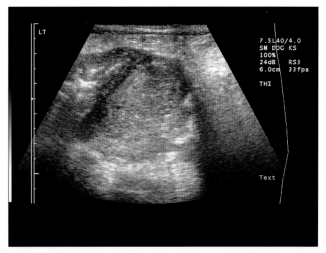

Figure 8.15.
Pancreatic abscess. This image shows the ultrasonographic image of a pancreatic abscess in a dog. The abscess is characterized by a large hypoechoic structure. In most cases, pancreatic abscesses are more echoic than pseudocysts. However, in some cases, an abscess and a pseudocyst cannot be differentiated ultrasonographically. In contrast to humans, pancreatic abscesses in dogs and cats are usually sterile. (Image courtesy of Dr. Kathy Spaulding, Texas A&M University, USA.)

8

8.3.4 Rare diseases of the exocrine pancreas

8.3.4.1 Pancreatic pseudocyst

A pancreatic pseudocyst is a complication of pancreatitis in human beings, but can also occur secondary to pancreatic trauma and pancreatic neoplasia.[14] Recently, several cases of pancreatic pseudocysts in dogs and cats have been described.[143,144] A pancreatic pseudocyst is a collection of sterile pancreatic juice, enclosed by a wall of fibrous or granulation tissue.[14] The clinical signs are usually nonspecific and mimic those of pancreatitis.[145] Vomiting was the most consistent clinical sign in both dogs and cats with a pancreatic pseudocyst. In some cases, a mass could be palpated in the cranial abdomen. On abdominal ultrasound, a cystic structure in close proximity to the pancreas could be identified (Figure 8.14).[145] In most cases described so far, the cystic structure was associated with the left lobe of the pancreas.[143] Aspiration of a pseudocyst is relatively safe and should be attempted for diagnostic and therapeutic purposes.[143] In contrast to the fluid from a pancreatic abscess, the drained fluid from a pancreatic pseudocyst should be of low cellularity. If measured, amylase and lipase activity of the aspirated fluid are usually very high. Pancreatic pseudocysts can be treated medically or surgically.[145] Surgical correction can involve extirpation of the pseudocyst, external drainage, or internal drainage.[146] However, internal drainage is the preferred method of surgical correction and in human patients with a pancreatic pseudocyst

extirpation is only recommended in cases where the pseudocyst is small. Medical management of pancreatic pseudocysts involves ultrasound-guided percutaneous aspiration and close monitoring of the size of the pseudocyst. This approach was successful in several cases described in the literature.[143] However, it seems prudent to consider surgical intervention in cases in which the clinical signs persist or when the size of the pseudocyst does not decrease significantly over time.

8.3.4.2 Pancreatic abscess

A pancreatic abscess is another complication of pancreatitis in human beings.[14] A pancreatic abscess is a circumscribed collection of pus, usually in close proximity to the pancreas, containing little or no pancreatic necrosis.[14] A bacterial infection may or may not be present. Cases of pancreatic abscesses have been described in dogs and in a single cat, and almost all the cases reported have been sterile.[22–24] The clinical signs are nonspecific, but may include vomiting, depression, abdominal pain, anorexia, fever, diarrhea, and dehydration.[145] In some patients, a mass in the cranial abdomen could be identified upon abdominal palpation.[22] Common clinicopathological findings are neutrophilia with a left shift, elevation of serum amylase and lipase activities, elevations of hepatic enzyme activities, and hyperbilirubinemia.[22,23] Abdominal ultrasound shows a hypoechoic structure that can be of variable size and may be irregular (Figure 8.15). Surgical drainage and aggressive antimicrobial therapy are the treatment of choice in human patients with a pancreatic abscess. Dogs and cats may also respond favorably to surgical drainage.[22] However, in one report only 56% of nine patients survived the immediate postsurgical period.[23] Thus, given the mixed results and the risks, difficulties, and expenses associated with anesthesia, surgery, and postoperative care, one should avoid surgical intervention unless there is clear evidence of an enlarging mass and/or sepsis in a patient that is not responding well to medical therapy. Also, based on the lack of identifiable infectious organisms, the need for antimicrobial therapy in small animals is questionable unless an organism can be identified upon bacterial culture. However, more patients will need to be studied before more definitive treatment recommendations for dogs or cats with a pancreatic abscess can be made.

8.3.4.3 Pancreatic parasites

Eurytrema procyonis. *Eurytrema procyonis*, the pancreatic fluke of the cat, can be found in the pancreatic ductular system of foxes, raccoons, and cats.[147] These parasites can lead to a thickening of the pancreatic ductular system and to pancreatic fibrosis. Even though a significant decrease of exocrine pancreatic secretion has been shown to occur, cats presenting with clinical signs of EPI secondary to *E. procyonis* infestation are extremely rare.[101] The diagnosis can be made by the detection of the characteristic eggs in fresh feces. Fenbendazole (30 mg/kg PO q 24 h for 6 consecutive days) has been recommended for therapy.[148]

Amphimerus pseudofelineus. The hepatic fluke of the cat, *A. pseudofelineus* can also infest the pancreas, and can lead to pancreatitis.[26] Diagnosis can be made on fecal examination by formalin-ethyl acetate sedimentation.[149] In one report, treatment with praziquantel (40 mg/kg PO q 24 h for three consecutive days) was successful in the management of an infestation with *A. pseudofelineus*, but concurrent symptomatic therapy for pancreatitis, as outlined above, also needs to be instituted in these cases.[149] The dose of praziquantel recommended for the treatment of this parasite is very high, but is similar to the dose recommended for schistosomiasis in people and praziquantel is considered to have a high therapeutic margin, when administered orally.

8.3.4.4 Pancreatic bladder

A pancreatic bladder, sometimes also referred to as a pancreatic pseudobladder, is an abnormal extension of the pancreatic duct.[150,151] Pancreatic bladders can be congenital or acquired. Only a few cats and no dogs with pancreatic bladders have been described in the literature.[151] These patients were presented with clinical signs compatible with biliary duct obstruction. Appropriate management has not been studied, but surgical removal may be of most benefit in cases presenting with clinical signs.

8.3.4.5 Pancreatolithiasis

Stone formation within the pancreatic duct system (pancreatolithiasis) has recently been reported in a single cat.[151] The cat presented with lethargy, vomiting, diarrhea, hematuria, and weight loss.[151] On abdominal ultrasound, there was a suggestion of the presence of two distinct gallbladders, but during an abdominal exploratory, a pancreatic bladder secondary to the obstruction of the duct system was diagnosed.[151] The stone was surgically removed and the pancreatic bladder was excised.[151] Initially, the patient did well, but after about 1 week the cat deteriorated significantly and was euthanized.[151] Pancreatolithiasis has previously been diagnosed in humans and cattle.

8.3.4.6 Pancreatic nodular hyperplasia

Pancreatic nodular hyperplasia (Figure 8.12) occurs quite frequently in older dogs and cats.[150] In a recent study, 81 of 101 dogs (80.2%) evaluated at necropsy showed nodular hyperplasia in at least one section.[43] The frequency of nodular hyperplasia was correlated with age, but not with pancreatic inflammation, fibrosis, and/or atrophy.[43] Disseminated small nodules can be found throughout the exocrine portion of the pancreas. These lesions may be visible during abdominal ultrasound, but differentiation from pancreatitis and pancreatic adenocarcinoma may be difficult.[44] During necropsy, pancreatic nodular hyperplasia can be differentiated from pancreatic adenomas by the absence of a capsule in cases of nodular hyperplasia.[152] Nodular hyperplasia does not lead to functional changes and does not cause any clinical signs. It is, therefore, most frequently diagnosed incidentally at necropsy examination of older dogs and cats.

Key Facts

- Pancreatitis occurs frequently in both dogs and cats and is the most common disease of the exocrine pancreas in both species.
- Pancreatitis can range in severity and can be subclinical or severe. Severe pancreatitis is associated with both local and systemic complications.
- When stringent criteria are applied abdominal ultrasound is highly specific for pancreatitis.
- Serum PLI concentration (Spec cPL™ in dogs and fPLI in cats) is both highly specific and sensitive for pancreatitis in small animals.
- Treatment of dogs and cats with pancreatitis is dependant on the severity of the disease and may include treatment of the underlying cause, if identified, supportive care, analgesia, antiemetics, nutritional support, plasma, and treatment of concurrent conditions. Also, patients with chronic pancreatitis may benefit from corticosteroid administration.
- Serum TLI concentration (cTLI in the dog and fTLI in the cat) is the diagnostic test of choice for EPI in both dogs and cats.
- Patients with EPI can often be successfully managed with pancreatic enzyme replacement therapy and if necessary, cobalamin supplementation, antibiotic therapy, and in some cases antacids.

8

References

1. Freudiger U. Krankheiten des exokrinen Pankreas bei der Katze. *Berl Münch Tierärztl Wschr* 1989; 102: 37–43.
2. Pandol SJ. Pancreatic physiology and secretory testing. In: Feldman M, Friedman LS, Sleisenger MH (eds.) *Gastrointestinal and liver disease*. Philadelphia, WB Saunders, 2002; 871–880.
3. Fyfe JC. Feline intrinsic factor (IF) is pancreatic in origin and mediates ileal cobalamin (CBL) absorption. *J Vet Intern Med* 1993; 7: 133 (abstract).
4. Carrière F, Laugier R, Barrowman JA et al. Gastric and pancreatic lipase levels during a test meal in dogs. *Scand J Gastroenterol* 1993; 28: 443–454.
5. Steer ML, Perides G. Pathogenesis: how does acute pancreatitis develop. In: Domínguez-Muñoz JE (ed.) *Clinical pancreatology for practicing gastroenterologists and surgeons*. Malden, Blackwell Publishing, 2005; 10–26.
6. Sahin-Tóth M. Biochemical models of hereditary pancreatitis. *Endocrinol Metab Clin North Am* 2006; 35: 303–312.
7. Bishop MA, Xenoulis PG, Suchodolski JS et al. Identification of three mutations in the pancreatic secretory trypsin inhibitor gene of Miniature Schnauzers. *J Vet Intern Med* 2007; 21: 614 (abstract).
8. Williams DA, Steiner JM. Canine pancreatic disease. In: Ettinger SJ, Feldman EC (eds.) *Textbook of Veterinary Internal Medicine*. St. Louis, Elsevier Saunders, 2005; 1482–1488.
9. Hänichen T, Minkus G. Retrospektive Studie zur Pathologie der Erkrankungen des exokrinen Pankreas bei Hund und Katze. *Tierärztliche Umschau* 1990; 45: 363–368.
10. Steiner JM, Newman SJ, Xenoulis PG et al. Comparison of sensitivity of serum markers in dogs with macroscopic evidence of pancreatitis. *J Vet Intern Med* 2007; 21: 614 (abstract).
11. Newman SJ, Steiner JM, Woosley K et al. Localization of pancreatic inflammation and necrosis in dogs. *J Vet Intern Med* 2004; 18: 488–493.
12. Watson PJ, Roulois AJ, Scase T et al. Prevalence and breed distribution of chronic pancreatitis at post-mortem examination in first-opinion dogs. *J Small Anim Pract* 2007; 28: 1–10.
13. DeCock HEV, Forman MA, Farver TB et al. Prevalence and histopathologic characteristics of pancreatitis in cats. *Vet Pathol* 2007; 44: 39–49.
14. Bradley EL. A clinically based classification system for acute pancreatitis. *Arch Surg* 1993; 128: 586–590.
15. Newman SJ, Steiner JM, Woosley K et al. Histologic assessment and grading of the exocrine pancreas in the dog. *J Vet Diagn Invest* 2006; 18: 115–118.
16. Hess RS, Kass PH, Shofer FS et al. Evaluation of risk factors for fatal acute pancreatitis in dogs. *J Am Vet Med Assoc* 1999; 214: 46–51.
17. Yadav D, Pitchumoni CS. Issues in hyperlipidemic pancreatitis. *J Clin Gastroenterol* 2003; 36: 54–62.
18. Xenoulis PG, Suchodolski SJ, Swin E et al. Correlation of serum triglyceride and canine pancreatic lipase immunoreactivity (cPLI) concentrations in Miniature Schnauzers. *J Vet Intern Med* 2006; 20: 750–751 (abstract).
19. DiMagno EP, Chari S. Acute pancreatitis. In: Feldman M, Friedman LS, Sleisenger MH (eds.) *Gastrointestinal and liver disease*. Philadelphia, WB Saunders, 2002; 913–941.
20. Matthiesen DT, Mullen HS. Problems and complications associated with endocrine surgery in the dog and cat. *Problems in Veterinary Medicine* 1990; 2: 627–667.
21. Westermarck E, Saario E. Traumatic pancreatic injury in a cat – a case history. *Acta Vet Scand* 1989; 30: 359–362.
22. Salisbury SK, Lantz GC, Nelson RW et al. Pancreatic abscess in dogs: Six cases (1978–1986). *J Am Vet Med Assoc* 1988; 193: 1104–1108.
23. Stimson EL, Espada Y, Moon M et al. Pancreatic abscess in nine dogs. *J Vet Intern Med* 1998; 9: 202 (abstract).
24. Simpson KW, Shiroma JT, Biller DS et al. Ante mortem diagnosis of pancreatitis in four cats. *J Small Anim Pract* 1994; 35: 93–99.
25. Dubey JP, Carpenter JL. Histologically confirmed clinical toxoplasmosis in cats: 100 cases (1952–1990). *J Am Vet Med Assoc* 1993; 203: 1556–1566.
26. Rothenbacher H, Lindquist WD. Liver cirrhosis and pancreatitis in a cat infected with *Amphimerus pseudofelineus*. *J Am Vet Med Assoc* 1963; 143: 1099–1102.
27. Möhr AJ, Lobetti RG, Van der Lugt JJ. Acute pancreatitis: a newly recognised potential complication of canine babesiosis. *J S Afr Vet Assoc* 2000; 71: 232–239.
28. Frick TW, Speiser DE, Bimmler D et al. Drug-induced acute pancreatitis: Further criticism. *Dig Dis* 1993; 11: 113–132.
29. Badalov N, Baradarian R, Iswara K et al. Drug-induced acute pancreatitis: an evidence-based review. *Clin Gastroenterol Hepatol* 2007; 5: 648–661.

8

30. Aste G, Di Tommaso M, Steiner JM et al. Pancreatitis associated with N-methyl-glucamine therapy in a dog with leishmaniasis. *Vet Res Commun* 2005; 29 Suppl 2: 269–272.

31. Hill RC, Van Winkle TJ. Acute necrotizing pancreatitis and acute suppurative pancreatitis in the cat. A retrospective study of 40 cases (1976–1989). *J Vet Intern Med* 1993; 7: 25–33.

32. Simpson KW. Current concepts of the pathogenesis and pathophysiology of acute pancreatitis in the dog and cat. *Comp Cont Ed Prac Vet* 1993; 15: 247–253.

33. Norman J. The role of cytokines in the pathogenesis of acute pancreatitis. *Am J Surg* 1998; 175: 76–83.

34. Ryan CP, Howard EB. Systemic lipodystrophy associated with pancreatitis in a cat. *Feline Pract* 1981; 11: 31–34.

35. Hess RS, Saunders HM, Van Winkle TJ et al. Clinical, clinicopathologic, radiographic, and ultrasonographic abnormalities in dogs with fatal acute pancreatitis: 70 cases (1986–1995). *J Am Vet Med Assoc* 1998; 213: 665–670.

36. Washabau RJ. Acute necrotizing pancreatitis. In: August JR (ed.) *Consultations in feline internal medicine.* St. Louis, Elsevier Saunders, 2006; 109–119.

37. Suter PF, Olsson SE. Traumatic hemorrhagic pancreatitis in the cat: A report with emphasis on the radiological diagnosis. *J Am Vet Radiol Soc* 1969; 10: 4–11.

38. Etue SM, Penninck DG, Labato MA et al. Ultrasonography of the normal feline pancreas and associated anatomic landmarks: a prospective study of 20 cats. *Vet Radiol Ultrasound* 2001; 42: 330–336.

39. Lamb CR. Pancreatic edema in dogs with hypoalbuminemia or portal hypertension. *J Vet Intern Med* 1999; 13: 498–500.

40. Saunders HM, Van Winkle TJ, Drobatz K et al. Ultrasonographic findings in cats with clinical, gross pathologic, and histologic evidence of acute pancreatic necrosis: 20 cases (1994–2001). *J Am Vet Med Assoc* 2002; 221: 1724–1730.

41. Forman MA, Marks SL, De Cock HEV et al. Evaluation of serum feline pancreatic lipase immunoreactivity and helical computed tomography versus conventional testing for the diagnosis of feline pancreatitis. *J Vet Intern Med* 2004; 18: 807–815.

42. Saunders HM. Ultrasonography of the pancreas. *Problems in Veterinary Medicine* 1991; 3: 583–603.

43. Newman SJ, Steiner JM, Woosley K et al. Correlation of age and incidence of pancreatic exocrine nodular hyperplasia in the dog. *Vet Pathol* 2005; 42: 510–513.

44. Hecht S, Penninck DG, Keating JH. Imaging findings in pancreatic neoplasia and nodular hyperplasia in 19 cats. *Vet Radiol Ultrasound* 2007; 48: 45–50.

45. Swift NC, Marks SL, MacLachlan NJ et al. Evaluation of serum feline trypsin-like immunoreactivity for the diagnosis of pancreatitis in cats. *J Am Vet Med Assoc* 2000; 217: 37–42.

46. Gerhardt A, Steiner JM, Williams DA et al. Comparison of the sensitivity of different diagnostic tests for pancreatitis in cats. *J Vet Intern Med* 2001; 15: 329–333.

47. Turner MA. The role of US and CT in pancreatitis. *Gastrointest Endosc* 2002; 56: S241-S245.

48. Spillmann T, Litzlbauer HD, Moritz A et al. Computed tomography and laparoscopy for the diagnosis of pancreatic diseases in dogs. *Proc 18th ACVIM Forum* 2000; 485–487.

49. Jaeger JQ, Mattoon JS, Bateman SW et al. Combined use of ultrasonography and contrast enhanced computed tomography to evaluate acute necrotizing pancreatitis in two dogs. *Vet Radiol Ultrasound* 2003; 44: 72–79.

50. Mansfield CS, Jones BR. Trypsinogen activation peptide in the diagnosis of canine pancreatitis. *J Vet Intern Med* 2000; 14: 346 (abstract).

51. Steiner JM, Broussard J, Mansfield CS et al. Serum canine pancreatic lipase immunoreactivity (cPLI) concentrations in dogs with spontaneous pancreatitis. *J Vet Intern Med* 2001; 15: 274 (abstract).

52. Steiner JM, Teague SR, Williams DA. Development and analytic validation of an enzyme-linked immunosorbent assay for the measurement of canine pancreatic lipase immunoreactivity in serum. *Can J Vet Res* 2003; 67: 175–182.

53. Steiner JM, Wilson BG, Williams DA. Development and analytical validation of a radioimmunoassay for the measurement of feline pancreatic lipase immunoreactivity in serum. *Can J Vet Res* 2004; 68: 309–314.

54. Steiner JM, Berridge BR, Wojcieszyn J et al. Cellular immunolocalization of gastric and pancreatic lipase in various tissues obtained from dogs. *Am J Vet Res* 2002; 63: 722–727.

55. Steiner JM, Rutz GM, Williams DA. Serum lipase activities and pancreatic lipase immunoreactivity concentrations in dogs with exocrine pancreatic insufficiency. *Am J Vet Res* 2006; 67: 84–87.

56. Nathens AB, Curtis JR, Beale RJ et al. Management of the critically ill patient with severe acute pancreatitis. *Crit Care Med* 2004; 32: 2524–2536.

57. Heinrich S, Schäfer M, Rousson V et al. Evidence-based treatment of acute pancreatitis – A look at established paradigms. *Ann Surg* 2006; 243: 154–168.

58. Kingsnorth A, O'Reilly D. Acute pancreatitis. *Br Med J* 2006; 332: 1072–1076.

59. Freeman LM, Labato MA, Rush JE et al. Nutritional support in pancreatitis: a retrospective study. *J Vet Emergency and Critical Care* 1995; 5:32–40.

60. Hansen B. Analgesics in cardiac, surgical, and intensive care patients. In: Kirk RW, Bonagura JD (eds.) *Current Veterinary Therapy XI.* Philadelphia, WB Saunders, 1992; 82–87.

61. De la Puente-Redondo VA, Tilt N, Rowan TG et al. Efficacy of maropitant for treatment and prevention of emesis caused by intravenous infusion of cisplatin in dogs. *Amer J Vet Res* 2007; 68: 48–56.

62. Balldin G, Ohlsson K. Trasylol prevents trypsin-induced shock in dogs. *Hoppe-Seylers Z Physiol Chem* 1979; 360: 651–656.

63. Satoh H, Harada M, Tashiro S et al. The effect of continuous arterial infusion of gabexate mesilate (FOY-007) on experimental acute pancreatitis. *J Med Invest* 2004; 51: 186–193.

64. Imrie CW, Benjamin IS, Ferguson JC. A single center double-blind trial of Trasylol therapy in primary acute pancreatitis. *Br J Surg* 1978; 65: 337–341.

65. Kitagawa M, Hayakawa T. Antiproteases in the treatment of acute pancreatitis. *JOP* 2007; 8: 518–525.

66. Logan JC, Callan MB, Drew K et al. Clinical indications for use of fresh frozen plasma in dogs: 74 dogs (October through December 1999). *J Am Vet Med Assoc* 2001; 218: 1449–1455.

67. Leese T, Holliday M, Heath D et al. Multicentre clinical trial of low volume fresh frozen plasma therapy in acute pancreatitis. *Br J Surg* 1987; 74: 907–911.

68. Leese T, Holliday M, Watkins M et al. A multicentre controlled clinical trial of high-volume fresh frozen plasma therapy in prognostically severe acute pancreatitis. *Annals of the Royal College of Surgeons of England* 1991; 73: 207–214.

69. Bourgaux JF, Defez C, Muller L et al. Infectious complications, prognostic factors and assessment of anti-infectious management of 212 consecutive patients with acute pancreatitis. *Gastroent Clin Biol* 2007; 31: 431–435.

70. Howes R, Zuidema GD, Cameron JL. Evaluation of prophylactic antibiotics in acute pancreatitis. *J Surg Res* 1975; 18: 197–200.

71. Lankisch PG, Lerch MM. The role of antibiotic prophylaxis in the treatment of acute pancreatitis. *J Clin Gastroenterol* 2006; 40: 149–155.

72. Isenmann R, Büchler MW, Friess H et al. Antibiotics in acute pancreatitis. *Dig Surg* 1996; 13: 365–369.

73. Mazaki T, Ishii Y, Takayama T. Meta-analysis of prophylactic antibiotic use in acute necrotizing pancreatitis. *Br J Surg* 2006; 93: 674–684.

74. Dellinger EP, Tellado JM, Soto NE et al. Early antibiotic treatment for severe acute necrotizing pancreatitis – A randomized, double-blind, placebo-controlled study. *Ann Surg* 2007; 245: 674–683.

75. Zhou YM, Xue ZL, Li YM et al. Antibiotic prophylaxis in patients with severe acute pancreatitis. *Hepatobiliary Pancreat Dis Int* 2005; 4: 23–27.

76. Johnson CD, Charnley R, Rowlands B et al. UK guidelines for the management of acute pancreatitis. *Gut* 2005; 54: 1–9.

77. Cook AK, Breitschwerdt EB, Levine JF et al. Risk factors associated with acute pancreatitis in dogs: 101 cases (1985–1990). *J Am Vet Med Assoc* 1993; 203: 673–679.

78. Pezzilli R, Fantini L. Diagnosis of autoimmune pancreatitis: clinical and histological assessment. *JOP* 2005; 6: 609–611.

79. Toomey DP, Swan N, Torreggiani W et al. Autoimmune pancreatitis. *Br J Surg* 2007; 94: 1067–1074.

80. Weiss DJ, Gagne JM, Armstrong PJ. Relationship between inflammatory hepatic disease and inflammatory bowel disease, pancreatitis, and nephritis in cats. *J Am Vet Med Assoc* 1996; 209: 1114–1116.

81. Sakai M, Harada K, Matsumura H et al. A case of feline pancreatitis. *J Vet Med Sci* 2006; 68: 1331–1333.

82. Karanjia ND, Lutrin FJ, Chang Y-B et al. Low dose dopamine protects against hemorrhagic pancreatitis in cats. *J Surg Res* 1990; 48: 440–443.

83. Sweiry JH, Mann GE. Role of oxidative stress in the pathogenesis of acute pancreatitis. *Scand J Gastroenterol* 1996; 31: 10–15.

84. Kraft W, Kaimaz A, Kirsch M et al. Behandlung akuter Pankreatiden des Hundes mit Selen. *Kleintierpraxis* 1995; 40: 35–43.

85. Braganza JM, Scott P, Bilton D et al. Evidence for early oxidative stress in acute pancreatitis. Clues for correction. *Inter J Pancreatology* 1995; 17: 69–81.

86. Kuklinski B. Akute Pankreatitis – eine "free radical disease". Letalitätssenkung durch Natriumselenit (Na2SeO3) –Therapie. *Zeitschrift für die gesamte Innere Medizin* 1992; 47: 165–167.

87. Virlos IT, Mason J, Schofield D et al. Intravenous n-acetylcysteine, ascorbic acid and selenium-based anti-oxidant therapy in severe acute pancreatitis. *Scand J Gastroenterol* 2003; 38: 1262–1267.

88. McCloy R. Chronic pancreatitis at Manchester, UK – Focus on antioxidant therapy. *Digestion* 1998; 59: 36–48.

89. McKay CJ, Curran F, Sharples C et al. Prospective placebo-controlled randomized trial of lexipafant in predicted severe acute pancreatitis. *Br J Surg* 1997; 84: 1239–1243.

90. Kingsnorth AN, Galloway SW, Formela LJ. Randomized, double-blind phase II trial of lexipafant, a platelet-activating factor antagonist, in human acute pancreatitis. *Br J Surg* 1995; 82: 1414–1420.

91. Abu-Zidan FM, Winsor JA. Lexipafant and acute pancreatitis: a critical appraisal of the clinical trials. *Eur J Surg* 2002; 168: 215–219.

92. Hartwig W, Werner J, Muller CA et al. Surgical management of severe pancreatitis including sterile necrosis. *J Hepatobiliary Pancreat Surg* 2002; 9: 429–435.

93. Büchler MW, Gloor B, Müller CA et al. Acute necrotizing pancreatitis: Treatment strategy according to the status of infection. *Ann Surg* 2000; 232: 619–626.

94. Ruaux CG, Atwell RB. A severity score for spontaneous canine acute pancreatitis. *Aust Vet J* 1998; 76: 804–808.

95. Domínguez-Muñoz JE. Early prognostic evaluation of acute pancreatitis: why and how should severity be predicted. In: Domínguez-Muñoz JE (ed.) *Clinical pancreatology for practicing gastroenterologists and surgeons*. Malden, Blackwell Publishing, 2005; 47–55.

96. Khwannimit B. A comparison of three organ dysfunction scores: MODS, SOFA and LOD for predicting ICU mortality in critically ill patients. *J Med Assoc Thai* 2007; 90: 1074–1081.

97. Banks PA. Medical management of acute pancreatitis and complications. In: Go VLW, DiMagno EP, Gardner JD et al. (eds.) *The pancreas: biology, pathobiology and disease*. New York, Raven Press, 1993; 593–613.

98. Kimmel SE, Washabau RJ, Drobatz KJ. Incidence and prognostic value of low plasma ionized calcium concentration in cats with acute pancreatitis: 46 cases (1996–1998). *J Am Vet Med Assoc* 2001; 219: 1105–1109.

99. Figarella C, De Caro A, Leupold D et al. Congenital pancreatic lipase deficiency. *J Pediatr* 1980; 96: 412–416.

100. Xenoulis PG, Fradkin JM, Rapp SW et al. Suspected isolated pancreatic lipase deficiency in a dog. *J Vet Intern Med* 2007; 21: 1113–1116.

101. Fox JN, Mosley JG, Vogler GA et al. Pancreatic function in domestic cats with pancreatic fluke infection. *J Am Vet Med Assoc* 1981; 178: 58–60.

102. Proschowsky HF, Fredholm M. Exocrine pancreatic insufficiency in the Eurasian dog breed – inheritance and exclusion of two candidate genes. *Anim Genet* 2007; 38: 171–173.

103. Moeller EM, Steiner JM, Clark LA et al. Inheritance of pancreatic acinar atrophy in German Shepherd dogs. *Am J Vet Res* 2002; 63: 1429–1434.

104. Wiberg ME, Saari SAM, Westermarck E. Exocrine pancreatic atrophy in German Shepherd dogs and Rough-coated Collies: An end result of lymphocytic pancreatitis. *Vet Pathol* 1999; 36: 530–541.

105. Westermarck E, Batt RM, Vaillant C et al. Sequential study of pancreatic structure and function during development of pancreatic acinar atrophy in a German Shepherd Dog. *Am J Vet Res* 1993; 54: 1088–1094.

106. Westermarck E, Wiberg M, Steiner JM et al. Exocrine pancreatic insufficiency in dogs and cats. In: Ettinger SJ, Feldman EC (eds.) *Textbook of Veterinary Internal Medicine*. St. Louis, Elsevier Saunders, 2005; 1492–1495.

107. DiMagno EP, Go VLW, Summerskill WHJ. Relations between pancreatic enzyme outputs and malabsorption in severe pancreatic insufficiency. *N Engl J Med* 1973; 288: 813–815.

108. Batchelor DJ, Noble PJ, Taylor RH et al. Prognostic factors in canine exocrine pancreatic insufficiency: prolonged survival is likely if clinical remission is achieved. *J Vet Intern Med* 2007; 21: 54–60.

109. Steiner JM, Williams DA. Serum feline trypsin-like immunoreactivity in cats with exocrine pancreatic insufficiency. *J Vet Intern Med* 2000; 14: 627–629.

110. Wiberg ME, Westermarck E. Subclinical exocrine pancreatic insufficiency in dogs. *J Am Vet Med Assoc* 2002; 220: 1183–1187.

111. Westermarck E, Wiberg M. Exocrine pancreatic insufficiency in dogs. *Vet Clin North Am Small Anim Pract* 2003; 33: 1165–1179.

112. Williams DA, Reed SD. Comparison of methods for assay of fecal proteolytic activity. *Vet Clin Path* 1990; 19: 20–24.

113. Williams DA, Batt RM. Sensitivity and specificity of radioimmunoassay of serum trypsin-like immunoreactivity for the diagnosis of canine exocrine pancreatic insufficiency. *J Am Vet Med Assoc* 1988; 192: 195–201.

114. Spillmann T, Wittker A, Teigelkamp S et al. An immunoassay for canine pancreatic elastase 1 as an indicator for exocrine pancreatic insufficiency in dogs. *J Vet Diagn Invest* 2001; 13: 468–474.

115. Spillmann T, Eigenbrodt E, Sziegoleit A. Die Bestimmung und klinische Relevanz der fäkalen pankreatischen Elastase beim Hund. *Tierärztliche Praxis* 1998; 26: 364–368.

8

8

116. Steiner JM, Pantchev N. False positive results of measurement of fecal elastase concentration for the diagnosis of exocrine pancreatic insufficiency in dogs. *J Vet Intern Med* 2006; 20: 751 (abstract).

117. Steiner JM, Rehfeld JF, Pantchev N. Serum CCK concentrations in dogs with severely decreased fecal elastase concentrations. *J Vet Intern Med* 2006; 20: 1520 (abstract).

118. Wiberg ME, Lautala HM, Westermarck E. Response to long-term enzyme replacement treatment in dogs with exocrine pancreatic insufficiency. *J Am Vet Med Assoc* 1998; 213: 86–90.

119. Westermarck E. Treatment of pancreatic degenerative atrophy with raw pancreas homogenate and various enzyme preparations. *J Vet Med A* 1987; 34:728–733.

120. Pidgeon G, Strombeck DR. Evaluation of treatment for pancreatic exocrine insufficiency in dogs with ligated pancreatic ducts. *Am J Vet Res* 1982; 43: 461–464.

121. Somogyi L, Toskes PP. Conventional pancreatic enzymes are more efficient than enteric-coated enzymes in delivering trypsin to the duodenum of chronic pancreatitis patients. *Gastroenterol.* 1998; 114: A500 (abstract).

122. Marvola M, Heinamaki J, Westermarck E et al. The fate of single-unit enteric-coated drug products in the stomach of the dog. *Acta Pharm Fenn* 1986; 95: 59–70.

123. Rutz GM, Steiner JM, Williams DA. Oral bleeding associated with pancreatic enzyme supplementation in three dogs with exocrine pancreatic insufficiency. *J Am Vet Med Assoc* 2002; 221: 1716–1718.

124. Perry LA, Williams DA, Pidgeon G et al. Exocrine pancreatic insufficiency with associated coagulopathy in a cat. *J Am Anim Hosp Assoc* 1991; 27: 109–114.

125. Rutz GM, Steiner JM, Bauer JE et al. Effects of exchange of dietary medium chain triglycerides for long-chain triglycerides on serum biochemical variables and subjectively assessed well-being of dogs with exocrine pancreatic insufficiency. *Am J Vet Res* 2004; 65: 1293–1302.

126. Westermarck E, Junttila J, Wiberg M. The role of low dietary fat in the treatment of dogs with exocrine pancreatic insufficiency. *Am J Vet Res* 1995; 56: 600–605.

127. Westermarck E, Myllys V, Aho M. Intestinal bacterial overgrowth in dogs with exocrine pancreatic insufficiency: Effect of enzyme replacement and antibiotic therapy. *J Vet Intern Med* 1991; 5: 131 (abstract).

128. DiMagno EP. Medical treatment of pancreatic insufficiency. *Mayo Clin Proc* 1979; 54: 435–442.

129. Proesmans M, De Boeck K. Omeprazole, a proton pump inhibitor, improves residual steatorrhoea in cystic fibrosis patients treated with high dose pancreatic enzymes. *Eur J Pediatr* 2003; 162: 760–763.

130. Lockhart AC, Rothenberg ML, Berlin JD. Treatment for pancreatic cancer: Current therapy and continued progress. *Gastroenterology* 2005; 128: 1642–1654.

131. Andrews LK. Tumors of the exocrine pancreas. In: Holzworth J (ed.) *Diseases of the cat.* Philadelphia, WB Saunders, 1987; 505–507.

132. Münster M, Reusch C. Tumoren des exokrinen Pankreas der Katze. *Tierärztl Prax* 1988; 16: 317–320.

133. Larsson MHMA, Dagli MLZ, Xavier JG et al. Obstructive jaundice caused by a metastatic adenocarcinoma of the pancreas in a cat. *Ars Veterinaria* 1989; 5: 113–116.

134. Brown PJ, Mason KV, Merrett DJ et al. Multifocal necrotising steatitis associated with pancreatic carcinoma in three dogs. *J Small Anim Pract* 1994; 35: 129–132.

135. Brooks DG, Campbell KL, Dennis JS et al. Pancreatic paraneoplastic alopecia in three cats. *J Am Anim Hosp Assoc* 1994; 30: 557–563.

136. Godfrey DR. A case of feline paraneoplastic alopecia with secondary *Malassezia*-associated dermatitis. *J Small Anim Pract* 1998; 39: 394–396.

137. Bennett PF, Hahn KA, Toal RL et al. Ultrasonographic and cytopathological diagnosis of exocrine pancreatic carcinoma in the dog and cat. *J Am Anim Hosp Assoc* 2001; 37: 466–473.

138. Zenoble RD, Crowell WA, Rowland GN. Adenocarcinoma and hypercalcemia in a dog. *Vet Pathol* 1979; 16: 122–123.

139. Lamb CR, Simpson KW, Boswood A et al. Ultrasonography of pancreatic neoplasia in the dog: A retrospective review of 16 cases. *Vet Rec* 1995; 137: 65–68.

140. Seaman RL. Exocrine pancreatic neoplasia in the cat: A case series. *J Am Anim Hosp Assoc* 2004; 40: 238–245.

141. Eloy R, Bouchet P, Clendinnen G et al. New technique of total pancreatectomy without duodenectomy in the dog. *Am J Surg* 1980; 140: 409–412.

142. Withrow SJ. Exocrine cancer of the pancreas. In: Withrow SJ, MacEwen EG (eds.) *Small Animal Clinical Oncology.* Philadelphia, WB Saunders, 2001; 321–323.

143. VanEnkevort BA, O'Brien RT, Young KM. Pancreatic pseudocysts in 4 dogs and 2 cats: Ultrasonographic and clinicopathologic findings. *J Vet Intern Med* 1999; 13: 309–313.

144. Hines BL, Salisbury SK, Jakovljevic S et al. Pancreatic pseudocyst associated with chronic-active necrotizing pancreatitis in a cat. *J Am Anim Hosp Assoc* 1996; 32: 147–152.

145. Coleman M, Robson M. Pancreatic masses following pancreatitis: Pancreatic pseudocysts, necrosis, and abscesses. *Compend Contin Educ Pract Vet* 2005; 27: 147–154.

146. Ephgrave K, Hunt JL. Presentation of pancreatic pseudocysts: implications for timing of surgical intervention. *Am J Surg* 1986; 151: 749–753.

147. Sheldon WG. Pancreatic flukes *(Eurytrema procyonis)* in domestic cats. *J Am Vet Med Assoc* 1966; 148: 251–253.

148. Roudebush P, Schmidt DA. Fenbendazole for treatment of pancreatic fluke infection in a cat. *J Am Vet Med Assoc* 1982; 180: 545–546.

149. Lewis DT, Malone JB, Taboada J et al. Cholangiohepatitis and choledochectasia associated with *Amphimerus pseudofelineus* in a cat. *J Am Anim Hosp Assoc* 1991; 27: 156–161.

150. Boyden EA. The problem of the pancreatic bladder. *Am J Anat* 1925; 36: 151–183.

151. Bailiff NL, Norris CR, Seguin B et al. Pancreatolithiasis and pancreatic pseudobladder associated with pancreatitis in a cat. *J Am Anim Hosp Assoc* 2004; 40: 69–74.

152. Jubb KVF. The Pancreas. In: Jubb KVF, Kennedy PC, Palmer N (eds.) *Pathology of Domestic Animals.* San Diego, Academic Press Inc., 1993; 407–424.

9 Diseases that affect more than one Organ of the Gastrointestinal Tract

9.1 Adverse Reactions to Food – Allergy versus Intolerance

ALBERT E. JERGENS, ELIZABETH R. MAY

9.1.1 Introduction

Adverse food reactions are recognized as being potential causes of various gastrointestinal and dermatological signs in dogs and cats. The true prevalence of these disorders is unknown. Accurate recognition of food-related reactions is required to avoid misdiagnosis and improper treatment of other primary gastrointestinal diseases, such as IBD. This chapter will provide a practical overview of the etiopathogenesis, clinical signs, diagnosis, management, and prognosis of adverse food reactions in companion animals.

9.1.2 Terminology

Adverse food reactions can be divided into two categories based on their etiology: immunological and non-immunological reactions (Figure 9.1).[1,2] Food allergy implies an immunological reaction following food intake. In contrast, food intolerance denotes non-immunological reactions to a food or food additive. Food idiosyncrasy, food toxicity, food poisoning, anaphylactic, pharmacological, and metabolic food reactions are all forms of food intolerance, which can be encountered clinically (Table 9.1). In a practical sense, food allergy and food intolerance may be associated with similar inciting food ingredients, clinical signs, diagnostic findings, and treatments, and may not be easily distinguishable.

9.1.3 Etiopathogenesis of food allergy

Both the intestinal mucosal barrier and the phenomenon of oral tolerance work synergistically to minimize the risk of food hypersensitivity reactions. The mucosal barrier consists of interrelated immunological and non-immunological components, which 1) block the penetration of ingested antigens (via an intact epithelial barrier, normal peristalsis, and a mucus glycocalyx coat); 2) promote the degradation of ingested antigens (via gastric acid, pancreatic enzymes, and brush border enzymes); and 3) facilitate antigen exclusion from the mucosa

(via antigen-specific secretory IgA [sIgA] in the gut lumen). Oral tolerance is defined as the specific local and systemic immunological unresponsiveness to an orally administered antigen.[3] This suppressor function is derived through the generation of antigen-specific regulatory T-lymphocytes (cellular immunity) and sIgA (humoral immunity), which is secreted onto the mucosal surface. Impairment of these mucosal defense mechanisms predisposes patients to food allergy.

The immunological mechanisms responsible for food allergy have not been fully elucidated but are likely to involve Type I (IgE-mediated) hypersensitivity responses. Without the development of oral tolerance to dietary antigens, an animal will develop a local IgE response towards that dietary antigen and

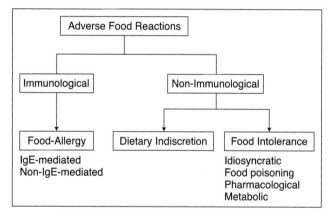

Figure 9.1:
Adverse food reactions. This figure shows the different types of adverse food reactions seen in veterinary patients.

Table 9.1: Types of adverse food reactions

Type of intolerance	Response
Food idiosyncrasy	Abnormal host response to a food substance or additive. Example is a reaction to food additives.
Food intoxication / poisoning	Abnormal host response to organisms contained in food or the presence of food toxins. Examples include aflatoxicosis and botulism.
Anaphylactic food reaction	Mimics real anaphylaxis, but is not mediated by immunological release of chemical mediators.
Metabolic food reaction	Affects metabolism of the host after food intake. Example is lactose (disaccharidase) intolerance.
Pharmacological food reaction	Drug-like effect of a food substance on the host. Example is chocolate toxicosis.

9

will become sensitized to it. Upon subsequent exposure to the sensitizing antigen, mast cell degranulation occurs, which in turn triggers the release of inflammatory mediators (e.g., pro-inflammatory cytokines) causing intestinal inflammation. These Type I responses occur within a few minutes to several hours after ingesting the offending antigen. More systemic (e.g., dermatological) reactions can occur when the antigen escapes from the gut and reaches sensitized basophils or IgE-bound mast cells in the skin. It has been suggested that non-IgE-mediated food hypersensitivity may also occur in dogs and cats.[4]

9.1.4　Food allergies

The specific dietary proteins a patient can develop an allergy towards have been poorly documented. In human beings with food allergy, food allergens are almost exclusively glycoproteins of a molecular mass range of 10–70 kDa.[5] There is no data defining the exact molecular mass of food allergens in dogs or cats. Factors such as stability and immunogenicity of the protein are likely to play an important role in defining the allergenicity of different dietary components. For example, allergens maintain their stability to a varying degree when treated with heat, acid, or proteases.[6] Furthermore, allergenicity can be influenced by food processing where protein denaturation destroys some epitopes (antigenic determinates) or exposes new ones, with a decrease or increase in allergenicity, respectively.[7]

Due to the large number of food proteins in commercial pet foods, it is difficult to identify specific food allergens. A meta-analysis of twelve different studies comprising 265 dogs, showed that two-thirds of the dogs, which developed dermatological lesions associated with adverse food reactions, were fed beef, dairy products, or wheat.[8] Adverse reactions to chicken, chicken eggs, lamb, or soy accounted for approximately 25% of the reported food allergies in dogs. Another study in dogs with food allergy showed that IgG was the single dominant antigen in cow's milk, beef, and lamb.[9] Rarely, dogs show adverse reactions to corn, pork, rice, or fish. Finally, in separate feline studies, it was shown that 80% of adverse food reactions (e.g., cutaneous lesions or GI signs) in cats were associated with diets containing beef, dairy products, or fish.[8]

Whether animals most commonly develop single or multiple food hypersensitivities has not been clearly established. According to Walton et al., multiple hypersensitivities are uncommon in dogs and cats.[10] In contrast, Harvey and Patterson showed that 35–48% of dogs with food hypersensitivity were allergic to more than one food component.[11,12] Similarly, Guilford et al. showed that 50% of cats with chronic gastrointestinal signs had food hypersensitivities towards multiple food allergens.[13] Cross-reactivity among food allergens has not been extensively investigated, but appears to be unlikely.

Clinical signs in dogs and cats

Canine or feline dietary hypersensitivity may manifest clinically as dermatological and/or GI signs. Surprisingly, dermatological rather than GI signs in response to food allergy appear to predominate in both species.

Food allergy in dogs

Food hypersensitivity reactions are responsible for approximately 1% of all skin diseases in dogs.[14] Food allergy is reported to be the third most common skin allergy after flea allergy and atopic dermatitis. There does not appear to be an age, gender, or breed predisposition. One-third of cases occur in young dogs less than one year of age. Some authors report that a contact time with the sensitizing food allergen must occur for 1–2 years before the first signs appear.[6] Dermatological manifestations typically occur as non-seasonal pruritic dermatitis, occasionally accompanied by GI signs. The pruritus varies in severity, but is often intense. Lesion distribution is similar to that seen with atopic dermatitis, where the face, feet, axillae, perineal region, rump, and ears are often affected (Figures 9.2, 9.3, and 9.4). Twenty to thirty percent of dogs with food allergy may have concurrent allergic disease, such as flea allergy or atopic dermatitis.[15] In some patients, otitis externa may be the only presenting complaint in dogs with food allergy. The GI manifestations of food allergy may include vomiting, diarrhea, weight loss, and abdominal discomfort.[4,6,15]

Food allergy in cats

As in dogs, food allergy is responsible for approximately one percent of all skin diseases in cats and represents a common cause for allergic dermatitis along with flea-allergy dermatitis.[14,16] Age and gender predispositions have not been reported. However, Siamese and Siamese-cross breed cats may be at an increased risk since they account for nearly one-third of all cases. Dermatological signs include 1) severe generalized pruritus without lesions; 2) miliary dermatitis; or 3) pruritus with self-trauma around the head, neck, and ears. Otitis externa may occur alone or in combination with other dermatological lesions. Gastrointestinal signs, such as vomiting or diarrhea are present in 10–15 percent of cases.[14]

Other disorders

Food-related immunological responses may contribute to the pathogenesis of several different enteropathies in the dog and cat (Table 9.2). In contrast to food allergy, these conditions are only associated with the GI tract in affected dogs and cats.

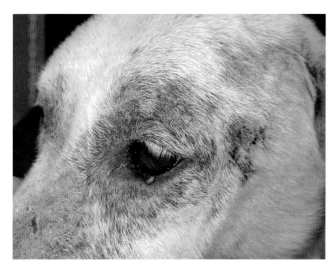

Figure 9.2:
Adverse food reaction. This figure shows periocular alopecia, hyperpigmentation, and excoriations secondary to intense pruritus resulting from an adverse cutaneous reaction to beef protein.

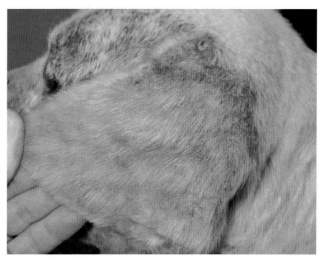

Figure 9.3:
Adverse food reaction. This figure shows erythema, alopecia, and excoriations on the ear lobe secondary to intense pruritus resulting from an adverse cutaneous reaction to beef protein.

9

Table 9.2: Role of food-related immunological responses in enteropathies

Disorder	Role of Food Allergens	Treatment(s)
Inflammatory bowel disease	Dietary antigens may contribute to GI inflammation	Elimination diet + immunosuppressive drugs
Gluten-sensitive enteropathy	Aberrant muscosal immune response to gliadin	Gluten-free diet
Protein-losing enteropathy of SCWT	Severe food allergy leads to enteritis and PLE	Elimination diet + immunosuppressive drugs

GI = gastrointestinal;
PLE = protein-losing enteropathy;
SCWT = Soft-coated Wheaten Terrier

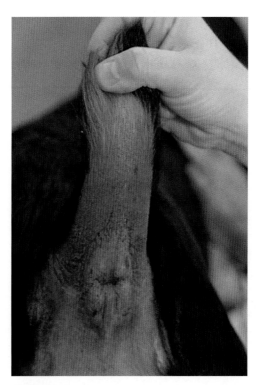

Figure 9.4:
Adverse food reaction. This figure shows perianal alopecia, erythema, lichenification, and hyperpigmentation secondary to intense pruritus resulting from an adverse cutaneous reaction to chicken protein.

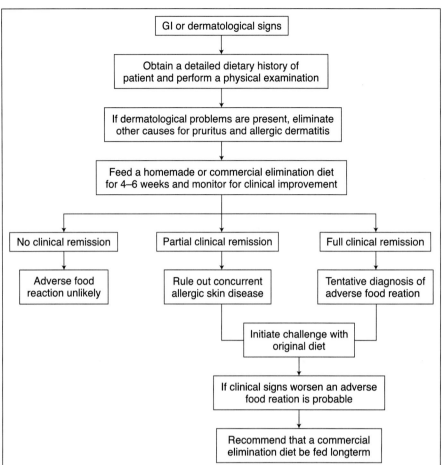

Figure 9.5:
Practical approach to elimination trials for the diagnosis of adverse food reactions (modified from Roudebush 2005[15]).

Diagnosis

A dietary elimination trial is the most important diagnostic tool in dogs and cats with suspected adverse food reactions. In-vitro testing (e.g., RASTs or ELISAs), biopsies, intradermal skin testing, or gastroscopic food sensitivity testing are unreliable for diagnosing food allergy.[6,15] Colonoscopic delivery of food allergens, Doppler ultrasound analysis of mesenteric arterial blood flow, and perinuclear antineutrophilic antibodies (pANCA) have been suggested as having some diagnostic utility in dogs with suspected food allergy.[17–19] However, further studies are necessary to confirm these preliminary findings.

Treatment of adverse food reactions

Concept of a dietary trial

The first step of a dietary trial is to discontinue the previous diet (offending foodstuff) and feed an elimination diet followed by a challenge with the patient's original diet (Figure 9.5). If clinical signs recur on the former diet and resolve on the elimination diet, a diagnosis of an adverse food reaction can be made. Provocation testing can help in identifying the offending antigen or antigens, but is often impractical in a clinical setting. A recommendation for an appropriate commercial elimination diet can then be made based on the results of the challenge studies.

Defining an elimination diet

The ideal elimination diet should 1) include a protein hydrolysate or a reduced number of novel, highly digestible protein sources; 2) avoid protein excess; 3) avoid additives and vasoactive amines; and 4) be nutritionally adequate for the animal's life stage and condition.[15] A variety of different diets may be fed including homemade elimination diets and commercial elimination diets.

A homemade elimination diet should consist of a single protein source and also a single carbohydrate source. This is because, even though carbohydrates are only poorly antigenic, every carbohydrate source does contain small quantities of a variety of proteins. Suggested food components in dogs include fish, rabbit, venison, rice, potatoes, and tofu; while, the use of baby food with protein sources such as lamb or rabbit and a carbohydrate source, such as rice is recommended in cats. Homemade diets are often advocated as the initial test food for dogs and cats with suspected food allergy. Caution is advised when feeding homemade diets for longer than 3 weeks, as they may be nutritionally inadequate.[15] Most commercial elimination diets are indicated for the long-term management of dogs and cats with adverse food reactions. These products are attractive because they are convenient, balanced, and nutritionally complete for either dogs or cats. Protein hydrolysate diets contain proteins that have been hydrolyzed into smaller peptides and amino acids, which reduces the antigenicity and allergenicity of the diet. The clinical superiority of one elimination diet versus another in the treatment of adverse food reactions has not been clearly established.

Duration of a dietary trial

The optimal duration of a dietary trial has been subject to considerable debate. Generally speaking, patients with dermatological signs will require longer elimination periods (6–10 weeks), while patients with GI signs will require shorter elimination periods (3–4 weeks). Cats with food allergy may respond to dietary trials in as short as 3–7 days.[13]

Interpreting dietary trials

A tentative diagnosis of an adverse food reaction can be made if the level of pruritus and/or the severity of GI signs markedly decrease subsequent to a dietary trial. However, a challenge with the original diet is necessary to confirm the diagnosis. Elimination trials may be difficult to interpret because of concurrent allergic skin disease. Thus, flea–allergy dermatitis and atopic dermatitis should be ruled out through appropriate diagnostic testing in partial responders.

Prognosis

The prognosis for adverse food reactions is generally good once the disorder is correctly identified and treated with a dietary elimination trial. In the author's (AEJ) experience, the offending food component is rarely identified since provocation testing is not permitted by most pet owners. Clients should be counseled that long-term (indefinite) feeding of a commercial elimination diet is usually required to maintain clinical remission.

9

🔑 Key Facts

- Adverse food reactions may be immunologically (i.e., food allergy) or non-immunologically (i.e., food intolerance) mediated.
- Dermatological signs (pruritic dermatitis) of food allergy predominate in both dogs and cats.
- A dietary elimination trial is the most important diagnostic tool in dogs and cats with suspected adverse food reactions.
- The prognosis for adverse food reactions is generally good once the disorder is correctly identified and treated with a dietary elimination trial.

References

1. Anderson JA. The establishment of common language concerning adverse reactions to foods and food additives. *J Allergy* 1986; 78: 140–144.
2. Halliwell REW. Comparative aspects of food intolerance. *Vet Med* 1992; 87: 893–899.
3. Crowe SE, Purdue MH. Gastrointestinal food hypersensitivity: basic mechanisms of pathophysiology. *Gastroenterology* 1992; 103: 1075–1095.
4. Day MJ. The canine model of dietary hypersensitivity. *Proc Nutr Soc* 2005; 64: 458–464.
5. Taylor SL, Lemanske RF, Bush RK et al. Food allergens: structure and immunologic properties. *Ann Allergy* 1987; 59: 93–99.
6. Verlinden A, Hesta M, Millet S et al. Food allergy in dogs and cats: a review. *Crit Rev Food Sci Nutr* 2006; 46: 259–273.
7. Guilford WG. Adverse reactions to food. In: Guilford, WG, Center SA, and Strombeck DR (eds.), *Strombeck's Small Animal Gastroenterology*. Philadelphia, WB Saunders, 1996; 436–450.
8. Roudebush P. Ingredients associated with adverse food reactions in dogs and cats. *Adv Small Anim Med Surg* 2002; 15: 1–4.
9. Martin A, Sierra MP, Gonzalez JL et al. Identification of allergens responsible for canine cutaneous adverse food reactions to lamb, beef and cow's milk. *Vet Dermatol* 2004; 15: 349–356.
10. Walton GS. Skin responses in the dog and cat to ingested allergens. *Vet Rec* 1967; 81: 709–713.
11. Harvey RG. Food allergy and dietary intolerance in dogs: a report of 25 cases. *J Small Anim Pract* 1993; 34: 175–179.
12. Paterson S. Food hypersensitivity in 20 dogs with skin and gastrointestinal signs. *J Small Anim Pract* 1995; 36: 529–534.
13. Guilford WG, Jones BR, Markwell PJ et al. Food hypersensitivity in cats with chronic idiopathic gastrointestinal problems. *J Vet Intern Med* 2001; 15: 7–13.
14. Muller GH, Kirk RW, Scott DW. Food hypersensitivity. In: Dison J (ed.) *Small Animal Dermatology*. Philadelphia, WB Saunders, 1989; 470–474.
15. Roudebush P. Adverse reactions to foods: allergies versus intolerance. In: Ettinger SJ, Feldman EC (eds.) *Textbook of Veterinary Internal Medicine*. Philadelphia, WB Saunders, 2005; 566–570.
16. Scott DW. Feline dermatology 1983–1985: the secret sits. *J Am Anim Hosp Assoc* 1987; 23: 255–274.
17. Allenspach K, Vaden SL, Harris TS et al. Evaluation of colonoscopic allergen provocation as a diagnostic tool in dogs with proven food hypersensitivity reactions. *J Small Anim Pract* 2006; 47: 21–26.
18. Kircher PR, Spaulding KA, Vaden S et al. Doppler ultrasonographic evaluation of gastrointestinal hemodynamics in food hypersensitivities: a canine model. *J Vet Intern Med* 2004; 18: 605–611.
19. Luckschander N, Allenspach K, Hall J et al. Perinuclear antineutrophilic cytoplasmic antibody and response to treatment in diarrheic dogs with food responsive disease or inflammatory bowel disease. *J Vet Intern Med* 2006; 20: 221–227.

9.2 Inflammatory Bowel Disease

EDWARD J. HALL, ALEXANDER J. GERMAN

9.2.1 Introduction

The collective term Inflammatory Bowel Disease (IBD) is used in canine and feline gastroenterology to describe patients affected by persistent or recurrent GI signs that have histological evidence of inflammatory infiltration of the GI mucosa.[1] However, the indiscriminate use of the term "IBD" in small animal gastroenterology is problematic. The condition can only be termed "idiopathic IBD" if no underlying cause for the inflammation can be found. A number of other diseases are recognized as being associated with chronic intestinal inflammation (Table 9.3). It is the duty of the clinician to rule out these known causes through systematic investigation before reaching a diagnosis of idiopathic IBD, which is, by definition, of unknown cause.

It seems likely that idiopathic IBD is actually a group of disorders and not a single disease entity, as variations of the histological appearance do exist. The histological nomenclature for IBD reports the predominant cell type present and forms the basis for its traditional classification (Table 9.4). Lymphoplasmacytic enteritis (LPE) is the most common form of idiopathic IBD reported in both dogs and cats and yet, even within this group, variations do exist in its distribution within the GI tract, its severity, its pattern within the lamina propria (i.e., villus, upper crypt, or lower crypt), and in the ratio of lymphocytes to plasma cells. A severe form has been reported in Basenjis. Isolated lymphoplasmacytic colitis (LPC) has been reported quite frequently by some authors, whereas others believe it usually occurs in concert with more diffuse intestinal inflammation (i.e., LPE).[2]

Eosinophilic (gastro-)enteritis (EGE) is less common than LPE, but is the second most frequently diagnosed variant of IBD. Granulomatous enteritis is considered rare, although a report of a condition called "regional enteritis" bears a strong resemblance to granulomatous enteritis in humans. Histiocytic ulcerative colitis is a rare condition seen almost exclusively in Boxers (see 6.4.2.1).

Neutrophilic infiltration is the hallmark of the variants of IBD occurring in humans, namely Crohn's disease (CD) and ulcerative colitis (UC). Yet predominantly neutrophilic infiltration is uncommon in idiopathic IBD in cats and rare in dogs.

Table 9.3: Causes of chronic intestinal inflammation

Chronic infection
Giardia
Histoplasma
Toxoplasma
Mycobacterium
Prototheca
Pythium and other zygomycetes

Pathogenic bacteria

Campylobacter spp., *Salmonella* spp., pathogenic *E. coli*

Food allergy

Associated with other primary GI diseases

Lymphoma
Lymphangiectasia
Idiopathic

Table 9.4: Histopathological classification of idiopathic inflammatory bowel disease

Histopathological description	Comment
Lymphoplasmacytic enteritis (LPE)	Most common form
Basenji enteropathy	Possibly a variant of LPE
Familial PLE and PLN in Soft-coated Wheaten Terriers	Possibly a variant of LPE
Lymphoplasmacytic colitis	May occur in isolation or with LPE
Eosinophilic enteritis (EE); eosinophilic gastroenteritis (EGE); eosinophilic enterocolitis (EEC); eosinophilic gastroenterocolitis (EGEC)	Marked increase in eosinophils noted
Granulomatous enteritis	Rare as idiopathic disease, but reported as a sequel of FIP infection in cats
Regional enteritis	Possibly the same as granulomatous enteritis
Neutrophilic enteritis	Rare in dogs, uncommon in cats
Histiocytic ulcerative colitis	Most common in Boxers Potential infectious etiology

CD is characterized by periods of remission, with relapses where initial neutrophilic inflammation is followed by granuloma formation. This disease can affect any part of the intestine but is typically localized to the terminal jejunum and ileum. It is further characterized by fistulous tract formation and intestinal obstruction due to granuloma formation, often necessitating surgical resection of affected tissue. In comparison, UC is restricted to the colon and differs histologically from CD as the neutrophilic inflammation is associated with ulceration and crypt abscessation. Thus, canine and feline IBD bear little resemblance histologically or clinically to IBD (i.e., CD and UC) in humans, but they may still share a common etiology.

9.2.2 Common principles of IBD

9.2.2.1 Etiology and pathogenesis

The underlying etiology of idiopathic IBD in small animals is, by definition, unknown. However, analogies have been drawn to IBD in humans and the breakdown of immunological tolerance to luminal antigens (bacteria and dietary components) is thought to be crucial in the pathogenesis of this disorder.[3]

The loss of tolerance probably results from disruption of the mucosal barrier, dysregulation of the immune system, disturbances in the intestinal microflora, or a combination of these events. Although the clinical benefit of dietary therapy in some patients with IBD suggests a role for diet-related factors, extrapolation from experimental rodent models of IBD and natural IBD in humans, suggest that antigens derived from the endogenous microflora are more important in the disease pathogenesis. In contrast to a specific, active immune response against an enteropathogen, the default response of the healthy mucosa to luminal antigens is tolerance. As the majority of antigens are derived from innocent dietary components or the GI microflora, the mounting of an active response to such ubiquitous antigens would be both wasteful and potentially harmful, since it could lead to uncontrolled inflammation.

Genetic factors are likely to contribute to the pathogenesis of IBD and in humans there are strong associations with the human major histocompatibility complex (human leukocyte antigen; HLA) genes.[4,5] In addition, a mutation of the *NOD2* gene is present in some human patients with CD.[6,7] The product of the *NOD2* gene detects bacterial lipopolysaccharide and can activate the pro-inflammatory nuclear transcription factor NF-κB. Aberrant immune responses to bacteria may therefore develop in affected individuals. Similar genetic factors predisposing to IBD are also likely to play a role in canine and feline IBD, given the recognized breed predispositions, although studies are lacking.

9

Whilst the mechanisms by which mucosal tolerance occurs have been well characterized, a fundamental question that remains unresolved is how the gut-associated lymphoid tissue (GALT) decides when to and when not to become tolerant. If idiopathic IBD does indeed represent a breakdown in mucosal tolerance to the endogenous bacterial flora, the reason why this occurs is also unresolved. Hence, in order to begin to understand the etiology and pathogenesis of IBD, an understanding of the normal small intestinal (SI) bacterial flora and its interaction with the intestinal immune system is essential.

Bacterial flora

The normal SI microflora is a diverse mixture of aerobic, anaerobic, and facultatively anaerobic bacteria, and plays an integral part in SI health. It influences a wide variety of functional parameters such as villus size, enterocyte turnover, brush border enzyme turnover, and intestinal motility. The digestion and absorption of fats, carbohydrates, amino acids (such as taurine), and vitamins (such as cobalamin and folate) are also affected by intestinal bacteria.

Bacterial numbers increase from duodenum to colon, but there is no consensus as to what constitutes a "normal" number of organisms in healthy animals. Some studies suggest that the proximal SI of healthy dogs can harbor up to 10^9 colony-forming units (CFU)/ml total bacteria, and these numbers are considerably higher than the numbers ($<10^5$ CFU/ml total bacteria) reported in healthy humans and initially extrapolated to dogs.[8] Yet, although the presence of a stable enteric flora is important for preventing colonization by pathogens, the absolute number of organisms is probably not crucial in the development of intestinal inflammation.

Mucosal immune system

The intestinal mucosa has a general barrier function, but it must also generate a protective immune response against pathogens, whilst remaining tolerant of harmless environmental antigens such as commensal bacteria and dietary components. Despite recent advances in our understanding of the structure and function of the immune system, it is still unclear as to how the immune system determines whether to respond to or to become tolerant of a particular antigen.[9] Yet it is believed that the host immune response to a bacterial organism is likely to be as important as its intrinsic pathogenicity, and an inability to tolerate a normal bacterial flora may be the mechanism underlying idiopathic IBD.

The GALT is the largest immunological organ in the body and its structure and function is complex. A more detailed review of its structure and function by the authors is available elsewhere.[10]

In brief, the inductive sites in the GALT comprise Peyer's patches (PPs), isolated lymphoid follicles, and the mesenteric lymph nodes (MLNs), whilst the effector sites consist of the intestinal lamina propria (LP) and the epithelium. The PPs are the main sites of induction of the immune response, and may also function as sites of B-lymphocyte development. Within the follicle-associated epithelium overlying a PP, a specialized population of antigen transport cells (microfold cells or M-cells) exists, acting as portals through which the underlying immune cells receive antigens. The MLNs receive afferent lymph from the intestine, and are also important in the generation of an immune response. The LP consists of a matrix of connective tissue with a large leukocyte population, composed principally of lymphocytes. Intra-epithelial lymphocytes (IELs) are located between the enterocytes.

B-lymphocytes are present within both the PPs and LP. In the PPs, the lymphocytes are located predominantly in the follicular regions, but in the LP they are largely represented by plasma cells around the intestinal crypts, and are mostly of the IgA isotype, secreting targeted, protective antibodies.

T-lymphocytes in the SI, are mostly of the conventional $\alpha\beta$ T-cell receptor type.[11] T-lymphocytes can be further subdivided on the basis of their expression of cell-surface markers, in particular CD4 and CD8 molecules. CD4$^+$ T-cells (classical helper T-cells) recognize an antigenic peptide presented by MHC class II molecules, particularly by macrophages and dendritic cells. In comparison, CD8$^+$ T cells (usually cytotoxic cells) are MHC class I restricted.

In the canine LP, the T-cells are most numerous in the upper villus regions and are mostly of the $\alpha\beta$, CD4$^+$ phenotype.[11–13] However, in the feline LP, CD8$^+$ T-cells outnumber the CD4$^+$ population.[14] Most LP lymphocytes are highly differentiated, implying that they are receiving continuous antigenic and mitogenic stimulation, probably from the endogenous microbial flora. The IELs are a heterogeneous population; most are CD8$^+$ but they can be either $\alpha\beta$ or $\gamma\delta$ in phenotype, depending on the species. The known functions of IELs include cytolytic activity and cytokine production, suggesting roles in epithelial surveillance and maintenance of mucosal immune homeostasis.

The CD4$^+$ T-cell population is a major cytokine-producing cell population, but different populations exist with different patterns of cytokine secretion, by which they can regulate the humoral and cell-mediated arms of the immune system. Two principal populations are postulated: a T-helper 1 (Th1) population that produces interleukin 2 (IL-2), interferon γ (IFN-γ), and tumor necrosis factor β (TNF-β), and a T-helper 2 (Th2) population producing IL-4, IL-5, IL-6, and IL-10.[15] Other populations with down-regulatory functions, which predominantly secrete tranforming growth factor β (TGF-β) or IL-10 respectively, have also been proposed.[16]

Although lymphocytes and plasma cells predominate in the intestinal mucosa, other immune cells are also present. Macrophages have functions including phagocytosis, antigen presentation, and immunoregulatory roles, mediated by the secretion of cytokines, chemokines, and inflammatory mediators including TNF-α, eicosanoids, and leukotrienes. Neutrophils are present in smaller numbers, although their numbers do increase during mucosal inflammation. Both mast cells and eosinophils can be found and actively produce chemical mediators (e.g., histamine, heparin, eicosanoids, and cytokines).

In addition to digestive functions, enterocytes have important immune functions. First, they are an important component of the mucosal barrier, controlling the uptake of antigens. Second, they may be capable of antigen presentation, through the expression of MHC II, and non-classical antigen-presenting molecules.[17] Finally, enterocytes can produce inflammatory mediators, chemokines and cytokines, and may regulate immune responses in both the epithelial and LP compartments.

Mucosal tolerance

Acquired immune responses develop after a series of steps involving antigen uptake, presentation to naïve lymphocytes, co-stimulation by helper cells, clonal expansion, homing to effector sites, and performance of effector functions. The specific mechanisms involved are described in detail elsewhere.[18] In the SI, a large array of cytokines is present, and can be grouped into pro-inflammatory, immunoregulatory, and chemokinetic cytokines. Many other cell types may also produce cytokines (see above), and consequently an overall cytokine environment exists, which determines the predominant type of immune response that develops.

Mucosal tolerance can result either from anergy/deletion (by apoptosis) of antigen-specific T-cells, or by active suppression through antigen-specific suppressor cells.[19] The CD4+ αβ T-cell subset that mediates active suppression either produces down-regulatory cytokines (e.g., TGF-β or IL-10) or functions through cell-cell interactions.[16] Furthermore, since TGF-β and IL-10 are also important in IgA production, generation of mucosal tolerance could potentially occur in parallel to a specific IgA response, which helps to maintain tolerance by immune exclusion.

As mentioned previously, the mucosal immune system must determine when to generate a specific immune response (e.g., towards a pathogen), and when to remain tolerant (e.g., to commensal bacteria or food components). The most workable hypothesis currently is the "danger theory", which is based on the supposition that the type of response depends upon the context in which the antigen is presented.[19] When the mucosa is invaded by a pathogen, cell damage leads to release of "danger signals" (i.e., inflammatory mediators, such as pro-inflammatory cytokines and chemokines). Hence the nature of the immune response generated changes from tolerance to active immune response and can either be Th1-dominated (i.e., cytotoxicity and IgG response) or Th2-dominated (i.e., IgE response). Such an immune response is aimed at eliminating the pathogen completely, but by-stander damage to host cells can occur, particularly if the danger persists, either because the mucosal barrier remains breached and the pathogenic insult continues unabated or because there is an inherent abnormality of the GALT. A state of chronic inflammation develops, which may lead to a breakdown in tolerance to harmless antigens (i.e., food components and commensal bacteria). The chronic inflammation ultimately leads to histological changes, which are generally similar regardless of the inciting cause.

Mucosal inflammation

A number of inciting causes (including infection, ischemia, trauma, toxins, neoplasia, and immune-mediated reactions) can cause a cellular and vascular response, collectively known as inflammation. The normal mucosa is usually tolerant of endogenous bacteria and food antigens, but can be considered to be in a state of "controlled inflammation". As postulated above, disruption of the mucosal barrier, dysregulation of the immune system, disturbances in the intestinal microflora, or a combination of these events can destabilize the system and may trigger uncontrolled inflammation.

Experimental rodent models of GI inflammation have permitted a better understanding of the pathogenesis of mucosal inflammation, and the mechanisms that trigger it.[3] These genetically engineered animals possess a variety of spontaneously arising or induced disruptions of the mucosal barrier, the mucosal immune system, or the endogenous microflora, all leading to chronic inflammation with a similar histological appearance. Whatever the model, the presence of an enteric flora is essential for the expression of disease and intestinal inflammation does not develop when the rodents are reared in a germ-free environment.[20] This final point demonstrates the importance of the endogenous flora in the pathogenesis of uncontrolled mucosal inflammation. This has been confirmed by studies showing that normal humans are tolerant to their own intestinal microflora, but that this tolerance is broken in patients with IBD.[21]

9.2.2.2　Clinical presentation

Idiopathic IBD is generally considered the most common cause of chronic vomiting and diarrhea in dogs and cats, but its true prevalence is unknown. In reality, the condition is most likely overdiagnosed, due to the ease of getting endoscopic intestinal biopsies, the difficulties in interpretation of histopathological specimens (particularly if collected endoscopi-

9

Table 9.5: Clinical signs associated with inflammatory bowel disease

Vomiting

- bile and/or food
- hair in cats
- grass in dogs
- hematemesis

Small intestinal-type diarrhea

- large volume
- watery
- melena

Large intestinal-type diarrhea

- hematochezia
- mucoid stool
- frequency and tenesmus

Abdominal discomfort/pain

Excessive borborygmus and flatus

Thickened bowel loops

Weight loss

Altered appetite or anorexia

Polyphagia

Eating grass or pica

Hypoproteinemia and/or ascites

cally), and the failure to adequately rule out other causes of mucosal inflammation. No apparent gender predisposition has been reported in dogs or cats, but in both species IBD is considered to be more common in middle-aged animals. IBD is uncommon in animals less than 6 months of age, when anatomical, infectious, and dietary causes of diarrhea are much more prevalent.

Although idiopathic IBD can potentially occur in any dog or cat breed, certain breed predispositions have been recognized. Examples include LPE in German Shepherd dogs and Siamese cats, EGE in German Shepherds, and lymphoproliferative enteropathy in Basenjis. A concurrent PLE and PLN has been reported in Soft-coated Wheaten Terriers. Shar Pei dogs often have severe LPE with hypoproteinemia and extremely low serum cobalamin concentrations. In cats, a syndrome, termed "triaditis", has been reported that is characterized by concurrent lymphoplasmacytic IBD, lymphocytic cholangitis, and chronic lymphocytic pancreatitis.[22]

Vomiting and diarrhea are the most common clinical signs in patients with IBD, but an individual patient may show some or all of the signs listed in Table 9.5. The clinical signs may wax and wane, and an obvious precipitating event may be evident (e.g., stress, acute GI infection, or dietary change). The appetite is often variable. Polyphagia may be present in the face of significant weight loss, whilst anorexia occurs with severe inflammation. Milder inflammation may not affect the appetite, although post-prandial pain can be significant even without other signs.

The nature of the GI signs can be correlated approximately with the region of the GI tract that is affected: vomiting and hematemesis are more common if gastric or upper SI inflammation is present, and in cats vomiting is often the predominant sign of SI IBD. Large intestinal (LI)-type diarrhea may be the result of colonic inflammation, or may result from prolonged SI diarrhea or the presence of agents that stimulate colonic secretion (e.g., bacteria, bacterial toxins, deconjugated bile acids, or hydroxylated fatty acids). Blood in the vomit or diarrhea is usually associated with more severe disease and, most often, eosinophilic inflammatory infiltrates.

Severe, chronic disease is associated with weight loss and PLE, even leading to hypoproteinemia and ascites. The measurement of fecal loss of alpha$_1$–proteinase inhibitor appears to be a sensitive test for PLE before hypoproteinemia develops. The serum concentrations of both albumin and globulin are reduced in most patients with PLE. Exceptions to the typical panhypoproteinemia are due to increased globulin production caused by immune system stimulation (e.g., immunoproliferative SI disease in the Basenji, see 9.2.5). Renal and hepatic causes of hypoalbuminemia can be eliminated by assay of serum bile acids concentrations and the urinary protein/creatinine ratio. Hypocholesterolemia and lymphopenia can also be seen in patients with PLE. Ionized hypocalcemia and hypomagnesemia have also been reported.

Physical examination findings may include edema, ascites, emaciation, thickened intestines, melena, and hematochezia (Figure 9.6). Thrombo-embolism and remote organ failure is a feature seen in some patients with PLE. Other systemic consequences of IBD, such as thrombocytopenia, can occur although reports are sparse.[23]

9.2.2.3 Diagnosis

Although the clinical signs and physical examination findings may be suggestive of IBD, ultimately intestinal biopsy is necessary for a definitive diagnosis. Since the term idiopathic IBD is restricted to cases in which intestinal inflammation is found without any obvious underlying cause, all other etiologies must be excluded before a diagnosis of IBD can be made. Therefore, before intestinal biopsies are collected, laboratory evaluation and diagnostic imaging must be performed. Such investigations are not intended to provide a definitive diagnosis of IBD, but to help eliminate the possibility of extra-intestinal disease (e.g., pancreatitis, hypoadrenocorticism, renal failure, and hepatic failure), anatomic intestinal disease (e.g., tumor or intussusception), or known causes of intestinal inflammation. Furthermore, by determining whether focal or diffuse intestinal disease is present, the most appropriate method of intestinal biopsy can be chosen.

Laboratory testing – Hematology

It is not unusual for the hematological examination to be completely unremarkable in animals with IBD. Occasionally, neutrophilia, with or without a left shift, is noted, and reactive atypical lymphocytes may be seen in patients with LPE. It has been suggested that eosinophilia is indicative of EGE, but it is not pathognomonic. If anemia is present, it may be a reflection of chronic inflammation or chronic blood loss. Anemia due to blood loss is usually strongly regenerative in nature and is initially, normocytic, normochromic. However, an iron deficiency anemia, characterized by microcytosis, hypochromasia, and thrombocytosis, may eventually develop.

Laboratory testing – Serum biochemistry profile

In many patients with IBD, the serum biochemistry profile is within normal limits. However, testing allows diseases of other organ systems to be recognized or excluded. Hypoalbuminemia and hypoglobulinemia are characteristic of a PLE, whilst hypocholesterolemia may suggest malabsorption. Furthermore, intestinal inflammation in dogs may cause a reactive hepatopathy with mild to moderate (2–4 fold) increases in liver enzyme (ALT, ALP) activities. In contrast, due to their shorter half-lives, any liver enzyme increases in cats are more likely to be the result of primary liver disease, although concurrent IBD and cholangitis are commonly seen in cats.

Laboratory testing – Fecal examination

Fecal examination by flotation techniques is very important in eliminating known parasitic causes of mucosal inflammation. For example, nematodes (e.g., *Trichuris*, *Uncinaria*, or *Ancylostoma*) and *Giardia* can be diagnosed by fecal smear and/or flotation. However, given that fecal examination and even a fecal ELISA for *Giardia* antigen may not always detect the presence of these important causes of intestinal inflammation and diarrhea, empirical treatment with fenbendazole is recommended in all cases.

Culture for bacterial pathogens such as *Salmonella* spp., *Campylobacter* spp., or *Clostridium* spp. is more problematic, as these

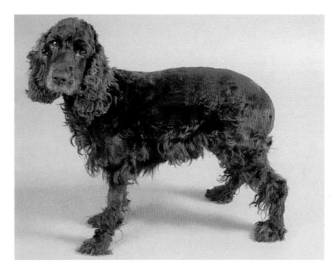

Figure 9.6:
Cocker Spaniel with PLE. An eight-year-old female Cocker Spaniel with a protein-losing enteropathy and signs of diarrhea, weight loss, and ascites associated with hypoalbuminemia (1.2 g/dl). The dog initially responded well to treatment with immunosuppressive doses of steroids, but after 3 months, as the dose of steroids was tapered, hypoproteinemia recurred and the dog was euthanized after developing severe dyspnea, suspected to be a result of pulmonary thromboembolism.

organisms can be found in the stools of healthy animals, and their presence in patients with IBD does not necessarily prove a causal relationship.

Significant intestinal protein loss probably develops in patients with IBD before hypoproteinemia occurs. Increased fecal α_1-proteinase inhibitor concentrations would be expected before PLE can be recognized clinically.

Laboratory testing – Serum folate and cobalamin concentrations

The measurement of serum folate and cobalamin concentrations is now commercially available for dogs and cats, and folate and cobalamin deficiency associated with IBD has been documented. As the serum concentrations of both of these water-soluble vitamins are affected by intestinal malabsorption, proximal, distal, or diffuse SI inflammation can result in decreased folate concentration, decreased cobalamin concentration, or both. Although such alterations are not pathognomonic, such deficiencies in IBD may require therapeutic correction. In particular, cobalamin deficiency may in itself have systemic metabolic consequences and may also cause intestinal dysfunction.[24] Also, anecdotal evidence suggests that the response to immunosuppressive therapy for IBD may be suboptimal until cobalamin deficiency is resolved.

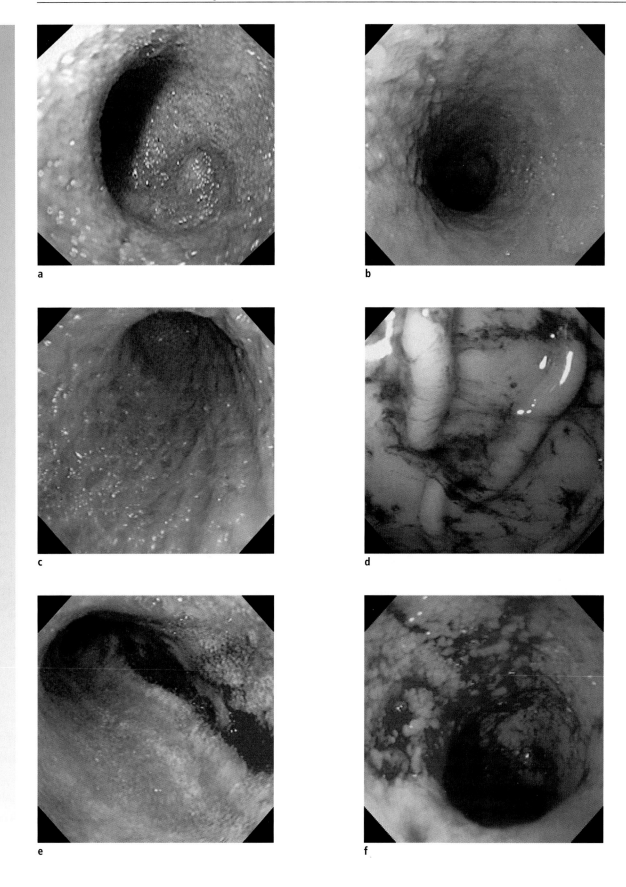

a

b

c

d

e

f

Diagnostic imaging

Radiographic and ultrasonographic studies are performed to document whether focal or diffuse disease is present, to document any anatomical GI disease, and to show any involvement of other abdominal organs. Used in conjunction with specific clinical signs and laboratory testing, the information from imaging studies enables an appropriate choice of a biopsy method (i.e., upper or lower GI endoscopy, or exploratory laparotomy) that will most likely lead to a definitive diagnosis.

Survey radiographs may be useful for identifying anatomical disease, whilst contrast studies rarely add further information. Ultrasonographic examination is superior to radiography for documenting focal intestinal disease. In addition, ultrasound-guided fine-needle aspiration can provide samples for cytological analysis.

Abdominal ultrasonography in IBD patients permits the evaluation of intestinal wall thickness, and can help document mesenteric lymphadenopathy.[25,26] It has been suggested that IBD is associated with increased intestinal wall thickness; however, this was not found to be true in a large case series.[27] In that case series, the intestinal wall thickness was only markedly increased if hypoproteinemia in a patient with PLE caused bowel wall edema. Furthermore, loss of the normal intestinal layering is indicative of neoplasia rather than IBD.

Intestinal biopsy

Intestinal biopsy is essential to prove the presence of intestinal inflammation and thus to confirm a diagnosis of IBD. Endoscopic biopsy is the simplest and least invasive method of specimen collection, although numerous limitations exist, including small sample size, superficial and often fragmented samples, and the fact that tissue can only be collected from the stomach, proximal SI, distal ileum, and colon. In some cases, exploratory celiotomy and full-thickness biopsy are necessary, although this is more invasive and wound healing can be problematic if severe hypoproteinemia is present and corticosteroids need to be given urgently. However, it may be more suitable for cats, given the tendency for concurrent hepatic and pancreatic involvement and the small size of endoscopic biopsies that can be achieved in this species.

The endoscopic appearance of the intestinal mucosa can give some clue as to the presence of intestinal inflammation. Increased granularity, irregularity, and friability with the presence of erosion, ulceration, and spontaneous hemorrhage are all potential markers of IBD (Figure 9.7). However, interpretation of the gross appearance of the mucosa is quite subjective, and obvious macroscopic changes are not invariably present despite histological evidence of even quite marked inflammation. Furthermore, similar changes are seen in other intestinal conditions, especially intestinal neoplasia.

The pattern of histopathological changes in biopsy specimens that is reported depends upon the type of IBD present (see above). Yet, while the histopathological assessment of intestinal biopsies remains the gold standard for the diagnosis of many intestinal diseases, it has marked limitations. For example, biopsy specimens can be normal by light microscopy in almost half of cats and dogs with chronic GI disease and suspected IBD. This suggests that either many patients do not have IBD and their disease is caused by functional rather than morphological abnormalities, or that sampling and interpretive problems occur.

A major problem of histopathological diagnosis is the poor agreement between histopathologists. This may be due to poor quality endoscopic biopsies, the subjective nature of interpretation of the degree of inflammation, the patchiness of inflammation, or the presence of edema (due to hypoproteinemia) leading to difficulties in assessing cell density.[28] In a recent study, even an incorrect diagnosis of lymphoma was made by a histopathologist assessing tissues from a healthy dog.[29]

The distinction of severe LPE from lymphoma can be difficult, particularly with endoscopic biopsies as the histological confirmation of lymphoma is made most readily when lymphocytic infiltration of muscle layers is seen on full-thickness surgical biopsy specimens.

Histopathological scoring schemes and standardized criteria (Table 9.6) have been suggested as a means of improving agreement, but marked variability in interpretation still exists. A WSAVA-sponsored GI Standardization Group has been established to try to resolve these inconsistencies, and a standard grading scheme that assesses architectural abnormalities in conjunction with changes in cellularity is being developed.[23]

9

Figure 9.7:
Endoscopic appearance of the intestine of patients with varying degrees of inflammatory bowel disease.
(a) Mild lymphoplasmacytic enteritis in a dog, showing increased granularity.
(b) Moderate lymphoplasmacytic enteritis in a cat, showing a classical "cobblestone" appearance.
(c) Severe lymphoplasmacytic enteritis in a dog, showing erosions and ulcers.
(d) Eosinophilic gastritis in a dog.
(e) Eosinophilic enteritis in the same dog as shown in d.
(f) Histiocytic ulcerative colitis in a Boxer, showing severe ulceration and hemorrhage.

Table 9.6: Criteria for the histological assessment of intestinal biopsies

Epithelium	Crypts and villi
■ enterocyte height	■ crypt abscessation
■ erosions	■ crypt depth
■ goblet cell number and size	■ crypt-villus ratio
■ intraepithelial lymphocyte density	■ mitotic index
	■ villus clubbing and fusion
	■ villus height and width

Lamina propria	Miscellaneous
■ immune cell density	■ edema
■ lymphangiectasia	■ fibrosis
■ predominant cell type	■ hyperemia or congestion
	■ infectious agents
	■ neoplasia

Alternate examinations of biopsy specimens are largely experimental, but can provide significant information. Examinations available in some institutions include electron microscopy, biochemical assays for brush border enzyme activities, immunocytochemical characterization of B-cells, T-cells, and their subsets (CD4, CD8, etc.) by histology and flow cytometry, immunocytochemical localization of MHC expression, assays for cytokine mRNA expression, and assessment of T-cell clonality.[11–13,30,31]

Ultimately, the primary clinician should interpret histopathology results cautiously and try to relate them to the clinical presentation. The results should be questioned if the histopathological diagnosis does not fit the clinical picture or the response to apparently appropriate therapy is poor. In some cases, repeat biopsy (e.g., by exploratory laparotomy) may be required.

In humans, activity indices are used to quantify disease severity in IBD patients, aiding the assessment of the response to treatment and allowing comparisons between published studies in the literature. Recently, an activity index has been suggested for canine IBD patients (Table 9.7) that may aid in disease classification in the future.[32]

9.2.2.4 Treatment

The treatment of IBD usually involves a combination of dietary modification, antibacterials, and immunosuppressive therapy, regardless of the histological type diagnosed. Most recommendations are based upon individual experience as objective information on efficacy is generally lacking. The authors recommend a staged approach to therapy whenever possible, except in seriously ill patients where immediate inter-

vention with immunosuppressive medication may be essential. Such a logical, staged approach involves initial treatment with antiparasitic agents to eliminate any occult endoparasite infestation. Sequential therapeutic trials with an exclusion diet and antibacterials should also be undertaken. Immunosuppressive medication is used only as a final resort. If the clinical signs are intermittent, the owners should keep a diary to provide objective information as to whether treatments produce genuine improvement. In addition, changes in the IBD activity index may provide objective evidence of treatment success or failure.

Intravenous fluid therapy should be given if the patient is dehydrated, but most patients with IBD have chronic disease and have reached a compensatory state, and so do not need fluid support. If PLE and hypoproteinemia are present, plasma transfusion may be indicated during the peri-operative period associated with intestinal biopsy. Diuretics may reduce ascites: spironolactone at 1–2 mg/kg PO q 12 h may be more effective than furosemide for treating ascites. Thromboembolism is present in some patients with PLE, and prophylactic low-dose aspirin at 0.5 mg/kg PO q 12 h has been advocated in dogs with PLE.

Diet and dietary supplements

The diets recommended for patients with IBD are either based on an easily digestible diet or on a single-source protein, single-source carbohydrate diet. Single-protein, single-carbohydrate source diets may be considered antigen-limited. Ideally, they contain a protein source that is novel to the patient and are true exclusion diets. An alternative approach is to use a diet containing hydrolyzed protein. The authors recommend that a full dietary trial should be employed in all cases of unexplained intestinal inflammation to exclude the possibility of an adverse food reaction. Most clients are willing to try this first, given concerns over the side-effects of immunosuppressive drugs, but in severely ill animals it may be necessary to give concurrent immunosuppressive therapy with the dietary trial, and then see if remission is maintained when the drug therapy is gradually withdrawn.

A novel, highly digestible diet will decrease intestinal antigenic load, and thus decrease mucosal inflammation. Such diets may also help to resolve any sensitivity to dietary components that may have arisen secondary to disruption of the mucosal barrier. After resolution of the inflammation, the original diet can be re-introduced without the fear of an acquired sensitivity. Well-cooked rice is the preferred carbohydrate source because of its high digestibility, but potato, corn starch, and tapioca are alternative options. It is probably appropriate that they are also gluten-free, although the prevalence of gluten-sensitivity in dogs and cats is unclear. If severe malabsorption is evident, fat restriction may reduce clinical signs. However, fat restriction is rarely necessary and may make it more difficult to resolve weight loss. Modification of the n3:n6 fatty acid ratio may also modulate the inflammatory response and have some benefit in treatment and maintenance of remission.[33,34] However, there have been no studies to prove a benefit of such modification in canine or feline IBD.

Prebiotics and probiotics

The modulation of the enteric flora with probiotics or prebiotics included in the diet may have benefits in targeting the pathogenesis of IBD. Prebiotics are substrates selectively used by a limited number of beneficial bacterial species, resulting in alterations in the luminal microflora. Non-digestible carbohydrates, such as lactulose, inulin, fructo-oligosaccharides (FOS), and mannanoligosaccharides are the most frequently used prebiotic agents.

A probiotic is an orally-administered living organism that exerts health benefits beyond those of basic nutrition.[35] Probiotics can directly antagonize pathogenic bacteria, but they also modulate mucosal immune responses, by stimulating either innate, phagocytic activity or a specific secretory IgA immune response.[36] At present, the most appropriate organisms to select are unknown, but are likely to vary between host species.

Vitamin supplementation

Folate malabsorption may accompany severe and prolonged IBD, and oral supplementation is easily achieved, with administration of approximately 1 mg folic acid per day.

Malabsorption of cobalamin is more common than that of folate in patients with IBD, and can have significant metabolic consequences. Cobalamin deficiency causes methylmalonic acidemia, which may, in part, cause the ill-thrift and poor appetite seen in many patients. In addition, experimental cobalamin deficiency causes intestinal mucosal pathology, and it seems logical that correction of a deficiency is necessary before an optimal response to therapy can be achieved. There are a number of anecdotal reports, particularly in cats, where significant improvement was only seen after cobalamin supplementation. Oral administration of vitamin B12 is ineffective and it must be given by parenteral injection. Weekly subcutaneous injections of between 250 μg (cats and small dogs) to 1 mg (large breed dogs) are given for 6 weeks, then every other week for 6 weeks, and another dose after a month. Serum cobalamin concentration is rechecked a month after the last dose and should be supranormal at that time, indicating that cobalamin supplementation can be discontinued. If serum cobalamin concentration is only within the reference range, or even subnormal, cobalamin supplementation should be continued.

Table 9.7: Criteria for assessment of the canine inflammatory bowel disease activity index (CIBDAI), as proposed by Jergens et al (2003)[32]

A. Attitude/activity

0 = normal
1 = slightly decreased
2 = moderately decreased
3 = severely decreased

B. Appetite

0 = normal
1 = slightly decreased
2 = moderately decreased
3 = severely decreased

C. Vomiting

0 = none
1 = mild (1 episode/week)
2 = moderate (2–3 episodes/week)
3 = severe (>3 episodes/week)

D. Stool consistency

0 = normal
1 = slightly soft feces or fecal blood, mucus, or both
2 = very soft feces
3 = watery diarrhea

E. Stool frequency

0 = normal
1 = slightly increased (2–3 times/day)
2 = moderately increased (4–5 times/day)
3 = severely increased (>5 times/day)

F. Weight loss

0 = none
1 = mild (<5% loss)
2 = moderate (5–10% loss)
3 = severe (>10% loss)

The scores for each of the six variables are added and a CIBDAI assigned as follows:

0–3 = clinically insignificant disease
4–5 = mild IBD
6–8 = moderate IBD
9 or greater = severe IBD

9

9

Antibacterial therapy

The use of antimicrobials in patients with IBD is justified, in part, by the potential to treat any undiagnosed enteropathogens or secondary SI bacterial overgrowth, and in part by the perceived importance of bacterial antigens in the pathogenesis of IBD (see above). In the authors' experience, metronidazole is the preferred antibacterial for small animals. Its efficacy may not just be related to its antibacterial activity, since there may be immunomodulatory effects on cell-mediated immunity. Other authors prefer other antibacterials, such as oxytetracycline and tylosin, that may also have immunomodulatory effects and have some efficacy in canine IBD. There have been recent reports that HUC in Boxers (see 9.2.9) is responsive to enrofloxacin.[37,38] This raises the possibility that this condition is not a variant of idiopathic IBD, but the consequence of a specific infection.

5-Aminosalicylic acid derivatives

Colitis can be treated with derivatives of 5-aminosalicylic acid (5-ASA) administered in a form that is only active in the colon, as long as the colitis is neither secondary to SI disease nor part of generalized IBD. Native 5-ASA is termed mesalazine, and slow-release enteric formulations are available for human patients. Premature release in the SI is likely to cause absorption and nephrotoxicity, but at the intraluminal pH in humans the majority of the 5-ASA is released in the colon. The safety of oral formulations of mesalazine in dogs and cats is unclear and they cannot be recommended for routine use. Mesalazine enemas and suppositories are safe, but not popular.

Sulfasalazine is the most commonly used preparation and is used at dosages of 10–30 mg/kg PO q 8–12 h in dogs and 10–20 mg/kg PO q 24 h in cats. It is a pro-drug with a diazo bond binding sulfapyridine to 5-ASA, which is cleaved by colonic bacteria to release free 5-ASA that acts locally in high concentrations in the colon as an anti-inflammatory agent. Hepatotoxicity can occur, but its major side-effect is keratoconjunctivitis sicca (KCS), and Schirmer tear tests should be performed on a regular basis. KCS is believed to be a complication of the sulfonamide-moiety, although it has also been seen with olsalazine, which contains no sulfonamide-moiety.

Olsalazine is a compound containing two 5-ASA molecules joined by a diazo bond. Again, free 5-ASA is released by colonic bacteria. Olsalazine was developed in an attempt to reduce the frequency of KCS, although occasional KCS is still reported with this drug. The dose is one half the dose of sulfasalazine as it contains twice the amount of active ingredient. Balsalazide is the newest pro-drug (4-aminobenzoyl-β-alanine-mesalamine), and is activated by the same mechanism as sulfasalazine, but its safety and efficacy have not been evaluated in small animals.

Immunosuppressive drugs

Undoubtedly, the most important therapy for idiopathic IBD is immunosuppression, although it should only be considered as a last resort. In human IBD, glucocorticoids and thiopurines (azathioprine, 6-mercaptopurine, etc.) are used most widely.[39]

Traditional glucocorticoid therapy

In dogs and cats, glucocorticoids are used most frequently, and prednisolone (or more commonly prednisone in the USA) is the drug of choice. Dexamethasone should probably be avoided since it has been shown to have a deleterious effect on enterocyte brush border enzyme expression in other species. In severe IBD, when oral absorption may be inadequate, prednisolone can be administered parenterally. The standard initial dosage of 1–2 mg/kg PO q 12 h, is given for 2 to 4 weeks, and then tapered slowly over the subsequent months. In most cases, the therapy can only be reduced to a low maintenance dose given q 48 h, but in the minority of cases it can be completely withdrawn.

In some cases, an initial response to steroids is followed by a relapse and lack of further response, even when the dosages are increased. Some of these cases probably represent either transformation to lymphoma, or an incorrect initial diagnosis. However, resistance to steroids may perhaps develop because of induction of the multiple drug resistance gene and expression of P glycoprotein.

Novel glucocorticoid therapy

When the highest glucocorticoid dose is administered, signs of iatrogenic hyperadrenocorticism (polyphagia, polydipsia/polyuria, pot-bellied appearance, and/or muscle wastage) are commonly observed, especially in dogs. However, most of these signs are transient and resolve as the dosage is reduced. If a relapse consistently occurs when the dosage is reduced, alternative drugs can be added to provide a "steroid-sparing" effect (see below). Alternatively, novel steroids with fewer side effects can be used.

An enteric-coated formulation of budesonide, a locally active steroid, has been used successfully in maintaining remission in human patients with IBD with minimal hypothalamic-pituitary-adrenal suppression, as 90% of the drug is metabolized during its first-pass through the liver after absorption. A preliminary study has shown an apparent efficacy of budesonide in dogs and cats with IBD, but limited information on the use of this drug is available.[40] Anecdotally, oral doses no greater than 3 mg/day in dogs and 1 mg/day in cats, or 1 mg/m²/day have been recommended. However, induction of ALP and development of a steroid hepatopathy have been seen, and hypothalamic-pituitary-adrenal suppression has been demonstrated in dogs.[41] Furthermore, the optimal dose of this drug has not yet been determined.

Azathioprine

Azathioprine at 2 mg/kg PO q 24 h is commonly used in dogs, in combination with prednisolone/prednisone, when the initial response to steroid therapy is poor or the side effects are marked and a steroid-sparing drug is required. However, its activity may show a delayed onset (up to 3 weeks) and, given its myelosuppressive potential, regular monitoring of the hemogram is necessary. Idiosyncratic bone marrow toxicity has been linked to the activity of the enzyme thiopurine methyltransferase (TPMT), the major enzyme involved in the degradation of 6-mercaptopurine (6MP), the active metabolite of azathioprine. However, there are other pathways of 6MP metabolism, and the correlation between toxicity and TPMT activity is not clear.[42] Azathioprine is not recommended for cats, partly because cats have very low activities of TPMT, and partly because the coated tablets cannot be split and need reformulation to a suitable size.

Other cytotoxic agents

Chlorambucil (2–6 mg/m² PO q 24 h until remission, then tapering) is a better choice of a cytotoxic immunosuppressive agent in cats. Other immunosuppressive cytotoxic drugs include methotrexate, cyclophosphamide, and cyclosporine (ciclosporin). Methotrexate is effective in the treatment of human CD, but it is not widely used in companion animals.[43] In dogs it often causes diarrhea when used for the treatment of lymphoma, but it is better tolerated in cats. Cyclophosphamide has few advantages over azathioprine and is rarely used. However, cyclosporine therapy may show promise for the future, given its T-lymphocyte specific effects and efficacy in canine anal furunculosis.[44,45] Unfortunately, it is expensive. Preliminary studies in dogs with IBD have shown variable efficacy (E. Hall, personal observation 2005).[46]

Novel therapies

New drugs are being used increasingly for human IBD patients, in an attempt to target the underlying pathogenetic mechanisms.[47] Novel immunosuppressive drugs, monoclonal antibody therapy, cytokines, transcription factors, and dietary manipulation are being trialed in human IBD patients (Table 9.8) and may be suitable for small animals with IBD in the future.

Mycophenolate mofetil has been used to treat human IBD, although its efficacy is variable.[48] Drugs that target TNF-α, (e.g., thalidomide and oxpentifylline) may be suitable for the treatment of canine IBD, because of the importance of this

9

Table 9.8: Novel therapies for human IBD[10]

Drug therapy	Proposed mechanism of action
Anti-rejection drugs	
Tacrolimus	Immunosuppressant macrolide
Mycophenolate	Inhibits lymphocyte proliferation, decreases IFN-γ production
Leukotriene antagonist	
Zileuton	Orally active inhibitor of 5-lipoxygenase
Thromboxane synthesis inhibitors	
Ridogrel	Inhibits thromboxane A2 synthase
Picotamide	Inhibits thromboxane A2 synthase and antagonizes TxA2 receptors.
Inhibitors of TNF-α expression	
Oxpentifylline	Inhibits TNF-α expression
Thalidomide	Inhibits TNF-α and IL-12 expression, reduces leukocyte migration, impairs angiogenesis
Bone marrow and stem cell transplantation	
Bone marrow grafts	Unknown; possibly immunomodulation
Cytokine manipulation	
Systemic IL-10 therapy	Down-modulatory cytokine
IL-10 production by genetically engineered probiotic	Down-modulatory cytokine
Anti-IL-2 monoclonal antibody (MAb)	Counteracts pro-inflammatory effects
Anti-IL-2R (CD25) MAb	Inhibits IL-2 effects
Anti-IL-12 MAb	Counteracts pro-inflammatory effects
Anti-IL-11 MAb	Down-regulates TNF-α and IL-1β
Recombinant IFN-α therapy	Anti-inflammatory, antiviral?
Anti-IFN-γ MAb	Immunomodulatory effect on Th1 cells
Anti-TNF-α MAb	Counteracts pro-inflammatory effects, induces inflammatory cell apoptosis
Manipulation of endothelial cell adhesion molecules	
ICAM-1 (antisense oligonucleotide)	Reduces immune cell trafficking
Anti-α4β7 MAb	Reduces immune cell trafficking
Transcription factor blockade	
NF-κB anti-sense oligonucleotide	Inhibits pro-inflammatory cytokine expression
ICAM-1 antisense oligonucleotide	Reduces immune cell trafficking
Other immune system modulations	
Anti-CD4 antibodies	Immunomodulation
Intravenous immunoglobulin	Saturates Fc receptors; possibly other mechanisms
T-cell apheresis	Immunomodulation
Verapamil	Inhibitor of P-glycoprotein (P-gp) and may reduce IL-2 production and T-lymphocyte proliferation

cytokine in disease pathogenesis. However, anti TNF-α monoclonal antibody therapy will only be suitable for canine and feline IBD if species-specific monoclonal antibodies can be made available.[49–51]

While some of these newer therapies hold promise for the future, the current treatment of idiopathic IBD in dogs and cats remains based on immunosuppression and its prognosis remains guarded.

9.2.3 Lymphoplasmacytic enteritis (LPE)

Idiopathic LPE is the most common histopathological form of idiopathic IBD that can be associated with mild inflammation up to severe infiltration. LPE is characterized by a mucosal infiltrate of lymphocytes and plasma cells (Figure 9.8). However, there are numerous other causes of lymphoplasmacytic infiltration of the SI, which must be excluded before a diagnosis of LPE can be confirmed. Furthermore, although LPE is most commonly reported, the lymphoplasmacytic inflammation may affect other regions of the GI tract, causing lymphoplasmacytic gastritis and/or colitis.

Pathogenesis

Idiopathic LPE is believed to reflect immune dysregulation and loss of tolerance to the enteric flora (see above). Specific alterations in immune cell populations in canine LPE have been documented, including increases in LP T-cells (especially CD4+ cells), IgG+ plasma cells, macrophages, and granulocytes. In cats, there is a marked up-regulation of MHC class II molecule expression. Increased concentrations of acute phase proteins (e.g., C-reactive protein) and marked alterations in cytokine mRNA patterns have been documented in canine LPE.[30] Increased expression of Th1 (IL-2, IL-12, and IFN-γ), Th2 (IL-5), proinflammatory (TNF-α), and immunoregulatory (TGF-β) cytokines has been documented, indicating that the mucosal immune response is upregulated in canine LPE.

Clinical signs

Clinical signs of LPE include diarrhea and weight loss. Also, chronic vomiting may be the predominant sign, especially in cats. LPE typically affects older animals, and the disease is uncommon (but not impossible) in individuals less than two years of age. Severe LPE is especially prevalent in German Shepherds, Shar Peis, Norwegian Lundehunds, and pure-bred cats. A very severe form of LPE (immunoproliferative disease), which often causes PLE, is recognized in Basenjis (see 9.2.5).[52] PLE, with or without concurrent PLN, has also been described in Soft-coated Wheaten Terriers (see 9.2.6).[53]

Diagnosis

The approach to diagnosing LPE is the same as for any other form of IBD (see above). Histopathological changes do not only include the presence of increased numbers of lymphocytes and plasma cells, but also architectural disturbances (see Table 9.4). Complete or partial villus atrophy may be present, while villus fusion and crypt abscessation may be noted in severe cases. The distinction between severe LPE and alimentary lymphoma is sometimes difficult, and discrepancies may exist between endoscopic biopsies and post-mortem examinations of the same patient. It is likely that such discrepancies arise either because both conditions are present concurrently in the GI tract or because low-grade lymphoma is initially misdiagnosed. Clonality studies would help resolve this dilemma and aid in the recognition of low grade lymphoma, but are not widely available. Alternatively, it has been hypothesized that prolonged intestinal inflammation may ultimately transform into lymphoma.

Treatment and prognosis

The treatment of LPE is the same as for idiopathic IBD (see above). First-line treatment usually involves dietary manipulation. Metronidazole may be effective alone in mild cases, especially in cats, with immunosuppression being reserved for cases that do not respond or for very sick animals. The prognosis for severe LPE is guarded, but some patients respond dramatically and can ultimately be weaned off all medications. Other cases, however, require persistent low dosage maintenance therapy.

9.2.4 Lymphoplasmacytic colitis (LPC)

Some veterinary gastroenterologists claim that LPC is the most common form of IBD, and that it occurs in isolation from LPE. However, this is not generally accepted, and may reflect a historical perspective from before the advent of flexible endoscopy, when it was possible to obtain colonic biopsy specimens through a rigid endoscope, but impossible to obtain SI biopsy specimens except by surgical biopsy. Thus, the discrepancy may reflect failure to perform upper GI endoscopy at the same time as colonoscopy, failure to recognize LPE histologically, and failure to perform serum folate and cobalamin assays as a marker for occult SI disease in animals with predominantly large bowel diarrhea. However, since the use of endoscopy to obtain SI biopsies has become routine, it has been shown that isolated LPC only occurs occasionally.[2]

The treatment of LPC is similar to that of LPE, but includes dietary modification with fiber and the use of 5-ASA derivatives. Prolongation of remission has also been reported after introduction of a hypoallergenic exclusion diet.

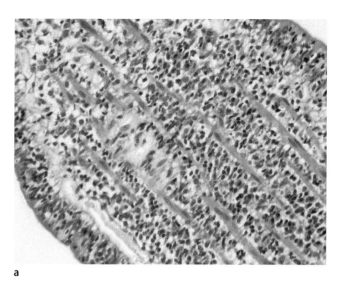
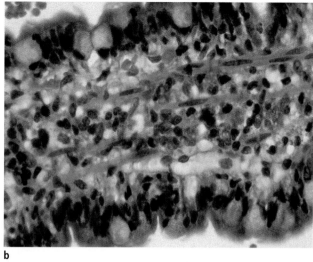

a   b

Figure 9.8:
Histological appearance of duodenal biopsy specimens taken from dogs with idiopathic IBD. **(a)** Lymphoplasmacytic enteritis (× 20) showing increased numbers of lymphocytes and plasma cells in the lamina propria. **(b)** Eosinophilic enteritis (× 40) showing a mixed population of inflammatory cells in the lamina propria of a villus, but with a significantly increased eosinophil component. (Stain: H&E).

9

9.2.5   Basenji enteropathy

Basenji enteropathy is a severe, hereditary form of LPE that has been well characterized in Basenjis, although the mode of inheritance remains unclear. It has been likened to immuno-proliferative small intestinal disease (IPSID) of humans as both conditions are associated with intense intestinal inflammation, but a typically associated gammopathy (alpha heavy-chain disease) and predisposition to lymphoma does not occur in Basenjis. The intestinal lesions in Basenjis are characterized by increases in CD4+ and CD8+ T-cells.[52,54]

Clinical signs

Lymphoplasmacytic gastritis, with hypergastrinemia and mucosal hyperplasia, causing vomiting may be seen in addition to the enteropathy. However, signs of chronic intractable diarrhea and emaciation are most common and usually progressive. PLE often occurs with consequent hypoalbuminemia, although edema and ascites are not common. In severe cases spontaneous intestinal perforation may occur.

Treatment

Treatment is generally unsuccessful, with progressive clinical signs and dogs dying within months of diagnosis. However, early aggressive combination treatment with prednisolone, antibiotics, and dietary modification (see above) may achieve remission in some cases.

9.2.6   Familial PLE and PLN in Soft-coated Wheaten Terriers

A unique clinical syndrome has been reported in Soft-coated Wheaten Terriers.[53] Affected dogs may present with signs of PLE, PLN, or both. A genetic basis is likely and, although the mode of inheritance is not yet clear, a common male ancestor has been identified.

Etiology and pathogenesis

The disease is probably immune-mediated, given the presence of inflammatory cell infiltration. Also, a potential role for food hypersensitivity has been suggested, since affected dogs have demonstrated adverse reactions during provocative food trials, and alterations in antigen-specific fecal IgE concentrations.[55,56] However, it can be speculated when considering the concurrence of intestinal and renal pathology, that this disease is not a failure of tolerance to bacterial antigens, but either a genetic defect in, or an autoimmune reaction to, a common protein/antigen. The brush border membrane of renal tubular cells resembles that of the enterocytes and even digestive enzymes, including the disaccharidases such as sucrase, are expressed in the kidney. Thus this condition is unlikely to remain in the idiopathic IBD category as more research is undertaken.

Clinical signs

Signs of PLE tend to develop at a younger age than PLN, and the clinical signs include vomiting, diarrhea, weight loss, and/or pleural and peritoneal effusions. Affected dogs are also at risk of thromboembolic disease.[57]

Diagnosis

Preliminary laboratory investigations, as in most dogs with PLE, demonstrate panhypoproteinemia and hypocholesterolemia. In contrast, hypoalbuminemia, hypercholesterolemia, proteinuria, and ultimately azotemia are seen with PLN. On histopathological examination of intestinal biopsies, there is evidence of intestinal inflammation, villus blunting, epithelial erosions, dilated lymphatics, and lipogranulomatous lymphangitis.

Treatment and prognosis

Treatment is similar to that described for general IBD (see above) including dietary modification and immunosuppression, but the prognosis is usually poor.

9.2.7 Eosinophilic enteritis (EE)

EE is reported to be the second most common form of IBD after LPE. It frequently involves the stomach (eosinophilic gastroenteritis, EGE), colon (eosinophilic enterocolitis, EEC), or both (eosinophilic gastroenterocolitis, EGEC). In addition, segmental EE has also been reported.[58] Histopathologically, variable mucosal architectural disturbances (e.g., villus atrophy) are present in conjunction with a mixed infiltrate of inflammatory cells with eosinophils predominating (Figure 9.8b). However, as with LPE, the diagnostic criteria vary between pathologists. The definition of EE may be based on subjective increases in mucosal eosinophil numbers despite increases in other inflammatory cells. More strict criteria require eosinophils to predominate in the LP. Other criteria include the presence of eosinophils between the epithelial cells of the villus and crypt, suggesting transepithelial migration. Nevertheless, there can be marked variation in the number of mucosal eosinophils in normal dogs and therefore this condition may be over-diagnosed.[12] As with other forms of IBD, a diagnosis of EE should only be made once other causes of eosinophilic infiltration have been eliminated. Parasitic and allergic diseases should always be considered as possible differential diagnoses.

Clinical signs

The condition can be seen in dogs and cats of any breed and age, although it is most common in younger adult animals. Boxers, German Shepherds, and Dobermans may be predisposed. EGE may also be associated with systemic eosinophilic disorders (i.e., hypereosinophilic syndrome) in both cats and dogs. The clinical signs reported depend on the area of the GI tract involved, and include vomiting, SI diarrhea, and LI diarrhea. Hematemesis, melena, or hematochezia may be seen as mucosal erosion and/or ulceration may occur more frequently in EE than in other forms of IBD. Severe EGE has rarely been associated with spontaneous perforation of the GI tract, but PLE and hypoproteinemia are commonly recognized.[59]

Pathogenesis

Eosinophil infiltration is likely to be the result of local and systemic production of cytokines and chemokines, such as IL-5 and members of the eotaxin family.[60] An eosinophilic mucosal infiltrate may be caused by dietary sensitivity, endoparasitism, or idiopathic EGE.

Diagnosis

The diagnosis of EGE is made by histopathological assessment of intestinal biopsies, and after exclusion of parasites and food allergy. Peripheral eosinophilia is neither pathognomonic for nor invariably present in EGE. It is probably more commonly seen in parasitism, hypoadrenocorticism, allergic cutaneous or respiratory disease, and mast cell neoplasia.

Treatment

Given that eosinophilic mucosal infiltrates may also be related to intestinal parasitism, empirical anthelmintic and antiprotozoal treatment is always advisable initially. If there is no response to treatment, a dietary trial with an exclusion diet should be instigated to eliminate the possibility of dietary sensitivity before considering immunosuppressive therapy. The prognosis for patients with idiopathic EGE is guarded, even with a good initial response to treatment, as recurrence is common.

9.2.8 Granulomatous enteritis

Granulomatous enteritis is an apparently rare form of IBD, and is characterized by mucosal infiltration with macrophages. The distribution of granulomata can be patchy. This condition is likely to be the same as regional enteritis in humans, where ileal granulomata have been reported.[61,62] In cats, a pyogranulomatous transmural inflammation has been associated with FIP infection. The condition in dogs does have some histological features common to human CD, but intestinal obstruction and fistula formation have not been noted. Conventional therapy for IBD (see above) is usually not effective and the prognosis is guarded, although a combination of surgical resection and anti-inflammatory treatment was reported to be successful in one case.[62]

9.2.9 Histiocytic ulcerative colitis (HUC)

This unusual form of IBD has been reported almost exclusively in Boxers but also sporadically in other breeds (see also 6.4.2.1). There are two reports of HUC in an ancestrally related breed, the French bulldog, and also recently HUC has been recorded in a Mastiff, an Alaskan Malamute, and a Doberman.[63] The disease is almost invariably restricted to the colon, although a case with SI involvement has also been observed (A. Boari, personal communication, 2004).

The colitis is characterized by accumulation of PAS-positive macrophages, although a mixed inflammatory response with T-cells and IgG plasma cells is usually present. The disease is rare and sporadic, and for many years it has been hypothesized that it is infectious in nature, although attempts at disease transmission have failed. However, recently the condition has been reported to be sensitive to enrofloxacin, again suggesting an infectious etiology.[37,38]

9.2.10 Proliferative enteritis

Proliferative enteritis is characterized by segmental mucosal hypertrophy of the intestine. It is most commonly seen in pigs, but a similar although very rare condition has been reported in dogs.[64] There may be an underlying infectious etiology and *Lawsonia intracellularis* infection has been implicated but not yet been proven. Other potential infectious causes include *Campylobacter* spp. or *Chlamydia*.

9

⚷ Key Facts

- IBD is a common cause of chronic vomiting and/or diarrhea in dogs and cats.
- Idiopathic IBD is diagnosed on the basis of histological evidence of inflammation and no identifiable underlying cause.
- The etiology of IBD is hypothesized to be a breakdown in mucosal tolerance to the normal enteric flora.
- Clinical signs of IBD reflect the type of inflammation, its anatomical site, its severity, and its chronicity.
- The mainstay of treatment of IBD is immunosuppression.

References

1. Hall EJ, German AJ. Diseases of the small intestine. In: Ettinger SJ, Feldman EC (eds.) *Textbook of Veterinary Internal Medicine*, 6th ed. Philadelphia, WB Saunders, 2005; 1332–1378.
2. Craven M, Simpson JW, Ridyard AE et al. Canine inflammatory bowel disease: retrospective analysis of diagnosis and outcome in 80 cases (1995–2002). *J Small Anim Pract* 2004; 45: 336–342.
3. Elson CO. Experimental models of intestinal inflammation: New insights into mechanisms of mucosal homeostasis. In: Ogra PL, Mestecky J, Lamm ME, Strober W, Bienenstock J, McGhee JR (eds.) *Mucosal Immunology*, 2nd ed. San Diego Ca, Academic Press, 1999; 1007–1034.
4. Karp LC, Targan SR. Ulcerative colitis: evidence for an updated hypothesis of disease pathogenesis. In: Ogra PL, Mestecky J, Lamm ME et al. (eds.), *Mucosal Immunology*, 2nd ed. San Diego Ca, Academic Press, 1999; 1047–1053.
5. Duchmann R, Zeitz M. Crohn's disease. In: Ogra PL, Mestecky J, Lamm ME et al. (eds.), *Mucosal Immunology*, 2nd ed. San Diego Ca, Academic Press, 1999; 1055–1080.
6. Hugot JP, Chamaillard M, Zouali H et al. Association of NOD2 leucine-rich repeat variants with susceptibility to Crohn's disease. *Nature* 2001; 411: 599–603.

7. Ogura Y, Bonen DK, Inohara N et al. A frameshift mutation in NOD2 associated with susceptibility to Crohn's disease. *Nature* 2001; 411: 603–606.
8. Johnston KL. Small intestinal bacterial overgrowth. *Vet Clin N Am Small Anim Pract* 1999; 29: 523–550.
9. Kelsall B, Strober W. Gut-associated lymphoid tissue antigen handling and T-lymphocyte responses. In: Ogra PL, Mestecky J, Lamm ME et al. (eds.), *Mucosal Immunology*, 2nd ed. San Diego Ca, Academic Press, 1999; 293–318.
10. German AJ, Hall EJ, Day MJ. Chronic intestinal inflammation and intestinal disease in dogs. *J Vet Intern Med* 2003; 17: 8–20.
11. German AJ, Hall EJ, Moore PF et al. Analysis of the distribution of lymphocytes expressing αβ and γδ T cell receptors, and the expression of mucosal addressin cell adhesion molecule-1 in the canine intestine. *J Comp Pathol* 1999; 121: 249–263.
12. German AJ, Hall EJ, Day MJ. Analysis of leucocyte subsets in the canine intestine. *J Comp Pathol* 1999; 120: 129–145.
13. Elwood CM, Hamblin AS, Batt RM. Quantitative and qualitative immunohistochemistry of T cell subsets and MHC class II expression in the canine intestine. *Vet Immunol Immunopathol* 1997; 58: 195–207.

14. Waly N, Gruffydd-Jones TJ, Stokes CR et al. The distribution of leucocyte subsets in the small intestine of normal cats. *J Comp Pathol* 2001; 124: 172–182.

15. Mosmann TR, Cherwinski H, Bond MW et al. Two types of murine helper T-cell clones. I. Definition according to profiles of lymphokine activities and secreted proteins. *J Immunol* 1986; 136: 2348–2357.

16. Groux H, OGarra A, Bigler M et al. A CD4+ T-cell inhibits antigen-specific T cell responses and prevents colitis. *Nature* 1997; 389: 737–742.

17. German AJ, Bland PW, Hall EJ et al. Expression of major histocompatibility complex class II antigens in the canine intestine. *Vet Immunol Immunopathol* 1998; 61: 171–180.

18. Mowat AM, Weiner HL. Oral tolerance: physiological basis and clinical applications. In: Ogra PL, Mestecky J, Lamm ME et al. (eds.) *Mucosal Immunology*, 2nd ed. San Diego Ca, Academic Press, 1999; 587–618.

19. Matzinger P. Tolerance, danger and the extended family. *Ann Rev Immunol* 1994; 12: 991–1045.

20. Madsen KL, Doyle JS, Jewell LD et al. Lactobacillus species prevents colitis in interleukin 10 gene-deficient mice. *Gastroenterology* 1999; 116: 1107–1114.

21. Duchmann R, Kaiser I, Hermann E et al. Tolerance exists towards resident intestinal flora but is broken in active inflammatory bowel disease (IBD). *Clin Exp Immunol* 1995; 102: 448–455.

22. Weiss DJ, Gagne JM, Armstrong PJ. Relationship between inflammatory hepatic disease and inflammatory bowel disease, pancreatitis, and nephritis in cats. *J Am Vet Med Assoc* 1996; 209: 1114–1116.

23. Jergens AE. Inflammatory bowel disease – current perspectives. *Vet Clin N Am Small Anim Pract* 1999; 29: 501–521.

24. Morgan LW, McConnell J. Cobalamin deficiency associated with erythroblastic anemia and methylmalonic aciduria in a Border Collie. *J Am Anim Hosp Assoc* 1999; 35: 392–395.

25. Baez JL, Hendrick MJ, Walker LM et al. Radiographic, ultrasonographic, and endoscopic findings in cats with inflammatory bowel disease of the stomach and small intestine: 33 cases (1990–1997). *J Am Vet Med Assoc* 1999; 215: 349–354.

26. Goggin JM, Biller DS, Debey BM et al. Ultrasonographic measurement of gastrointestinal wall thickness and the ultrasonographic appearance of the ileocolic region in healthy cats. *J Am Anim Hosp Assoc* 2000; 36: 224–228.

27. Rudorf H, O'Brien R, Barr FJ et al. Ultrasonographic evaluation of the small intestinal wall thickness in dogs with inflammatory bowel disease from the UK. *J Small Anim Pract*, in press

28. Willard MD, Lovering SL, Cohen ND et al. Quality of tissue specimens obtained endoscopically from the duodenum of dogs and cats. *J Am Vet Med Assoc* 2001; 219: 474–479.

29. Willard MD, Jergens AE, Duncan RB et al. Interobserver variation among histopathologic evaluations of intestinal tissues from dogs and cats. *J Am Vet Med Assoc* 2002; 220: 1177–1182.

30. German AJ, Helps CR, Hall EJ et al. Cytokine mRNA expression in mucosal biopsies from German Shepherd dogs with small intestinal enteropathies. *Dig Dis Sci* 2000; 45: 7–17.

31. Vernau WM, Moore PF. An immunophenotypic study of canine leukemias and preliminary assessment of clonality by polymerase chain reaction. *Vet Immunol Immunopathol* 1999; 69: 145–164.

32. Jergens AE, Schreiner CA, Frank DE et al. A scoring index for disease activity in canine inflammatory bowel disease. *J Vet Intern Med* 2003; 17: 291–297.

33. Hawthorne AB, Daneshmend TK, Hawkey CJ et al. Treatment of ulcerative colitis with fish oil supplementation: a prospective 12 month randomised controlled trial. *Gut* 1992; 33: 922–928.

34. Belluzzi A, Brignola C, Campieri M et al. Effect of an enteric-coated fish-oil preparation on relapses in Crohn's disease. *N Engl J Med* 1996; 334: 1557–1560.

35. Wagner RD, Warner T, Roberts L et al. Colonization of congenitally immunodeficient mice with probiotic bacteria. *Infect Immunity* 1997; 65: 3345–3351.

36. Mitsuyama K, Toyobaga M, Sata M. Intestinal microflora as a therapeutic target in inflammatory bowel disease. *J Gastroenterol* 2002; 37 suppl. 14: 73–77.

37. Hostutler RA, Luria BJ, Johnson SE et al. Antibiotic-responsive histiocytic ulcerative colitis in 9 dogs. *J Vet Intern Med* 2004; 18: 499–504.

38. Davies DR, O'Hara AJ, Irwin PJ et al. Successful management of histiocytic ulcerative colitis with enrofloxacin in two Boxer dogs. *Aust Vet J* 2004; 82: 58–61.

39. Travis S. Recent advances in immunomodulation in the treatment of inflammatory bowel disease. *Eur J Gastroenterol Hepatol* 2003; 15: 215–218.

40. Stewart A. The use of a novel formulation of budesonide as an improved treatment over prednisone for inflammatory bowel disease. *Proceedings of the 15th ACVIM Forum*, 1997; p. 662 (abstract).

41. Tumulty JW, Broussard JD, Steiner JM et al. Clinical effects of short-term oral budesonide on the hypothalamic-pituitary-adrenal axis in dogs with inflammatory bowel disease (IBD). *J Am Anim Hosp Assoc* 2004; 40: 120–123.

42. Salavaggione OE, Kidd L, Prondzinski JL et al. Canine red blood cell thiopurine S-methyltransferase: companion animal pharmacogenetics. *Pharmacogenetics* 2002; 12: 713–724.

43. Fraser AG. Methotrexate: first-line or second-line immunomodulator? *Eur J Gastroenterol Hepatol* 2003; 15: 225–231.

44. Sandborn WJ. Cyclosporine therapy for inflammatory bowel disease – definitive answers and remaining questions. *Gastroenterology* 1995; 109: 1001–1003.

45. Hawthorne AB. Ciclosporin and refractory colitis. *Eur J Gastroenterol Hepatol* 2003; 15: 239–244.

46. Allenspach K, Rufenacht S, Sauter S. et al. Pharmacokinetics and clinical efficacy of cyclosporine treatment of dogs with steroid refractory inflammatory bowel disease. *J Vet Intern Med* 2006; 20: 239–244.

47. Forbes A. Alternative immunomodulators. *Eur J Gastroenterol Hepatol* 2003; 15: 245–248.

48. Neurath MF, Wanitschke R, Peters M et al. Randomised trial of mycophenolate mofetil versus azathioprine for treatment of chronic active Crohn's disease. *Gut* 1999; 44: 625–628.

49. Ehrenpreis ED, Kane SV, Cohen LB et al. Thalidomide therapy for patients with refractory Crohn's disease: an open-label trial. *Gastroenterology* 1999; 117: 1271–1277.

50. Bauditz J, Haemling J, Ortner M et al. Treatment with tumour necrosis factor inhibitor oxpentifylline does not improve corticosteroid dependent chronic active Crohn's disease. *Gut* 1997; 40: 470–474.

51. D'Haens G, Van Deventer S, Van Hogezand R et al. Endoscopic and histological healing with infliximab anti-tumor necrosis factor antibodies in Crohn's disease: A European multicenter trial. *Gastroenterology* 1999; 116: 1029–1034.

52. Breitschwerdt EB, Halliwell WH, Foley CW et al. A hereditary diarrhetic syndrome in the Basenji characterized by malabsorption, protein losing enteropathy and hypergammaglobulinemia. *J Am Anim Hosp Assoc* 1980; 16: 551–560.

53. Littman MP, Giger U. Familial protein losing enteropathy (PLE) and/or protein losing nephropathy (PLN) in Soft-coated Wheaten Terriers (SCWT); 222 cases (1983–1997). *J Vet Intern Med* 2000; 14: 68–80.

54. Lothrop Jr CD et al. Immunological characterization of intestinal lesions in Basenji dogs with inflammatory bowel disease. *Proceedings of the 15th ACVIM Forum*, 1997; 662 (abstract).

55. Vaden SL, Sellon RK, Melgarejo LT et al. Evaluation of intestinal permeability and gluten sensitivity in Soft-coated Wheaten Terriers with familial protein-losing enteropathy, protein-losing nephropathy, or both. *Am J Vet Res* 2000; 61: 518–524.
56. Vaden SL, Hammerberg B, Davenport DJ et al. Food hypersensitivity reactions in Soft-coated Wheaten Terriers with protein-losing enteropathy or protein-losing nephropathy or both: gastroscopic food sensitivity testing, dietary provocation, and fecal immunoglobulin E. *J Vet Intern Med* 2000; 14: 60–67.
57. Kovacevic A, Lang J, Lombardi CW. Thrombosis of the pulmonary trunk in a Soft-coated Wheaten Terrier as a complication of a protein-losing nephropathy; a case report. *Kleintierpraxis* 2002; 47: 549–552.
58. Regnier A, Delverdier M, Dossin O. Segmental eosinophilic enteritis mimicking intestinal tumors in a dog. *Canine Pract* 1996; 21: 25–29.
59. Van der Gaag I, Happé RP, Wolvekamp WTC. Eosinophilic enteritis complicated by partial ruptures and a perforation of the small intestine in a dog. *J Small Anim Pract* 1983; 24: 575–581.
60. Baggiolini M. Chemokines and leucocyte traffic. *Nature* 1998; 392: 565–568.
61. Bright RM, Jenkins C, DeNovo R et al. Chronic diarrhea in a dog with regional granulomatous enteritis. *J Small Anim Pract* 1994; 35: 423–426.
62. Lewis DC. Successful treatment of regional enteritis in a dog. *J Am Anim Hosp Assoc* 1995; 31: 170–173.
63. Stokes JE, Kruger JM, Mullaney T et al. Histiocytic ulcerative colitis in three non-Boxer dogs. *J Am Anim Hosp Assoc* 2001; 37: 461–465.
64. Cooper DM, Gebhart CJ. Comparative aspects of proliferative enteritis. *J Am Vet Med Assoc* 1998; 212: 1446–1451.

9.3 Gastrointestinal Lymphoma

KEITH P. RICHTER

9.3.1 Feline gastrointestinal lymphoma

Epidemiology

Lymphoma is the most frequently diagnosed canine and feline cancer, and the most common GI neoplasm in both dogs and cats.[1–5] There are several anatomical locations for lymphoma and the GI tract is regarded by some authors as the most common site in the cat.[6–10] Gastrointestinal tract lymphoma accounts for 32% to 72% of total lymphoma cases. However, other forms of lymphoma (i.e., leukemic, mediastinal, and multicentric) also have each been reported to be the most common form of lymphoma in cats by other authors.[11–14] These discrepancies in the reported incidence of the various forms of lymphoma may be due to the differences in classification schemes used, a change in incidence over time, differences in FeLV subtypes in various geographical areas, and a decreased incidence of non-gastrointestinal forms since the introduction of a FeLV vaccine.[15] The apparent increase in the proportion of GI location over time has been elucidated by comparing incidences in the same institutions over different time periods. For example, in the New England area, the proportion of lymphomas in cats that were classified as GI lymphomas increased from 8% in 1979, to 18% in 1983, and 32% in 1996.[9,11,16] Likewise, in the New York City area, the proportion of GI lymphomas in cats increased from 27% in 1989 to 72% in 1995.[8,14]

The association between FeLV and lymphoma in cats is well established. The incidence of FeLV antigenemia in cats with GI lymphoma ranges from 0% to 38%.[10,13,17–21] However, such estimation of FeLV infection rate is significantly influenced by the method of testing. Underestimation of FeLV incidence with immunohistochemistry (IHC) versus PCR has been suggested.[13] In one study, PCR testing detected FeLV viral nucleic acid sequences in up to 63% of cats with GI lymphoma, whereas only 38% of cats were positive using IHC.[13] Generally, cats with leukemia or mediastinal lymphoma tend to be young and FeLV positive, while those with GI lymphoma are typically older and FeLV negative.[6,10,16,17,20,21] An association between lymphoma and FIV has also been proposed. Cats infected with FIV, FeLV, or both were determined to have 5.6, 62.1, and 77.3 times the relative risk of developing lymphoma respectively, when compared to retrovirus-negative cats.[22]

Gross pathological findings

The gross appearance of feline GI lymphoma varies with the specific anatomical location. Many segments of the GI tract, including the liver, may be involved. There can be a focal mass or diffuse infiltration. In some cases, especially with low-grade lymphocytic lymphoma, the gross appearance may be normal. When a focal alimentary tract mass is present, there is usually transmural thickening, with or without mucosal ulceration

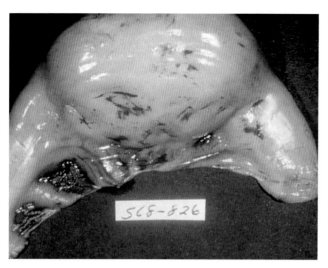

Figure 9.9:
Intestinal lymphoma. This figure shows a solitary mass located in the small intestine of a cat, which was diagnosed as a high-grade lymphoma on histopathology.

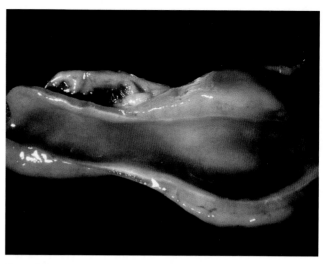

Figure 9.10:
Intestinal lymphoma. This figure shows the cut surface of the solitary mass shown in Figure 9.9.

9

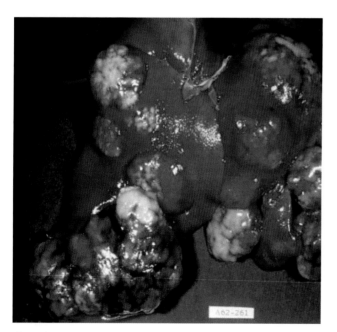

Figure 9.11:
Hepatic lymphoma. Multifocal hepatic nodules in a cat with high-grade hepatic lymphoma.

(Figures 9.9 and 9.10). Mural thickening is often eccentric, resulting in preservation of the lumen, though a functional obstruction may develop (Figures 9.9 and 9.10). This contrasts with intestinal carcinoma, which frequently results in a mechanical obstruction due to a decreased luminal diameter, often appearing as a "napkin ring". With diffuse infiltration, the intestinal wall may be visibly and/or palpably thickened. Mesenteric lymphadenopathy is usually overt, grossly or on ultrasonographic examination. Intussusception can develop secondary to intestinal lymphoma, with the jejunum being the most common location. In one study, lymphoma was associated with intussusception in seven of twenty cats (35%).[23]

Hepatic involvement can have a variable appearance. In some cases, the liver appears to be grossly normal, whereas in others there may be an enhanced lobular pattern, a mottled appearance, or a gross nodular appearance (Figure 9.11).

In summary, the appearance of lymphoma is extremely variable in all the regions of the GI tract. In light of how commonly this neoplasm develops in cats, lymphoma should be considered as a differential diagnosis in patients with normal or grossly abnormal organ appearance.

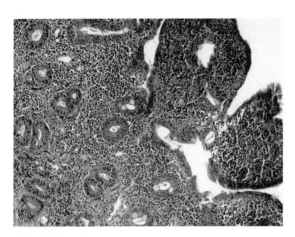

Figure 9.12:
Intestinal lymphoma. This image shows duodenal mucosa from a 14-year-old female Maine Coon cat presented for chronic diarrhea and weight loss. There is severe villous blunting and the lamina propria is infiltrated with monomorphic lymphocytes with large nuclei, typical of feline alimentary lymphoma. (H&E, magnification 200×; image courtesy of Dr. Thomas Bilzer, University of Düsseldorf, Germany.)

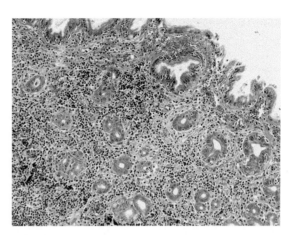

Figure 9.13:
Inflammatory bowel disease. This image shows duodenal mucosa from a 6-year-old female English Setter with chronic diarrhea. The villi are blunted, there are moderate epithelial lesions, and the propria is infiltrated severely by lymphocytes and plasma cells, intermingled with polymorphic granulocytes. The dog was diagnosed with IBD and was successfully managed for a period of more than 1 year by corticosteroid administration. (H&E, magnification 200×; image courtesy of Dr. Thomas Bilzer, University of Düsseldorf, Germany)

9

Histopathology and immunohistochemistry

There are different grades of GI lymphoma, commonly referred to as low-grade (lymphocytic or small cell), high-grade (lymphoblastic, immunoblastic, or large cell), and intermediate grade.[24] Less common descriptions, such as large granular lymphocytic lymphoma also exist.[25–28] Most published reports are of either undetermined grade or predominately high-grade lymphomas, although more recently low-grade lymphocytic lymphoma was described in a large case series.[17,20,21] In the latter study, 50 of 67 cats (75%) diagnosed with GI lymphoma had low-grade, lymphocytic lymphoma. The criteria used to classify lymphoma as lymphocytic have been described.[17] However, these criteria have recently been questioned based on the difficulty in interpreting small endoscopic biopsies, the difference in opinion between pathologists, and a lack of characterization using immunohistochemical methods.[29] Consequently, further studies are needed to define specific criteria for differentiating lymphocytic lymphoma, lymphocytic inflammation, and T-cell infiltrative disease, and to correlate such classifications with clinical outcome. While it is customary to consider that there is a continuum from IBD to lymphoma, there is little supporting data for this notion (Figures 9.12, 9.13, and 9.14).

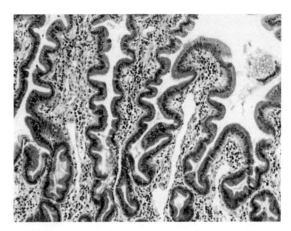

Figure 9.14:
Normal intestinal mucosa. Duodenal mucosa from a healthy 7-year-old female Labrador Retriever showing normal villi and mucosal texture and a mild lymphoplasmacytic infiltration of the propria. (H&E, magnification 200×; image courtesy of Dr. Thomas Bilzer, University of Düsseldorf, Germany)

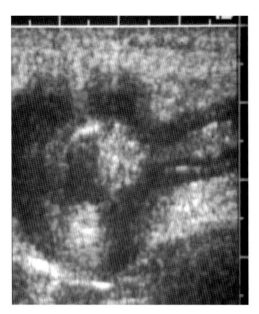

Figure 9.15:
Small intestinal mass. This figure shows an ultrasonographic image of a focal small intestinal mass in a cat, which was diagnosed as lymphoma.

Recently, IHC has been used to better characterize feline lymphoma. Characterization of the normal feline small intestinal diffuse mucosal associated lymphoid tissue (MALT) has been described in SPF cats, and immunophenotyping has been applied to feline lymphomas.[24,29–35] In some studies, intestinal lymphomas were more likely to be of B-cell rather than of T-cell phenotype, whereas other studies describe a predominantly T-cell phenotype.[21,24,29,33] Also, in a limited number of studies, the immunophenotype did not appear to correlate with response to chemotherapy treatment or survival.[10,21,36] Thus, further study is necessary to determine the clinical value of immunophenotyping.

Clinical findings

Signalment

Male cats appear to be predisposed to GI lymphoma.[6,17,20,21] While a breed predilection is not apparent, most cats are DSH.[17,18,20,21] The reported median age ranges from 9 to 13 years in different studies, with an age range spanning from 1 to 18 years.[6,12,17–21]

Clinical signs and physical examination findings

Irrespective of the grade of GI lymphoma, the clinical signs include weight loss, anorexia, vomiting, diarrhea, lethargy, and polydipsia/polyuria. Importantly, many cats have minimal or no vomiting and/or diarrhea, with anorexia, weight loss, or both as the only historical findings.[17,20] Therefore, when confronted with these signs in a geriatric cat with an otherwise unrewarding initial evaluation, GI lymphoma should be considered as a differential diagnosis. Physical examination findings may include poor body condition, thickened intestinal loops, and/or a palpable abdominal mass. The presence of an abdominal mass is more suggestive of high-grade lymphoma.[17,20] Notably, many cats may have a normal abdominal palpation.

Ancillary test findings

Laboratory findings are generally non-contributory, with mild anemia and/or hypoalbuminemia most commonly seen. Abnormalities on plain abdominal and thoracic radiographs are also uncommon and usually nonspecific. An abdominal ultrasound examination may be helpful in many cases, and is considered more sensitive than radiography.[37,38] Lesions can be nodular (focal or multifocal) or diffuse.[37] While the most common ultrasonographic abnormality observed is thickening of the gastric or intestinal wall, other important findings include loss of normal intestinal wall layering, a localized mass effect associated with the intestine (Figure 9.15), decreased intestinal wall echogenicity, regional hypomotility, regional lymphadenopathy, and ascites.[18,37,38] Endoscopy can be an effective tool for diagnosing GI mucosal lymphoma in people, as well as in dogs and cats, when involved areas are within the endoscopic retrieval zones.[17,39,40] In one study, endoscopy was performed in 61 of 67 cats with GI lymphoma, and was the main ancillary test leading to the definitive diagnosis, with a histological diagnosis reached in 56 cases.[17] Most gross endoscopic findings are nonspecific, with considerable overlap with IBD and other GI diseases. In many cases the endoscopic appearance can be grossly normal.

Treatment (Table 9.9)

Reports of treatment strategies for feline GI lymphoma are fairly limited and only some of these reports give specific results for cats with GI lymphoma, but rather address the treatment of feline lymphoma in general.[8,11,14,17,19–21,36] In addition, the outcome in different forms of GI lymphoma remains ill-defined because many reports do not describe the histological grades or the results of complete anatomical staging, and different combinations of chemotherapeutic agents were used in different studies.

Table 9.9: Summary of reports describing the treatment of feline gastrointestinal lymphoma

Primary author	Number of cats	Number (and %) with GI involvement	Grade	Treatment protocol	Percent CR	Median remission duration	Median survival of those in CR	Overall median survival Time
Cotter[11]	7	7 (100)	NR	C,V,P	86	19 weeks	NR	26 weeks
Jeglum[19]	14	14 (100)	NR	C,V,M	NR	NR	NR	12 weeks
Mooney[14]	103	28 (27)	NR	C,V,P,L	62	NR	7 months	NR
Mauldin[8]	132	95 (72)	NR	C,V,P,D,L,M	67	21weeks	NR	30 weeks
Zwahlen[21]	21	21 (100)	NR	C,V,P,D,L,M	38	20 weeks	41.5 weeks	40 weeks
Malik[36]	60	14 (23)	NR	C,V,P,D,L,M	80	NR	27 weeks	17 weeks
Mahony[20]	28	28 (100)	89% HG, 11% LG	C,V,P	32	NR	NR	7 weeks
Fondacaro[17]	29	29 (100)	100% LG	P,Cl	69	20.5 months	22.8 months	17 months
Fondacaro[17]	11	11 (100)	100% HG	C,V,P or C,V,P,L,D	18	18 months	18 months	11 weeks

CR = complete remission; NR = not reported; C = cyclophosphamide; V = vincristine; P = prednisone; M = methotrexate; L = L-asparaginase; D = doxorubicin; Cl = chlorambucil; HG = high grade; LG = low grade.

Cotter et al. described seven cats with GI lymphoma treated with cyclophosphamide, vincristine, and prednisone (CVP).[11] Six cats achieved complete remission with a median remission duration of 19 weeks, and a median survival time of 26 weeks. Jeglum et al. reported 14 cats with GI lymphoma treated with cyclophosphamide, vincristine, and methotrexate.[19] These cats had a median survival time of 12 weeks. Mooney et al. described 103 cats with lymphoma, of which 28 (27%) had GI lesions.[14] These were treated with CVP plus L-asparaginase and methotrexate, with 62% achieving a complete remission for a median survival time of 7 months. Cats achieving partial and no remission had median survival times of 2.5 and 1.5 months, respectively. The specific response of cats with GI lymphoma was, however, not described. At the same institution, Mauldin et al. described 132 cats, of which 95 (72%) had a GI lesion.[8] These cats were treated with CVP plus doxorubicin, methotrexate, and L-asparaginase. Sixty seven percent achieved a complete remission, with a 21-week disease-free interval. The overall median survival time was 30 weeks. Though the specific responses of those cats with GI lesions were not described, anatomical location was not found to be a prognostic factor in this study. Zwahlen et al. described 21 cats with GI lymphoma of unknown grade, treated with a similar protocol (CVP plus doxorubicin, L-asparaginase, and methotrexate).[21] Of these cats, 38% achieved a complete remission, 57% a partial remission, and 5% had stable or progressive disease. The median disease-free interval was 20 weeks, and the median survival time 40 weeks. For those achieving a complete remission, the disease-free interval was 40 weeks, but the median survival was only 41.5 weeks. Sixty cats with lymphoma in Australia treated with a similar protocol achieved a median survival period of 17 weeks, and of 48 cats achieving a complete remission, the median survival was 27 weeks.[36] Of these 48 cats, only 14 had GI lesions. Four of the fourteen cats

(29%) survived for longer than one year. Mahony et al. described 28 cats, 25 of whom had high-grade GI lymphoma, treated with CVP.[20] The overall median survival time was only 7 weeks, whereas the median disease-free interval of those achieving a complete remission (32%) was 30 weeks. These findings are in agreement with those of Fondacaro et al., who described 11 cats with high-grade lymphoma treated with CVP or CVP with doxorubicin and L-asparaginase, where only 18% achieved a complete remission (both cats that responded received doxorubicin), with a median survival of 11 weeks.[17] Other chemotherapy agents have not been extensively studied in cats with GI lymphoma. In a phase 1 trial of the oral alkylating agent lomustine (CCNU), two of six cats with GI lymphoma had only a partial response.[41]

These findings contrast with those of cats having low-grade lymphoma. Fondacaro et al. described 50 cats with low-grade GI lymphoma, 36 of which were treated with chemotherapy.[17] Twenty-nine cats with lymphocytic lymphoma were treated with prednisone (10 mg/cat/day) and high-dose pulse chlorambucil (Leukeran®; 15 mg/m² of body surface area, orally, once daily for 4 days, repeated every 3 weeks). Sixty-nine percent of the cats achieved a complete clinical remission, with a median disease-free interval for cats that achieved complete remission of 20.5 months (range: 5.8–49.0 months). The median survival time for all cats was 17 months (range: 0.3–50.0 months), with a median survival time of 22.8 months for cats that achieved complete remission (range: 10.0–50.0 months). Twelve of the twenty cats that achieved a complete remission were "rescued" with cyclophosphamide at a dosage of 225 mg/m² of body surface area, orally, every three weeks. These cats had a median disease-free interval of 24 months and a median survival time of 29 months. Seven cats were alive at the time of data collection; all but one of these cats had received a rescue treatment with cyclophosphamide. Adverse reactions to chlorambucil or cyclophosphamide were rare, but included vomiting, diarrhea, anorexia, lethargy, and neutropenia. None of the affected cats required hospitalization or discontinuation of therapy.

Some conclusions and recommendations can be made from these studies. In general, response to chemotherapy for high-grade GI lymphoma is poor, whereas the clinical response for low-grade lymphoma is good. For cats with high-grade GI lymphoma, combining doxorubicin with other agents in a multi-agent protocol, such as CVP and L-asparaginase is associated with longer remission and survival times, when compared with single-agent doxorubicin or CVP alone. For cats with low-grade lymphoma, excellent results can be achieved with oral prednisone and high-dose pulse chlorambucil therapy.[17] However, it is unknown whether these cats would do better with a more aggressive multi-agent protocol. Lastly, chemotherapy is generally well tolerated by cats. Self-limiting anorexia, vomiting, diarrhea, and myelosuppression may be observed in some patients. It may also be difficult to distinguish some of these chemotherapy-related side effects from active or progressive lymphoma.

The role of surgery in the treatment of GI lymphoma has been discussed previously.[17,20,21,36] These studies have shown either no effect or a negative effect of surgical intervention on disease-free interval and survival. However, this effect is most likely not due to the surgical intervention itself, but is more likely due to the fact that cats requiring surgery (i.e., those with GI obstruction) have shorter survival periods due to the severity of their disease. The main indications for surgery are partial or complete intestinal obstruction, intestinal perforation, or to obtain biopsy specimens for a definitive diagnosis.

It is believed that some patients with transmural focal disease are at risk for perforation when treated with cytotoxic chemotherapy that induces a rapid response. Surgery may result in dehiscence at intestinal anastomosis sites, and may require a delay in the initiation of chemotherapy to allow proper wound healing. Following resection of a focal GI or mesenteric mass, chemotherapy is still warranted since most cases have diffuse or multifocal microscopic involvement and lymphoma can be considered a systemic disease in most cases.

Prognostic factors

Few prognostic factors have been described for cats with GI lymphoma. Fondacaro et al. reported that histological grade was a strong indicator of outcome.[17] Compared to cats with high-grade lymphoma treated with a multi-agent chemotherapy regimen, cats with low-grade lymphoma treated with oral prednisone and chlorambucil had a significantly better remission rate (69% versus 18%) and survival time (17.0 months

versus 2.7 months). Since other studies did not compare low-grade and high-grade lymphomas, this finding has not been further verified. Low-grade and high-grade GI lymphomas in many ways represent different disease entities, and must be considered separately. Thus, statements about feline GI lymphoma may in some cases be overly generalized.

In the majority of studies, the most significant prognostic indicator for a positive outcome was initial response to chemotherapy.[7,8,10,14,17,20,21,36] In general, cats that survive the initial induction period and achieve remission generally also have a better long-term outcome. Though this may seem intuitively obvious, it may give clinicians and owners encouragement to continue chemotherapy treatment in cats that attain a complete remission. Otherwise there is no consistent association with any patient or tumor characteristic that is predictive of outcome (including sex, immunophenotype, clinical stage, age, and body weight). In most recent studies, FeLV virus antigenemia was not found to be a negative prognostic factor.[8,20,21,36] Some studies also showed little benefit of an exhaustive "staging evaluation", since very few factors have enough of an impact on prognosis to make their determination helpful.[8,20,21,36]

Recently, investigators have looked at molecular markers as prognostic factors. However, argyrophilic nucleolar organizer region (AgNOR) frequency and proliferating cell nuclear antigen labeling index (PCNA-LI) showed no correlation with response to chemotherapy or survival.[10,42] Similarly, the immunophenotype of tumor cells also does not seem to correlate with outcome in cats.[10,21,36] This is in contrast to dogs, where a T-cell phenotype has long been recognized as a negative prognostic factor for response to therapy and survival. Concentration of serum alpha$_1$-acid glycoprotein, an acute phase protein, has recently been evaluated in cats with lymphoma, and was not shown to be useful in predicting the response to treatment or survival.[43] The limitations of many studies published include incomplete staging, inconsistent grading, multiple non-sampled GI locations, lack of prospective randomization to different chemotherapy protocols, lack of control (untreated) patients, and lack of confirmation of remission through follow-up biopsies. Prospective, controlled, and randomized cohort studies with large numbers of cats aimed at investigating the response of each grade of GI lymphoma to single agent chemotherapeutic regimens seem warranted. Furthermore, additional studies to correlate clinical outcome with immunophenotyping and molecular markers are needed.

9.3.2 Canine gastrointestinal lymphoma

Gastrointestinal lymphoma in the dog appears to be less common than in the cat and much less has been published about it.[44–46] Gastrointestinal lymphoma accounts for approximately 5–20% of all canine lymphomas and is the most common extranodal form.[44–46] The majority of canine GI lymphomas are primary, with involvement in descending order of frequency of the small intestine, liver, regional lymph nodes, stomach, and colon.[44,45] Occasionally, the GI tract can be involved concurrently with thoracic or peripheral sites as a manifestation of multicentric disease.[44] A wide range of ages and breeds is affected.[44,45] In two studies, the age ranged from 1.5 to 14.7 years (means 6.7 and 7.7 years).[44,45] In one of these studies, 90% of dogs were male, while 48% were male in the other study.[44,45] Reported clinical signs in descending order of frequency were depression, vomiting, anorexia, diarrhea, weight loss, icterus, and tenesmus.[44] Vomiting and diarrhea often occur together, and blood is visibly present in approximately 50% of cases.[44] Generally, clinical signs are chronic and progressive, with acute exacerbations occasionally seen. The physical examination findings may include poor body condition, the presence of an abdominal mass, abdominal pain, and hepatomegaly. Laboratory findings commonly reflect hepatic involvement when present, including increases in serum hepatic enzyme activities and serum bilirubin concentration. Other laboratory findings are usually nonspecific, with anemia and hypoalbuminemia being the most common abnormalities (each occurring in approximately 30% of dogs).[44] Plain abdominal radiographs may reveal hepatosplenomegaly and an abdominal mass if present.[44] Upper GI barium series may reveal mucosal irregularities, luminal filling defects, and irregular wall thickening, suggesting infiltrative disease.[44] Ultrasonography may demonstrate an abdominal mass, gastric or intestinal wall thickening, ascites (suggesting peritonitis), and/or hepatic abnormalities.

Gross pathological findings are variable and are dependent on organ involvement. Most commonly, there are soft to firm cream-colored masses in the submucosa, which may extend into the lumen and transmurally into the serosa.[45] Some cases may also show diffuse disease. In one series of 15 cases, all the tumors originated from the submucosa, with most of the lesions consisting of diffuse infiltrates of non-cleaved cells.[44] In this case series, lymphoplasmacytic inflammation was common both adjacent to as well as distant from the areas of lymphoma.[44] The junctional region between neoplastic and non-neoplastic tissue was not sharply demarcated, and often an inflamed mucosa was found to overlay a submucosal region of lymphoma.[44] Thus, there is a risk of missing the diagnosis of lymphoma and erroneously diagnosing IBD when biopsies are obtained endoscopically. In another study, epitheliotropism was common, with neoplastic lymphocytes infiltrating the superficial mucosal epithelium.[45] In this study, immunohistochemical staining determined that most canine GI lymphomas are primarily of T-cell origin.[45]

Therapy for canine GI lymphoma is generally unrewarding. Since several segments of the GI tract are usually involved, surgical therapy alone is rarely effective as the sole treatment. As with other forms of lymphoma, a multi-agent chemotherapy protocol that incorporates doxorubicin is most effective, though only a small percentage of dogs with a GI lymphoma achieve a complete and/or durable remission with chemotherapy.[44,46]

⚷ Key Facts

- Gastrointestinal lymphoma is a common cause of anorexia and weight loss in older cats, with or without vomiting and/or diarrhea.
- Most cats with GI lymphoma are FeLV and FIV negative.
- Low-grade gastrointestinal lymphoma in cats may be more common than previously thought and appears to be more responsive to chemotherapy than high-grade lymphoma.
- The most significant prognostic indicator for gastrointestinal lymphoma in cats is the initial response to chemotherapy, with patients that survive the initial induction period generally achieving long-term remission.
- Gastrointestinal lymphoma in the dog may originate from the submucosa, which can make endoscopic diagnosis more difficult.
- Gastrointestinal lymphoma in the dog often responds poorly or transiently to chemotherapy treatment.

9

References

1. Brodey RS. Alimentary tract neoplasms in the cat: A clinicopathologic survey of 46 cases. *Am J Vet Res* 1966; 27 (116): 74–80.
2. Loupal VG, Pfeil C. Tumoren im Darmtrakt der Katze unter besonderer Berücksichtigung der nicht-hämatopoetischen Geschwülste. *Berl Münch Tierärztl Wschr* 1984; 97: 208–213.
3. Ogilvie GK, Moore AS. Lymphoma in cats. *Managing the Veterinary Cancer Patient*. Trenton, Veterinary Learning Systems, 1995; 249–259.
4. Schmidt RE, Langham RF. A survey of feline neoplasms. *J Am Vet Med Assoc* 1967; 151 (10): 1325–1328.
5. Vail DM, MacEwen EG. Feline lymphoma and leukemias. In: Withrow SJ, MacEwen EG (eds.) *Small Animal Clinical Oncology*, 3rd ed. Philadelphia, WB Saunders, 2001; 590–611.
6. Gabor LJ, Malik R, Canfield PJ. Clinical and anatomical features of lymphosarcoma in 118 cats. *Aust Vet J* 1998; 76 (11): 725–732.
7. Kristal O, Lana SE, Ogilvie GK et al. Single agent chemotherapy with doxorubicin for feline lymphoma: A retrospective study of 19 cases (1994–1997). *J Vet Intern Med* 2001; 15: 125–130.
8. Mauldin GE, Mooney SC, Meleo KA et al: Chemotherapy in 132 cats with lymphoma: 1988–1994. *Proc Vet Cancer Soc 15th Annual Conference*, Tucson, 1995; 35–36.
9. Moore AS, Cotter SM, Frimberger AE et al: A comparison of doxorubicin and COP for maintenance of remission in cats with lymphoma. *J Vet Intern Med* 1996; 10 (6): 372–375.
10. Vail DM, Moore AS, Ogilvie GK et al. Feline lymphoma (145 cases): Proliferation indices, cluster of differentiation 3 immunoreactivity, and their association with prognosis in 90 cats. *J Vet Intern Med* 1998; 12: 349–354.
11. Cotter SM. Treatment of lymphoma and leukemia with cyclophosphamide, vincristine, and prednisone: II. Treatment of cats. *J Am Anim Hosp Assoc* 1983; 19: 166–172.
12. Court EA, Watson ADJ, Peaston AE. Retrospective study of 60 cases of feline lymphosarcoma. *Aust Vet J* 1997; 75 (6): 424–427.
13. Jackson ML, Haines DM, Meric SM et al. Feline leukemia virus detection by immunochemistry and polymerase chain reaction in formalin-fixed, paraffin-embedded tumor tissue from cats with lymphosarcoma. *Can J Vet Res* 1993; 57: 169–276.
14. Mooney SC, Hayes AA, MacEwen EG et al. Treatment and prognostic factors in lymphoma in cats: 103 Cases (1977–1981). *J Am Vet Med Assoc* 1989; 194 (5): 696–699.
15. Hardy WD Jr. Hematopoietic tumors of cats. *J Am Anim Hosp Assoc* 1981; 17: 921–940.
16. Francis DP, Cotter SM, Hardy WD et al. Comparison of virus-positive and virus-negative cases of feline leukemia and lymphoma. *Cancer Res* 1979; 39: 3866–3870.
17. Fondacaro JV, Richter KP, Carpenter JL et al. Feline gastrointestinal lymphoma: 67 cases (1988–1996). *Eur J Com Gastroenterol* 1999; 4 (2): 5–11.
18. Hittmair K, Krebitz-Gressl E, Kubber-Heiss A et al. Feline alimentary lymphosarcoma: Radiographical, ultrasonographical, histological and virological findings. *Eur J Compan Anim Pract* 2001; 11 (2): 119–128.
19. Jeglum KA, Whereat A, Young K. Chemotherapy of lymphoma in 75 cats. *J Am Vet Med Assoc* 1987; 190 (2): 174–178.
20. Mahony OM, Moore AS, Cotter SM et al. Alimentary lymphoma in cats: 28 cases (1988–1993). *J Am Vet Med Assoc* 1995; 207 (12): 1593–1597.
21. Zwahlen CH, Lucroy MD, Kraegel SA et al: Results of chemotherapy for cats with alimentary malignant lymphoma: 21 Cases (1993–1997). *J Am Vet Med Assoc* 1998; 213 (8): 1144–1149.
22. Shelton GH, Grant CK, Cotter SM et al. Feline immunodeficiency virus and feline leukemia virus infections and their relationships to lymphoid malignancies in cats: A retrospective study (1968–1988). *J Acquir Immune Defic Syndr* 1990; 3: 623–630.
23. Burkitt JM, Drobatz KJ, Hess RS et al. Intestinal intussusception in twenty cats. *J Vet Intern Med* 2001; 15 (3): 313 (abstract).
24. Gabor LJ, Canfield PJ, Malik R. Immunophenotypic and histological characterization of 109 cases of feline lymphosarcoma. *Aust Vet J* 1999; 77 (7): 436–441.
25. Darbes J, Majzoub M, Breuer W et al. Large granular lymphocyte leukemia / lymphoma in six cats. *Vet Pathol* 1998; 35: 370–379.
26. Endo Y, Cho KW, Nishigaki K et al. Clinicopathological and immunological characteristics of six cats with granular lymphocyte tumors. *Com Immun Microbiol Infect Dis* 1998; 21: 27–42.
27. Kariya K, Konno A, Ishida T. Perforin-like immunoreactivity in four cases of lymphoma of large granular lymphocytes in the cat. *Vet Pathol* 1997; 34: 156–159.
28. Wellman ML, Hammer AS, DiBartola SP et al. Lymphoma involving large granular lymphocytes in cats: 11 Cases (1982–1991). *J Am Vet Med Assoc* 1992; 201 (8): 1265–1269.
29. Charney SC, Valli VE, Kitchell BE et al. Histopathological, phenotypic, and molecular assessment of feline infiltrative enteric disease – a pilot study. *Proc Vet Cancer Soc Mid-Year Conference*, Galena, IL, 2002; 18 (abstract).
30. Roccabianca P, Woo JC, Moore PF. Characterization of the diffuse mucosal associated lymphoid tissue of feline small intestine. *Vet Immunol Immunopathol* 2000; 75: 27–42.
31. Barrs VR, Beatty JA, McCandlish IA et al. Hypereosinophilic paraneoplastic syndrome in a cat with intestinal T cell lymphosarcoma. *J Small Anim Pract* 2002; 43: 401–405.
32. Callanan JJ, Jones BA, Irvine J et al. Histologic classification and immunophenotype of lymphosarcomas in cats with naturally and experimentally acquired feline immunodeficiency virus infections. *Vet Pathol* 1996; 33: 264–272.
33. Jackson ML, Wood SL, Misra V et al. Immunohistochemical identification of B and T lymphocytes in formalin-fixed, paraffin-embedded feline lymphosarcomas: Relation to feline leukemia virus status, tumor site, and patient age. *Can J Vet Res* 1996; 60: 199–204.
34. Krecic MR, Black SS. Epitheliotropic T-cell gastrointestinal tract lymphosarcoma with metastases to lung and skeletal muscle in a cat. *J Am Vet Med Assoc* 2000; 216 (4): 524–529.
35. Rojko JL, Kociba GJ, Abkowitz JL et al. Feline lymphomas: immunological and cytochemical characterization. *Cancer Res* 1989; 49: 345–351.
36. Malik, R, Gabor LJ, Foster SF et al. Therapy for Australian cats with lymphosarcoma. *Aust Vet J* 2001; 79 (12): 808–817.
37. Grooters AM, Biller DS Ward H et al: Ultrasonographic appearance of feline alimentary lymphoma. *Vet Radiol Ultrasound* 1994; 35 (6): 468–472.
38. Penninck DG, Moore AS, Tidwell AS et al. Ultrasonography of alimentary lymphosarcoma in the cat. *Vet Radiol Ultrasound* 1994; 35 (4): 299–304.
39. Arista-Nasr J, Jimenez A, Keirns C et al. The role of the endoscopic biopsy in the diagnosis of gastric lymphoma: A morphologic and immunohistochemical reappraisal. *Hum Pathol* 1991; 22 (4): 339–348.
40. Roth L, Leib MS, Davenport DJ et al. Comparisons between endoscopic and histologic evaluation of the gastrointestinal tract in dogs and cats: 75 Cases (1984–1987). *J Am Vet Med Assoc* 1990; 196 (4): 635–638.
41. Rassnick KM, Gieger TL, Williams LE et al. Phase I evaluation of CCNU (lomustine) in tumor-bearing cats. *J Vet Intern Med* 2001; 15: 196–199.
42. Rassnick KM, Mauldin GN, Moroff SD et al. Prognostic value of argyrophilic nucleolar organizer region (AgNOR) staining in feline intestinal lymphoma. *J Vet Intern Med* 1999; 13: 187–190.

43. Correa SS, Mauldin GN, Mauldin GE et al. Serum alpha 1-acid glycoprotein concentration in cats with lymphoma. *J Am Anim Hosp Assoc* 2001; 37: 153–158.

44. Couto CG, Rutgers HC, Sherding RG et al. Gastrointestinal lymphoma in 20 dogs. A retrospective study. *J Vet Intern Med* 1989; 3: 73–78.

45. Coyle KA, Steinberg H. Characterization of lymphocytes in canine gastrointestinal lymphoma. *Vet Pathol* 2004; 41: 141–146.

46. Vail DM, MacEwen EG, Young KM. Canine lymphoma and lymphoid leukemias. In: Withrow SJ, MacEwen EG (eds.) *Small Animal Clinical Oncology,* 3rd ed. Philadelphia, WB Saunders, 2001; 558–590.

9.4 Neuroendocrine Tumors of the Gastrointestinal Tract

JÖRG M. STEINER

9.4.1 Introduction

The GI tract is the largest endocrine organ of the body, but little is known about it.[1] Traditionally, mechanisms of cell-to-cell communication have been divided into autocrine, paracrine, neurocrine, endocrine, and spermiocrine mechanisms, but this division is not entirely clear in the GI tract. Almost all regulatory substances synthesized in the GI tract are peptides, but several of them function as endocrine, neurocrine, paracrine, and even autocrine peptides.

In 1902, secretin was discovered as the first GI hormone, and in fact the first hormone overall.[1] Since then, a large number of GI regulatory peptides have been identified (Table 9.10).[1,2] Many of these regulatory peptides are considered true hormones, although currently only six meet all the physiological criteria for a hormone: insulin, glucagon, gastrin, secretin, cholecystokinin (CCK), and motilin. The main functions of the more important regulatory peptides are listed in Table 9.11.[2]

In general, endocrine disorders are due to a lack (e.g., hypoadrenocorticism) or overabundance (e.g., hyperadrenocorticism) of a hormone. To date, the only syndrome known to be due to the lack of a GI hormone is diabetes mellitus, which is due to an absolute or relative insulin deficiency. Surprisingly, a lack of other GI regulatory peptides has not been identified as causing specific syndromes in any species. However, there is no reason to believe that a lack of GI regulatory peptides could not lead to clinical disease; therefore, it appears likely to be only a matter of time before such syndromes are discovered. Many chronic GI diseases are considered idiopathic, and it is possible that some of these conditions are caused by GI regulatory peptide deficiency.

Disorders related to an overabundance of GI regulatory peptides are well recognized and are caused by neuroendocrine tumors (NETs). The prevalence of GI NETs in humans is low, with about 3–4 cases per million population. Approximately 55% of these NETs are carcinoids, 25% insulinomas, 10% gastrinomas, 2% vasoactive intestinal polypeptidomas (VIPomas), 2% glucagonomas, less than 1% somatostatinomas, and the remaining 5–6% non-functioning tumors or pancreatic polypeptidomas. Similar epidemiological data are not available for dogs and cats and many of these GI NETs have not yet been described in veterinary patients. To date, GI NETs described in dogs and cats are limited to insulinomas, gastrinomas, glucagonomas, carcinoids, and a single case of a pancreatic polypeptidoma.

9.4.2 Insulinoma

Introduction

An insulinoma is a functional beta cell tumor causing hyperinsulinism. Insulinomas occur infrequently in dogs and are rare in cats.[3–5] Insulinoma cells produce a wide variety of regulatory polypeptides, such as insulin, pancreatic polypeptide, somatostatin, glucagon, serotonin, gastrin, and ACTH.[6] Despite the variety of polypeptides produced by insulinoma cells, almost all of the patients diagnosed with an insulinoma show only clinical signs of hyperinsulinism. Insulinomas in humans are sometimes seen in concert with other endocrine neoplastic lesions, a condition known as multiple endocrine neoplasias (MEN). Recently, a cat with MEN has been described.[5] This cat was diagnosed with a parathyroid gland adenoma, an adrenal gland cortical adenoma, and an insulinoma.

Pathogenesis

The etiology of insulinomas remains unknown and risk factors for insulinomas have not been described. Beta cells take up glucose through an insulin-independent process and the intracellular glucose concentration of the islet cells mirrors the se-

9

Table 9.10: Gastrointestinal regulatory peptides
This table shows a list of the most prominent groups of gastrointestinal regulatory peptides. It should be pointed out that there are many more regulatory peptides in the gastrointestinal tract; however, their physiological relevance is less well understood.

Regulatory peptide family	Members of regulatory peptide family
Gastrin-cholecystokinin family	■ cholecystokinin ■ gastrin
Secretin/glucagon/vasoactive intestinal polypeptide family	■ gastric inhibitory peptide (GIP) ■ glicentine ■ glucagon ■ glucagon-like peptide 1 ■ glucagon-like peptide 2 ■ growth hormone-releasing factor (GRF) ■ oxyntomodulin ■ peptide HI/HM ■ secretin ■ vasoactive intestinal polypeptide (VIP)
Pancreatic polypeptide family	■ neuropeptide Y (NPY) ■ pancreatic polypeptide (PP) ■ peptide YY (PYY)
Tachykinin/bombesin family	■ gastrin-releasing peptide (GRP) ■ GRP decapeptide ■ neuromedin B ■ neuromedin K ■ substance K ■ substance P
Opioid peptide family	■ adrenocorticotrophic hormone (ACTH) ■ β endorphin ■ β neoendorphin ■ dynorphin ■ [leu]-enkephalin ■ Leumorphin ■ melanocyte stimulating hormone (MSH) ■ [met]-enkephalin
Insulin family	■ insulin ■ insulin-like growth factor I
Epidermal growth factor family	■ epidermal growth factor ■ transforming growth factor α (TGFα)
Somatostatin family	■ somatostatin
Calcitonin family	■ calcitonin ■ calcitonin gene-related peptide
Miscellaneous regulatory peptides	■ endothelin ■ galanin ■ motilin ■ neurotensin ■ thyrotropin-releasing hormone (TRH)

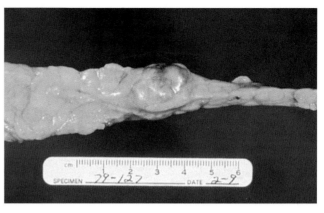

Figure 9.16:
Insulinoma. This figure shows an insulinoma in a dog. Note the small size of the tumor. (Courtesy of Dr. Thomas J. Van Winkle, University of Pennsylvania, Philadelphia, PA.)

rum glucose concentration. In normal subjects, insulin secretion from beta cells is suppressed when the blood glucose concentration falls below approximately 60 mg/dl. At the same time, secretion of the counterregulatory hormones (immediate response: catecholamines and glucagon; delayed response: cortisol and growth hormone) increases. Insulinomas do not respond appropriately to a falling blood glucose concentration. This results in hypoglycemia, which in turn can result in central nervous system (CNS) abnormalities. Glucose uptake into the CNS is by facilitated diffusion and is also non-insulin-dependent, so that glucose uptake is low at times of hypoglycemia. In addition, the CNS utilizes glucose as its primary energy source, and cannot utilize fatty acids and ketone bodies as can other tissues, including the peripheral nervous system. Clinical signs of hyperinsulinism also include signs induced by an increased discharge of the sympathetic nervous system, which is part of its counterregulatory response. However, insulinoma patients apparently adjust to repeated or chronic states of hypoglycemia as they can tolerate extremely low blood glucose concentrations without showing any clinical signs.

In addition to the degree of hypoglycemia, the rate of decrease in blood glucose concentration, and the duration of hypoglycemia all determine the extent of the clinical signs.

Table 9.11: Main functions of important gastrointestinal regulatory peptides
This table shows an alphabetical listing of the most important regulatory peptides of the gastrointestinal tract, their location and cell type of secretion, their most important functions, and the stimulatory and inhibitory factors for their secretion.

Regulatory peptide	Location of secretion	Cell type	Most important functions	Stimulatory factors	Inhibitory factors
cholecystokinin	duodenum, jejunum	I	■ stimulation of pancreatic enzyme secretion ■ gallbladder contraction ■ regulation of pancreatic growth	■ fat, fatty acids, proteins, amino acids, H$^+$ ■ bombesin, GRP	■ somatostatin
gastric inhibitory polypeptide (GIP)	duodenum, jejunum	GIP	■ inhibition of gastric acid secretion ■ stimulation of intestinal fluid secretion ■ stimulation of insulin release	■ all major classes of nutrients in the gut ■ bombesin	
gastrin	stomach, duodenum	G	■ stimulation of gastric acid secretion ■ trophic effect on acid-secreting gastric mucosa ■ stimulation of pepsinogen secretion	■ stomach distension ■ digested proteins and amino acids ■ bombesin, GRP, Ca^{++}	■ luminal acidification ■ somatostatin
glucagon	pancreas	A	■ stimulation of glycogenolysis ■ stimulation of gluconeogenesis from lactate, amino acids, and glycerol	■ hypoglycemia ■ high concentration of amino acids or low concentration of free fatty acids in plasma	■ hyperglycemia
insulin	pancreas	B	■ stimulation of peripheral glucose uptake ■ stimulation of glycogen synthesis ■ stimulation of lipogenesis ■ stimulation of DNA, RNA, and protein synthesis	■ hyperglycemia ■ glucagon	■ hypoglycemia
motilin	duodenum, jejunum	M	■ initiates phase III of the migratory motor complex	■ cyclic release during the fasting state ■ intraluminal lipids	
neurotensin	ileum, colon	N	■ inhibition of gastric acid secretion	■ intraluminal lipids ■ bombesin	
opioids	entire GI tract		■ inhibition of intestinal water and electrolyte secretion ■ modulation of GI motility	■ unknown	
oxyntomodulin	ileum, colon	L	■ inhibition of gastric acid secretion ■ stimulation of intestinal mucosal growth	■ intraluminal glucose and lipids	
pancreatic polypeptide (PP)	pancreas	F	■ inhibition of pancreatic enzyme and fluid secretion	■ intraluminal proteins ■ vagal stimulation	
peptide YY	ileum, colon	L	■ inhibition of pancreatic secretion ■ inhibition of gastric acid secretion ■ inhibition of gastric emptying	■ intraluminal lipids ■ bombesin	
secretin	duodenum, jejunum	S	■ stimulation of pancreatic bicarbonate secretion	■ duodenal acidification	
somatostatin	entire GI tract	D	■ inhibition of gastric and pancreatic secretions ■ inhibition of intestinal amino acid and glucose absorption ■ inhibition of intestinal motility	■ intraluminal lipid, protein, and bile	
tachykinins	entire GI tract		■ regulation of GI motility ■ transmission of pain impulses	■ luminal distension	
vasoactive intestinal polypeptide (VIP)	entire GI tract		■ relaxation of smooth muscle ■ vasodilation ■ stimulation of pancreatic and intestinal secretion	■ vagal stimulation	

9

Table 9.12: Breed distribution of dogs with insulinoma
This table shows the breed distribution of 222 canine patients with insulinoma and the breed distribution of the canine population seen at the Veterinary Hospital at the University of Pennsylvania (VHUP) for the period 1991–1992.[3] Boxers, Irish Setters, German Shorthaired Pointers, and Weimaraners appear to be predisposed. The 222 cases compiled were seen at several different veterinary institutions. Thus, the hospital population of VHUP is not a statistically valid reference population and the percentages are shown in parentheses.

Breed	Number of dogs	% of all cases of insulinoma	% of VHUP population
Mixed Breed	62	28.6	(26.5)
Boxer	21	9.7	(1.2)
German Shepherd	18	8.3	(6.6)
Irish Setter	17	7.8	(0.6)
Golden Retriever	10	4.6	(4.9)
Miniature Poodle	9	4.1	(2.5)
Labrador	8	3.7	(6.2)
German Shorthaired Pointer	7	3.2	(0.4)
Collie	6	2.8	(0.9)
Standard Poodle	6	2.8	(1.1)
Weimaraner	6	2.8	(0.4)
West Highland White Terrier	6	2.8	(0.8)
Basset	5	2.3	(0.8)
Other breeds	36	16.6	(47.1)

(Table re-printed with permission from: Steiner JM, Bruyette DS. Canine insulinoma. *Compend Contin Educ Pract Vet* 1996; 18: 13–24.)

Table 9.13: Incidence of clinical signs reported in 113 canine insulinoma patients[3]

Clinical Sign	Number of patients	% of patients
seizures	77	68
collapse	38	34
generalized weakness	37	33
posterior weakness	37	33
depression / lethargy	21	19
ataxia	21	19
muscle fasciculation	20	18
bizarre behavior	17	15
polyphagia	12	11
exercise intolerance	11	10
shaking / trembling	11	10
polyuria / polydipsia	8	7
weight gain	7	6
all other clinical signs were reported with a frequency of less than 5%		

(Table re-printed with permission from: Steiner JM, Bruyette DS. Canine insulinoma. *Compend Contin Educ Pract Vet* 1996; 18: 13–24.)

Pathology and natural behavior

Insulinomas most commonly appear as tan nodules in the pancreas (Figure 9.16). They are generally small (i.e., 1 cm in diameter or less). Most often they appear to be singular, but in a series of 129 dogs, 14% had multiple masses.[3] On histopathology, the tumor cells appear as normal islet cells, forming irregular nests and cords with a variable pattern of dense stromal proliferation.

Malignant tumors are defined as tumors which are locally invasive and/or form distant metastasis. In many neoplastic diseases, the malignant potential of a tumor can be successfully predicted by histopathological evaluation. However, this is not the case for insulinomas and other endocrine neoplasias, as these neoplasias often lack many of the typical features of malignancy. Thus, estimation of the malignant potential of insulinomas based on histopathological findings can be misleading and should not be attempted.

Signalment

Insulinomas mainly occur in older dogs and cats. The mean age of 233 dogs reported in the literature was 8.9 years with a range of 3.5 to 14 years in 128 dogs.[3] The sex distribution of 133 dogs with insulinoma showed 45% males and 55% females.[3] Table 9.12 shows the breed distribution of 222 dogs with insulinoma.[3]

Clinical presentation

Dogs presenting with insulinomas generally present with two types of clinical signs: neuroglycopenic signs, such as weakness, ataxia, depression, or seizures or signs related to an increased discharge of the sympathetic nervous system, such as behavioral changes, shaking, trembling, and muscle fasciculations.[3,4] The incidence of clinical signs reported in 113 dogs with insulinoma is shown in Table 9.13.[3] Most patients with insulinoma show only intermittent clinical signs, and will have a rather unremarkable physical examination. A few patients will present in status epilepticus or even comatose. Due to the age of the affected population, a number of geriatric abnormalities may be evident that are unrelated to the presence of an insulinoma. Rather rare are those patients presenting with peripheral polyneuropathies. Subclinical polyneuropathy appears to be more common than symptomatic disease.

Diagnosis

A fasting blood glucose concentration should be part of the workup of a patient with clinical signs suggestive of hypoglycemia, preferably during times when the patient is symptomatic. Most dogs diagnosed with an insulinoma will present with a low blood glucose concentration, even in the absence of clinical signs. If hypoglycemia is confirmed, the causative relationship between the observed clinical signs and the hypoglycemia needs to be established. This is best accomplished by demonstrating Whipple's triad, which consists of 1) demonstrating a subnormal blood glucose concentration, 2) presence of clinical signs of hypoglycemia, and 3) cessation of clinical signs with resolution of hypoglycemia. After Whipple's triad has been established, the cause of hypoglycemia must be identified. A basic workup should include a complete blood count, a chemistry profile, and a urinalysis. In insulinoma patients these basic parameters will usually be within normal limits. Infrequently reported abnormalities include mild elevations in liver enzymes. Radiographs of the thorax and abdomen are usually within normal limits, but may be helpful to exclude other causes of hypoglycemia. Abdominal ultrasound is a valuable tool in patients with suspected insulinoma. Even though only a small percentage of insulinomas can actually be visualized by this method, it is very helpful for assessing the patient for the presence of organ metastasis or mesenteric lymphadenopathy.

Many tests have been employed in human and veterinary patients with a suspected insulinoma. The single most reliable test for an insulinoma is the demonstration of an inappropriately high serum insulin concentration in the face of hypoglycemia, also referred to as insulin-glucose pair. Serum for the determination of insulin concentration needs to be collected at the time of the hypoglycemia. This is accomplished by serial blood glucose measurements while food is withheld from the animal. It is best to start early in the morning with the patient being closely monitored throughout the day. Blood glucose concentration is measured every 30–60 minutes. When the blood glucose falls below 60 mg/dl, a sample for the measurement of serum insulin concentration is drawn and the animal is fed. It is important to verify blood glucose concentrations measured by a glucometer through the use of a chemistry analyzer. Interpretation of the insulin-glucose pair is straight forward if the insulin concentration exceeds the reference range (the reference range is dependant on the laboratory used) in the face of hypoglycemia. However, the serum insulin concentration may be within the reference range and still be inappropriately high with respect to the blood glucose concentration. Several ratios have been evaluated to help document inappropriate insulin secretion: glucose-insulin ratio, insulin-glucose ratio, and the amended insulin-glucose ratio. Unfortunately, none of these ratios improve the diagnostic accuracy in either humans or dogs with a suspected insulinoma and the use of these ratios is not recommended. An insulin-glucose pair is the single most reliable test to diagnose an insulinoma as the cause of hypoglycemia.

A variety of provocative tests have been suggested to aid in the diagnosis of an insulinoma. These include the glucagon toler-

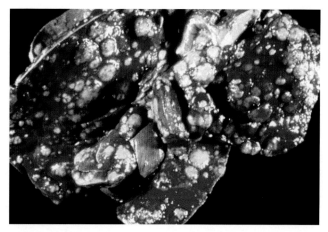

Figure 9.17:
Insulinoma metastases in the liver. This figure shows a liver with diffuse dissemination of metastatic lesions of an insulinoma in a dog. (Courtesy of Dr. Thomas J. Van Winkle, University of Pennsylvania, Philadelphia, PA.)

9

ance test, the IV glucose tolerance test, the tolbutamide tolerance test, the L-leucine test, the oral glucose tolerance test, the epinephrine stimulation test, and the calcium infusion test. All of these tests are time consuming, expensive, and, at least in people, have lower sensitivities than a simple insulin-glucose pair. In addition, some of these tests put the patient at risk for severe hypoglycemia. In cases where the cause for the hypoglycemia can not been determined, and the evaluation of serum insulin and glucose concentrations have been equivocal, the measurement of serum insulin and glucose should be repeated whilst food is withheld from the patient.

Staging

As with any other neoplastic disease, patients with an insulinoma should be staged. Unfortunately, the available modalities to stage canine and feline insulinoma patients are limited. Abdominal ultrasound is inconsistent in detecting the primary tumor, but can be helpful in demonstrating evidence of local extension and distant metastasis of the disease. Currently, the most reliable staging tool in veterinary patients appears to be abdominal exploration.

In a compilation of 129 abdominal exploratories of canine insulinoma patients, 66 (51%) of the dogs had metastatic disease detected during the exploratory laparotomy.[3] Of those, 29 (22%) had metastatic lesions in the liver (Figure 9.17), 19 (15%) had metastases to regional lymph nodes, 7 (5%) had metastatic lesions in both liver and lymph nodes, and 11 (8%) had metastatic lesions in other locations.[3]

Treatment

Emergency treatment

Patients presenting for clinical signs of hypoglycemia need to be treated as quickly as possible. If hypoglycemia has been documented, a dextrose bolus (0.5 g/kg as a 25% solution IV over approximately one minute) should be administered and a dextrose constant rate infusion should be initiated. Suitable infusion solutions are 5% dextrose or balanced electrolyte solutions with added dextrose. It is important to note that the goal of emergency therapy is to eliminate the clinical signs of hypoglycemia rather than to restore euglycemia. If neuroglycopenic signs persist, cerebral edema should be suspected and treatment using mannitol and corticosteroids should be considered. If seizures still persist, diazepam or other anticonvulsants may be indicated.

Pancreatic surgery

Surgical exploration is the treatment of choice for the management of canine and feline patients with an insulinoma. It is crucial to stabilize the blood glucose concentration of the patient prior to surgery. Also, the surgeon should be aware that handling of the tumor can lead to increased insulin release. In contrast, removal of the tumor may suddenly lower plasma insulin concentrations. Therefore, blood glucose must be monitored closely throughout the procedure.

In order to stage the disease, a careful abdominal exploratory should be performed, and biopsies of suspicious lymph nodes or areas within the liver should be obtained.

Identification of the insulinoma can be difficult. In a compilation of 129 abdominal exploratories of canine patients with a suspected insulinoma, a pancreatic nodule could not be identified in 26 patients (20%).[3] Even though some of these cases might have had a rarely described diffuse infiltration of the pancreas, further evaluation of localization techniques seems warranted in canine insulinoma patients. Some investigators have suggested the intravenous infusion of methylene blue.[7] However, this procedure has only been described in five patients and the drug can cause a Heinz body hemolytic anemia, so further investigation of this technique is necessary. In human medicine, a variety of localization techniques have been described and compared. Currently, endoscopic ultrasonography and somatostatin receptor scintigraphy (SRS) are considered the most sensitive modalities in human insulinoma patients.[8] Other modalities include intraoperative ultrasonography, CT, MRI, selective arteriography, intraoperative quick frozen sections, and transhepatic venous sampling.

The majority of localization techniques reported in the human literature are either very expensive or of limited availability in veterinary medicine. Thus, intraoperative inspection and palpation remain the primary mode of localization of an insulinoma in veterinary patients. However, other modalities may be employed. Intraoperative ultrasonography is technically feasible and relatively inexpensive, but has never been systematically evaluated for the localization of insulinomas in small animals. However, the author believes that it should be considered in cases where intraoperative visualization and palpation are unsuccessful. It also can be utilized to scan the liver for possible metastasis. The use of CT has recently been evaluated for the localization of insulinomas in dogs and was able to visualize the primary tumor in 10/14 (71%) patients.[9] This was superior to transabdominal ultrasound, which was successfully used to identify the primary tumor in 5/14 (36%).[9]

Somatostatin receptor scintigraphy, that is the intravenous administration of ^{111}In-DTPA-D-Phe^1-octreotide (OctreoScan, Mallinckrodt Medical) followed by planar scintigraphy or single-photon emission CT, has also been evaluated in canine insulinoma patients.[9–11] In one study, the primary lesion was identified in all five dogs evaluated.[10] However, in two other studies the insulinoma was only identified in 6/14 (43%) and 4/17 (24%) dogs.[9,11] This discrepancy can be explained by the fact that the tumor was positive for somatostatin receptor subtype 2 (sst2), one of the somatostatin receptor subtypes to which octreotide preferentially binds to, in all five dogs in the first study, but only in 7/17 (41%) dogs in one of the other two studies.[10,11] Thus, while SRS may be useful to identify and/or localize an insulinoma in some cases, if the tumor does not express sst2, the tumor may not be able to be visualized with this modality.

Extreme care should be exercised at all times when handling the pancreas. After localization of the insulinoma, it can be removed by enucleation, partial pancreatectomy, and total pancreatectomy +/– duodenectomy. While the surgical technique for total pancreatectomy has been described for the dog, this procedure is associated with a high postsurgical morbidity and mortality, and should thus only be considered if there are no other options. Local enucleation has been shown to result in shorter survival times than partial pancreatectomy, and should therefore only be considered if the tumor is in the body of the pancreas, or very proximally in the right lobe.[12] Thus, the surgical procedure of choice is partial pancreatectomy (Figure 9.18). If the tumor cannot be localized on abdominal exploratory, a small pancreatic biopsy should be taken to evaluate the pancreas for diffuse infiltration histopathologically. Since the right and left lobes are involved with equal frequencies and occult insulinomas are probably most common in the pancreatic body, random removal of pancreatic tissue should not be performed.

The most common postoperative complication of pancreatic surgery is acute pancreatitis. However, the risk of postoperative pancreatitis can be minimized by aggressive fluid therapy during anesthesia and gentle handling of the pancreas during surgery. Other common postoperative complications are hypoglycemia and hyperglycemia. Persistent hypoglycemia indicates that the insulinoma has not been completely removed. The patient either has to be re-explored, or medical therapy has to be instituted. Hyperglycemia, if present, is most often transient, but some patients may require insulin therapy to control the hyperglycemia.

Chemotherapy

If surgical exploration is not an option or if it does not lead to removal of the entire insulinoma, chemotherapy can be considered. Streptozotocin is a nitrosurea compound isolated from *Streptomyces achromogenes*. The drug has been used in approximately 20 dogs with insulinoma.[13,14] Streptozotocin is highly nephrotoxic and can also be hepatotoxic. Therefore, pre- and post-treatment diuresis is crucial. In addition, the mean duration of normoglycemia in treated dogs was not significantly longer than in untreated controls in one study of 17 dogs. Thus, further studies are needed to evaluate the clinical usefulness of streptozotocin for the treatment of canine insulinoma.

Alloxan is an unstable uric acid derivative that has two effects, selective cytotoxicity of islet cells and stimulation of hepatic gluconeogenesis. The use of alloxan has been described in five canine insulinoma patients.[15] Two of the five patients developed hyperglycemia for several months without any additional medical therapy. Alloxan, like streptozotocin, is also nephrotoxic and concurrent fluid therapy should be instituted for several days in order to minimize renal toxicity. The use of several other chemotherapeutic drugs has been reported in the human literature, but no data are available for veterinary species.

Radiation therapy

Successful treatment of insulinomas with radiation therapy has been described in isolated human patients. However, to date, data for canine or feline patients are not available.

Symptomatic therapy

Antihypoglycemic therapy

Symptomatic therapy should be instituted in insulinoma patients when surgical exploration is not an option or is not successful. The dog should be fed a high protein, high fat, high complex carbohydrate diet divided into multiple small feed-

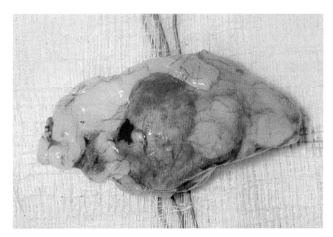

Figure 9.18:
Insulinoma. An insulinoma after surgical removal by partial pancreatectomy. Size and appearance of this tumor are typical. (Re-printed with permission from Steiner JM, Bruyette DS. Canine insulinoma. *Compend Contin Educ Pract Vet* 1996; 18: 13–24.)

9

ings (4–6 per day). If the patient shows signs of weakness, a small amount of food should be offered immediately. Owners should also be familiarized with the clinical signs of hypoglycemia and instructed that if signs occur, dextrose solution (e.g., Karo-Syrup or honey) should be applied onto the gums of the patient. Excitement should be avoided and exercise should be limited to short leash walks.

Glucocorticoids should be administered if frequent feedings alone will not control the clinical signs. Cortisol is an endogenous counterregulatory hormone to insulin. It increases peripheral lipolysis and protein catabolism, increases hepatic gluconeogenesis and glycogenolysis, and decreases peripheral glucose utilization. It also decreases the sensitivity of insulin receptors in the periphery. Prednisone or prednisolone can be started at an oral dose of 0.25 mg/kg twice a day. If clinical signs of hypoglycemia cannot be controlled, the dose can be increased up to 2–3 mg/kg twice per day. The development of iatrogenic Cushing's and GI side effects (e.g., gastritis, gastric ulceration, or colitis), may warrant the discontinuation of steroid therapy, and additional medical therapy may be required.

Antihormonal therapy

Another therapeutic option for insulinoma patients is the treatment with agents that depress insulin secretion. Several such agents are available. Diazoxide is a non-diuretic benzothiadiazine that has anti-hypertensive as well as hyperglycemic properties. Its hyperglycemic action is due to a depression in insulin release from beta-cells. Diazoxide does not impair insulin synthesis and it is not cytotoxic to beta cells. Survival times in insulinoma patients treated with diazoxide are rather short. However, this might be due to the fact that in most reports, diazoxide was only administered after previous medical and surgical therapy had failed. A few long-term responders have been reported, the longest being 18 months.[16] The recommended starting dose is 5 mg/kg orally twice per day, but the dose can be gradually increased to 30 mg/kg twice a day. Since the drug is metabolized in the liver and excreted by the biliary system and the kidneys, dosing should be carefully evaluated for patients with hepatic or renal disease. Also, care should be taken to avoid hyperglycemia. Thiazide diuretics enhance the effects of diazoxide and hydrochlorothiazide can be added to the therapeutic protocol (2–4 mg/kg PO q 24 h). In order to decrease the frequency of GI side effects, the drug should be administered together with a meal.

Somatostatin (i.e., octreotide acetate) decreases several polypeptides of the gastroenteropancreatic system, including insulin. Octreotide consistently suppresses plasma insulin concentrations in canine insulinoma patients, while it has no effect on counterregulatory hormones, suggesting that it maybe useful in the treatment of canine insulinoma.[17] However, of approximately 20 dogs described in the literature that have been treated with octreotide only 50% showed a clinical response.[11,18] As with SRS, the limited response of canine insulinoma patients to octreotide may be due to a lack of sst2 expression of the insulinoma cells. Doses of 20–100 µg octreotide SC q 8–12 h have been described in the literature.[11,18]

Prognosis

The long-term prognosis for dogs with insulinoma is grave, although the short-term prognosis is good. In a compilation of 114 dogs with an insulinoma, which had been treated with surgery and with symptomatic therapy after recurrence of clinical signs, the mean survival was 11.5 months.[3] Results may be more favorable as 31 dogs were alive and asymptomatic at their last follow-up visit, and time to relapse or death could not be determined. It should also be noted that the mean age of dogs presenting with an insulinoma is 9 years, and therefore many patients may die for other reasons. In one study, the mean survival of canine insulinoma patients without metastatic disease at the time of diagnosis was 17 months, while it was only 8.4 months for dogs that did have metastatic disease.[19] Thus, detection of distant metastases at the time of the abdominal exploratory may serve as a prognostic indicator. Age and serum insulin concentrations at the time of diagnosis have also been proposed as prognostic indicators, but supportive data are not available.[19]

9.4.3 Gastrinoma

Introduction

A gastrinoma is a rare tumor in small animals, having been reported in only 25 dogs and 5 cats, compared to approximately 250 dogs and four cats with an insulinoma.[20–22]

Gastrinomas are most commonly single nodules of small size (Figure 9.19). However, multiple masses have also been reported. In humans, gastrinomas are ultimately malignant, but most grow slowly. When gastrinomas were first described in humans, most were localized in the pancreas, but to date over 50% of gastrinomas in humans have been found outside the pancreas, with most of those being found in the duodenum.[23] This is probably due to improved localization techniques. By sharp contrast, gastrinomas have not been localized in the duodenum in either dogs or cats, although tumors could not be accurately located in many cases. Recently, a bile duct carcinoma in a cat was shown to stain positive for gastrin.[24]

Gastrinomas synthesize and release excessive quantities of gastrin (Figure 9.20), leading to gastric acid hypersecretion, hypertrophy of the gastric mucosa, and eventually gastric and duodenal ulceration (Figure 9.21).[23,25] Persistent hyperchlorhydria also leads to a decrease in duodenal pH, which in turn leads to mucosal injury and inactivation of digestive enzymes with subsequent maldigestion.

Clinical presentation

Gastrinomas usually develop in middle-aged to older dogs (age range 3.5–12 years in 21 dogs reported) and cats (age range of five reported cats: 8–12 years).[22] In dogs, females are anecdotally more commonly affected than males (69% vs. 31%), but this may be a reflection of the small number of cases reported.

The most common clinical signs observed in 25 of the reported cases included vomiting (92%), weight loss (88%), anorexia (72%), lethargy (64%), and diarrhea (60%). In addition, polydipsia, melena, and abdominal pain were noted in approximately 25%, and hematemesis, hematochezia, fever, and ravenous appetite in approximately 10% of cases each. Clinical signs in cats are similar with vomiting, weight loss, and poor body condition being reported most consistently.

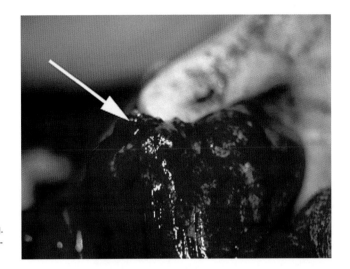

Figure 9.19:
Gastrinoma. This figure shows a small tumor (arrow) in the pancreas of a dog. This tumor is barely visible and was identified as a gastrinoma by immunohisto-chemistry. (Courtesy of Dr. Kenneth W. Simpson, Cornell University, Ithaca, NY.)

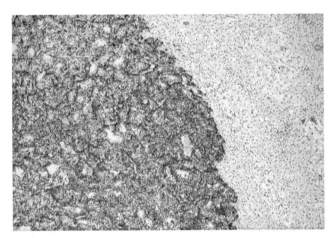

Figure 9.20:
Immunohistochemistry of a gastrinoma. This image shows a pancreatic tumor that was stained for gastrin. Note the massive degree of brown staining on the left side of the picture. The brown stain shows the presence of gastrin, identifying this pancreatic tumor as a gastrinoma. (Courtesy of Dr. Kenneth W. Simpson, Cornell University, Ithaca, NY; magnification: 10×.)

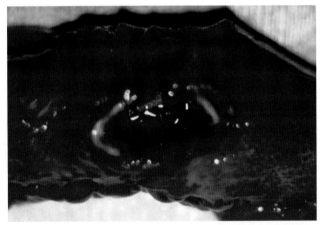

Figure 9.21:
Duodenal perforated ulcer. This figure shows a perforated ulcer in the duodenum of a dog. This dog was diagnosed with a pancreatic tumor that stained positive for gastrin, identifying it as a gastrinoma. (Courtesy of Dr. Kenneth W. Simpson, Cornell University, Ithaca, NY.)

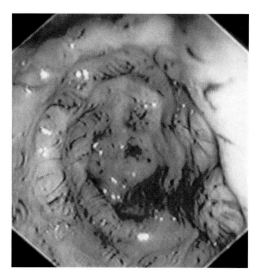

Figure 9.22:
Esophageal ulceration. This image shows an endoscopic view of severe ulceration of the distal esophageal mucosa in a dog with a gastrinoma. (Courtesy of Dr. Kenneth W. Simpson, Cornell University, Ithaca, NY)

9

Routine laboratory tests do not reveal any specific changes, but up to 50% of affected dogs and cats have a regenerative anemia, indicating ongoing blood loss. Many patients also show a neutrophilia with a left shift. Hypoproteinemia with hypoalbuminemia, hypokalemia, increased serum hepatic enzyme activities, hypochloremia, and hyperglycemia are also common. More serious changes may occur if complications, such as pyloric obstruction due to mucosal hypertrophy, or ulcer perforation with peritonitis occur.

Survey abdominal radiographs are unremarkable in most cases. Upper GI contrast radiography, which is rarely performed these days, may reveal plaque-like defects in the stomach or duodenum, indicating ulceration. In the small number of dogs described, abdominal ultrasonography failed to locate the primary lesion, but abdominal ultrasound may be useful for identifying metastatic lesions. Of the five cats diagnosed with a gastrinoma, two were evaluated by transabdominal ultrasound and in one of these cases the tumor was identified during a repeat ultrasound examination.[22] Gastroduodenoscopy allows for direct visualization of esophageal (Figure 9.22), gastric, and duodenal lesions, but cannot identify the underlying cause of these lesions. In human gastrinoma patients, sensitivities and specificities of different localization techniques for gastrinoma have been compared. Abdominal ultrasonography, CT, MRI, or selective angiography all have a rather low sensitivity for the diagnosis of the primary lesion.[23] However, these modalities are all useful in identifying metastatic lesions. Much more promising for localization of the primary lesion are endoscopic ultrasonography and SRS, which successfully identify the primary lesion in almost all human patients. SRS is the most sensitive technique for localization of both the primary tumor and metastatic lesions in human gastrinoma patients.[23] Currently, endoscopic ultrasonography is not routinely available in veterinary practice. The diagnosis of a gastrinoma by SRS using ^{111}In-DTPA-D-Phe[1]-octreotide (OctreoScan, Mallinckrodt Medical) has recently been reported in a single dog.[26]

Diagnosis

Although rare, gastrinomas should be ruled out in all patients with a history of chronic vomiting, weight loss, anorexia, or diarrhea when an alternative diagnosis cannot be arrived at. Also, a gastrinoma should be considered in patients with severe peptic ulcer disease without any predisposing risk factors.

A definitive diagnosis of gastrinoma, short of histopathological confirmation, is difficult. A species-specific assay for gastrin is not available, but several assays developed for use in humans have been validated for dogs and cats.[27] Few veterinary laboratories currently offer serum or plasma gastrin measurements (current reference range for dogs: 10–40 ng/L). According to the diagnostic recommendations for humans, a presumptive diagnosis of a gastrinoma can be made when the 24-hour fasting serum gastrin concentration is ten times the upper limit of the reference range. This recommendation is rather conservative and reflects the high prevalence of chronic atrophic gastritis in humans, which can cause severely elevated serum gastrin concentrations in humans. In dogs and cats, differential causes of elevated serum gastrin concentrations are chronic renal failure, gastric outlet obstruction, small intestinal resection, immunoproliferative enteropathy of Basenji dogs, gastric dilation / volvulus, and administration of proton-pump inhibitors. All of these differential diagnoses are considerably more easy to rule out than atrophic gastropathy in humans.[2] Therefore, in dogs and cats, a less than 10-fold elevation of serum gastrin concentration may be sufficient to diagnose a gastrinoma if other differential diagnoses have been carefully ruled out.

In cases where serum gastrin concentrations are less markedly elevated, provocative testing may be useful. Secretin can be injected intravenously at a dose of 2 U/kg after withholding food from the patient for a 24-hour period. Blood samples are collected at 0, 2, 5, 10, 15, and 20 minutes. An increase of serum gastrin concentration to greater than 200 ng/L or a two-fold increase of the serum gastrin concentration at any time point is considered diagnostic for a gastrinoma.[20] Alternatively, calcium is administered intravenously at a dose of 5 mg/kg/h, followed by serial measurements of serum gastrin concentrations at 0, 15, 30, 60, 90, and 120 minutes. A two-fold increase at any time point is diagnostic for a gastrinoma. In humans, the calcium challenge test is less sensitive than the secretin challenge test.

Treatment

Symptomatic therapy is started in most cases before a definitive diagnosis can be established and should be continued for several weeks after definitive therapy. The mainstay of symptomatic treatment of human gastrinoma patients are proton-pump inhibitors. The proton-pump inhibitor omeprazole has also been successfully used in the management of canine and feline patients with a gastrinoma (0.7 mg/kg PO q 24 h).[20,22,28] Initially, sucralfate, a mucosal protectant that adheres to the exposed proteins of the ulcer, should be added to the treatment protocol (1 g per dog PO q 8 h; 0.25–0.5 g per cat PO q 8 h). Histamine₂ antagonists, such as ranitidine or famotidine, at double the standard dose are used if omeprazole is ineffective. Octreotide, a long-acting somatostatin analogue, acts by inhibiting gastrin release and by decreasing gastric acid secretion directly and may inhibit tumor growth, thus affording more than just symptomatic relief. It has been used successfully in two canine gastrinoma patients (2–20 μg/kg SC q 8 h).[18,20] These two dogs survived for 10 and 14 months, respectively, compared to a reported mean survival time of 5.5 months for other dogs with gastrinoma.[20]

Before initiating definitive treatment, the patient should be staged, which involves the localization of the primary lesion and the search for metastatic disease. Metastatic lesions serve as a long-term prognostic indicator, and approximately 85% of all dogs and cats with a gastrinoma have metastatic disease at the time of diagnosis. After localization of the primary tumor and after widespread metastatic disease has been excluded, an exploratory laparotomy should be performed. Even if the primary tumor can be identified easily, the rest of the pancreas and abdominal cavity should be carefully inspected for additional primary or metastatic lesions. This should include careful palpation of the duodenum. If a primary lesion cannot be identified, intraoperative ultrasonography or illumination of the duodenal wall with an endoscope may be useful. In cases where a primary lesion can still not be identified, biopsy samples of pancreas, lymph nodes, and the liver should be collected. Some authors have recommended partial pancreatectomy of the right lobe of the pancreas if a primary lesion can not be identified, as 60% of all gastrinomas in small animals have historically been identified in the right lobe and only 7% in the left lobe of the pancreas.[2] However, this statistic is based on only 15 dogs and may not reflect the true localization distribution.

If the primary tumor can be identified, it is removed by partial pancreatectomy. The tumor should be submitted for histopathological examination and immunohistochemical staining for regulatory peptides most commonly found in GI NETs. Metastatic lesions, which are present in most cases, should only be removed if this is possible without radical excision. Postoperatively, the patient should not be given anything per os for 24 to 48 hours, followed by the gradual re-introduction of water and an easily digestible low-fat diet.

If the primary tumor cannot be localized and removed during surgery or if extensive metastatic disease is present, an alternative therapeutic approach should be considered. The use of chemotherapy has not been reported in dogs or cats with a gastrinoma and it has a low success rate in human patients. Radiation therapy using OctreoScan® has been successfully used in humans with a response rate of up to 50%, but has not been attempted in veterinary species.[23] Also, medical therapy as described above may prove useful.

Prognosis

The long-term prognosis for dogs and cats with a gastrinoma is grave. However, with appropriate medical management the short-term prognosis and quality of life can be good. Several canine and feline gastrinoma patients have been successfully managed for more than 1 year after diagnosis.[22] With increasing awareness leading to earlier diagnosis, improved localization and staging techniques, and advanced treatment options, survival times are likely to increase further.

9.4.4 Glucagonoma

Introduction

In 1974, the first series of nine human patients with a glucagon-producing pancreatic tumor was reported. To date, only seven cases of canine glucagonoma have been conclusively diagnosed, and this syndrome has not yet been reported in a cat.[2,29]

Clinical presentation

Glucagonomas in humans are associated with typical skin lesions characterized by marked erythema, destruction of the superficial epidermis, and a tendency to heal and progress to other areas of the body. These skin lesions are descriptively termed necrolytic migratory erythema (NME).[30] Similar skin lesions have been reported in several dogs and have been descriptively termed superficial necrolytic dermatitis (SND).[31] However, approximately 90% of canine patients with SND are diagnosed with hepatic disease, diabetes mellitus or, less commonly, other conditions.

9

9

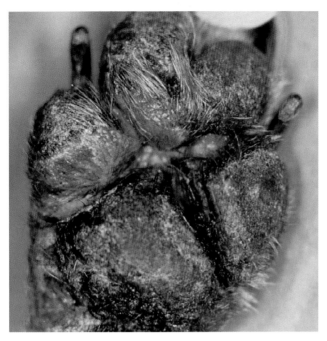

Figure 9.23:
SND foot pad. This dog shows severe crusting lesions on his foot pads with significant interdigital ulceration. A biopsy must be collected to confirm the presence of SND. Most dogs with SND do not have a glucagonoma, but have hepatic disease instead. (Courtesy of Dr. Sandy Merchant, Louisiana State University, Baton Rouge, LA.)

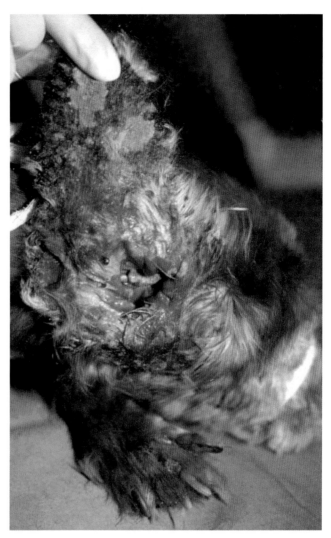

Figure 9.24:
SND ear. This figure shows severe crusting and ulceration on the concave pinna of a dog. A biopsy must be collected to confirm the presence of SND. (Courtesy of Dr. Sandy Merchant, Louisiana State University, Baton Rouge, LA.)

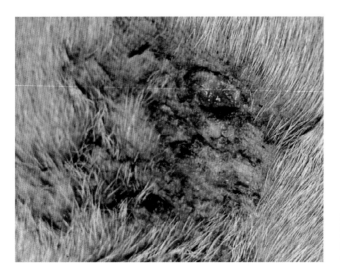

Figure 9.25:
SND skin. This image is a close-up of crusting with ulceration on a pressure point area of a dog. A biopsy must be collected to confirm the presence of SND. (Courtesy of Dr. Sandy Merchant, Louisiana State University, Baton Rouge, LA.)

Human patients with glucagonoma present with NME, weight loss, diabetes mellitus, glossitis, stomatitis, cheilitis, and a tendency for thromboembolic disease. The small number of dogs diagnosed with a glucagonoma have had crusting and scaling skin lesions, most commonly of the footpads, hocks, abdomen, elbows, perineum, nose, and mucocutaneous junctions (Figures 9.23, 9.24, and 9.25). These canine patients also exhibited depression, peripheral lymphadenopathy, and anorexia. Hyperglycemia was reported in 4 of 7 dogs, but was mild in most cases. Also, in some dogs, diabetes mellitus was diagnosed after the diagnosis of the glucagonoma. It is, therefore, appropriate to suspect a glucagonoma in dogs presenting with SND that do not show evidence of hepatic disease, even if they do not concurrently present with diabetes mellitus.

Diagnosis

Most dogs with a glucagonoma are hypoaminoacidemic. Measurement of serum or plasma glucagon concentrations may be helpful in confirming a diagnosis. While an assay has been validated for use in domestic animals, to the author's knowledge, no veterinary endocrine laboratory currently offers this assay. However, samples can be submitted to a human laboratory for assay. In such cases, the laboratory must be contacted for special submission instructions. Caution is advised in interpreting high serum or plasma glucagon concentrations, as they have also been reported in human patients with other conditions, such as chronic renal failure, diabetic ketoacidosis, starvation, acute pancreatitis, hyperadrenocorticism, and sepsis.[30]

If a glucagon assay is not available, the diagnosis of SND is confirmed by histopathology and other potential causes are ruled out. An exploratory laparotomy should then be considered for definitive diagnosis and treatment.

Treatment

The same treatment guidelines for localization and surgical exploration discussed for other NETs also apply for glucagonomas. As for gastrinomas, metastatic disease at the time of diagnosis is common in dogs with a glucagonoma. Since most patients with a glucagonoma have hypoaminoacidemia preoperatively, total or partial parenteral nutrition may improve the overall condition of the patient. An exploratory laparotomy was performed in four of the seven dogs diagnosed with a glucagonoma and a mass was removed in three, two of which died or were euthanized within 3 days after surgery for pancreatitis. One dog survived for 9 months before the skin lesions returned and the patient was euthanized.[32]

Medical management should be considered if abdominal exploration is not an option in cases of a metastatic glucagon-oma or in recurrent cases. Medical therapy can include exogenous insulin, intravenous infusion of essential amino acids and fatty acids, zinc supplementation, and octreotide therapy.[2] However, more clinical information is needed before more specific treatment recommendations can be given.

9.4.5 Pancreatic polypeptidoma

GI NETs secreting pancreatic polypeptide have been described in humans.[30] Although not yet associated with a distinct clinical syndrome, watery diarrhea, diabetes mellitus, weight loss, decreased gastric acid secretion, peptic ulceration, flushing, rashes, and acute psychosis have been described in human patients with a pancreatic polypeptidoma.[30]

Only one dog with a suspected pancreatic polypeptidoma has been reported in the veterinary literature.[33] This dog presented for chronic vomiting, anorexia, weight loss, and lethargy. A concurrent insulinoma was diagnosed on the basis of hypoglycemia in the face of a high serum insulin concentration. Baseline serum gastrin concentration was seven-times the upper limit of the reference range, but did not rise after secretin or calcium challenge. Serum pancreatic polypeptide concentration was 3,500-times the upper limit of the reference range. Multiple pancreatic tumors removed at exploratory laparotomy showed a strongly positive immunoreactivity for pancreatic polypeptide and a positive reaction for insulin, but no reaction for gastrin or other GI regulatory peptides. It should, however, be noted that approximately 75% of NETs of the GI tract stain positive for pancreatic polypeptide, although the clinical syndrome in these patients is caused by other neuroendocrine substances.[33] Thus, it remains uncertain whether there truly was a cause-effect relationship between the extremely high serum pancreatic polypeptide concentration and the clinical signs observed in this patient.

9.4.6 Carcinoids

Gastrointestinal carcinoids are a heterogeneous group of tumors arising from the diffuse neuroendocrine system of the GI tract. In human patients, carcinoids have been reported to secrete a variety of regulatory substances such as histamine, serotonin, gastrin, somatostatin, tachykinins, peptide YY, pancreatic polypeptide, calcitonin, CCK, motilin, and bombesin.

Human gastric carcinoids often secrete large amounts of histamine, which leads to a syndrome characterized by flushing, hypotension, lacrimation, cutaneous edema, and bronchoconstriction. In comparison, small intestinal carcinoids often secrete serotonin and lead to flushing, diarrhea, and bronchoconstriction.

Gastrointestinal carcinoids have been reported in dogs and cats.[34,35] Recently, gastric carcinoids have been described in both a dog and a cat. Both patients were old and presented for chronic vomiting. The dog also showed weakness, ataxia, and coughing. It later deteriorated and was euthanized. The cat was surgically treated and remained free of clinical signs for 21 weeks, but then presented with clinical signs of chronic renal failure.

Signs of flushing, hypotension, or bronchoconstriction have not been reported in dogs or cats diagnosed with a GI carcinoid. This may reflect a lack of synthesis of these regulatory substances by canine and feline GI carcinoids, secretion of different regulatory substances, or a relative resistance of dogs and cats to high plasma histamine and serotonin concentrations.

Careful evaluation of future cases, including the measurement of urinary histamine and serotonin metabolite excretion, immunohistochemical behavior, and ultrastructural studies of the tumor cells, are required for a better understanding of this disease in dogs and cats.

9.4.7 Other neuroendocrine tumors of the gastrointestinal tract

Several other GI NETs, including VIPomas, somatostatinomas, and GRFomas, have been reported in human patients, but have not yet been identified in dogs or cats.[30]

9

Key Facts

- Insulinoma is the most common NET in dogs, followed by gastrinoma. All other NETs of the GI tract are extremely rare in dogs. All GI NETs are extremely rare in cats.
- An insulinoma should be suspected in a patient with hypoglycemia with an increased serum insulin concentration.
- Insulinomas are ultimately malignant in most dogs. However, many dogs can be successfully managed for more than 1 year.
- Localization of NETs of the GI tract can be challenging.
- If a gastrointestinal NET has been identified, the treatment of choice is removal of the tumor and medical management of the clinical syndrome.

References

1. Rehfeld JF. A centenary of gastrointestinal endocrinology. *Horm Metab Res* 2004; 36: 735–741.
2. Zerbe CA, Washabau RJ. Gastrointestinal endocrine disease. In: Ettinger SJ, Feldman EC (eds.) *Textbook of Veterinary Internal Medicine*. Philadelphia, WB Saunders, 2000; 1500–1508.
3. Steiner JM, Bruyette DS. Canine insulinoma. *Compend Contin Educ Pract Vet* 1996; 18: 13–24.
4. Kraje AC. Hypoglycemia and irreversible neurologic complications in a cat with insulinoma. *J Am Vet Med Assoc* 2003; 223: 812–814.
5. Reimer SB, Pelosi A, Frank JD et al. Multiple endocrine neoplasia type I in a cat. *J Am Vet Med Assoc* 2005; 227: 101–104.
6. Hawkins KL, Summers BA, Kuhajda FP et al. Immunocytochemistry of normal pancreatic islets and spontaneous islet cell tumors in dogs. *Vet Pathol* 1987; 24: 170–179.
7. Fingeroth JM, Smeak DD. Intravenous methylene blue infusion for intraoperative identification of pancreatic islet-cell tumors in dogs. *J Am Anim Hosp Assoc* 1988; 24: 175–182.
8. Plöckinger U, Rindi G, Arnold R et al. Guidelines for the diagnosis and treatment of neuroendocrine gastrointestinal tumours – A consensus statement on behalf of the European Neuroendocrine Tumour Society (ENETS). *Neuroendocrinology* 2004; 80: 394–424.
9. Robben JH, Pollak YW, Kirpensteijn J et al. Comparison of ultrasonography, computed tomography, and single-photon emission computed tomography for the detection and localization of canine insulinoma. *J Vet Intern Med* 2005; 19: 15–22.
10. Garden OA, Reubi JC, Dykes NL et al. Somatostatin receptor imaging in vivo by planar scintigraphy facilitates the diagnosis of canine insulinomas. *J Vet Intern Med* 2005; 19: 168–176.
11. Vezzosi D, Bennet A, Rochaix P et al. Octreotide in insulinoma patients: efficacy on hypoglycemia, relationships with Octreoscan scintigraphy and immunostaining with anti-sst2A and anti-sst5 antibodies. *Eur J Endocrinol* 2005; 152: 757–767.
12. Mehlhaff CF, Peterson ME, Patnaik AK et al. Insulin-producing islet cell neoplasms: Surgical considerations and general management in 35 dogs. *J Am Anim Hosp Assoc* 1985; 21: 607–612.
13. Moore AS, Nelson RW, Henry CJ et al. Streptozocin for treatment of pancreatic islet cell tumors in dogs: 17 cases (1989–1999). *J Am Vet Med Assoc* 2002; 221: 811–818.
14. Bell R, Mooney CT, Mansfield CS et al. Treatment of insulinoma in a Springer Spaniel with streptozotocin. *J Small Anim Pract* 2005; 46: 247–250.
15. Meleo K. Management of insulinoma patients with refractory hypoglycemia. *Probl Vet Med* 1990; 2: 602–609.
16. Parker AJ, O'Brian D, Musselman EE. Diazoxide treatment of metastatic insulinoma in the dog. *J Am Anim Hosp Assoc* 1982; 18: 315–318.
17. Robben JH, Van den Brom WE, Mol JA et al. Effect of octreotide on plasma concentrations of glucose, insulin, glucagon, growth hormone, and cortisol in healthy dogs and dogs with insulinoma. *Res Vet Sci* 2006; 80: 25–32.

18. Lothrop CD. Medical treatment of neuroendocrine tumors of the gastroenteropancreatic system with somatostatin. In: Kirk RW (ed.) *Current Veterinary Therapy*. Philadelphia, WB Saunders, 1989; 1020–1024.

19. Caywood DD, Klausner JS, O'Leary TP et al. Pancreatic insulin-secreting neoplasms: Clinical, diagnostic, and prognostic features in 73 dogs. *J Am Anim Hosp Assoc* 1988; 24: 577–584.

20. Simpson KW, Dykes NL. Diagnosis and treatment of gastrinoma. *Seminars in Veterinary Medicine & Surgery (Small Animal)* 1997; 12: 274–281.

21. Liptak JM, Hunt GB, Barrs VR et al. Gastroduodenal ulceration in cats: eight cases and a review of the literature. *J Feline Med Surg* 2002; 4: 27–42.

22. Diroff JS, Sanders NA, McDonough SP et al. Gastrin-secreting neoplasia in a cat. *J Vet Intern Med* 2006; 20: 1245–1247.

23. Pisegna JR. Zollinger-Ellison syndrome and other hypersecretory states. In: Feldman M, Friedman PA, Sleisenger MH (eds.) *Gastrointestinal and liver disease*. Philadelphia, WB Saunders, 2002; 782–796.

24. Patnaik AK, Lieberman PH, Erlandson RA et al. Hepatobiliary neuroendocrine carcinoma in cats: A clinicopathologic, immunohistochemical, and ultrastructural study of 17 cases. *Vet Pathol* 2005; 42: 331–337.

25. Lurye JC, Behrend EN. Endocrine tumors. *Vet Clin North Am Small Anim Pract* 2001; 31: 1083–1101.

26. Altschul M, Simpson KW, Dykes NL et al. Evaluation of somatostatin analogues for the detection and treatment of gastrinoma in a dog. *J Small Anim Pract* 1997; 38: 286–291.

27. Gabbert NH, Nachreiner RF, Holmes-Word P et al. Serum immunoreactive gastrin concentrations in the dog. Basal and postprandial values measured by radioimmunoassay. *Am J Vet Res* 1984; 45: 2351–2353.

28. Brooks D, Watson GL. Omeprazole in a dog with gastrinoma. *J Vet Intern Med* 1997; 11: 379–381.

29. Allenspach K, Arnold P, Glaus T et al. Glucagon-producing neuroendocrine tumour associated with hypoaminoacidemia and skin lesions. *J Small Anim Pract* 2000; 41: 402–406.

30. Jensen AL, Norton JA. Pancreatic endocrine tumors. In: Feldman M, Friedman PA, Sleisenger MH (eds.) *Gastrointestinal and liver disease*. Philadelphia, WB Saunders, 2002; 988–1016.

31. Gross TL, O'Brien TD, Davies AP et al. Glucagon-producing pancreatic endocrine tumors in two dogs with superficial necrolytic dermatitis. *J Am Vet Med Assoc* 1990; 197: 1619–1622.

32. Torres SM, Caywood DD, O'Brien TD et al. Resolution of superficial necrolytic dermatitis following excision of a glucagon-secreting pancreatic neoplasm in a dog. *J Am Anim Hosp Assoc* 1997; 33: 313–319.

33. Zerbe CA, Boosinger TR, Grabau JH et al. Pancreatic polypeptide and insulin-secreting tumor in a dog with duodenal ulcers and hypertrophic gastritis. *J Vet Intern Med* 1989; 3: 178–182.

34. Carakostas MC, Kennedy GA, Kittelson MD et al. Malignant foregut carcinoid tumor in a domestic cat. *Vet Pathol* 1979; 16: 607–609.

35. Sykes GP, Cooper BJ. Canine intestinal carcinoids. *Vet Pathol* 1982; 19: 120–131.

9

Subject Index